# Leddy & Pepper's Conceptual Bases of Professional Nursing

# Leddy & Pepper's Conceptual Bases of Professional Nursing

## SIXTH EDITION

**Lucy Jane Hood, RN, DNSc**
*Associate Professor*
*St. Luke's College*
*Kansas City, Missouri*

**Susan Kun Leddy, PhD, RN**
*Professor Emerita*
*School of Nursing*
*Widener University*
*Chester, Pennsylvania*

 **LIPPINCOTT WILLIAMS & WILKINS**
A **Wolters Kluwer** Company

Philadelphia • Baltimore • New York • London
Buenos Aires • Hong Kong • Sydney • Tokyo

*Senior Acquisitions Editor:* Quincy McDonald
*Managing Editor:* Helen Kogut
*Editorial Assistant:* Marivette Torres
*Production Project Manager:* Cynthia Rudy
*Director of Nursing Production:* Helen Ewan
*Senior Managing Editor / Production:* Erika Kors
*Art Director:* Joan Wendt
*Manufacturing Coordinator:* Karin Duffield
*Production Services / Compositor:* Schawk, Inc.
*Printer:* R. R. Donnelley–Crawfordsville

6th edition

9 8 7 6 5 4 3 2 1

**Library of Congress Cataloging-in-Publication Data**

Hood, Lucy J.
    Leddy & Pepper's conceptual bases of professional nursing / Lucy Jane Hood, Susan Kun Leddy.—6th ed.
        p. ; cm.
    Includes bibliographical references and index.
    ISBN 0-7817-6100-X (alk. paper)
    1. Nursing.  2. Nursing—Philosophy.  I. Leddy, Susan. II. Pepper, J. Mae.  III. Title.
IV. Title: Leddy and Pepper's conceptual bases of professional nursing. V. Title:
Conceptual bases of professional nursing.
    [DNLM: 1. Nursing Theory. 2. Nursing—trends.  WY 86 H776L 2006]
RT41.H66 2006
610.73—dc22

                                                                        2005021548

Care has been taken to confirm the accuracy of the information presented and to describe generally accepted practices. However, the authors, editors, and publisher are not responsible for errors or omissions or for any consequences from application of the information in this book and make no warranty, express or implied, with respect to the content of the publication.

The authors, editors, and publisher have exerted every effort to ensure that drug selection and dosage set forth in this text are in accordance with the current recommendations and practice at the time of publication. However, in view of ongoing research, changes in government regulations, and the constant flow of information relating to drug therapy and drug reactions, the reader is urged to check the package insert for each drug for any change in indications and dosage and for added warnings and precautions. This is particularly important when the recommended agent is a new or infrequently employed drug.

Some drugs and medical devices presented in this publication have Food and Drug Administration (FDA) clearance for limited use in restricted research settings. It is the responsibility of the health care provider to ascertain the FDA status of each drug or device planned for use in his or her clinical practice.

IN MEMORY
**J. Mae Pepper**
January 18, 1936–March 19, 1997

For 20 years, Mae was my colleague, coauthor, mentor, and friend. We met in 1977, when Mae joined the faculty at Mercy College in Dobbs Ferry, New York. Mae's previous teaching experience at the University of North Carolina-Chapel Hill, New York University, and Bronx Community College, as well as her vision, wisdom, and dedication, was crucial to the development and accreditation of our new baccalaureate program for registered nurses and to the subsequent development of the first master's program at the College.

Mae held the position of Chairperson of the Nursing program from 1981 until her sudden death in March 1997 from a ruptured aortic aneurysm. Although she talked for years about leaving administration in order to do more scholarly work, she continued to serve as Chair out of a sense of duty and responsibility. She was devoted to the students and faculty, and very conscientious in her service to the College and many civic and professional organizations.

Mae found time to read voraciously, listen to music, care for animals, and to enjoy outdoor white-water rafting, camping, and bird watching. She loved her garden, was a careful craftsperson in her furniture refinishing, and liked to go to garage sales and flea markets looking for collectibles. Mae had a good sense of humor and loved a good time. I remember a trip we took to a convention in Las Vegas. Mae "knew" which slot machines were ready to pay off and she won over $900. Devoted to her friends and family, she willingly gave time and attention to anyone who asked.

Mae was an irreplaceable, intellectual mentor as well as a friend. She was a great listener, and her counsel was always wise and kind. Mae lived her belief in mutuality, genuineness, and respect for others. She is missed greatly.

# Reviewers

**Joyce Bruce, RN, BN, MSA**
Faculty Primary Care Nurse
    Practitioner Program
Nursing Division
SIAST Wascana Campus
Regina, Saskatchewan, Canada

**Mary Cook, PhD, RN**
Associate Professor
California University of Pennsylvania
California, Pennsylvania

**Lucille Gambardella, PhD, RN, CS,
    APN-BC**
Chair and Professor, Nursing
Wesley College
Dover, Delaware

**Linda P. Grimsley, RN, DSN**
Chair, Department of Nursing
Albany State University
Albany, Georgia

**Ginny Wacker Guido, JD, MSN, RN,
    FAAN**
Associate Dean and Director,
    Graduate Studies
University of North Dakota,
    College of Nursing
Grand Forks, North Dakota

**Karen Johnson Karner, EdD, RN, CS**
Professor of Nursing
East Stroudsburg University
East Stroudsburg, Pennsylvania

**Jacqollyne Keath, RPN, RN, CPMHN(C)
    MA, PhD**
Nurse Educator
Health Sciences, Department of
    Psychiatric Nursing
Douglas College
New Westminster, British Columbia, Canada

**Mary L. Kinnaman, PhD(c), MN, BSN**
Clinical Instructor
University of Missouri–Kansas City,
    School of Nursing
Kansas City, Missouri

**Judith MacIntosh, RN, BN, MScN, PhD**
Professor of Nursing
University of New Brunswick
Fredericton, New Brunswick, Canada

**Francine M. Parker, RN, MSN**
Assistant Professor of Nursing
AUM School of Nursing
Auburn, Alabama

**Joan Propst, EdD, RN, CS**
Professor of Nursing; Director, RN-to-BSN
    Degree Completion Program
Alderson-Broaddus College
Philippi, West Virginia

**Karen S. Ward, PhD, RN, COI**
Professor and Associate Director for
　Online Programs
Middle Tennessee State University
Murfreesboro, Tennessee

**Lillian Wise, RN, DSN**
Coordinator of RN-to-BSN/MSN Track
School of Nursing
Troy State University
Montgomery, Alabama

# Preface

Twenty-five years ago, Susan Leddy and Mae Pepper realized the need for a professional development textbook for registered nurses who were returning to school to earn baccalaureate degrees in nursing. This edition builds on the previous contributions that Leddy and Pepper have made in earlier editions. Continued efforts have been made to make *Conceptual Bases of Professional Nursing* more "user-friendly" and to engage the reader in the learning process by the addition of vignettes based on real life experiences, reflection questions scattered throughout the chapters, and Internet exercises. The conclusions found in the fifth edition have been renamed "Summary and Significance to Practice" to capture the importance of chapter content to professional practice. To further expand the use of content, the chapters end with exercises entitled "From Theory to Practice" to help readers link content to daily professional practice. To promote the use of nursing research in practice, research briefs appear in the majority of the chapters.

## ⊕ ORGANIZATION

Based on reviews received from faculty using the fifth edition of *Conceptual Bases of Professional Nursing,* several changes were made in the organization of the book. The sixth edition is organized into the following sections:

- Section I, Exploring Professional Nursing
- Section II, The Changing Health Care Context
- Section III, Professional Nursing Roles
- Section IV, Glimpsing the Future of Professional Nursing

Additional changes include:

- New content on the Canadian and Mexican health care systems and the history of health care insurance in the United States (Chapter 9)
- Newly expanded content on nursing management and leadership theories and approaches (Chapter 19)
- A new chapter to help nurses understand quality improvement processes (Chapter 20)

The previous chapter on Career Development has been separated into two chapters—Career Options for Professional Nurses and Developing a Professional Nursing Career—with newly expanded content on general nursing and advanced nursing career opportunities.

As Mae Pepper and Susan Leddy noted in the preface to the third edition, "During these changing times, we have been pleased with the utilization of our book in many educational settings, particularly in baccalaureate and graduate programs. Although the first edition of the book was targeted for upper division RN baccalaureate programs, we have become aware of its utilization in generic baccalaureate programs, masters programs, and practice settings. . . ." It is our hope that this sixth edition of *Conceptual Bases of Professional Nursing* will continue to make a contribution to the profession.

*L.J.H. & S.K.L.*

# Preface to the First Edition

In the last quarter century, nursing has moved decisively toward becoming a scientific discipline. It has begun to develop and test its own theoretical bases, to promote scholarly development of its professional practitioners, and to apply its own theory to its practice. Although progress in attaining control of its own practice has been slow and is still not completely accomplished, a clearer picture of the special service offered to society by the profession is emerging. As the autonomous body of knowledge that is called nursing is developed and disseminated, and as the profession assumes accountability to the public it services by requiring excellence in the education of its practitioners and the delivery of its services, control of its practice is more likely to be completely accomplished. Acknowledging the absolute necessity for the profession to practice from its own body of knowledge, we have recognized the need to emphasize the conceptual bases from which professional nursing is practiced.

*Conceptual Bases of Professional Nursing* represents our efforts to present an overview and synthesis of professional concepts that we believe to be basic to the development of professional practitioners. This book was originally conceived to assist the registered nurse engaged in baccalaureate nursing education to become resocialized into the full professional role. In the process of writing, however, it seemed to us that the contents of this book could serve as a useful resource to all professional nursing education programs; to facilitate resocialization in "second step" programs; to serve as a resource at multiple points in the educational development of students in first professional degree programs; and to provide a professional review with a consistent framework in the early part of the education of graduate students from diverse baccalaureate nursing programs.

The book is organized into four sections. Section 1 addresses the nature of the profession through exploration of historical influences, philosophical perspectives, factors that influence socialization into the profession, and the development of a professional self concept by the practitioner. Section 2 focuses on theoretical bases of professional nursing, with separate chapters related to scientific thought and theory development, the research process, theories applicable to nursing, and models of nursing. Section 3 addresses concepts relevant to the delivery of professional nursing, the health process, the health care delivery system, and accountability. Finally, in Section 4, the components and roles of professional nursing are considered. These include nursing process; communication and helping relationships; leadership; and the roles of change agent, client advocate, and contributor to the profession. Future perspectives are then projected briefly.

The book has been written as an integrated text with a common framework and liberal use of cross-references; however, each chapter can "stand alone," and thus the content can be read in any order. If the contents are assigned in a different sequence from that presented, however, we would encourage an early review of our conceptual framework for nursing, which is found at the end of Chapter 2.

We have been fortunate to have received feedback from a number of our professional colleagues. Special appreciation is expressed to Sharron Humenick, Donea Shane, Roanne Dahlen, Carolyn Lansberry, Hanna Jacobson, and Carol Lofstedt, who all critiqued parts of the manuscript; however, we take full responsibility for the philosophical and conceptual views expressed.

We could not have completed this book without the support and tangible assistance provided by Ed and Carol, to whom we express our heartfelt appreciation and love.

The contents of this book reflect the current synthesis of ideas, knowledge, and values that we began to articulate seven years ago, as we struggled with the development of a new curriculum. Our conceptions are continuing to evolve. We eagerly anticipate the debate and dialogue we hope this book will engender, in order to further the development and refinement of nursing science.

*Susan Leddy, R.N., Ph.D.*
*J. Mae Pepper, R.N., Ph.D.*

# Contents

What does it mean to be a nurse? To persons outside of the profession, being a nurse means taking care of persons who are ill or injured. Since its beginning, the profession of nursing has struggled to attain professional status. In today's world, nursing has yet to clearly define the unique contributions it makes to health care delivery. Nurses offer a valuable service to society and make differences in the lives of those with whom they serve. Learning the art and science of nursing requires time and perseverance. However, professional nursing offers its members many diverse opportunities to help others. Sometimes, unfortunately, nurses place their own health in jeopardy in order to help others in need.

# Exploring Professional Nursing

# The Professional Nurse

## KEY TERMS AND CONCEPTS

Socialization
Resocialization
Role Theory
Role
Role Conflict
Returning-to-School Syndrome
Professional Self-Concept
Novice-to-Expert Model
Professional Nursing Roles
Caregiver
Colleague
Client Advocate
Teacher
Counselor
Critical Thinker
Change Agent
Coordinator
Characteristics of a Profession
Associate Degree
Diploma
Baccalaureate Degree
Differentiated Competencies
Graduate Nursing Education
Postgraduate Nursing Education
Critical Thinking
Creative Thinking
Reflective Thinking
Autonomy

## LEARNING OUTCOMES

By the end of this chapter, the learner will be able to:

**1** Identify strategies for thriving in the nursing education environment.

**2** Specify a process for socialization into the profession.

**3** Outline a process to develop a professional self-concept.

**4** Identify characteristics of a profession.

**5** Explain how the nursing profession meets the characteristics of a profession.

**6** Discuss ways for nurses to attain professional status.

State Boards of Nursing
Professional Organizations
General Purpose Nursing Organizations
Specialized Nursing Organizations
National League for Nursing
American Association of Colleges of Nursing
National Council of State Boards of Nursing
American Nurses Association
International Council of Nurses
Sigma Theta Tau International
National Student Nurses' Association
Ethical Codes
Licensure

**VIGNETTE**

Sue graduated from an associate's degree nursing program. She has been working on a medical–surgical unit at the local community hospital as a night charge nurse. A bachelor of science in nursing (BSN) student who will graduate soon has been working with Sue. Sue thinks that perhaps she should go back to school and earn her BSN. While speaking with her nurse manager, Sue says, "I am a good nurse, even though I don't have a BSN. I don't see how more education will make me more professional or improve my patient care, but I see where it may make my charge nurse position secure." What assumptions has Sue made related to the importance of education in nursing practice? How would you respond to her? What are your assumptions about BSN and higher education for nurses?

The words "nurse," "nourish," and "nurture" all come from the Latin root "nutrire" (*Merriam-Webster's Collegiate Dictionary,* 1994). Persons not employed in health care frequently consider all caregivers "nurses." Nurses provide many different services to health care consumers in a variety of settings. Some things nurses do on a daily basis offer a unique contribution to health care, whereas others can be done by other health team members. Is nursing an art, a science, or both? What are the unique contributions that nurses make to health care delivery? The profession of nursing struggles with defining itself as an art or a science.

Professional nursing offers a specialized service to society. Professional nurses use a broad approach when considering holistic health needs of the people they serve. According to the American Nurses Association *Social Policy Statement* (1995, p. 5), the following four features distinguish professional nursing practice:

1. Nurses use a problem-focused orientation when attending to all ranges of human responses to health and illness.
2. Nurses integrate health-related knowledge to client subjective and objective data after gaining an understanding of the individual's or group's experience.
3. Nurses apply scientific knowledge to diagnose and treat human responses.
4. Nurses provide a caring relationship with clients to facilitate health and healing.

Thus, nurses provide a more comprehensive approach to client care than all of the other health team members.

Because of the broad nature of the discipline, nurses assume multiple roles while meeting health care needs of clients. They serve as caregivers when providing direct client care. They assume the role of teacher when providing education to unlicensed personnel, instructing clients how to manage health-related problems and providing persons with health promotion strategies. When working to reform public policy, modify work processes, or transform workplace environments, nurses become change agents. They accept the role of coordinator when assuming supervisory and managerial responsibilities. Finally, nurses act as counselors, providing emotional support for persons experiencing mental or spiritual distress. Successful professional nurses have the ability to assume all the various nursing roles. They execute them competently, and with genuine concern and compassion. To execute the multiple roles of professional nursing effectively, some nurses embark on a journey of lifelong learning that might include returning to formal educational settings.

## ● CHALLENGES TO THE RETURNING PROFESSIONAL NURSING STUDENT

Nurses who return to school assume the role of student, which results in many lifestyle changes. Unless the nurse is single and independent, family members make sacrifices. Money once used for recreation is spent on tuition, student fees, books, and other school supplies. Nurses in school find that they have much less time to spend with family and friends. Families and friends have different reactions to the nurse returning to school. They may feel neglected at times and do things to derail the educational process. Sometimes family members enjoy their new independence and view it as an opportunity to become more self-sufficient. Communication between the new student, family, and friends enables all involved parties to understand how roles will be altered and what sacrifices will need to be made in order to achieve academic success (Dunham, 2001).

Along with families and friends, employer and school responsibilities may be challenging to the nurse who works. Employers may not support educational endeavors either financially or by permitting work schedule changes. Coworkers may add to the difficulties by refusing, or complaining loudly about, work schedule changes, although some coworkers may find the schedule changes highly beneficial (especially if the nurse assumes more than the allotted number of weekend or late shifts). In addition, some coworkers may become jealous of the nurse's academic accomplishments. However, other colleagues may feel proud that one of their own has returned to school to make a different contribution to the profession.

Part of the toll of returning to school is entering into unfamiliar learning situations. The once-confident professional nurse may question the ability to thrive in an academic setting and to learn new things. The overconfident nurse does not realize what he or she does not know and may pretend to know everything. The educational process is designed to change persons. During times of change, persons frequently encounter feelings of discomfort.

### Skills for Educational Success

When students assume responsibility for learning, they reap maximum benefits from the educational process. Education can be viewed as the cultivation of intelligence (Martinez, 2000). To make professional transitions, nurses focus their educational efforts on refining previously learned skills while establishing theoretical foundations for professional practice. Theory-based practice enables professional nurses to understand complex situations and anticipate potential complications in clinical settings. Learners need a variety of skills to be successful in the educational process.

#### Communication Skills (Reading, Listening, Speaking, and Writing)

In ideal educational situations, students and faculty interact with each other as colleagues. Faculty design educational experiences, but students bear the responsibility for learning. Unfortunately, some students bring patterns of behaviors and communication with them from previous and less than ideal educational settings. In traditional education, faculty serve as authoritarian experts who may create oppressive climates, engage in polemic discussions, and set educational goals without student input. In educative-caring education, faculty hold equal status with students, create liberating climates, engage in illuminating dialogues, and set educational goals focused on innovative, participatory learning (Bevis & Watson, 2000). Egalitarian interactions with faculty members provide students with experience in establishing collegiality. Sometimes long-term friendships result when students and faculty members connect.

### Reading

Reading constitutes a major component of the continuing education experience. Success in any program requires reading assigned material. Nursing faculty identify aliteracy (the ability to read, but refusal to do so) as a major obstacle for students. Along with academic success, reading stimulates the release of neurotrophins, which are growth factors that stimulate neuron proliferation and brain vascularization and also may be responsible for strengthening neural pathways (Martinez, 2000).

Finding time to read remains a challenge in today's busy world and especially for nursing students juggling multiple roles. Students studying printed and electronic media need effective reading skills. Trying to read and digest each word printed on a page (or screen) is inefficient reading. Often, beginning and returning students strive to remember every detail from assigned readings. When students master the skill of reading for major ideas within a passage, reading becomes more efficient (Dunham, 2001).

### Listening and Speaking

Returning nursing students come with well-refined listening skills because they have used them in a variety of clinical practice situations to establish therapeutic relationships with clients and professional relationships with other health team members. In educational settings, effective speaking and listening are essential. Students listen to faculty members as they share their nursing expertise. When faculty ask questions, students are forced to think and respond quickly. Taking time to think before responding to questions enables students to organize their thoughts and select the best words to use. Many programs require that students give oral classroom presentations. Although oral presentations may be stressful for some students, they provide opportunities for nurses to refine public speaking skills.

Asking questions is essential to avoid making errors in the education and health care settings. Most persons (including faculty) welcome questions from students. However, fear prevents some students from asking questions. Question formulation also requires having the skills to communicate what is not fully understood. If a person cannot formulate a clear question, there is no shame in admitting that one does not understand. Sometimes, the most difficult task to master is learning what question needs to be asked.

### Writing

Along with refined speaking and listening skills, professional nurses need effective writing skills. Professional nurses use writing skills to document client care, develop clinical practice policies, compose e-mail messages and letters, publish articles, develop budgets, and submit change proposals. Handwritten communication continues to provide essential client care documentation in practice situations without computerized charting. Writing requires nurses to use critical and reflective thinking (Broussard & Oberleitner, 1997).

Written course assignments provide opportunities to refine writing and thinking skills. Most writers make multiple drafts of their works. Success on written assignments requires understanding the purpose of the assignment, setting a timeline for completion by the designated deadline, allowing time for multiple drafts, and having a trusted friend or family member proofread the work.

Once the purpose of the assignment is understood, sometimes students find selecting and limiting topics challenging. Topic refinement becomes an essential step because of the enormous volume of information available on nursing topics. Using computerized or printed indexes available at the library streamlines the collection of information. The amount of information to be collected varies, depending on the nature of the assignment. Students who encounter difficulty in finding information on a topic can seek assistance from a librarian, which will save time and reduce frustration in obtaining relevant information for assignments (Dunham, 2001).

Authors develop nonfiction prose using description, narration, exposition, and argumentation. Authors use description to create a dominant impression. When story telling is the goal, narration serves as an effective tool. Exposition is used when authors want to show the how and why of something. Authors use the following tools for expository writing:

1. Exemplification (provide illustrations or examples for a concept).
2. Process analysis (give step-by-step instructions to do something).
3. Compare/contrast (outline similarities and differences).
4. Analogy (compare something unknown with something familiar).
5. Classification (place into groups based on common features).
6. Definition (explain the meaning of something).
7. Causal analysis (outline cause-and-effect relationships).

Finally, writers use arguments to present objective rationale to support a position (Fondiller, 1992).

Most educational or collegiate teaching programs select a standard format for preparing written assignments. Students enrolled in specific programs should purchase the publication manual for the selected format. Students also may find Internet sites that provide assistance with questions related to a specific format for written assignments.

Before putting ideas in a specific format, a writer should create an outline, which provides an effective means for verifying that ideas have been solidified, all required material has been collected, thoughts have been organized, headings are related to the work, no gaps are present in the work, and proper support is available for the main points (Fondiller, 1992).

Finally, authors select words to convey messages clearly. Reading serves as a vehicle to expand vocabulary that can be used in writing (Fondiller, 1992; Martinez, 2000). Dictionaries and thesauri provide a rich source of words for use in writing. Many dictionaries provide summaries of grammatical rules for written language. When writing is done using a word processing program, many writers use spelling and grammar checking features. Some writers find it useful to read written passages aloud (Dunham, 2001). However, nothing supersedes proofreading by another person to verify that what is written clearly communicates desired ideas.

## Professional Image and Physical Appearance

Besides effective communication, physical appearance plays a role in projecting a professional image. Nursing caps were removed in the 1970s and nurses quickly abandoned their white uniforms for different colored scrub suits and dresses. Clean, pressed scrub suits and dresses present a professional appearance. However, some printed fabrics used by scrub manufacturers may fail to project a desired professional image.

Because nurses work at promoting health, cleanliness and safety become priorities when preparing for professional practice. Clean uniforms, manicured natural nails, and clean shoes decrease the spread of infections. Dangling earrings and necklaces serve as hazards for nurses if they encounter confused or combative clients. Tongue piercing impairs the clarity of a nurse's speech. Visible body piercing and extensive tattooing might create distress for some clients.

## Organizational Skills for Educational and Professional Success

Scholastic success requires organizational skills. Nursing programs in higher education settings provide support services to help students succeed. Previously learned organizational skills transfer readily for effective balancing of personal and professional responsibilities. Key organization skills for success include managing information, refining test-taking skills, and managing personal time.

### Managing Information

Sifting through volumes of information in printed or electronic media is challenging for all nursing professionals, not just students. Scientific discoveries and changes in health care delivery systems surface quickly. Reliable information sources include governmental, university, and nonprofit organizations. Peer-reviewed journals provide more reliable information than do other types of journals. Caution should be exercised when considering information from for-profit sources. Alexander and Tate (1998) offer techniques for evaluating web-based resources. They outline five criteria for critiquing website information because websites can be a "virtual soapbox" for any person or organization. The following six aspects of a website should be assessed before using information from it in assignments:

1. Accuracy: reliability and freedom from error.
2. Authority: the qualifications of the author(s) and whether or not any fact-verifying procedures are used.
3. Objectivity: freedom from biases or attempts to sway the viewers.
4. Currency: dates of initial and updated information entry.
5. Coverage: the breadth and depth of topic coverage.
6. Verification: information on the website does not conflict with other scientific-based publications.

Alexander and Tate (1998) also caution that hyperlinks may send viewers to websites of lesser quality and suggest always viewing the home page of the information source to verify the credibility of the source. Finally, Alexander and Tate caution website users about the instability and susceptibility of web pages to unauthorized and accidental changes.

Students and professional nurses spend much time sorting through large volumes of mail, e-mail, publications, advertisements, and professional information. Going through information immediately as it arrives eliminates clutter. Setting priorities for action enables students and nurses to meet deadlines for professional (license renewal, assignment deadlines, renewal of insurance policies) and personal obligations (family life, community service, holidays, birthdays, and anniversaries). Time spent organizing personal libraries and files saves time. Discarding obsolete and unused items on a regular basis keeps resources current, and filing items facilitates finding them when they are needed (Dunham, 2001).

### Refining Test-Taking Skills

Testing serves as a means for validating student learning and professional competence. Test items come in a variety of forms: multiple choice, true/false, matching, short answer, and essay. Most nursing students find test taking stressful. Test experiences may affect current test performance. Adequate test preparation increases the chance of a favorable performance. Many students find establishment of a study schedule helpful. Optimal test preparation includes reading all required class readings, attending class, asking questions during class, taking notes, reviewing learning objectives for each class, reviewing class materials frequently, attending test reviews (if available), and talking with faculty members to verify understanding of course content before the examination. Some students also find participating in a peer study group helpful, while others prefer to study alone. Depending on how they learn best, some students make audiotapes of class sessions (if permitted), outline readings, recopy notes, and create study cards (Dunham, 2001). Nothing allays test anxiety better than adequate preparation.

Some students become overly anxious during examinations. Sometimes test anxiety impedes performance. However, every person uses different techniques to alleviate stress. Some ways to alleviate test anxiety include arriving 15 minutes early to the testing site, practicing relaxation techniques (deep breathing exercises, visualizing success, guided imagery), skimming notes and textbooks, and talking with classmates. Some students find peer interaction increases test anxiety (Dunham, 2001). Complementary health practices such as aromatherapy (smelling the essential oil of mandarin [citrus reticulate] that evokes feelings of calmness, thereby allaying anxiety) may be useful (Leddy, 2003). For some students, a bit of stress may be needed for optimal performance.

### Managing Personal Time

Time becomes a premium when assuming a student role (especially for the nurse returning to school who has employment and family responsibilities). Balancing professional, student, and family responsibilities is an art. Family members may often feel neglected as nurses (and students) fulfill professional obligations. Some nurses and students find it useful to schedule special time to attend to the needs of family and friends. Taking such breaks helps nurses and students maintain mental and spiritual health (Dunham, 2001).

Learning to say no and asking for help without feeling guilty are essential time-management techniques. Delegation of household tasks (such as cooking, cleaning, and laundry) to others frees time for study while providing the family member with an opportunity to learn or refine life survival skills (Dunham, 2001). Success in education requires a team effort. Finally, networking with one's colleagues can result in time-saving techniques. For example, students enrolled in a BSN program published a book containing quick, easy recipes and sold the cookbooks for a fundraiser. Students who purchased the book used the recipes and cooked healthy, appetizing meals for their families in 30 minutes or less.

## ⬥ SOCIALIZATION AND RESOCIALIZATION INTO THE NURSING PROFESSION

Becoming a member of the nursing profession and being educated to assume advanced nursing practice roles requires socialization and resocialization. **Socialization** is the process of making someone ready for a particular societal role. Professional socialization expands the definition of socialization to include the "formation and internalization of a professional identity congruent with the professional role" (Lynn, McCain, & Bass, 1989, p. 232). Professional socialization for nurses begins in an educational setting and is followed by a resocialization process in the work setting. **Resocialization** occurs when someone adapts a role to a new setting. Throughout a nursing career, the professional nurse has many socialization and resocialization experiences.

Socialization has been described as "a process that produces attitudes, values, knowledge, and skills required to participate effectively as an individual or group member" (Kozier & Erb, 1988, p. 47). This definition highlights an inherent conflict: Is socialization a process, or is it an outcome? Many authors (Conway, 1984; Hinshaw, 1976; Kozier & Erb) refer to socialization as a continuing, interactive, lifelong process. They describe socialization as adaptation to the changing roles that characterize human development and professional growth. This view emphasizes the longitudinal and fluid nature of socialization and implies that the educational setting should provide the learner with initial skills for professional practice. These skills will be further developed or modified in the course of continuing education and practice in changing roles.

Traditionally, the study of socialization has emphasized the ways in which external factors, such as family, peers, school, and other institutions, affect a person's development. Professional socialization addresses the processes by which a person develops a professional identity and the process whereby other members of the profession accept the individual. Any significant change in the environment, such as starting work in the practice setting, changing from a hospital to a community-based position, or returning to school, stimulates a resocialization process. Thus, resocialization is a lifelong occurrence. Nurses can reduce the discomfort of resocialization by becoming actively involved in change processes required for successful professional transitions.

Many students choose educational mobility as an alternative route toward professional nursing. These students start health careers as unlicensed care providers then become practical/vocational nurses or become technical nurses before entering an upper division collegiate nursing program (baccalaureate or higher degree). At each level of education, resocialization is needed to help the nurse synthesize a changed theoretical foundation for practice and adapt to new professional role expectations.

Returning nursing students bring a rich source of information to educational programs. They have developed a sense of self as a nurse if they have been either licensed practical nurses (LPNs) or registered nurses (RNs). Because of experience in client care settings, they possess a sense of self as a nurse; know how to use current health care–related technology; understand governmental and accrediting agency regulations; know how to interact with other health care professionals and unlicensed team members; have encountered human suffering and death; coped with personal fears, anxiety, concerns, and shortcomings; worked within an organization; seen others who model lifelong learning; and acknowledge the inevitability of change (Diekelmann & Rather, 1993).

Although nurses returning to school bring much knowledge and expertise with them, they still face the process of resocialization. Most of the time nurses experience a transformation in the way they practice after earning a new degree. However, in some cases, resocialization may be ineffective and students may finish programs with more knowledge, but without changes in an internalized professional self-image.

## Role Theory

**Role theory** serves as the basis for socialization. A **role** is defined as "a set of expectations that are associated with a position you hold in society" (Hamilton & Keifer, 1986, p. 3). In professional socialization, emphasis shifts from preparation for life in society to preparation for particular expectations or roles. Because roles are viewed as separate and discontinuous, it is assumed that stress occurs when a person assumes a new role or new expectations within an existing role (Bradby, 1990). For example, when getting married, a woman assumes the new role of wife. In addition, new expectations might be assumed in an existing homemaker role. As adults, nursing students often hold multiple roles that sometimes compete for attention. These roles may include employee, spouse, parent, or care provider for an aging parent. When new roles are assumed (becoming a "student" again), students must adjust how they met the responsibilities for all selected roles. **Role conflict** arises when roles assumed by a person compete with each other for time and attention (Bradby, 1990). The newly acquired student role competes with practicing nurses when school demands detract attention from other roles.

Most students enter nursing with a service orientation. They want to do things that will help sick people. In contrast, the professional educational image of the nurse is generally of one who defines clients in terms of health and maintaining health; views the relationship between the nurse and clients therapeutically and analytically; approaches technical mastery of tools and procedures from the viewpoint of knowledge principles that guide their use; uses critical inquiry processes to creatively manipulate knowledge in relation to clients' concerns; and accepts responsibility/accountability for patient care decisions (Hinshaw, 1976, p. 5). Clearly, the socialization process involves changes in knowledge, attitudes, values, and skills. These changes can be associated with conflict and strong emotional reactions.

### Questions for Reflection 1-1

1. What potentially competing roles may surface as I return to school?
2. Why is it important to identify potentially competing roles?
3. List your roles in order of priority. Why do you think you listed them in this order?

## Shane's Returning-to-School Syndrome

Shane (1980) describes the positive and negative emotional states experienced by RNs who return to school for baccalaureate education. She labels these states the **"returning-to-school syndrome."** The first phase, the honeymoon, is positive. Nurses identify similarities between previous education and the present experience, and these similarities tend to reinforce the original role identity as a nurse. The nurse feels energetic about learning new things.

The next stage, conflict, is characterized by turbulent negative emotions. Conflict arises during the first nursing theory or clinical nursing course when faculty challenge the nurse to change ways of thinking and/or practicing. Feelings of professional inadequacy may emerge during this stage and may be expressed by angry outbursts or feelings of helplessness or depression.

Successful resolution of conflict results in the next stage, the beginning of reintegration. A struggle to hold on to cherished beliefs about practice occurs and frequently nurses wonder why they decided to pursue a higher degree. Hostile feelings toward the nursing program and faculty are common in this stage. Shane (1980, p. 123) indicates that

the length of time any individual spends in the hostility phase and the mode of resolution probably depends on the overall resiliency of the individual, the intensity of the emotions and experiences she is feeling, and the interpretation and guidance provided by those significant others (faculty, peers, family) surrounding her.

Finally, the ability to integrate the original culture of work with the new culture of school results in a positive resolution of the returning-to-school syndrome. Nurses recognize that a transformation has occurred. They notice that their clinical practice has forever changed and relate this to personal and professional growth. Newly acquired theoretical knowledge guides practice. The previous and new conceptualizations of nursing practice have blended together. Learning new things enables these nurses to embrace change, which fosters a new curiosity to learn more.

Throughout a nursing career, every time a nurse changes positions a process of resocialization into another working environment is required. Nurses have the flexibility to change specialty areas and organizational positions. Changing to a new practice arena or position may mean, despite years of clinical experience and additional specialized education, the nurse must serve time as a novice before resuming nursing practice as an expert. By recognizing the various stages of socialization and resocialization processes, nurses can identify sources of actual and potential feelings of discomfort and work effectively by steering the processes of change.

### Questions for Reflection 1-2

Thinking back to Sue in the vignette, answer the following questions:

1. What assumptions can you identify that Sue has made about the benefit of seeking a baccalaureate degree in nursing?
2. What personal transitions will be required of Sue to successfully work through resocialization using Shane's Returning-to-School Syndrome? Why are these transitions important?

## ● DEVELOPMENT OF A PROFESSIONAL SELF-CONCEPT

As a person develops patterns of behavior, the self-system becomes organized and strives to actualize itself, although it is continually undergoing change, being repatterned, and affecting the environment in a significant way. The self-system interacts symbiotically with the environment. These interactions with the environment provide the conditions from which a view of the self emerges—the self-concept. As a person, the nurse continually interacts with the personal environment; as a professional, the nurse continually interacts with the professional environment. Because human beings develop personal selves first, those personally organized sets of behaviors form the basis of the selves brought into the profession. Thus, the personal self highly influences the emerging professional self.

The development of the **professional self-concept** (how a person perceives oneself as a nurse) follows the same path as that of development of the personal self. In every profession, the professional has significant others. Every nurse has had different significant others during her or his various stages of growth and development. When initially starting a career, beginning nursing students may view faculty members as significant others. Novice nurses may identify experienced nursing colleagues and/or nurse managers as significant others. Sometimes, other members of the health care team may be identified as significant others.

The identified significant others in professional self-development are determined to some degree by the nurse's adjustments to changing situations. The professional nurse moves in and out of new situations. Adjusting to the perceived expectations of the significant others in each situation, the nurse tries to be the kind of person the situation demands. Highly related to how successful the nurse is in moving in and out of changing situations is the nurse's personal self-view and the nurse's sensitivity to the professional significant others. The personal self-concept cannot be separated from the professional self-concept, although the professional significant others are different from the personal significant others.

## The Professional Self

To a great extent, the kind of professional a person becomes depends on the person's self-system. The professional self-system emerges from the personal self.

One's self-concept "results from previous interpersonal relationships" (Simms & Lindberg, 1978, p. 9) and affects one's future relationships. "A person's view of self controls the roles he or she will be able to assume" (Simms & Lindberg, p. 9). One's self-system determines one's personal characteristics, and these personal qualities enable one to carry out professional roles. Successful implementation of professional nursing roles and tasks reinforce one's perception of the professional self. Repeated successes in practice solidify the concept of being a competent professional nurse. Throughout professional careers, nurses experience transitions that require achievement of professional developmental tasks. Because the development of a professional self requires interactions with others in the profession, separating the developmental from the socialization processes may be impossible.

## Benner's Novice-to-Expert Model

Benner (1984) devised a model of stages from novice to expert that has relevance for experienced nurses. Benner's (1984) **novice-to-expert model** describes stages in the progression of patient care expertise that can result from practice nursing experience

**TABLE 1-1**

## Benner's Stages from Novice to Expert

|  | Stage I | Stage II | Stage III | Stage IV | Stage V |
|---|---|---|---|---|---|
| Title | Novice | Advanced beginner | Competent | Proficient | Expert |
| Experience level | Graduate | New graduate | 2–3 years in same setting | 3–5 years | Extensive |
| Characteristics of performance | Is inflexible Exhibits rule-governed behavior | Formulates principles Needs help with priority setting | Plans Feelings of mastery | Perceives "wholes" Interprets nuances | Has an intuitive grasp |

*Source:* Benner, P. (1984). *From novice to expert* (pp. 21–34). Menlo Park, CA: Addison-Wesley.

(Table 1-1). This model, based on work by Dreyfus and Dreyfus (1996), suggests three general aspects of skilled performance:

1. Movement from reliance on abstract principles to use of past concrete experience as paradigms
2. Change in perception of the demand situation from a compilation of equally important bits of information to a more or less complete whole in which only certain parts are relevant
3. Passage from a detached observer to an involved performer who is engaged in the situation

Stage one, the novice stage, corresponds to the student experience in nursing school. Because no background understanding exists, the novice depends on context-free rules to guide actions. Although this approach enhances safety, "rule-governed behavior is extremely limited and inflexible" (Benner, 1984, p. 21).

The new nursing graduate demonstrates marginally acceptable performance as an advanced beginner in stage two. The advanced beginner relies on basic theory and principles and believes that "clinical situations have a discernible order" (Benner et al., 1996, p. 54). The advanced beginner can formulate principles for actions, but because all actions are viewed as equally important, help is needed for priority setting.

The competent practitioner, who has reached stage three, typically has worked in the same setting for 2 to 3 years. The competent practitioner is consciously aware of long-range goals and can engage in deliberate planning based on abstract and analytical contemplation. As a result of this planning activity, the practitioner has a feeling of mastery and the ability to cope with contingencies and feels efficient and organized.

By stage four, which requires 3 to 5 years of experience, the nurse is a proficient practitioner. The proficient nurse perceives situations as "wholes," rather than as accumulations of aspects, and performance is guided by maxims. Actions do not need to be thought out, and meanings are perceived in relation to long-term goals. In addition, the proficient practitioner can interpret nuances in situations and recognize which aspects of the situation are most significant.

Finally, the fifth stage, the expert practitioner, is achieved only after extensive experience. The expert has an intuitive grasp of situations and thus does not have to think through actions analytically. In fact, the expert is so skilled at grasping the situation as a whole that she or he often is unable to think in terms of steps.

### Professional Nursing Roles

Benner (1984, p. 6) identifies that nurses use 31 different competencies as they engage in clinical practice. She organizes them into the following seven domains upon which **professional nursing roles** are based:

1. "The helping role" provides the foundation for the roles of **caregiver** (provider of direct client care)**, colleague** (helpful team member), and **client advocate** (person looking out for the client's best interests).
2. "The teaching–coaching function" provides the foundation for the roles of **teacher** (provider of education and information) and **counselor** (one who provides emotional support and encouragement).
3. "The diagnostic and patient monitoring function" provides the foundation for the caregiver, and **critical thinker** (someone who uses complex thought processes) roles.
4. "Effective management of rapidly changing situations" provides the foundation for the caregiver, **change agent** (person who initiates and guides the change process) and **coordinator** (person who manages, leads and verifies that things get done) roles.
5. "Administration and monitoring of therapeutic interventions and regimens" provides the foundation for the caregiver and change agent roles.
6. "Monitoring of and ensuring the quality of health care practices" provides the foundation for the roles of coordinators, client advocates, and change agents.
7. "Organizational and work role competencies" provides the foundation for the client advocate, change agent, and coordinator roles.

Benner states that experience is absolutely necessary for the development of professional expertise.

## ● CHARACTERISTICS OF A PROFESSION

**Characteristics of a profession** (what differentiates a professional from a technician) have been debated for many years. *The Flexner Report* issued by the Carnegie Foundation in 1910 served as the criteria for determining medicine as a profession. Since the 1950s, the nursing profession has been compared to sociological theories that define "a profession." To be classified as a profession, the following characteristics should be met:

1. Authority to control its own work
2. Exclusively unique body of knowledge
3. Extensive period of formal training

4. Specialized competence
5. Control over work performance
6. Service to society
7. Self-regulation
8. Credentialing systems to certify competence
9. Legal reinforcement of professional standards
10. Ethical practice
11. Creation of a collegial subculture
12. Intrinsic rewards
13. Public acceptance (Freidson, 1994; Miller, Adams, & Beck, 1993)

Although considered a profession for many years, an assessment of the characteristics of a profession reveals that nursing fails to meet all required criteria. Nursing is more accurately classified as an "emerging profession." Table 1-2 outlines the characteristics of a profession and how the profession of nursing fulfills them. The nursing profession does use a specialized knowledge base, has autonomy and control over its work, requires specialized competence, regulates itself, possesses a collegial subculture, and has public acceptance (Freidson, 1994; Miller, Adams, & Beck, 1993). Unfortunately, nursing fails to have a standardized education for entry into the profession. Like many other professions, professional nursing requires that its members have intelligence, deep personal commitment, mutually shared values, and specialized skill to make autonomous decisions to serve society.

## Intellectual Characteristics

Because nurses make decisions that affect clients' lives, nurses must have the intellectual capability to master scientific concepts, understand the impact of self on others, use this information in clinical practice, and understand potential consequences for alternative actions (American Association of Colleges of Nursing, 1998). Professional nurses possess the following three intellectual characteristics:

1. A body of knowledge on which professional practice is based.
2. A specialized education to transmit this body of knowledge to others.
3. The ability to use the knowledge in critical and creative thinking.

Because of the global nature of professional nursing to meet client care needs, nurses frequently use knowledge that originated in other professional disciplines. However, they use critical and creative thinking to adapt this knowledge to the realm of professional nursing practice.

### Body of Knowledge

Professional practice is based on a body of knowledge derived from experience (leading to expertise) and research (leading to theoretical foundations for knowledge and practice). State Nurse Practice Acts specify minimal education requirements to obtain RN status. In most states, a minimum of a 2-year, associate of arts degree in nursing serves as the educational qualification to take the registered nursing licensing examination. Professional nursing education includes a liberal education along with specialized education in the arts and sciences of nursing with increased emphasis on theory

TABLE 1-2

## How Nursing Meets Characteristics of a Profession

| Professional Characteristic | How Nursing Meets the Criteria or Characteristic |
|---|---|
| Authority to control its own work | Nurses work for physicians or health care agencies unless engaged in private advanced nursing practice. |
| Exclusive body of specialized knowledge | Nursing pulls from a variety of fields to provide holistic nursing care. Nursing research generates new scientific knowledge for practice. |
| Extensive period of formal education and training | Currently, there are three levels of education entry into professional nursing practice: associate degree, diploma, and baccalaureate nursing programs. |
| Specialized competence | Nurses demonstrate assessment skills; possess an understanding of pharmacology, various branches of physical sciences, patho-physiology, diagnostic tests, surgical procedures; and have skills to manage the technical equipment used in client care. Many nurses hold certification in specialized areas of nursing practice. |
| Control over work performance | Nurses make independent judgments based on client situations and area of practice. Some nurses work in organizations that use shared governance and quality management frameworks. |
| Service to society | Nursing care focuses on the client system. Caring for others serves as a major theme for most nursing theories. Nurses receive middle-income pay for taking care of others. |
| Self-regulation | Nurses abide by the Nurse Practice Act of the state in which they practice. Individual state boards of nursing regulate nursing practice. |
| Credentialing systems to certify competence | Nurses take the National Certification Licensing Exam developed by nurses which measures minimum competence for safe nursing practice. Nurses obtain certification in specialized areas of nursing practice from nurse specialty organizations. Some states require continuing education for continued licensure. |
| Legal reinforcement of professional standards | All nurses are held liable for their actions based on what the reasonable and prudent nurse would do in a given client care situation. Individual state boards of nursing have the power to restrict the practice of nursing within a state. |
| Ethical practice | The American Nurses' Association has published *The Nurses' Code of Ethics*, last updated in 2001. |
| Creation of a collegial subculture | Professional nursing organizations offer networking opportunities, shared governance and clinical practice partnership models, and they enhance collegiality among staff nurses and nursing administration. |
| Intrinsic rewards | Many nurses derive a deep personal satisfaction from making a difference in the lives of clients and families one person at a time. Some nurses view the profession as an opportunity to practice religious beliefs on a daily basis. |
| Public acceptance | Nursing was ranked as the most honest and ethical profession of all the professions (The Gallup Organization, 2003).[a] |

[a]The Gallup Organization (2003). Nursing ranks first as the most honest and ethical profession. Available online at http://www.gallup.com/poll/content/login.aspx?ci=14236. Accessed Feb. 1, 2004.

and utilization of research (American Association of Colleges of Nursing, 1998). Most states require graduate collegiate education for nurses who assume advanced practice nursing roles. Professional nurses practice using a theoretical approach that facilitates clinical decision-making. This knowledge base contributes to nursing judgments based on solid, scientific rationale for modifying actions to meet the demands of specific client situations. Associate degree and diploma nursing education programs often emphasize scientifically substantiated methods for responding to specific client situations. This limited approach to education could explain why many nurses seem unwilling or unable to apply knowledge to clinical problem-solving, thereby contributing to dependence in practice. Frequently, nurses (especially novices) seek the "right" answer and do things the way they have always been done. For example, pain medications may be withheld because "4 hours have not passed since the last dose of medication."

Liberal arts education serves as a hallmark of professional education. A liberal education "leads to a greater personal and professional contribution to nursing and society" (Bottoms, 1988, p. 124). All college majors have liberal arts requirements. Liberal arts courses foster the development of thinking and communication skills, cognizance of historical contributions, understanding of science, exploration of personal values, appreciation of the fine arts and sensitivity of human diversity (American Association of Colleges of Nursing, 1998). Knowledge and skills derived from a liberal education enhances the nurse's ability to adapt knowledge and skills to novel situations while arming nurses with tools to better communicate and appreciate clients and other health care providers. In addition, courses in disciplines other than nursing provide opportunity for future nurses to interact with other students who may be pursuing health care careers.

Whether nursing has a unique body of knowledge or applies knowledge borrowed from the fields of medical, behavioral, or physical science has been a matter of debate. In the early days of nursing, nurses derived knowledge through intuition, tradition, experience, or by borrowing it from other disciplines (Kalisch & Kalisch, 2004). However, the nursing profession uses nursing models and frameworks as a foundation for practice. The models and frameworks have provided guidance for nurse researchers to substantiate scientifically the unique contributions that nurses make for attainment of positive outcomes for consumers of health care.

## Specialized Education

Before entering the nursing field, nurses receive specialized education to provide safe client care. Currently, candidates with three levels of nursing education qualify to take the same registered nursing licensing examination, the National Council of State Boards of Nursing Licensure Examination (NCLEX-RN). These three programs (associate degree, diploma, and baccalaureate degree) accept high school graduates as students.

**Associate degree** programs educate students in the community college setting. Students usually take 2 years of coursework that focus on the technical aspects of professional nursing. In 2002, there were 780 associate degree nursing programs (Bureau of Labor Statistics, 2004).

**Diploma** programs provide nursing education in primarily the hospital setting. Diploma nursing students attend school for 3 years and take courses focused on professional nursing.

Diploma nursing programs emphasize the scientific aspects of nursing practice, provide more hours of clinical instruction than other programs, and graduate nurses adept at following policies and procedures rather than relying on theory to meet clinical practice demands. In 2004, there were 68 diploma nursing programs in the United States (All Nursing Schools, 2004).

**Baccalaureate degree** programs educate students in collegiate and university settings. Baccalaureate programs may be traditional or accelerated in nature. The traditional baccalaureate nursing student receives a well-rounded education over 4 years. Courses in nursing may be integrated with other fields of study. In baccalaureate programs, nursing majors frequently take the same courses as other health profession majors. To meet the current demand for more professional nurses, some colleges and universities developed accelerated baccalaureate nursing programs. These programs admit students with previous college degrees and provide them with concentrated study in the field of nursing for 12 to 18 months. In 2002, there were 1,678 BSN programs, 1,100 of which were accelerated BSN programs (Bureau of Labor Statistics, 2004).

Education for other health care professions (pharmacists, social workers, physical therapists, occupational therapists, chaplains, and physicians) requires post-baccalaureate education. Some leaders in nursing have proposed requiring a master's degree (or even a doctorate) as the educational entry level for professional nursing. Advanced practice nurses hold master's or higher degrees. Efforts during the mid-1980s resulted in **differentiated competencies** for associate degree-prepared nurses (ADNs) and baccalaureate degree-prepared nurses (BSNs). The agreed upon role competencies appear in Table 1-3 (Primm, 1987). ADN competencies center around providing nursing care to persons with similar alterations in health in structured settings while using developed policies, procedures, and protocols. BSN competencies include independent thinking and providing nursing care to persons with complex and differing health alterations within a variety of structured or unstructured settings. They are prepared to provide nursing care to persons in the community setting and work with communities to develop community-based health programs. BSNs also assume responsibility for developing research-based care protocols, assume nursing management positions, and coordinate care for persons with complex, interactive health care needs.

**Questions for Reflection 1-3**

1. Do I agree with the table of differentiated competencies for associate degree- and baccalaureate degree-prepared nurses?
2. Why or why not?

In the 1990s, the PEW Health Professions Commission (1995, p. 34) proposed focusing "associate preparation on the entry-level hospital setting and nursing home practice, baccalaureate on the hospital-based care management and community-based practice, and master's degree for specialty practice in the hospital and independent practice as a

TABLE 1-3

## Differentiated Practice for AD- and BSN-Prepared Nurses

| AD-Prepared Nurses | BSN-Prepared Nurses |
| --- | --- |
| Provide direct care to individual clients with common, well-defined nursing diagnoses while considering clients' familial relationships. | Provide direct care to clients with many different nursing diagnoses using nursing process to define individualized and complex interactive nursing diagnoses while considering the client relationships within a family and community. |
| Practice within a structured setting that is a geographic or situated environment where policies, procedures, and protocols provide provisions for health care. | Practice within structured or nonstructured settings for families, groups, aggregates, and communities. The lack of formalized policies and protocols necessitates the use of independent nursing decisions. |
| Use basic therapeutic communication skills with a focal client group and coordinate efforts with other health team members to meet client-focused needs. | Use complex communication skills with clients, collaborate with other health team members, and assume an accountable charge role for client care in a variety of settings. |
| Recognize the focal client's need for information and modify standardized teaching plans. | Assess client information needs and design individualized client teaching plans. |
| Acknowledge that nursing research influences nursing practice and assist in standardized data collection procedures. | Collaborate with nursing researchers to incorporate nursing research findings into nursing practice. Develop research-based nursing protocols. |
| Organize client care aspects for which the nurse is responsible. | Manage comprehensive client care for clients for whom the charge nurse is responsible. |
| Maintain accountability for own practice and aspects of care delegated to peers, licensed practical (vocational) nurses, and unlicensed assistive personnel. | Maintain accountability for own practice and aspects of care delegated to other nursing personnel consistent with their levels of education, licensure, and expertise. |
| Plan and implement nursing care consistent with the overall admission to post-discharge plan within a specified work period. | Plan nursing care on identified needs of clients from admission until after discharge. |
| Practice within the legal and ethical parameters of nursing. | Practice within the legal and ethical parameters of nursing. |

primary care provider." The Commission also emphasized the importance of strengthening career mobility paths within the nursing profession for ADN and diploma nursing school graduates (PEW Health Professions Commission, 1998). The three educational levels qualifying persons to take the licensing examination are outlined in Table 1-4. Over the past few years, approximately 60% of persons entering the nursing profession start with associate degrees. The education level disparity among nurses and other health team members sometimes creates friction. Contributions of the professional nurse to client care may be discounted if the nurse does not have a bachelor's degree. Multiple entry levels into the nursing profession compound the struggle for nursing to attain a professional stature.

TABLE 1-4

## Graduations from Baccalaureate, Associate Degree, and Diploma Nursing Programs

| Years | Baccalaureate | | Associate Degree | | Diploma | | Total Number |
|---|---|---|---|---|---|---|---|
| | Number | Percent of Total | Number | Percent of Total | Number | Percent of Total | |
| 1960–1961 | 4,031 | 13% | 917 | 3% | 25,071 | 84% | 30,019 |
| 1965–1966 | 5,488 | 16% | 3,349 | 10% | 26,072 | 74% | 34,909 |
| 1970–1971 | 9,856 | 21% | 14,534 | 31% | 22,065 | 48% | 46,455 |
| 1975–1976 | 22,579 | 29% | 34,625 | 45% | 19,861 | 26% | 77,065 |
| 1980–1981 | 24,370 | 33% | 36,712 | 50% | 12,093 | 17% | 73,985 |
| 1985–1986 | 25,170 | 33% | 41,333 | 54% | 10,524 | 14% | 77,027 |
| 1990–1991 | 19,264 | 27% | 46,794 | 65% | 6,172 | 8% | 72,230 |
| 1993–1994 | 28,912 | 30% | 58,839 | 62% | 7,118 | 8% | 94,870 |
| 1994–1995 | 31,254 | 32% | 58,749 | 61% | 7,049 | 7% | 97,052 |
| 1995–1996 | 32,413 | 34% | 56,641 | 60% | 5,703 | 6% | 94,757 |
| 1997 | 31,828[a] | 35% | 52,396[a] | 59% | 5,240[a] | 6% | 89,437[a] |
| 1998 | 30,142[a] | 35% | 49,045[a] | 60%[a] | 3,978[a] | 5% | 83,165[a] |
| 1999 | 28,107[a] 37,548[b] | 37% | 45,255[a] | 59% | 3161[a] | 4% | 76,523[a] |
| 2000 | 26,048 | 36% | 42,685 | 60% | 2,679 | 4% | 71,412 |
| 2001 | 24,832 | 36% | 41,567 | 60% | 2,310 | 4% | 68,759 |
| 2002 | 25,821 | 36.5% | 42,382 | 60.5% | 2,425 | 3% | 70,692 |
| 2003 | 26,630 | 34.7% | 47,423 | 61.8% | 2,565 | 3.5% | 76,618 |
| 2004 | 30,648 | 35.1% | 53,275 | 61.3% | 3,162 | 3.6% | 87,085 |

[a]Total number of graduates taking NCLEX for the first time in 1997, 1998, and 1999 online data from the National Council of State Boards of Nursing. *Statistics on 1999 first time NCLEX pass rates according to degree type.* 2000. Available at http://www.ncsbn.org/research1999licstats/ 20%lic20%exam20%statistics/20%reportson-line.pdf. National Council of State Board of Nursing Inc. *2000 Licensure and Examination Statistics.* Available at http://www.ncsbn.org/pdfs/2000_lic_exam_statistics_report_on-line.pdf Does not represent the number of registered nurses completing BSN degrees. Crawford, L., Marks, C., Gawel, S. & White, E.(2002). *NCSBN Research Brief, 2001 Licensure & Exam Statistics, 4,* 32. Crawford, L., Marks, C., Gawel, S. & White, E. (2003). *NCSBN Research Brief, 2002 Licensure & Exam Statistics, 13,* 29. NCSBN (2004). Statistics on NCLEX Pass Rates 2003 Available at http://www.ncsbn.org/pdfs/Table_of_Pass_Rates_203.pdf, Accessed January 29, 2005; NCSBN (2005). Statistics of NCLEX Pass Rates 2004. Available at http://www.ncsbn.org/pdfs/Table_of_Pass_Rates_2004.pdf Accessed January 29,2005.
[b]Data reported by American Association of College of Nursing. February 17, 2000. Fall 1999 nursing enrollments. Online news release available at http://www.aacn.nche.edu/Media/NewsReleases200Feb17.htm.

Adapted from National League for Nursing (NLN). (1982). *Nursing data book* (pp. 39, 56). New York: Author; National League for Nursing (NLN). (1996). *Nursing data review* (p. 43). New York: Author; and Louden, D. (1997). In, *Nursing data source 1997; Vol. 1. Trends in contemporary RN nursing education.*

## Research Brief 1-1

Aiken, L. H., Clarke, S. P., Cheung, R. B., Sloane, D. M., & Silber, J. H. (2003). Educational levels of hospital nurses and surgical patient mortality. *Journal of the American Medical Association, 290,* 1617–1623.

This longitudinal study looked at the outcomes of 232,342 persons who were hospitalized for general, orthopedic, or vascular surgery in 168 nonfederal Pennsylvania hospitals.

> Data were collected regarding surgeon board certification status and institutional characteristics (size, teaching versus nonteaching, level of technology, staffing patterns). In addition, nurses were sent surveys for data related to educational level, age, employment status (full- vs. part-time), patient loads, and years of experience.
>
> In the study, nurses holding bachelor's degrees in nursing constituted less than 20% to greater than 50% of study hospital nursing workforces. Results indicated (after adjusting for institutional variables, staffing patterns, surgeon certification, and demographic characteristics of the nurses) a 5% decrease in the likelihood of patients dying within 30 days of hospital admission and of failure to rescue the patients for medical emergencies with each 10% increase of proportion of baccalaureate-prepared nurses.
>
> Implications for this study demonstrate that when hospitals are staffed with higher proportions of RNs holding bachelor's degrees, clients are less likely to die within 30 days of hospital admission and are more likely to have better responses to situations when needing to be rescued within the confines of the hospital. More studies are needed to validate the findings of this report as well as to identify if any other additional benefits to having baccalaureate-prepared nurses providing patient care in hospitals.

Graduate nursing education programs offer advanced education for nurses interested in pursuing careers as advanced practice nurses (certified nurse midwifery, nurse practitioners, clinical specialists), or in nursing education, nursing administration, or nursing informatics. Most **graduate nursing education** programs offer a master's degree. A master's degree in nursing can usually be completed within 3 years if a student assumes a full-time plan of study. Most programs give students up to 7 years to complete graduate work.

**Postgraduate nursing education** leads to a doctorate in nursing. Nurses enrolled in these programs generate new nursing knowledge by executing original nursing research studies. Doctoral nursing programs prepare nurse researchers and collegiate faculty. Some doctoral nursing programs offer clinical doctorates to prepare nurses for a specific area such as clinical practice and nursing education. Many have residency requirements making full-time employment difficult. However, grants and scholarships are available for nurses interested in doctoral work. Although the process of nursing education seems complex, faculty challenge students to refine thinking processes and practice critical thinking.

## Using Knowledge by Critical Thinking

Critical thinking has cognitive and affective characteristics. **Critical thinking** imposes standards (Paul, 1992) and prevents nurses from engaging in illogical thinking. As critical thinkers, nurses "exhibit these habits of mind: confidence, contextual perspective, creativity, flexibility, inquisitiveness, intellectual integrity, intuition, open-mindedness, perseverance and reflection. Practicing nurses have cognitive skills of analyzing, applying standards, discriminating, information seeking, logical reasoning, predicting, and transforming knowledge" (Scheffer & Rubenfeld, 2000, p. 357). Professional nurses use critical thinking as they practice in order to make the best possible clinical decisions.

### Creative Thinking

Considered an essential component of critical thinking (Scheffer & Rubenfeld, 2000), creative thinking generates alternative approaches to clinical situations. **Creative thinking** requires an ability to think outside of what usually is done and results in novel approaches to client care. If not tempered with critical thinking, solutions generated with creative thinking may be hazardous. For example, nurses follow care standards when providing client care. Suppose a nurse uses an alternative health treatment such as therapeutic touch to reduce client pain that results in deep relaxation and hypotension. If the hypotension results in the client fainting when getting out of bed after the therapeutic touch session and sustains an injury, the nurse is accountable for the adverse result. Because the institution has no policy related to nurse use of therapeutic touch, the hospital may determine that the nurse practice deviated from the standard of care, and terminate his or her employment. Nurses engage in creative thinking when confronted with clients who have complex integrative health problems that require individually designed plans to attain desired outcomes.

### Reflective Thinking

**Reflective thinking** is engaging in purposeful analysis about what one is currently doing and about what one has done (Schon, 1987). Reflection plays a key role in professional nursing practice. Consider the following clinical situation: Ms. S. has advanced cancer and lives in constant pain. Because the pain is unbearable, Ms. S's physician orders patient-controlled analgesia with morphine. Ms. S is fearful that the morphine will not ease her pain and that she will lose consciousness. Her fear and anxiety have resulted in increased muscle tension. As the nurse initiates the morphine drip, she remembers the pharmacologic action and potentially adverse effects of the morphine. She decides to stay and talk with Ms. S, while giving her detailed instructions on how to use the device for assuming control of medication for pain. As the nurse talks with Ms. S., she performs a back massage knowing the theoretical benefits of human touch and the physiologic response to muscle massage. When thinking about and using theory in daily practice, nurses engage in reflection in action (Schon, 1983). Reflection in action occurs when nurses think about theoretical and scientific principles while delivering client care (Clarke, James, & Kelly, 1996; Kim, 1999; Powell, 1989).

Schon (1983, 1987) advocates for reflection on action, another form of professional reflection. Reflection on action occurs when the professional practitioner considers practice aspects other than the moment of the action (Clarke et al., 1996; Schon, 1987). While the nurse plans a report for the next nurse who will be providing care to Ms. S., she reviews which interventions were effective and considers other interventions to try. Reflection on action enables the practitioner to develop a deeper understanding of practice and provides a vehicle to learn from experience (Clarke et al.; Schon). Journal writing also provides practice with reflection on action. When professional nurses reflect-in action and reflect-on-action, they generate purposes for clinical decisions they make in practice.

## Independent Clinical Decision Making

Professional nurses make independent decisions to solve problems as they work with clients, families, and communities. Sometimes, nurses tend to act hastily based on both inadequate information and insufficient time to generate alternative approaches. Consider the following situation.

*Problem:* Which of the following actions would you take with a patient whose visitors insist on staying beyond the visiting hours established by hospital policy?

1. Possible Action 1: Tell the patient and the visitors that the visitors must leave.
2. Possible Action 2: Allow the visitors to stay for an additional hour.
3. Possible Action 3: Explore the reasons why the visitors want to stay and the significance of having the visitors spend time with the patient. Base the decision on the result of information generated.

*Discussion:* The nurse uses critical thinking to realize that collecting more information surrounding the situation would result in a better decision. Perhaps, the visitors have arrived from out of town and have no place to stay. Maybe the client has not seen them in a long time or the client may be afraid to be left alone in the hospital the night before a potentially life-threatening procedure. When nurses use critical thinking and logical reasoning to support actions taken, they make effective clinical decisions.

## Nursing Process

Nurses use nursing process, a systematic thinking method to process information about specific client care situations. Basically, nursing process is a problem-solving approach that consists of five steps: assessment, diagnosis, planning, implementation, and evaluation. Figure 1-1 depicts the steps of nursing process. Assessment consists of collecting subjective (what clients say) and objective (measured or verifiable by another) information about clients. Nurses then categorize data into clusters to determine nursing diagnoses (an actual or potential client response) upon which a care plan is developed. After the care plan is implemented (executed), nurses evaluate the effectiveness of the plan and start the process again with assessment. Effective use of nursing process requires critical, creative, and reflective thinking.

## Service to Society

Since the beginning, nursing has been associated with serving others. Many students still enter nursing "to help people," an image of the nurse shared with the public. However, the intrinsic motivation "to care" is only one way to look at caring emphasized in the nursing literature. Morse, Bottorff, Neander, and Solberg (1991, p. 122) have identified the following five conceptualizations of caring: (1) caring as a human trait, (2) caring as a moral imperative, (3) caring as an affect, (4) caring as an interpersonal interaction, and (5) caring as a therapeutic intervention. Obviously, caring encompasses more than just intuitive concern for others. Several theories of nursing use caring as a major concept or central theme.

Professional service to society requires impeccable integrity, individual responsibility for ethical practice, and lifelong commitment. Some nurses view nursing as a job, rather than a professional career. Approximately 80% of employed nurses work full time and 10% of nurses hold two nursing jobs (Bureau of Labor Statistics, 2004). Many nurses leave the profession (permanently or temporarily) to pursue personal interests or to raise a family. Some nurses work to supplement family income, and others work because they are sole or primary income providers for a family. Sometimes, professional commitments

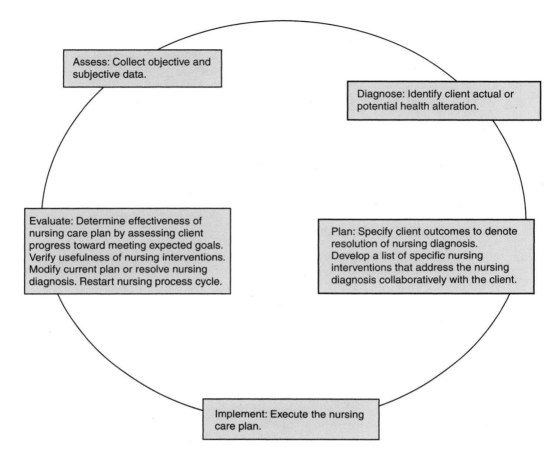

**Figure 1-1**
Nursing process as a continuous cycle.

become secondary to other concerns. Nurses needing job security avoid confronting less-than-ideal nursing practice situations. Employing agencies occasionally exploit these nurses. Regardless of difficulties, such as high client-to-nurse ratios, rotating shifts, and floating, some nurses make do and maintain the status quo. However, other nurses in similar circumstances strive to always do what is best for clients.

Service to others involves ethical and legal responsibilities. Nurses must have the integrity to do what is right, often in situations that cause real moral dilemmas. Codes for nurses have been developed by the International Council of Nurses (ICN) and the American Nurses Association (ANA). These codes emphasize that nursing care recipients have basic rights and that the nurse's primary responsibility is to the client.

Service to society requires legal assurances that practitioners are competent. Credentialing systems, such as licensure, provide a means to certify minimal competence for safe practice by a person legally permitted to use the title "registered nurse." State nurse practice acts also provide legal reinforcement against incompetence by specifying the legal definition of nursing practice, minimal education preparation for licensure, and penalties for illegal, unethical, or negligent practice. Upon initial state licensure, the nurse receives a copy of a state Nurse Practice Act. Copies of a specific Nurse Practice Act can be obtained in print form from the State Board of Nursing (a fee usually is charged) or copies may be downloaded from State Board of Nursing websites. When litigation occurs, courts of law hold nurses accountable for what a usual and prudent nurse would do in a particular client care situation. Most nurses would do whatever it would take to keep clients safe.

Along with protecting clients within their care, nurses advocate for clients to ensure that health care access, equity, and quality are not compromised by a system emphasizing cost control. Some professional nurses work to change public policies to increase access to health care for persons who cannot afford health insurance. Other professional nurses provide primary health care services to disadvantaged persons in nurse-managed health centers.

## Autonomy and Self-Regulation

**Autonomy** means that practitioners have control over their functions in the work setting. Autonomy involves independence, a willingness to take risks, and accountability for one's actions, as well as self-determination and self-regulation.

In the United States, each state has a nursing board that governs practice that occurs within its borders. **State Boards of Nursing** regulate professional nursing practice by issuing professional licenses to qualified individuals, revising state Nurse Practice Acts, and disciplining nurses failing to comply with specified rules contained within Nurse Practice Acts. Nurses hold most of the positions on State Boards of Nursing. Advanced practice RNs have legal authority to prescribe medications granted to them by Nurse Practice Acts. Although RNs must rely on other health team members before administering medications, nurses may independently institute interventions such as therapeutic communication, application of ice or heat, massages, and other noninvasive therapies. Some nurses make decisions to institute medical therapies if they have sets of standing orders. In 1978, the State Boards of Nursing saw a need for a united approach to nursing licensure and education. They formed the National Council of State Boards of Nursing (NCSBN), which has developed licensure examinations for professional and practical nursing.

As in the United States, Canadian legislation to regulate nursing practice is passed by the provincial and territorial governments. In all provinces (except Ontario), the regulation of professional nurse registration lies with the professional nursing association at the provincial/territorial levels. In Ontario, the College of Nurses of Ontario assumes responsibility for the regulation of professional practice. Canadian nursing regulatory bodies determine educational and practice standards along with defining the scope of nursing practice. They also specify who may use the title of RN and outline mechanisms for professional discipline. Finally, the regulatory bodies also approve educational programs to prepare persons for entry into practice and establish continuing educational and competency requirements for members of the nursing profession (Brunke, 2003).

Because the profession of nursing defines nursing practice, sets practice standards, and has established mechanisms to discipline members failing to meet practice standards, nursing fulfills the element of autonomy and self-regulation. In some cases, the regulatory bodies also provide a means for professional nurses to engage in activities resulting in the creation of a collegial subculture, another hallmark of a profession.

# A Collegial Subculture (Accrediting, Professional, and Student Nursing Organizations)

## Professional Nursing Organizations

Like other professions, nursing has **professional organizations** that set standards, advocate, and provide networking opportunities for members. Professional nursing organizations foster the development of collegial relationships among nurses. International and national professional nursing organizations develop standards for professional practice. American nursing organizations offer certification programs for advanced nursing practice. Professional nursing organizations can be divided into two categories: **general purpose nursing organizations** (that address the issues and concerns of all nurses) and **specialized nursing organizations** (that address specific issues and concerns of nurses practicing within a specific specialized practice arena). Participation in a specialty nursing organization links nurses who practice in a particular area and creates subcultures of nurses with common interests inside the nursing profession. Each nursing organization specifies its mission, goals, and constituency. Numerous professional organizations exist. Some nurses believe that membership in specialty organizations better fit their professional needs than membership in a general nursing organization. Unfortunately, only about 10% of professional nurses belong to the American Nurses Association (DeLeskey, 2003). Some argue that if all professional nurses would join a single, general purpose nursing organization, nurses would become more influential in health care policy formation and in the delivery of health care. The following discussion presents some of the major broad purpose organizations.

## National League for Nursing

The **National League for Nursing** (NLN) strives to improve and advance the quality of nursing education so that the nursing workforce will be prepared to meet the health care needs of diverse populations in the continuously changing health care environment (NLN, 2002). In 2002, the NLN determined the following broad goals to achieve its mission by providing leadership in:

1. Setting standards that advance excellence and innovation in nursing education (p. 1, paragraph 3)
2. Promoting the professional growth and continuous quality improvement of educators who prepare the nursing workforce (p.1, paragraph 4)
3. Promoting evidence-based teaching in nursing and ongoing development of research that informs and improves nursing education (p.1, paragraph 5)
4. Serving as the authority in providing and interpreting comprehensive nursing workforce supply information (p. 2, paragraph 1)
5. Developing and providing comprehensive services to the nursing community that evaluate and assess educational outcomes and practice competencies for quality nursing care (p. 2, paragraph 2)
6. Advocating for all types of academic and lifelong learning programs in nursing (p. 2, paragraph 3)

The NLN served as the only national accrediting body for all basic and graduate nursing programs in the United States from 1952 to 1995. During this time, the NLN became very prescriptive in its requirements for program accreditation resulting in limited opportunities for nursing programs to engage in creative ways to change nursing education to meet the demands of the future. Accredited programs sometimes felt obligated to purchase tests from the NLN because they measured specific criteria for accreditation. In 1996, the NLN established an accrediting commission as an independent entity for accrediting nursing education programs. The NLN accredits associate degree, diploma, baccalaureate, and upper degree nursing programs.

Along with its accreditation activities, NLN provides consultation services, continuing education programs, analysis of statistical data related to nursing education and nursing manpower resources, various examination and testing services, information about legislative affairs affecting nursing, journals, continuing education seminars, and a variety of information packages to affect nursing image and recruitment. NLN Agency membership is available to nursing education institutions, nurses, other health care professionals and anyone interested in improving the quality of nursing education or health care services. NLN offers separate councils for each type of nursing programs. Because of its inclusive nature, some would argue that NLN perhaps serves as a major obstacle in the nursing profession's ability to define a standardized education entry level.

### American Association of Colleges of Nursing

The **American Association of Colleges of Nursing** (AACN) membership consists exclusively of deans and directors of baccalaureate and higher degree nursing programs. In 1997, AACN established two separate entities: a commission for baccalaureate and higher degree program accreditation called the Commission on Collegiate Nursing Education, and an alliance of all professional nursing organizations to streamline credentialing of advanced practice nurses. Criticisms of AACN include aggravating tensions among education programs offering various nursing degrees, limiting membership to deans and directors, and emphasizing the importance of the baccalaureate degree as a minimal entry level for professional nursing (Gelman, Bellack, & Berkman, 1999).

### National Council of State Boards of Nursing

The **National Council of State Boards of Nursing** (NCSBN) and individual State Boards of Nursing (SBN) bear the responsibility for protecting the public from fraudulent and unsafe nursing practice. The NCSBN assumes the responsibility for development and administration of the professional nursing licensing examination (NCLEX) (Bower, 1999). Along with licensure examination, the NCSBN keeps records on nursing license suspensions, tracks professional nursing demographics, and spearheads an effort toward interstate licensure. State governors usually appoint SBN members. Each SBN accredits nursing programs within a given state. In collaboration with the American Nurses Association and other advanced nursing practice groups, the NCSBN and SBN set guidelines for licensure of advanced practice nurses at state levels (Bower, 1999).

### American Nurses Association

The **American Nurses Association** (ANA), the oldest professional nursing organization in the United States, was officially established in 1911 (Flanagan, 1976). Membership criteria require professional nursing licensure. When professional nurses join the national organization, they obtain membership at the state and local district levels. The ANA represents nurses in all 50 states, the District of Columbia, Guam, and the Virgin Islands. Individual nurses also may join individual state nurses associations.

The ANA offers a wide variety of services to members and plays a key role in promoting healthy workplaces for nurses. The ANA participates in the following activities:

- Accredits continuing education programs;
- Provides voluntary individual certification for areas of specialized and advanced practice through the American Nurses' Credentialing Commission;
- Supplies data for research and analysis;
- Engages in public policy analysis, political education, governmental relations maintenance, and political action activities;
- Implements economic and general welfare programs;
- Determines and publishes standards for professional nursing practice for nursing practice in general and for specialty areas of nursing practice;
- Develops and publishes social policy statements and an ethical code for nurses;
- Publishes handbooks, the newsletter, *The American Nurse*, and the journal, *American Journal of Nursing*;
- Holds membership in the International Council of Nurses; and
- Offers special services for members, including discounted malpractice insurance, retirement plans, and reduced rates for conference attendance.

The ANA established the American Nurses Credentialing Commission as a separately incorporated center for credentialing services. Eleven certification boards bear responsibility for programs and policies relating to a specialty area of nursing practice. Eight of the boards officially recognized the American Board of Nursing Specialty Organizations as meeting national standards for advanced practice and specialty certification.

Through the ANA's Congress on Nursing Economics and Nursing Practice, standards and programs are developed for nursing education, practice, research, organized nursing services, economic security, employment, and human rights. ANA participates in national nursing issues through membership in various national nursing councils that meet regularly to discuss issues and concerns related to specialty practice areas, such as computer applications, community health nursing, medical–surgical nursing, mental health nursing. The ANA also sponsors activities of The American Academy of Nursing, a group of distinguished nurses that have made major contributions to the nursing profession and The American Nurses Foundation, a program that provides funding for nursing research and other projects to advance the nursing profession. ANA is also a member organization of The International Council of Nurses.

### The International Council of Nurses
The **International Council of Nurses** (ICN) unites national nursing organizations from 120 nations into a single confederation. The founders included nurses from nursing organizations in Great Britain, Canada, Germany, Scandinavia, and the United States. Since 1899, the ICN has worked to preserve the professional welfare of nurses, address interests of women and improve global health. The mission of the ICN is "to represent nursing worldwide, advancing the profession and influencing health policy" (ICN, 2001). The ICN addresses a wide array of nursing concerns including nursing regulatory issues, global standardization and credentialing of nurses, human rights, ethics, socioeconomic welfare of nurses, occupational safety, health policy formation, career development, and position statements on health issues.

The ICN serves as an advocate for nurses and for all people of the world. Current efforts by the ICN focus on establishing a global definition of professional nursing practice, addressing the global shortage of nurses, credentialing nursing competence, measuring the value of professional nursing contribution on client outcomes, addressing a variety of global health issues, and furthering advanced nursing practice. The organization has advised the United Nations on global health issues. The ICN has published position statements that have been presented to governments to consider when making health care policy decisions.

### Sigma Theta Tau International

Four nursing students at the University of Indiana formed Sigma Theta Tau in 1922. **Sigma Theta Tau International** (STTI) became an international honor society for nurses in 1985. In 2004, the organization had 130,000 members in more than 383 chapters; members reside in 75 countries. International chapters are located in Australia, South Korea, Canada, Pakistan, Taiwan, and Brazil. STTI holds membership in the Association of College Honor Societies.

To become a member, a nurse must demonstrate superior scholastic achievement, professional leadership potential, or marked achievement in the nursing field. Organizational membership occurs exclusively by invitation. In addition to student members, community members may be inducted. STTI contributes to the advancement of nursing via small grants, conferences, and publications. The organization publishes the printed journal, *The Journal of Nursing Scholarship* and the electronic journal, *The Online Journal of Knowledge Synthesis*. STTI also sponsors writer's seminars, has a media development program, and bestows awards for outstanding contributions to nursing practice, research, education, creativity, leadership, career development, professional goals, and chapter programming. Individual chapters present educational programs awards and scholarships. In 1989, STTI dedicated The Center for Nursing Scholarship and the Virginia Henderson International Nursing Library, a state-of-the-art electronic library and information resource center (Vance, 1999). Through promotion of nursing scholarship and leadership, STTI hopes to shape the nursing profession into the future.

### National Student Nurses' Association

The **National Student Nurses' Association** (NSNA) is an inclusive student association with members from associate degree, diploma, and baccalaureate nursing programs. The student members finance and run the organization. As an autonomous organization, NSNA goals, according to the group's mission statement (1994), are to

- Organize, represent, and mentor students preparing for initial licensure as RNs, as well as those nurses enrolled in baccalaureate completion programs;
- Promote development of the skills that students will need as responsible and accountable members of the nursing profession; and
- Advocate for high quality nursing care for all persons.

NSNA offers a variety of activities and services to implement its mission. The Association participates on committees of the NLN, ANA, and the ICN. The NSNA Foundation administers a scholarship program and publishes the journal *Imprint*, the newsletter *NSNA News*, and a variety of reports and handbooks. As members of NSNA, students enjoy discounts on health insurance, publications, conference attendance fees, and state board review courses.

**Questions for Reflection 1-4**

1. Am I currently a member of a professional nursing organization? Why or why not?
2. If you are a member of an organization: How would I go about recruiting another nurse to join a professional nursing organization?
3. If you are not a member of an organization: What factors prevent you from joining one?
4. Is a nurse more professional if he or she holds membership in a professional organization? Why or why not?

## Ethical Practice

Ethical professional practice has been defined by several of the broad purpose nursing organizations (ICN, ANA, and NSNA) by published **ethical codes** (statements defining honest, honorable, humane, and fair practice). Ethics permeates all areas of professional practice. Nurses with solid professional identities who have been socialized into a variety of clinical settings possess strong individual and professional values. Values provide the foundation for ethical dimensions of professional practice. Caring emerges as a shared value within the nursing profession. Clients trust nurses with their lives. Professional nurses must never violate this sacred trust. Nurses serve as caregivers and client advocates. Sometimes, these duties conflict with each other. Nurses have a duty to the individual, society, and their profession (Bandman & Bandman, 1995; Bower, 1999). As science and technology advance and resources dwindle, nurses confront difficult, complex, and conflicting issues as they practice. Ethical systems provide nurses with a set of values and behaviors to use when situations arise without clearly right or wrong answers. By studying ethics, nurses identify their own biases and values. A code of ethics assists nurses to make decisions when confronted with ethical dilemmas.

Nurses frequently encounter ambiguity as they practice. Issues arise that have conflicting values, rights, and obligations. Bandman and Bandman (1995, p. 46) state, "Effective nurses function as moral agents." When acting as moral agents, nurses assume responsibility and accountability for attempts to do no harm. Nurses assume responsibility for action when they assume blame or credit for their own actions. Accountability encompasses the ability to provide sound reasons, explanations, and defenses for actions taken (Sullivan & Christopher, 1999). Nurses encounter many practice situations with multiple correct actions and answers. When this occurs, nurses agonize about which of the imperfect and alternative choices would serve the best interests of the client. Table 1-5 identifies some common ethical dilemmas encountered by nurses in clinical practice.

For ethical decision-making, nurses use several codes of ethics. Common principles appear in original versions of the International Council of Nurses Code for Nurses, Ethical Concepts Applied to Nursing (1973), and the American Nurses Association Code for Nurses with Interpretive Statements (2001). Nurses can read specific ethical codes online. Despite recent updates to ethical codes, all contain the following common principles: (1) respect for human dignity and uniqueness, (2) protection of confidential

TABLE 1-5

## Ethical Issues Encountered by Professional Nurses in Practice

| Ethical Principle | Definition | Practice Dilemma(s) |
| --- | --- | --- |
| Sanctity of human life | Human life as the most important characteristic of being human | Quality versus quantity of life<br>Pro-choice versus pro-life<br>Capital punishment<br>Withholding life saving treatments<br>Euthanasia and assisted suicide |
| Autonomy | Individual freedom to make rational and unconstrained decisions | Lack of client knowledge about available treatments<br>Coercive power<br>Paternalism<br>Cognitively impaired individuals<br>Individual decisions that interfere with another person's rights |
| Veracity | Truth-telling | Whistleblowing<br>Concealing a chemical or physical abuse pattern<br>Falsification of legal document to cover errors<br>Covering up reasons<br>Informed consent |
| Distributive justice | Allocation of limited resources | Managed care<br>Reduced access to care based on inability to pay for services<br>Judicious use of high-tech equipment for prolonging life<br>Deciding who gets resources based on fitness, cost-benefit analysis, equal chance, equal share, or equal consideration |
| Respect for personal beliefs | Accepting individual beliefs as a basis for decision making | Religious preferences not to subject self or family to "impure" acts<br>Conflicts of research evidence on personal health habits |
| Nonmalfeasance | Do no harm | Securing court orders for life-saving therapies<br>Withholding therapy<br>Assisted suicide<br>Right to leave clients alone |
| Beneficence | Do only good | Balancing what is morally right with what is legal and practical. Highly individualized for each situation and shares actions with many of the principles presented above. |
| Confidentiality | Keeping privileged information private | Reporting health problems that interfere with safe driving to state officials<br>Telling families about poor prognoses before informing clients<br>Disclosing alternative lifestyles |
| Fidelity | Keeping promises | Not keeping one's word<br>Failing to follow up with what one says one will do |
| Justice | Treating people fairly | Treating clients differently based on their ability to pay or other sociocultural characteristic<br>Singling out special clients for extra nursing care<br>Denying health care access to anyone |

information, (3) acts to safeguard persons receiving nursing care, (4) responsibility and accountability for nursing actions, (5) maintenance of nursing competence, (6) use of informed judgment, (7) participation in research and other activities to generate new nursing knowledge, (8) participation in activities to improve and implement nursing standards, (9) integrity of the nursing profession, and (10) collaboration with other health care professionals and citizens. Ethical codes define professional standards but fail to state specific guidelines for nursing actions in a given situation. Ethical codes are morally, not legally, binding.

## Societal Acceptance: Legal Reinforcement of Professional Standards

Society holds professional nurses accountable for abiding by standards of professional nursing practice. The legal system protects consumers from unsafe nursing practice. Along with licensure, the legal system holds nurses responsible for professional actions. **Licensure** refers to "a form of credentialing whereby permission is granted by a legal authority to do an act, without such permission, action would be illegal, trespass, a tort, or otherwise not allowable" (Loquist, 1999, p.105). A professional nursing license is a legal document that certifies that an individual has met minimal standards for qualified practice. As a state function, licensure protects citizens from unsafe or incompetent health care providers. Upon licensure, nurses become registered in a particular state to practice professional nursing. Registration denotes the "enrolling or recording the name of a qualified individual on an official roster by an agency of government" (Loquist, 1999, p. 15).

Requirements for licensure as a RN appear in each state's Nurse Practice Act (NPA). Most NPAs contain information related to reasons for licensure, nursing definitions, licensure requirements, licensure exemptions, reasons for license revocation, endorsement provisions for nurses licensed in other states, development of a State Board of Examiners, nursing board responsibilities, and penalties for practicing nursing without a license or not in accordance with the state NPA (Kelly & Joel, 1995).

All states use the National Council Licensure Examination for Registered Nurses (NCLEX-RN) as criteria for professional licensure. The test focuses on client needs and nursing process. Although licensure is permanent (unless it is revoked for illegal or immoral behavior), registration must be renewed periodically (usually every 1 to 2 years) by paying a fee to each state in which current registration is desired.

Licensure as a RN carries with it the responsibility for safe and competent practice. If injury, unnecessary suffering, or death should occur as a result of care delivered by a nurse, the nurse may be held legally responsible. States expect all licensed professional nurses to act reasonably and prudently and judge their actions compared with a nurse with the same education and experience within a given situation.

Nurses must know and function within the legal parameters of nursing practice in the state where nursing services are offered. If nurses have ethical or legal concerns about medical treatment or client situations, they must share them with medical and institutional authorities. Because nurses are responsible for client well-being, they may refuse to execute a treatment, but must not attempt to circumvent the physician by interfering with treatment without the physician's knowledge. Nurses and physicians must collaborate, not compete with each other.

## Future Work for the Nursing Profession to Attain Full Professional Status

Because the nursing profession fails to meet all characteristics of a profession, nursing can be thought of as an emerging profession. Several barriers to fulfilling all criteria for professional stature have occurred. First, professional nursing has multiple levels of education for entry into the profession. Most professions have a single, specialized plan of study before persons can enter them. Many recipients of nursing services do not know the differences in educational preparation. To them, a nurse is a nurse.

Along with an inconsistent educational entry level, many nurses have become specialists in a particular area of practice (e.g., oncology, cardiology, critical care. . . .). Frequently, some of these nurses find themselves having to choose between joining a specialty or general purpose nursing organization because of limited time and monetary resources. Other nurses may not even join a professional organization (DeLeskey, 2003). By failing to unite, nurses reduce their political effectiveness when issues that address health care delivery, client safety, and professional nursing practice arise. The lack of working collectively also may create opportunity for others to exploit nurses.

In addition, society tends to devalue nurses more than other health team members. Although nurses hold the lives of other persons in their hands as they take care of the basic human needs of clients, sometimes clients view them as "hired" help. In a capitalistic society, the amount of money received for a service is based on its perceived value. Professional nurses tend to receive much less compensation when compared to other professional members of the health care team. In 2004, average salaries for RNs working as staff nurses earn an average of $49,600; nurse managers earn $67,100; nursing faculty earn $52,000, and advanced practice nurses earn $72,400 (Robinson & Mee, 2004). In comparison, based on 2002 data, physicians and surgeons earned a mean income of $150,153; hospital administrators earned $83,590; pharmacists earned $75,140; physical therapists earned $60,110; dental hygienists earned $57,790; and postsecondary educators earned $54,960 (Horrigan, 2004). The disparity in salary could be related to the fact that all of the above health team members (with the exception of dental hygienists) have received at least a master's degree in their practice area. Because of lower salaries, many nurses work more than one job (U.S. Bureau of Labor Statistics, 2004), thereby creating more demands on the nurse's time.

Professional nurses must work together to showcase the contributions they make to society while developing methods to overcome the barriers from attaining full status as a profession. Currently, 2.3 million RNs make contributions to health care delivery in the United States (U.S. Bureau of Labor Statistics, 2004). Professional nursing has more numbers than any of the other members of the interdisciplinary health team. If efforts by the profession were channeled toward cooperation rather than competition, nurses could make substantial contributions toward the betterment of health for all.

## ◯ SUMMARY AND SIGNIFICANCE TO PRACTICE

Because the nursing profession fails to meet all criteria for a profession, nursing is sometimes referred to as an emerging profession. The process of becoming a professional nurse involves change and growth throughout various stages of a career. For some nurses, nursing practice serves primarily as a way to earn money. Other nurses display a genuine commitment to serving clients and the profession. Sometimes, a nurse vacillates between thinking of nursing as a job and thinking of it as a professional career of which to be proud. Over time, being a professional nurse may become embedded into one's personal identity and being. Through educational and occupational experiences, the nurse develops attitudes, beliefs, and skills as knowledge expands and deepens. A nurse should expect continuous growth and development within a professional career. Any change in clinical specialty practice area and formal education results in a process of resocialization. The professional nurse assumes many roles when engaged in clinical practice. Effective implementation of the roles associated with professional nursing practice requires deep commitment, broad knowledge base, refined communication, networking skills, and keen insight into one's personal values, strengths, and weaknesses.

## FROM THEORY TO PRACTICE

1. What advice would you give to Sue as she enters a baccalaureate nursing program? Why do you think each piece of advice you will give her is important?
2. Has your perception of professional nursing changed since reading the chapter? Why or why not?
3. What do you think is a major barrier to nursing achieving status as a profession? Why do you think this is a major barrier? What steps could the nursing profession take to eliminate this barrier to attaining full status as a profession?
4. Do you belong to a professional nursing organization? Why or why not?

## WWW INTERNET EXERCISES

This chapter has provided a broad overview of the profession of nursing. These Internet Exercises will enhance your understanding of the chapter material and help you appreciate what it means to be a professional nurse.

1. Visit the website www.nursingworld.org, the official website of the American Nurses Association. Analyze the benefits and costs of membership and view the most recent form of the ANA's Code of Ethics with Interpretive Statements.
2. Using the search engine of your choice, type in any specialized area of nursing practice and see if you can find a professional nursing organization to support nurses practicing in that field of nursing. Analyze the benefits and costs of membership. Compare and contrast two professional nursing organizations.
3. Visit the website www.ncsbn.org. Identify key issues surrounding safe nursing practice. Discover what states have enacted the multistate compact for professional nursing practice. While there, visit your State Board of Nursing website using the hyperlinks and identify key information about license renewal, announcements, and news.

## WWW INTERNET RESOURCES

American Nurses Association: http://www.nursingworld.org. Read about ANA history, membership services, and current issues affecting professional nursing.

Sigma Theta Tau International: http://www.nursingsociety.org. Read about Sigma Theta Tau history, membership criteria, membership services, efforts to promote nursing scholarship, and visit the Virginia Henderson Library.

National League for Nursing: http://www.nln.org. Learn about NLN history, membership services, and standards for professional and vocational nursing program accreditation, testing services, and research initiatives.

American Association of Colleges of Nursing: http://www.aacn.nche.edu. Read about AACN's history and mission and get a hyperlink to the Commission for Credentialing of Nursing Education for program accreditation standards for baccalaureate and graduate nursing educational programs.

The National Council of State Boards of Nursing: http://www.ncsbn.org. Read about the history of nursing licensure, current status of multistate compact licensure agreements, test plan for licensure, license revocation guidelines, and statistics related to nurses and find hyperlinks to individual state nursing boards.

The International Council of Nurses: http://www.icn.ch. Read about the history of the profession's global efforts to unite all nurses and improve health care for all global citizens. Review the ICN Code of ethics and find numerous position papers on professional practice issues.

## REFERENCES

Aiken, L. H., Clarke, S. P., Cheung, R. B., Sloane, D. M., & Silber, J. H. (2003). Educational levels of hospital nurses and surgical patient mortality. *Journal of the American Medical Association, 290,* 1617–1623.

Alexander, J., & Tate, M.A. (1998). *Web resource evaluation techniques.* Chester, PA: Widener University.

All Nursing Schools (2004). All Diploma RN Programs. Available at http://www.allnursingschools .com/find/results.php?st=&prog=diploma-nursing.html. Accessed June 25, 2005.

American Association of Colleges of Nursing (1998). *The essentials of baccalaureate education for professional nursing practice.* Washington, DC: Author.

American Nurses Association. (1995). *Social policy statement.* Kansas City: Author.

American Nurses Association. (2001). *Code for nurses with interpretive statements.* Washington, DC: American Nurses Publishing.

Bandman, E. L., & Bandman, B. (1995). *Nursing ethics through the life span* (3rd ed.). East Norwalk, CT: Appleton & Lange.

Benner, P. (1984). *From novice to expert.* Menlo Park, CA: Addison-Wesley.

Benner, P., Tanner, C., & Chesla, C. (Eds.). (1996). *Expertise in nursing practice: Caring, clinical judgment, and ethics.* New York: Springer.

Bevis, E. O., & Watson, J. (2000). *Toward a caring curriculum: A new pedagogy for nursing.* Sudbury, MA: Jones & Bartlett.

Bottoms, M. S. (1988). Competencies of a liberal education and registered nurses' behavior. *Journal of Nursing Education, 27,* 124–130.

Bower, F. L. (1999). The role of professional organizations (pp. 345–354). In E. J. Sullivan (Ed.), *Creating nursing's future.* St. Louis: Mosby.

Bradby, M. (1990). Status passage into nursing: Another view of the process of socialization. *Journal of Advanced Nursing, 15,* 1220–1225.

Broussard, P. C., & Oberleitner, M. G. (1997). Writing and thinking: A process to critical understanding. *Journal of Nursing Education, 7,* 334–336.

Brunke, L. (2003). Canadian provincial and territorial professional organizations and colleges (pp. 143–160). In M. McIntyre, & E. Thomlinson (Eds.), *Realities of Canadian Nursing.* Philadelphia: Lippincott Williams & Wilkins.

Bureau of Labor Statistics (2004). *Occupational Outlook Handbook 2004–2005.* Available at http://stats.bls.gov/oco/.

Clarke, B., James, C., & Kelly, J. (1996). Reflective practice: Reviewing the issues and refocusing the debate. *International Journal of Nursing Studies, 33,* 171–180.

Conway, M. E. (1984). Socialization and roles in nursing. In H. H. Werley & J. J. Fitzpatrick (Eds.), *Annual review of nursing research* (Vol. 1, pp. 183–208). New York: Springer.

Crawford, L., Marks, C., Gawel, S., & White, E. (2002). *NCSBN Research Brief 2001 Licensure and Examination Statistics* (Vol. 4).

Crawford, L., Marks, C., Gawel, S., & White, E. (2003). *NCSBN Research Brief 2002 Licensure and Examination Statistics* (Vol. 13).

DeLeskey, K. (2003). Factors affecting nurses' decisions to join and maintain membership in professional associations. *Journal of PeriAnesthesia Nursing, 18,* 8–17.

Diekelmann, N. L., & Rather, M. L. (Eds.). (1993). *Transforming RN education: Dialogue and debate.* New York: National League for Nursing.

Dreyfus, H. L., & Dreyfus, S. E. (1996). The relationship of theory and practice in the acquisition of skill. In P. Benner, C. A. Tanner, & C. A. Chesla (Eds.), *Expertise in nursing practice: Caring, clinical judgment, and ethics* (pp. 29–47). New York: Springer.

Dunham, K. S. (2001). *How to survive and maybe even love nursing school!* Philadelphia: F. A. Davis.

Flanagan, L. (1976). *One strong voice.* Kansas City, MO: The Lowell Press.

Fondiller, S. H. (1992). *The writer's workbook.* New York: National League for Nursing Press.

Freidson, E. (1994). *Professionalism reborn: Theory, prophecy and policy.* Chicago: The University of Chicago Press.

Gelman, S.B., Bellack, J.P., Berkman, A.K. (1999). Educational accreditation. Chapter 24 (pp. 226–240). In E. J. Sullivan (Ed.), *Creating nursing's future.* St. Louis: Mosby.

Hamilton, J. M., & Kiefer, M. E. (1986). *Survival skills for the new nurse.* Philadelphia: J. B. Lippincott.

Hinshaw, A. S. (1976, November). *Socialization and resocialization of nurses for professional nursing practice* (pp. 1–15). National League for Nursing Publication No. 15-1659. New York: National League for Nursing.

Horrigan, M. (2004). Employment projections to 2012: Concepts and context. *Monthly Labor Review, 127,* 3–22.

International Council of Nurses (1973). *ICN code for nurses: Ethical concepts applied to nursing.* Geneva: Author.

International Council of Nurses (2001). About ICN. Available at http://wwwicn.ch/abouticn.htm. Accessed June 25, 2005.

Kalisch, P., & Kalisch, B. (2004). *The advance of American nursing: A history* (4th ed.). Philadelphia: Lippincott Williams & Wilkins.

Kelly, L. Y., & Joel, L. A. (1995). *Dimensions in professional nursing* (7th ed.). New York: McGraw-Hill.

Kim, H. S. (1999). Critical reflective inquiry for knowledge development in nursing practice. *Journal of Advanced Nursing, 29,* 1205–1212.

Kozier, B., & Erb, G. (1988). Concepts and issues in nursing practice. Menlo Park, CA: Addison-Wesley.

Leddy, S. K. (2003). *Integrative health promotion.* Thorofare, NJ: Slack.

Loquist, R. S. (1999). Regulation: Parallel and powerful. In Milstead, J. A. (Ed.), *Health policy and politics: A nurse's guide.* Gaithersburg, MD: Aspen.

Lynn, M. R., McCain, N. L., & Boss, B. J. (1989). Socialization of RN to BSN. *Image, 21,* 232–237.

Martinez, M. E. (2000). *Education as the cultivation of intelligence.* Mahwah, NJ: Lawrence Erlbaum Associates.

*Merriam-Webster's Collegiate Dictionary* (10th ed.). (1994). Springfield, MA: Merriam-Webster.

Miller, B. K., Adams, D., & Beck, L. (1993). A behavioral inventory for professionalism in nursing. *Journal of Professional Nursing, 9,* 290–295.

Morse, J. M., Bottorff, J., Neander, W., & Solberg S. (1991, Summer). Comparative analysis of conceptualizations and theories of caring. *Image, 23,* 119–126.

National Council of State Boards of Nursing (2000). *Statistics on 1999 first time NCLEX pass rates according to degree type.* Available at http://www.ncsbn.org/research1999/licstats/%20lic20%statistics/%20reportson-line.pdf. Accessed February 7, 2004.

National Council of State Boards of Nursing (2001). *2000 Licensure & Examination Statistics.* Available at http://ww.ncsbn.org/pdfs/2000lic_exam_statistics_report_on-line.pdf. Accessed February 7, 2004.

National League for Nursing (NLN). (2002). *About NLN*. Available at http://www.nln.org/aboutnln/ourmission.htm. Accessed June 25, 2005.

Paul, R. (1992). *Critical thinking: What every person needs to survive in a rapidly changing world* (2nd rev. ed.). Santa Rosa, CA: The Foundation for Critical Thinking.

PEW Health Professions Commission (1995). *Critical challenges: Revitalizing the health professions for the 21st century.* University of California: San Francisco Center for the Health Professions.

PEW Health Professions Commission (1998). *Recreating health professional practice for a new century.* University of California: San Francisco Center for the Health Professions.

Powell, J. H. (1989). The reflective practitioner in nursing. *Journal of Advanced Nursing, 14,* 824–832.

Primm, P. L. (1987). Differentiated practice for ADN- and BSN-prepared nurses. *Journal of Professional Nursing, 3,* 218—225.

Robinson E. & Mee, C. (2004). Nursing 2004 salary survey. *Nursing 2004, 34,* 36–39.

Scheffer, B. K., & Rubenfeld, M. G. (2000). A consensus statement on critical thinking in nursing. *Journal of Nursing Education, 39,* 352–359.

Schon, D. (1983). *The reflective practitioner.* London: Temple Smith.

Schon, D. A. (1987). *Educating the reflective practitioner: Toward a new design for teaching and learning in the professions.* San Francisco: Jossey-Bass.

Shane, D. L. (1980). The returning-to-school syndrome. In S. Mirin (Ed.), *Teaching tomorrow's nurse* (pp. 119–126). Wakefield, MA: Nursing Resources.

Simms, L. M., & Lindberg, J. (1978). *The nurse person.* New York: Harper & Row.

Sullivan, M. C., & Christopher, M. M. (1999). Ethical issues. Chapter 25 (pp. 241–251). In E. J. Sullivan (Ed.), *Creating nursing's future.* St. Louis: Mosby.

Tanner, C. A., Benner, P., Chesla, C., & Gordon, D. R. (1993). The phenomenology of knowing the patient. *Image, 25,* 273–280.

The Gallup Organization (2003). Nursing ranks first as the most honest and ethical profession. Available at http://www.gallup.com/subscription/?mf&c_14141. Accessed Feb. 1, 2004.

United States Department of Labor. (2003). *National Employment and Wage Data from the Occupational employment Statistics survey by occupation, 2002.* Available at http://www.bls.gov/neews.release/ocwaget01.htm.

Vance, C. (1999). Nursing in the global arena. Chapter 35 (p. 334). In E. J. Sullivan (Ed.), *Creating nursing's future.* St. Louis: Mosby.

# CHAPTER 2

# The History Behind the Development of Professional Nursing

## KEY TERMS AND CONCEPTS

Ancient Nursing Practice
Roots of Holistic Nursing Practice
White Magic
Deaconess Movement
Roman Matrons
Early Christian Nurses
Nurses from Religious Orders
Kaiserworth
Florence Nightingale
Careful Nursing
Mary Seacole
Civil War Nursing
Public Health Nursing
State Registration
Work Redesign
Case Management
Consilience

## LEARNING OUTCOMES

By the end of this chapter, the learner will be able to:

1  Trace the history of nursing from ancient to current times.

2  Outline key societal trends that affected recruitment and retention of nurses in the workforce.

3  Explain the parallels of past history to current nursing practice.

4  Describe how history could be used to address current and future nursing issues.

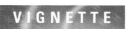

**VIGNETTE**

Martha, Carol, and Joe received an assignment to give a class presentation on nursing history that could be used to prepare the nursing profession for a future challenge. At first, they view this assignment as just more busywork. However, as they explore the history of nursing, they come to appreciate historically significant events and persons. They acknowledge that the profession may need to look at history to solve current and future problems.

As modern health care increases in scientific and technological complexity, people realize its limitations. Advances in technology permit measurement of previously unmeasured dimensions of the human species. Increasingly, the field of health care, especially medicine, has initiated targeted efforts to explain the interrelationships of health, longevity, multiculturalism, socioeconomics, and spirituality. In many ways, nursing forged a path to holistic health care even before it became popular. An examination of nursing history provides professional nurses with an understanding of the profession's unique place within the health care arena and how history may have answers for today's problems.

## ✦ NURSING IN ANCIENT CIVILIZATIONS (BEFORE AD 1)

Humans learned how to care for each other from observing animals treating themselves and each other. Humans observed uninjured animals bringing food to injured companions and offspring. By watching animals, human learned a variety of therapies such as licking of wounds (a form of an antiseptic dressing), applying pressure to control bleeding (from apes), amputating extremities when ensnared in traps (from rats), licking salt (from deer, cows, and antelope), wrapping wounds in spiral fashion (from birds), applying splints (from snipe), traveling great distances to soak in healing water (from deer), ventilating living space (cutting slits in tents to let in fresh air), and entombing the dead (from bees). Because some of the treatments could not be performed independently, ancient man observed that animals relied on each other at times (Nutting & Dock, 1935a).

### Primitive Man

The earliest of men believed in a spirit world. Some primitive cultures developed the belief of a soul that existed independently of the body. Human tragedy, including illness, was blamed on the spirit world. To please the spirits, certain members of society possessed special powers that could ease suffering, enhance healing, and cure diseases. Techniques used by early healers included pummeling (a form of massage), administrating herbs to induce vomiting, exposing persons to strong odors or smoke, squeezing, starving, purging, applying roots or balms to the skin, or twisting the body into various positions. Along with touch, the medicine magician frequently provided the person with warm applications and other healing ceremonies with various effects such as drumming, smoking, and chanting to drive out evil spirits (Nutting & Dock, 1935a).

### The East

As persons organized societies, the need for someone to care for the very young, injured, infirmed, and aging members emerged. Many years before the Christian era, the ancient Hindi linked hygiene to health. Details of nursing are recorded in Lesson IX of *Charada-Samhita*. This Indian record describes the following four qualifications for a nurse: (1) knowledge of drug preparation, (2) cleverness, (3) devotion to patients, and (4) purity of body and mind (Nutting & Dock, 1935a). These early nurses were primarily men and nursing was viewed as a sacred service that only the purest of body and mind could perform (Nutting & Dock; Kalisch & Kalisch, 2004; Jamieson & Sewall, 1954).

In the 3rd century BC, King Asoka expanded the community institutions for caring for the sick travelers in hospitals that were described as spacious and roomy mansions that were protected from strong winds, breezes, smoke, sun, dust, or malodorous scents. In **ancient nursing practice,** the sick were cared for by a body of attendants (men) noted for their purity and cleanliness of habits, full of kindness, having cleverness and great skills in all kinds of service. Along with good nutrition, ventilation, and a clean environment, the attendants read stories, chanted hymns, played musical instruments, and conversed with the infirmed while attending to all their needs (Nutting & Dock, 1935a). In many cases, nursing interventions that occurred in ancient times serve as the **roots of holistic nursing practice.**

Along with India, ancient Buddhist texts from Ceylon possess equally touching accounts of good deeds and philanthropy. These texts contain allusions to "thousands" of priestesses whose duties included the care of the sick (Nutting & Dock, 1935a).

## China

Chinese civilization began around 3000 BC on the banks of the Yellow River. The Chinese valued women over men and a woman's worth was determined only by the number of sons that she could produce. Young married women were treated as slaves until they produced one or more sons. However, old women who bore many sons were given high positions in society and were revered. The ancient Chinese developed the concept of yin (the passive, negative feminine energy force) and yang (the active, positive, masculine energy force). They defined health as a balance of the two energy forces. Before 2000 BC, the Chinese practiced dissection, performed acupuncture, and prescribed herbal therapies to enhance health and cure illness. They used baths to reduce fever, bloodletting to remove evil spirits from the body, and outlined detailed principles of physical examination (look, listen, ask, and feel) (Jamieson & Sewall, 1954).

## Egypt

The oldest written recordings about medicine and nursing come from Egypt on papyrus and date to 3000 BC. The Ebers Papyrus outlines over 700 therapies derived from minerals, plants, and animals. The compounded prescriptions were made up in forms of decorations, pills, tablets, injections, infusions, lozenges, powder, potions, inhalations, lotions, ointments, and plasters (Kalisch & Kalisch, 2004; Nutting & Dock, 1935a). Because of the sacredness of temples, dying persons were placed on the street so that persons walking by could give them advice. The art of medicine in ancient Egypt consisted of two branches: the theurgic class devoted themselves to magical cures, and the practitioners used natural cures. Along with disease treatment, the Egyptians practiced public hygiene and sanitation. Egyptians had ordinances specifying practices for neighborliness. In all records from Egypt, there is no evidence of hospitals and nursing. However, there is mention of temple priestesses without reference to their duties (Nutting & Dock).

## Babylonia

The Babylonians experienced a vastly different lifestyle than the Egyptians. They believed that numbers possessed magical powers and displayed a great interest in astrology. They devised the first calendar (Jamieson & Sewall, 1954). Illness was viewed as punishment for displeasing and sinning against the gods. The Babylonians left a record of medicine that outlined surgical procedures, methods to banish demons, and ways to avoid evil spirits. In 1900 BC, Hammurabi developed a code that provided the first sliding scale for payment of fees and divided the public into three classes. The law specified that citizens compensate each other for transgressions equally. Therefore, a surgeon may have his hands amputated if he performed unsuccessful surgery (Nutting & Dock, 1935a; Jamieson & Sewall, 1954).

## Assyria

The Assyrian civilization began about 2300 BC. Like other ancient cultures, the Assyrians credited the good and evil spirits for human conditions. Failure to abide by cultural mandates resulted in severe punishment, including mutilation and death. Medical practices centered on sacred rites for banishment of evil spirits or severe punishment for sins (Jamieson & Sewall, 1954).

## Persia

In a Persian epic dated 642 to 242 BC, three kinds of physicians were mentioned. One healed by the knife, another by exorcism and incantations, and a third by using plants. Although there is no mention of nurses, there are descriptions of many procedures, many of which fall within the domain of current nursing practice (Nutting & Dock, 1935a).

## Palestine

Sanitary measures from Egypt became part of the Hebrew culture during the period of enslavement. The ancient Hebrews adopted natural cures, but rejected the magical therapies. The Old Testament outlines food inspection, tree preservation, vital statistic records, and infectious disease quarantine followed by fumigation. Rabbis declared that every Hebrew had an obligation to show sympathy, cheer, aid, and relieve the sick as an incumbent duty. One of the seven acts of charity mentioned in rabbinical literature is to visit the sick. The ancient Hebrews built rest houses for travelers and the destitute, which were connected to the sick house (Nutting & Dock, 1935a).

## Greece

Like Egypt, Greece traced medical arts to divine myths. In the *Iliad*, Homer identifies Asklepios, the father of Machaon and Podalirius, as the "blameless physician." The Greeks also divided the healing arts into two branches with one retaining priestly powers and the other having medical functions. Temples of Asklepios were reported to exist as early as 1134 BC. Hospitality was a sacred obligation in Greek culture. The "xenodochion" served as a municipal inn for strangers, the poor, and sick in large Greek cities (Nutting & Dock, 1935a).

Besides the public xenodochion, "iotrions" were established where surgery was performed and dispensaries were located. Only persons who could be cured were admitted to the iotrions or temples for healing services. The temples had a place devoted to the sick called the "abaton." Ruins reveal that the abaton contained a large room with an altar surrounded by smaller rooms that could accommodate one person. Along with priests, the abaton was staffed with key bearers, clerks, bookkeepers, and a class of workers who were sometimes physicians, bath attendants, slaves, and priestesses who carried baskets of mysteries and holy things. Because of the ancient belief that death and birth pollute locales, the terminally ill were left on the street to die (Nutting & Dock, 1935a).

In the golden age of Greece, the great physician Hippocrates practiced. He outlined the role of physician as assisting nature to bring about a cure. Hippocrates set standards for bathing, bandaging, and other cures. Although he provided no treatise on nursing, his work specified that his assistants were coworkers (Nutting & Dock, 1935a; Kalisch & Kalisch, 2004).

## Rome

The Greeks introduced the Romans to medicine sometime in the third century BC. Before then, Romans believed that lost health could only be restored by the good will and peace of the gods, especially Apollo. Roman construction of drains, aqueducts, good roads, sewage systems, and proper cemeteries, as well as an organized system of medical help, enhanced public health for the Romans. Nero organized a Roman medical service and appointed a superintendent of court physicians. Slaves of rich families cultivated knowledge of practical medicine. Many slaves earned freedom by curing owners with their skills. The Romans reserved the best medical and nursing care for the soldiers. Wounded soldiers were carried to private homes, tents, or a separate building to be cared for by women and old men of irreproachable behavior (Nutting & Dock, 1935a; Kalisch & Kalisch, 2004).

## Northern Europe

In northern Europe, the ancient Teutons revered their wise women. These ancient women went out early and late in the day to gather herbs, which they knew had medicinal and remedial qualities. This practice may have been the earliest prototypes of the witch of myth and legend. As time progressed, various superstitions followed both wise women and the medicine men. According to Finnish mythology, the ancient healers practiced **"white magic"** that was primarily medicinal in nature. However, society grew to believe that these persons with special healing powers also had connections to evil spirits and could use "black magic" that caused natural catastrophes or human illness, and injury (Nutting & Dock, 1935a).

## Germany

Like the northern Europeans, the Gauls and Germans highly regarded women. They believed that women could communicate with the gods more easily than men. These women possessed great knowledge and skill in medicine and surgery. German women established expertise in treating wounds from war, providing obstetrical care and treating animals (Nutting & Dock, 1935a).

### Questions for Reflection 2-1

1. Are any ancient nursing interventions used to tend to the ill and infirmed today?
2. Why do you think that some ancient nursing interventions and medical therapies had to be "rediscovered"?

## ⬤ NURSING IN THE EARLY CHRISTIAN ERA (AD 1–500)

### Roman Matrons

Women from well-established Roman families enjoyed dignified and respected positions in society. When the personal-contract or free marriage system was established in the Roman Empire, wives became coequals, retained legal independence, and maintained control of her property. The earliest women workers in the Church that were concerned with nursing were the deaconess and widows. The virgin, presbyteress, canoness, and nun appeared later. A large share of the nursing duties were performed by men in these times. Early converts to Christianity, especially the ladies of leisure, viewed comforting the afflicted as a sacred duty. Women joined the **deaconess movement** and attended to the sick in their homes. In AD 60, Phoebe, a deaconess and a friend of St. Paul, assumed clerical and secular duties. She became the first parish worker, friendly visitor, and district nurse and is credited as the mother of visiting nursing (Nutting & Dock, 1935a).

Early church deacons and deaconesses sought out those in need, established a system of visiting nurses, and sometimes brought the ill into their homes for care. As home hospitals were organized, the deaconate became associated with the work of nursing. Eventually, the bishops followed their example, and kept open their homes to tend to the sick. As congregations grew and more poor persons joined them, individual homes were too small to accommodate the vast numbers of persons needing help. The Christian xenodochium, or home for strangers, was opened. The institution contained a section for the ordinary traveler and one for the poor and infirmed. As early as the second century, Roman converts to Christianity transformed their homes into places to care for the sick and poor. **Roman matrons** organized and delivered care to these persons in need. Nutting and Dock credit this work to the matrons named, Marcella, Paula, Eustochia, Blesilla, Proba, Laeta, Lucina, Fabiola, Principia, Ansella, Lea, Melanie, Albina and others. Nursing the sick was seen as proper penance for past sins and solace for unhappy lives (Nutting & Dock, 1935a).

Between the years of AD 249 and 263, an extensive epidemic hit Rome resulting in many deaths of the deaconate. In AD 350, another epidemic hit the city of Edessa, where wealthy inhabitants in desperation freely gave money to Ephren to provide care for the ill. St. Ephren used the donations to build the first hospital. Along with the matrons, widows, old men, and the disenfranchised provided nursing care.

In the 5th century, Justinian granted the bishops authority over hospitals. With great zeal, the bishops built shelters, hospices, foundling asylums, and nosocomia (nursing hospitals) within the confines of monasteries. A glorious record of the religious nursing orders of men and women flourished for a thousand years. Through religious order life, women found freedom from social fetters and distasteful arranged marriages. They were free to conduct satisfying work and cultivate intellectual desires (Nutting & Dock, 1935a; Jamieson & Sewall, 1954).

## Advances in Greece

Although the **early Christian nurses** were instrumental in the development of modern nursing, other groups played a key role in the advancement of nursing practice. In AD 100, Areateus emphasized the necessity of strict cleanliness of bedclothes, use of powders on moist skin, and mouth washes for patients who were not allowed to drink. He also specified environmental guidelines for persons suffering from a variety of illnesses. For fevers, the room should be light and airy and the patient should be lightly covered and receive only liquids for nourishment. Excitable patients should be kept in a small, undecorated room, with constant temperature. He outlined strategies for pain control that included hot baths, fomentations, hot water bladders, light massage, plasters and salves. Music was also used to soothe and lull persons in distress. In AD 138, the Greeks established a maternity hospital and a home for the dying (Nutting & Dock, 1935a).

## ● NURSING IN THE MIDDLE AGES (500–1500)

As the church gained influence and power, the monasteries provided service to society. Religious men and women through service gained societal status. In 1190, the first mention of a nursing uniform surfaced when a Bavarian monk insisted that religious women needed to wear distinctive dress to be recognized when out in public as they performed charitable acts, including tending the ill. As monasteries flourished as centers of learning, nuns became distinguished for work in academia and service. By the 13th century, monks and nuns were said to have higher medical knowledge than the rest of society (Nutting & Dock, 1935a).

The Lateran Council in 1123 forbade monks and priests to practice medicine. The Benedictine sisters, however, actively continued to expand the knowledge of medicine and practiced medicine and nursing. Monks and nuns conjointly cared for the sick. The monks cared for men; the nuns cared for women. The nuns took charge of the hospital while the monks served as priests (Nutting & Dock, 1935a).

Perhaps Hildegarde, a nun, heralded the beginning of female dominance in nursing. She possessed extraordinary intellectual powers and amassed great knowledge of medicine and nursing that she gained through her observation and management of patients. Between 1151 and 1159, she wrote volumes devoted to medical works that include accurate physiology related to reproduction, circulation, and the nervous system. Although her work primarily addresses the art of medicine, she wrote about key nursing principles (Nutting & Dock, 1935a).

## The Crusades and Nursing Knights

During the Crusades, hospitals were built on the routes to and in Jerusalem where men delivered care to travelers and battle-scarred warriors. The Knights Hospitallers of St. John of Jerusalem were purely a nursing order, but later became devoted to military service. The Teutonic Knights had both nursing and military duties. The Knights of

St. Lazarus were a nursing order from the great hospital built by St. Basil in AD 329 who also later assumed military duties. Along with the Knights of St. Lazarus, there were Sisters of St. Lazarus. In England, the Order of St. John consisted of men devoted to charitable work including formation of cottage hospitals and convalescent homes and providing nurse's training for the poor (Nutting & Dock, 1935a; Kalisch & Kalisch, 2004).

In the 11th century, two hospitals were built in England: one to care for lepers, and another to care for persons suffering from other ailments. Brothers attended to the sick men and sisters attended to the sick women. The hospital for lepers (St. Giles) was run by an order of nuns known as the Poor Clares. Around 1148, ladies of noble birth added attending the sick as an expressed duty (Nutting & Dock, 1935a).

## Religious Orders of Nursing for Women

In the 12th century, French nursing became part of the manual labor performed by several orders of Roman Catholic sisters. Besides Catholic orders of sisters devoted to nursing, secular orders of sisterhood also emerged. In France, one hospital staffed itself with women who were either widowed or repenting from a previously impure life (Nutting & Dock, 1935a). **Nurses from religious orders** provided a more structured approach to the care of the ill and infirmed.

In Paris, the Augustinian order or nuns provided nursing care for the hospital. The Augustinian order routinely handed down information of how to care for the sick from one to another. Many of the wealthy families sent a son or daughter for religious service during these times. In 1212, the Church passed statutes to regulate the nursing orders. Nursing orders for both men and women were decreed to take permanent vows of poverty, chastity, and obedience. By 1368, conflict among the various orders resulted in corruption and greed. Funds dedicated by the Church were used for war. Morale of the men and women caring for the sick became demoralized because of no respite from the unrelenting toil. Religious orders, especially the sisters, accumulated much money and many possessions and focused their efforts to manage them. An epidemic of syphilis spread and hospitals became centers of infection. During this time, many persons left monasteries and convents taking whatever they could carry, further depleting resources for the care of the infirmed (Nutting & Dock, 1935a).

## ⬤ NURSING IN THE RENAISSANCE AND COLONIAL AMERICA (1500–1860)

In 1505, King Louis XII decreed that jurisdiction of the hospitals be temporarily removed from the canons of Notre Dame and be placed with secular directors. In 1526, the rectors of a hospital (located in Lyons, France) directed hospital staff to wear a white uniform because the women came to work in scandalous apparel. In 1562, the dress changed from white to a black dress, white linen apron, and unstarched white cap. By the middle of the 16th century, the rectors introduced stringent regulations and required nursing service members to become part of a religious order. The male nurses (who were brothers) wore a blue robe and a silver cross. At this time, a woman left nursing only to marry or to care for aging parents. Also during this time, two notable nursing orders of men flourished. They worked in hospitals, visited the sick at home, and distributed herbal medications (Nutting & Dock, 1935a).

Similar degeneration of religious life occurred in England. The control of hospitals became the responsibility of the cities. Philanthropy and state aid emerged as the major funding sources. Religious orders were replaced with ordinary lay servants and attendants who had little knowledge of how to care for the infirmed. A matron who had some knowledge of how to run a hospital supervised them. The matron was responsible for finding persons to care for the sick. Frequently, the matron found the care attendants from jails and debtor prisons. Under this system, nursing suffered great degradation. City hospitals became like crowded prisons with small rooms, undecorated walls, and small windows. Patients received care from heartless attendants and sisters (also called servant nurses) who were required to work 12 to 48 hours without a break. Charles Dickens's description of the untrustworthy and drunken Sairey Gamp depicted the quality of nursing of the times. In some cases, patients nursed each other as the servant nurses slept (Nutting & Dock, 1935a).

As the New World was settled, the French and Spanish opened hospitals. The Jesuits opened a hospital for settlers and the Canadian Indians. The Indians shared remedies for scurvy with the French. Likewise, the Jesuits shared their knowledge of medicines with the Indians. As hospital labors for the nuns grew heavier, the native women quickly grasped the concept of charitable practice and brought great physical strength to patient care (Nutting & Dock, 1935b).

Before 1524, Cortez built the hospital of the Immaculate Conception in the current location of Mexico City. The nursing staff consisted primarily of a brotherhood. In 1531, the second oldest hospital of the new world was founded in Santa Fe where a community of over 30,000 Native Americans practiced hospitality and charitable works (Nutting & Dock, 1935b).

In the New England colonies, the growth of hospitals was slow. Frequently, the captain of the ship served as deacon and his wife assumed midwife responsibilities. Early treatment for illness in the English colonies consisted of prayer and superstitious practices. When hospitals opened in New York and Philadelphia, inmates provided nursing services (Jamieson & Sewall, 2004).

The 1700s marked the beginning of hospital reform. After becoming a prisoner of war in France, John Howard embarked on a crusade as a prison reformer. His work evolved into work on hospital reform (Jamieson & Sewall). In 1789, John Howard wrote about the state of hospitals throughout Europe and England. He reported inconsistent conditions in the hospitals across Europe. He noted that the hospitals staffed by religious orders tended to be quiet, neat, and clean with careful attention to patient hygiene and infection prevention measures. He also described secular hospitals where patients were dirty, infected with pests, and had no bed linens (Nutting & Dock, 1935b).

## ✦ THE MOVEMENT OF NURSING TO A RESPECTABLE PROFESSION (1820–1917)

Twenty-five years after Howard's death, Stephen Grellet (a French-American) toured English prisons that housed French military prisoners. When he observed the conditions, he was appalled at the living conditions of children who had been born in prison. He consulted Elizabeth Fry, an English friend, to help the infants. Mrs. Fry founded a program for the women prisoners to make goods and sell them. The women used the income generated to provide care for their children. Mrs. Fry traveled throughout

Europe to set up similar programs. During her travels, Mrs. Fry became acquainted with **Kaiserworth,** a training program for nurses. Mrs. Fry referred **Florence Nightingale** to Kaiserworth upon learning of Florence's interest in nursing (Jamieson & Sewall, 1954 Nutting & Dock, 1935b).

In 1821, Pastor Fliedner arrived in Kaiserworth, Germany, to find himself the pastor of a financially depressed congregation. Like Mrs. Fry, he possessed a profound interest in prison reform. Along with his efforts of successful prison reform, Pastor Fliedner founded a hospital for two purposes. First, he wanted to care for the sick and second, he wanted to provide a field for deaconess instruction. In 1836, Gertrud Reichardt, a physician's daughter who helped with her father's practice, became the first probationer. Under the leadership of Fredrike Fliedner (the Pastor's wife), the hospital tended the sick and probationers received clinical and theoretical instruction on the art of nursing. Upon completion of their education, the newly ordained deaconesses provided relief work for the poor, imprisoned, or those who needed help (Jamieson & Sewall, 1954; Nutting & Dock, 1935b).

The deaconesses from Kaiserworth established an honorable reputation that spread worldwide. Kaiserworth deaconesses established themselves in Europe and the Middle East. In 1850, Fliedner took several deaconesses to Pittsburgh, Pennsylvania, where they staffed a hospital. The movement progressed to Milwaukee where the Deaconess Home and Hospital was founded.

In 1831, a group of Irish women under the leadership of Catherine McAuley formed the Religious Sisters of Mercy and provided nursing services throughout Ireland and the world. The Irish sisters devised a system of **careful nursing** that comprised "physical care and emotional consolation provided from a spiritual perspective" (Meehan, 2003, p. 99). In the realm of careful nursing, nurses provided nursing services using great tenderness, gentleness, kindness, and patience with each client encounter. Patients received highly skilled care from nurses who practiced with spiritual love, sought to create an environment of calmness, created restorative environments, strove for perfection in keeping patients safe and comfortable, provided health education, collaborated with physicians and other health care providers (including physicians), and took care of themselves. During the Asian cholera epidemic of 1832, there was a substantially lower mortality rate among recipients of nursing services from McAuley and her colleagues (Meehan, 2003).

At the end of the 18th century, nursing manuals began to appear. Some contained common sense information and some were scientifically based. J. D. Phahler's manual gave specific examples of instruction of how to arrange and care for a sick room, procedures for various treatments, instructions for use of equipment, and maintenance of written records. Along with procedures, Dr. Phahler's manual emphasized the importance of attending to patient psychological needs. Dr. Franz May's manual provided more general approaches to patient care and also emphasized the importance of maintaining the health of the caregivers. Dr. May also established a course of instructions for care attendants in Mannheim, Germany. Other educational programs opened in Germany. An evangelical hospital in Germany supplied nurses' training. In 1836, Pastor Gossner favored the word *Pfelegerin* (nurse) to title care attendants in Prussia (Nutting & Dock, 1935b).

During the American Revolutionary War, Catholic nuns were the only organized group of nurses. Women followed husbands to the battlegrounds and provided nursing care to soldiers who were wounded or infirmed. Many homes and barns became hospitals. In 1786, the Quakers established the Philadelphia Dispensary, which was financed through public donations. Physicians from the Dispensary practiced disease prevention. In New York, a residential insane asylum was founded in 1798. In Canada, the Augustinian nuns from France opened with the establishment of hospitals, visiting nurse programs, schools and orphanages (Nutting & Dock, 1935b; Jamieson & Sewall, 1954).

Along with the establishment of hospitals and asylums, Protestant and Catholic sisterhoods were founded. Mother Elizabeth Seaton established the first American order of nuns, the Catholic Sisters of Charity in 1809. The Catholic Sisters of Mercy emigrated from Ireland. Finally, the Reverend William Passavant founded a hospital in 1848 and staffed it with deaconesses from Kaiserworth (Jamieson & Sewall, 1954).

The Nursing Society of Philadelphia was founded in 1836 and primarily provided home maternity service. The Nursing Society selected its nurses from applicants who displayed stable character and who had experience as familial heads. In 1850, the Society opened a home and school where systematic instruction was given on cooking and obstetrics. Students were also exposed to clinical practice in homes (Jamieson & Sewall, 1954).

## The Birth of Nursing as a Profession

Efforts at social reform flourished in the late nineteenth century. The reform of nursing evolved from efforts to reform prisons and hospitals. Florence Nightingale led the efforts to reform patient care and sowed the seeds of establishing nursing as a profession. Florence Nightingale was born into an English family who were established members of the "good society." Mr. Nightingale delighted in teaching Florence Latin, Greek, and other languages, mathematics, science, and reading. From her diary entries about accompanying her mother to hospitals, Florence identified her life passion. However, Mrs. Nightingale expressed concern about the possibility of her delicate daughter keeping company with drunken, immoral nurses and tending to the needs of people with unhealthy bodies in prison-like, dirty, smelly hospitals. Eventually, Florence's parents gave in to her desire and Florence entered a nurse's training program in an English hospital when she turned 25 years old. Florence did not practice nursing full-time after her training, but continued to travel with her parents.

During European trips, Florence explored the option of starting a community of trained nurses after visiting with nuns in Rome. Mrs. Fry, a friend of the Nightingale family informed Florence about Kaiserworth upon learning about her interest in nursing. She attended Kaiserworth in 1850 and 1851, where she was instructed in the art of nursing (Kalisch & Kalisch, 2004; Jamieson & Sewall, 1954; Nutting & Dock, 1935b).

At the age of 34, Florence attained a position as the superintendent of a small institution on Harley Street in London that provided shelter to homeless women and nursing services to sick governesses. After a cholera epidemic, the British became involved with the Crimean War and discovered that they had no sisters to assist with injured and infirmed troops as their enemies. In 1854, the British government appointed Florence as the Superintendent of the Nursing Staff. She and 38 other women (including Joanna Bridgeman, a colleague of Catherine McAuley) went to Scutari where they found two hospitals in deplorable condition. Florence pleaded with her friends in England to send money and supplies. After providing a clean, well-ventilated environment along with the provision of nutritious meals for the patients, the mortality rate declined from 40% to 2% (Kalisch & Kalisch, 2004; Jamieson & Sewall, 1954; Meehan, 2003).

Power, admiration, and fame came to Florence. Before long, army nursing under Florence Nightingale evolved into a health service where both the physical and psychosocial needs of the ill were considered. She wrote letters for soldiers, employed wives who had accompanied spouses to the battlefield, and made night rounds in the wards with a lamp.

During the Crimean War, Nightingale met **Mary Seacole,** a Jamaican nurse volunteer who also nursed the soldiers. Seacole also saw the need for holistic outreach nursing services to civilians who had been injured or displaced because of the war. She set up a hotel where she provided shelter, relaxation, and excellent food. When guests became ill, she prescribed medicines that had been learned from her grandmother and mother. After the war, Mary Seacole dedicated her life to elevating nursing to a respectable profession (Wheeler, 1999).

In 1855, important British citizens established the "Nightingale fund" to enable Florence to establish a school to train an elite group of women in the art of nursing. Nightingale expected these women to teach nursing to the entire world. Besides establishing a formalized program of nursing education, Florence continued her efforts at reforming hospitals, public health, and nursing (Jamieson & Sewall, 1954; Nutting & Dock, 1935b).

Along with Florence Nightingale, several American women influenced the reform of health care and nursing. In 1893, Lillian Wald and Mary Brewster opened a Nurses' Settlement House in New York City. They used the term "public health nurse" to describe the trained nurses who responded to nursing needs outside of the hospital. These nurses responded to calls from individuals as well as physicians to provide home nursing services. The program provided services regardless of the ability of recipients to pay. In 1895, Wald and Brewster moved to larger accommodations that became known as the Henry Street Settlement House. By 1900, 20 district nursing organizations employed 200 nurses across the United States (Roberts, 1954).

## Questions for Reflection 2-2

1. Did you know about the contributions of others to professional nursing in the 19th century?
2. Why do you suppose these contributions were overlooked?

## The Birth of Formal Nursing Education

Efforts to standardize training for nursing occurred in the Victorian era, a time characterized by exaggerated chivalry and etiquette. Upper- and middle-class women led circumscribed lives, were considered property of their fathers or husbands, had no independent rights, and were considered incapable of intellectual development. Some even thought that education would damage reproductive organs. Women from lower classes, who had to work, found socially acceptable employment as retail clerks, factory workers, governesses, or domestic servants. Nursing, on the other hand, was considered an unacceptable profession and reserved for women paupers from workhouses or those who served prison time for drunkenness, vagrancy, or prostitution.

However, the example of Florence Nightingale's service in the Crimean War elevated the profession. Society began thinking of nursing as an art that ". . . must be raised to the status of a trained profession" (Kjervik & Martinson, 1979, p. 22). Graduates of Nightingale's program in England traveled abroad to establish professional nursing schools.

Although she established a theoretical model for nursing practice, Nightingale proposed that nurses should follow protocol rather than use independent thinking. She emphasized that nurses should be taught how to carry out physician orders. To maintain discipline among nurses, Nightingale delineated a strict nursing service hierarchy. Good character superseded intellectual ability when the Nightingale nursing school selected applicants into the program. Education received by nurses in Nightingale's school focused on teaching nurses what to do, how to do it, following physician's orders, knowing why, training the nurse's senses, and linking these things with reflection to decide what should be done (Kalisch & Kalisch, 2004).

## Civil War Nursing

As nursing became more acceptable, women volunteered during the Civil War to be nurses. American women transformed the ballrooms of their homes into wards for the injured and infirmed soldiers; this resulted in the birth of **Civil War Nursing.** Dorothea Dix was appointed as the Superintendent of Female Nurses in the Union Army, founded the first American Army nursing corps, and was given full power to organize human and material resources to care for sick and injured soldiers. She appointed 3,214 nurses and placed eight to 20 of them in each Union hospital.

Along with nurses from the Army Nursing Corps, female volunteers and family members also provided nursing services to Civil War casualties. Louisa May Alcott wrote about her tragic experiences caring for soldiers. Mother Bickerdyke diligently searched to find living soldiers who had been wounded in battle but had been placed among the dead. Clara Barton used her own resources to provide necessities and supplies to care for those injured or displaced on both sides of the battle. In her writings, Jane Stuart Woolsey noted that the hospitals run by Roman Catholic nuns were cleaner and had better outcomes while praising the devotion and virtue of all nurses (Kalisch & Kalisch, 2004). Along with female volunteers, the Young Men's Christian Association (YMCA) members volunteered to serve as nurses (Jamieson & Sewall, 1954).

In Confederate states, most of the nursing care was delivered by Southern "matrons" who volunteered their services despite having no formal education. Efforts made by these women focused on cooking, making bandages and sewing. However, many times Southern mansion owners opened their doors and provided care to sick and injured soldiers. Slaves and plantation mistresses and daughters worked together at times (Kalisch & Kalisch, 2004).

## American Hospital Training Programs and Diploma Schools

In the United States, nursing training programs started simultaneously with the acceptance and availability of college education for upper-class women. As medical education moved into the postgraduate university, nursing education became established as apprenticeship training under the control of physicians and hospitals. The first nursing training programs were established in 1872 and 1873 in Boston, New Haven, and New York City. By 1880, 15 programs existed. Within a decade, programs proliferated to 432 and had graduated 3,465 nurses (Burgess, 1928).

The early hospital training schools had some autonomy in setting the nursing program of study. They rapidly became dependent on hospitals for financial support as they lacked independent budgets and endowed funds. Eventually, they became nursing service departments within the affiliated hospitals. Students worked 7 days a week, 50 weeks annually, for 1 to 2 years in exchange for on-the-job training, a few lectures, and a small allowance. Staffing the hospitals with students and faculty proved financially advantageous and hospitals without training programs quickly established them. From 1880 to 1926, the number of hospital-based nursing programs increased from 15 to 2,155 (Burgess, 1928).

## The American Public Health Movement

As the field of **public health nursing** grew, basic principles specific to the specialty emerged. Reform efforts indicated a need to provide nursing services to all who were sick without considering ability to pay, religious affiliation, or ethnic background. To provide consistency in service, the district nurses acknowledged the need to keep formal client records. To avoid duplication of services and prevent gaps in fulfilling client needs, the nurses learned the importance of cooperation with other groups that provided community care. During the public health movement, the family rather than the individual surfaced as the basic care unit (Spradley, 1990). The challenges of managing these activities proved burdensome for the district nurses with the narrowly focused education received in hospital-based nursing education programs. Some nurses acknowledged the limitations of their education and sought additional education in institutions of higher learning.

Public health nursing prospered from 1900 until the outbreak of World War I. The patient home served as the major location for nursing practice, as hospitals had become places to receive charity, contract infection, and die. As news of Nightingale's successes spread, hospitals began practicing principles of hygiene and nursing became a respectable career.

## Other Social Reform Movements

Following the Civil War, numerous social reform movements emerged. William Booth founded the Salvation Army to protect the poor, ex-prisoners, old, young, and any who were miserable and had fallen from the grace of God. Jane Adams established the Hull House in Chicago that provided day care, kindergarten, and library services to immigrant women and children. Christian Associations of young men and women were formed to build character and provide community services. Medicine experienced reforms that emphasized science and invention over superstitious practices such as bloodletting. Finally, word of these and many more movements became known throughout the world from the invention of the telegraph and telephone (Jamieson & Sewall, 1954; Kalisch & Kalisch, 2004).

## ● NURSING DURING THE EARLY 20TH CENTURY, THE WORLD WARS, AND POST–WORLD WAR II ERA (1890–1960)

The hospital and medical reform movement resulted in changes in the nursing care of patients. Physician demand for educated nurses caused the untrained attendants who had dominated hospital nursing to be replaced with nursing students. Because of the lack of trained nurses, graduates of nursing programs found themselves in supervisory positions, or as home private duty nurses. Hospitals with nursing students used them as staff or contracted their services with families and pocketed the money for services rendered. The typical private nursing case lasted 3 weeks and required the nurse to live with the family, to be available for 24 hours a day. The average wage earned was $1200 per month. The nurse remained idle if not on a private case. As nurses aged, they lacked the stamina required for all night vigils and the hard work required for safe, effective patient care (Goldmark, 1923).

North Carolina led the efforts to **state registration** of nurses in 1903 by establishing guidelines for professional registration. Requirements included graduation from an established diploma nursing school. New Jersey and New York quickly followed. By 1912, 29 states and the District of Columbia had registration requirements for nurses. To renew initial registration, nurses were given a 3-year grace period to practice then they were required to write a licensing exam that emphasized dietetics, patient comfort, skilled handling of patients, and general management (Dock, 1912).

The United States entered the First World War in 1917. Unmarried trained nurses entered the Army and Navy Nurse Corps. Along with trained nurses, volunteers from well-to-do families served as nurses' aides at their own expense after taking intensive Red Cross courses. The government launched a publicity campaign to recruit women into nursing. Advertisements glamorizing nursing appeared in newspapers and magazines. However, on the battlefields, the nurses encountered the horrors of injuries sustained from bullets and poisonous gas. At times, the ratio of nurse to patient rose to as high as 1 to 60. Frequently, nurses were required to perform actual surgery to save lives. Finally, the flu epidemic of 1918 to 1919 compounded the need for more nurses at home and abroad (Kalisch & Kalisch, 2004).

Nursing sustained an image problem in the 1920s. Movies became available and cinema portrayals were unrealistic and unflattering to the profession. Reduced prestige for the profession resulted from the fact that 95% of nurses were women, most nursing leaders were unmarried, renewed emphasis of the woman's place in the home as devoted wife and mother by society, and portrayal of nurses as an altruistic self-sacrificing profession in a time that focused on frivolity and self-indulgence.

### Proliferation of Nursing Education Programs

The proliferation of nursing programs resulted in widespread variance in nursing education quality. Linda Richards, a graduate of a Canadian nursing program and the first trained American nurse, led reforms at a minimum of 12 major American nursing programs (Jamieson & Sewall). Isabel Hampton Robb questioned the qualifications of nursing faculty and spearheaded the first educational program for nursing faculty at Teacher's College in New York in 1901 (Dock, 1912). Widespread concerns about the safety of nursing and medical care arose among the public. Reforms in nursing education followed reforms in medical education. In 1910, *The Flexner Report* broadcasted problems with the quality of medical education and resulted in drastic reforms (Flexner, 1910). Nursing leaders of the time hoped that results from *The Flexner Report* would result in nursing education reforms. *The Goldmark Report* of 1923 and other studies and surveys done at the time indicated that the root of most of the difficulties related to nursing training stemmed from the nursing schools' dual purpose of providing education and nursing service. Unfortunately, these studies resulted in limited reform.

## Baccalaureate Programs

In 1893, the School of Medicine at Howard University established the first nursing diploma program within a university setting. The program, designed for African American students lasted only 1 year before being assumed by Freedmen's Hospital. The University of Texas recognized nursing in the early 1890s and gave an endowed professorial chair to Hanna Kindborn who lectured to both nursing and medical students (Dock). In 1909, the University of Minnesota established a 3-year diploma nursing program within the College of Medicine. In subsequent years, colleges adopted the pattern of combining academic and professional courses that led to both a diploma and a Bachelor of Science degree in nursing. Students attended academic courses at the university and received professional nursing courses using the apprenticeship model at the hospital (Dock; Jamieson & Sewall). In 1909, Dr. Richard Olding Beard instituted a plan to make nursing a college major at the University of Minnesota (Jamieson & Sewall, 1954).

Early baccalaureate nursing programs failed to be established on an independent basis. In 1923, Yale University established an independent nursing program that had its own dean and endowed funds. Other universities that established baccalaureate nursing programs included Case Western Reserve University (1923), the University of Chicago (1925), and Vanderbilt University (1930). As nursing education moved to the collegiate setting, physicians voiced opposition to the overeducated, whose high intelligence and theoretical knowledge could handicap the prospective nurse (Kalisch & Kalisch, 2004). The American Nurses Association (ANA), the oldest professional nursing organization in the United States, was officially established in 1911 (Flanagan, 1976).

By the 1920s, most trained nurses were employed as private duty nurses. However, with the advent of technological advances in patient care, more patients were being hospitalized for treatment and surgery. Public acceptance of going to the hospital for acute and serious illnesses reduced the demand for private duty nurses who worked in home settings (Kalisch & Kalisch, 2004). The hospitals relied on student nurses to care for patients despite graduates of nursing programs remaining unemployed and in dire financial straights. In 1939, the National League for Nursing (NLN) reported that the typical hospital connected with a school of nursing during 1938 employed an average of ten graduate nurses for general duty or bedside nursing (National League for Nursing, 1939, p. 898).

During the Great Depression, some hospitals' staff consisted of trained nursing graduates willing to work for room and board. As the economic state improved, some hospitals kept these trained nurses as staff members despite resistance from other hospitals. As scientific knowledge related to medical practice increased, the demand for hospitals to employ graduate nurses increased. A limited number of nurses found employment with the new aviation industry as nurse-stewardesses. Other nurses participated in the Civil

Work Administration (CWA) and Works Progress Administration (WPA) programs and became employed in public hospitals, clinics, and in public health agencies. Health insurance started to fill the empty public hospital beds. Cinematographers portrayed nurses as attractive young women who placed professional duties over personal desires (Kalisch & Kalisch, 2004).

By World War II, graduate nurses had become accepted members of hospital staffs. When hospitals discovered that hiring graduate nurses could cut costs, many nursing schools closed. However, as news of war loomed in Europe, the government took steps to promote the entry of young women into nursing. Recruitment methods included advertisements in printed media and the Nurse Cadet Program (Kalisch & Kalisch, 2004). As registered nurses joined the military, a civilian nurse shortage resulted. Hospitals employed civilian workers who held certificates from the Red Cross and hired the volunteers who had been helping nurses with nonprofessional duties.

After World War II, the United States experienced a great time of economic growth. Companies offered health insurance as a fringe benefit for workers. Insurance reimbursement of hospital care resulted in a proliferation in the number of hospitals and expansions of well established ones. Because of this, hospitals also became profitable and provided a central location for proliferating medical technology. However, the nursing shortage increased as more hospital beds became available. Workplace reforms led to an 8-hour day, 40-hour workweek. Also, many nurses left practice to pursue marriage, better pay outside the profession, and more autonomous positions in industry or public health.

## Associate Degree Programs

*The Brown Report* (1948) and *The Ginzberg Report* (1949) specified that professional nursing education should be removed from hospitals and transferred to the collegiate setting. In 1951, Mildred Montag published a doctoral dissertation that proposed education for the technical nurse to occur in community college settings. She proposed that the technical nurse education would be a terminal degree and that technical nursing would attain a unique and semiprofessional identity (Montag, 1951). Upon graduation, the technical nurse would be completely prepared for hospital of nursing home employment. After a decade of research on the concept, community college nursing programs flourished. Eventually, the majority of graduate nurses came from community nurse settings. Graduates of associate degree programs wrote the professional nursing licensure examination, as did graduates from diploma and baccalaureate nursing programs.

## ● NURSING IN THE MODERN ERA (1960–1999)

### The 1960s

In the early 1960s, the health care system consisted primarily of independent, not-for-profit hospitals, small independent physician offices, and neighborhood pharmacies and medical supply stores. By working independently or in small practices, physicians enjoyed autonomy and control over patient care. Hospitals recruited physicians to join medical staffs. Private insurance companies or patients reimbursed physicians based on fee-for-service payment systems. Persons unable to afford care sought health care services in local government-managed hospitals and clinics. Society and nurses viewed nursing as being subservient to the physician.

In the 1960s, the National League for Nursing denied accreditation of hospital diploma schools that used students to staff hospitals. Hospital-based diploma schools remained the dominant educational pattern for registered nursing until the early 1970s. Table 2-1 highlights historical events that have resulted in multiple entry points into the nursing profession.

**TABLE 2-1**

### Historical Events Resulting in Multiple Educational Programs for Entry Into Professional Nursing

| Event | Date |
| --- | --- |
| First school for training practical nurses opens | 1897 |
| Daughters of the American Revolution serve as the examining board for military nurses | 1898 |
| North Carolina becomes the first state to require registration of nurses | 1903 |
| 1,006 hospital-based nursing training programs and 90 mental health institution–based nursing programs | 1911 |
| *The Goldmark Report* proposes that additional education beyond the basic diploma is needed for the practice areas of public health, nursing education, and supervision | 1923 |
| University of Minnesota starts a baccalaureate degree nursing program | 1909 |
| Apprenticeship approach dominates nursing educations | 1920s |
| 25 programs of nursing granted A.B. or B.S. degrees in nursing with Yale opening the first separate university nursing department in 1924 | 1926 |
| 11 practical nursing programs in the United States | 1930 |
| 1,472 hospital-based education programs, 70 collegiate nursing education programs, 36 practical nursing programs | 1936 |
| Development of crash programs to train nursing aides to alleviate nursing shortage of World War II | 1941 |
| *The Brown Report* ranked nursing as important to society as teachers; ranks collegiate nursing education as equal to other professional education programs | 1948 |
| Accreditation programs for practical and professional nursing schools | 1952 |
| 296 practical nursing programs | 1954 |
| Birth of associate degree nursing programs in community colleges | 1958 |
| 797 hospital-based, 218 associate degree, and 210 baccalaureate degree nursing education programs | 1966 |
| 288 hospital-based, 742 associate degree, and 402 baccalaureate degree nursing programs | 1982 |
| 60 hospital-based, 890 associate degree, and 661 baccalaureate degree nursing programs | 2003 |

*Sources:* Kalisch, P. A., & Kalisch, B. J. (2004). *The advance of American nursing* (4th ed.). Philadelphia: Lippincott Williams & Wilkins.

Biomedical advances proliferated leading to expensive technologies to save lives. Complex surgical procedures, new pharmaceuticals, and new technology increased the cost of health care delivery. This increased the need for highly skilled and educated nurses. By this time, employers offered health care insurance as a standard benefit to workers. In 1965, the government introduced Medicare and Medicaid to provide health care coverage to the poor and elderly. Improved insurance coverage meant improved access to health care services for the employed and elderly citizens. Demand for hospital care and physician services increased. Hospital admissions rose and along with it the need for highly educated, clinically competent professional nurses for patient care. Americans became enamored with advances in health care. With the growing popularity of television, two fictional medical programs, *Ben Casey* and *Dr. Kildare,* attracted viewers. In these programs, nurses primarily were depicted as handmaidens to physicians. Occasionally, a nurse who sought to marry a physician or was nosy by nature received airtime. An episode of *Perry Mason* featured a story about a private duty nurse murdering her patient.

## The 1970s

Inflation and unemployment increased in the 1970s. Consumers revolted against tax increases. To decrease the economic burden of supplying health care, the government employed mechanisms to monitor health care delivery to Medicare and Medicaid recipients. Although ineffective, mechanisms such as utilization review to reduce lengths of hospital stays and physician peer review programs became common practice. Hospitals and physicians were required to participate in these programs or lose Medicare and Medicaid reimbursement.

Insurance providers also carried increased risks as consumers and employers exerted pressure on them to keep premiums from rising. Because Blue Cross had been accused of simply passing on increased hospital costs to its participants, they legally separated from the American Hospital Association in 1972. In 1974, the Employment Retirement Security Act added incentives to business to self-insure employees. A few, for-profit, investor hospitals were established, but medical and hospital care proceeded as usual. Therefore, the need for professional nurses continued.

During this era, community colleges prospered as society placed emphasis on equal opportunity for all American citizens to education. Community college-based nursing programs flourished. Associate degree-prepared nurses successfully passed the professional nursing licensure examination and soon filled vacant nursing positions where they provided effective nursing care services. Costs for hospital-based nursing education programs continued to rise.

The 1970s also saw increases in graduate nursing education. Graduate nursing education programs proliferated and offered advanced study in clinical specialty areas, nursing education, and nursing administration. Nurse practitioner programs were started to improve health care delivery while reducing costs. Nursing research became a hallmark of advanced nursing education and practice.

Compared to medical research, nursing research has also been hampered by inadequate financial support. Between 1971 and 1981, the government awarded the National Center for Nursing Research $40 million. During the same period, the National Institutes of Health (NIH) received $1.7 billion for general biomedical research. However, the NIH noted the importance for nursing research and established the National Center for Nursing Research.

Television and movies increased in popularity. Positive images of nurses surfaced on television shows such as *Julia, Nurse, Emergency,* and *MASH.* In *Emergency,* Nurse Dixie, a fictional emergency department nurse, had collegial relationships with paramedics, physicians, and fellow nurses; performed telephone triage and complex nursing procedures; and even disagreed with physicians. Margaret Houlihan of *MASH* was portrayed as a competent, caring professional who had many personal problems. Nurses as persons with rigid and cold personalities were depicted in the 1975 movie *One Flew Over the Cuckoo's Nest.* Some less-than-flattering images of nurses in the media appear in Table 2-2.

**TABLE 2–2**

## Less-than-flattering Images of Nurses in the Media

| Image | Example(s) |
|---|---|
| Rigid and cold personality | Nurse Ratchet in *One Flew Over the Cuckoo's Nest* (1975 movie)<br>Major Margaret Houlihan in *MASH* (1969 movie and 1972–1983 TV show) |
| Intense drive to satisfy sexual needs | "Hot Lips" Houlihan in *MASH* (movie and TV show)<br>*Nightingales* (1988–89 TV show)<br>Margaret on *Becker* (2000–04) |
| Sex objects | *Nightingales* (1988–89 TV show)<br>*Pearl Harbor* (2001 movie)<br>Various soap operas |
| A goal to marry a physician and flirtatious relationships with male physicians | Nurse Hathaway in *ER* (1993–2005 TV show)<br>Nurse characters in *Diagnosis Murder* (1994–2001 TV show)<br>Nancy Nichol, clinic nurse in *Doc* (2001–2005 TV show) |
| Dysfunctional lives | Suicide attempt by Nurse Hathaway during the *ER* TV show pilot<br>*ER's* Nurse Abby, a chain smoker and alcoholic<br>*MASH's* Major Houlihan's intermittent drinking binges<br>Margaret's marital woes on *Becker* (2000–04 TV show) |
| Selfless martyr | Hanna in *The English Patient* (1996 movie) |
| Complicity | Phillip Seymour Hoffman in *Magnolia* (1999 movie) |
| Men in nursing as being effeminate | Ben Stiller's role as the male nurse in *Meet the Parents* (2000 movie) |
| Nurses kill or injure patients | *Dateline* (TV show)<br>Series of three articles published by *The Chicago Tribune* in September 2000 |
| Temporary and agency nurses as engaging in illegal and unethical behavior | Bogdanich's 1991 report in the *The Wall Street Journal* |

*Sources:* Berens, M. J. (2000), accessed March 18, 2001. Nursing mistakes kill, injure thousands. *The Chicago Tribune.* Available online http://www.chicagotribune.com/news/specials/chi-000910nursing1.1,2682439.story?ctrack-1?cset=true Bogdanich, W. (1991, November 1). Danger in white: The shadowy world of 'temp' nurses. *The Wall Street Journal,* pp. B1, B4; Muff, J. (1988). Of images and ideals: A look at socialization and sexism in nursing. In A. H. Jones (Ed.), *Images of nurses: Perspectives from history, art, and literature* (pp. 197–220). Philadelphia: University of Pennsylvania Press.

## The 1980s

Costs for health care continued to skyrocket during the 1980s, despite a weak economy. More expensive and sophisticated diagnostic equipment and treatments became common as new advances in health care were discovered and consumers demanded them. In 1983, Medicare introduced a prospective payment system known as diagnosis-related groups. The goal of the program was to reduce cost rate increases for hospital care in Medicare participating institutions by reducing hospital length of stays. Employers selected health insurance programs offering preferred provider organizations that negotiated reduced costs for services offered by hospitals and ambulatory health care-providing organizations. By the end of the decade, hospitals experienced decreased profits, as beds remained empty. Hospitals consolidated resulting in a decreased demand for hospital nurses.

As the number of hospital beds declined, inpatient acuity increased substantially, thereby requiring that highly skilled nurses care for patients. Primary nursing became the dominant nursing care delivery system. Primary nursing brought the professional nurse back to the bedside. In primary nursing, the registered nurse planned individualized care, implemented the plan, and also provided health education for hospitalized patients and families. Persons were sent home to recover from surgery and illnesses once their conditions stabilized. An increased demand for nurses working in home health and ambulatory health care surfaced.

Media portrayals of nurses were less than flattering. Soap operas and the prime time television show, *Nightingales*, depicted nurses and nursing students as sex objects. In a coordinated effort with the ANA, professional nurses instituted a boycott of sponsors of *Nightingales*, which resulted in its cancellation.

## The 1990s

By 1990, "95% of insured employees were enrolled in some form of managed care, including fee-for-service plans with utilization management, preferred provider organization or HMOs" (Bodenheimer & Grumbach, 1995, p. 87). Hospitals, physicians, and insurance companies joined forces and created integrated health care networks. Large surpluses of specialist physicians with a shortage of generalists were predicted. Physicians increasingly formed large practices, while commercial companies dominated insurance coverage through managed care plans. For-profit companies took control of many nursing homes, home health care companies, and multihospital system networks. Physicians lost control of medical practice. Third-party payers dictated reimbursement rates to hospitals. Eighty-five million Americans remained uninsured, underinsured, or enrolled in Medicaid (Ginsberg, 1995). Insurance providers employed management tactics to avoid enrolling potentially high users of health care services.

As hospital and home health care agencies lost profits, efforts to control costs of services resulted in reducing professional nursing staff even as the acuity level of inpatients continued to rise. Use of unlicensed assistive personnel (UAP) became popular despite evidence that registered nurses improved patient care quality (Brooten & Naylor, 1995). The change in skill mix reduced professional nurse positions and further devalued the contributions of registered nurses to client care (Buerhaus, 1995).

Patient-focused care and **work redesign** efforts were developed. Greenberg (1994) outlined the following four key elements of patient focused care:

1. Patients with similar diagnoses are grouped on the same units.
2. Ancillary and support services are decentralized to the nursing unit.
3. Staff are cross-trained shifting from specialized to generalized care providers.
4. Patient care teams of cross-trained providers give the majority of care for the specified patient group.

In efforts to improve quality of care by minimizing variance in care-providing procedures, hospitals instituted clinical pathways. The clinical paths also standardized the hospital length of stay for persons having the same procedures or hospital admissions for the same illness. Standardized paths reduced the individualization of nursing care plans.

Work redesign effort expanded the responsibility and job scope for nonprofessional staff. UAP replaced registered and licensed vocational (practical) nurses. With minimal on-the-job training, UAP perform the basic tasks of patient hygiene, ambulation, vital signs, and intake–output determination while assuming phlebotomy, EKG testing, bladder catheterization, and simple dressing changes in some institutions. In addition, some institutions assign social workers, housekeeping personnel, dietary workers, respiratory therapists, and clinical laboratory staff to a nursing department under the supervision of a nurse manager. As a result, the registered nurse (RN) role changed from one of direct care provider to one requiring delegation of patient care to others. Instead of spending time with patients, the RN now supervised care provided by UAP. The RN role shifted to one of manager who focused efforts at patient outcome evaluation.

### Questions for Reflection 2-3

1. How do you think the expanded use of unlicensed personnel in health care settings has affected professional nursing practice?
2. What are the consequences of increased use of unlicensed care providers for the nursing profession?
3. What are the consequences of increased use of unlicensed care providers for clients?

To assure efficient and effective use of health care resources without sacrificing client satisfaction and care quality, health care providers and insurers developed **case management** systems. Case management systems varied in setting and implementation. Table 2-3 outlines seven common components contained in all case management models.

Social workers served as the first case managers. However, when they realized their limitations to see the entire patient situation, health care institutional administration and social workers turned to nurses for assistance. In addition, case management required thought processes frequently used by nurses in clinical practice. Early efforts at case management improved patient outcomes, increased consumer satisfaction with care and decreased health care costs (Cohen & Cesta, 2001).

TABLE 2-3

## Common Components of Case Management Systems

| Component | Description |
|---|---|
| Client identification and outreach services | Case managers receive clients through referrals, interviews, and networking. |
| Client assessment and diagnosis | Case managers perform comprehensive holistic client assessments to identify physical, psychological, sociocultural, and spiritual problems. |
| Planning of services and resource identification | Case managers determine what services will be used in collaboration with the client. The case manager then assumes the responsibility for planning and coordinating the services. |
| Linking clients to required services | Case managers serve as brokers to expedite and follow through with the coordination and planning of services for theclient. |
| Coordination and implementation of services | Case managers verify that the identified needs are met and abide by formal agreements made with the service providing agencies by keeping extensive documentation and records focused on the efficiency, effectiveness, and quality of case managed care services. |
| Service delivery monitoring | Case managers collaborate with interdisciplinary team members who are providing client services and verify that the client is receiving appropriate, quality services from the agencies. |
| Client advocacy | Case managers work on behalf of the client to assure that the client is receiving services contracted for, making progress in the delineated program, and receiving satisfactory services. |
| Evaluation of services and outcomes | Case managers bear responsibility for specific and general client outcomes. They continuously monitor and reassess services being provided. Prompt identification of need for change or problems ensures timely intervention and replanning. |

Research in nursing continued to be hampered by inadequate financial support. In 1993, the National Institute for Nursing Research (NINR) was established with the purpose of identifying nursing research priorities, distributing grants to nurse researchers and disseminating findings of nursing research to the public and other health professions. In 2000, NINR received $90 billion to achieve its mission.

### Research Brief 2-1

Davis, L., Mohay, H., & Edwards, H. (2003). Mothers' involvement in caring for their premature infants: An historical overview. *Journal of Advanced Nursing, 42,* 578–586.

The investigators reviewed published literature from 1960 to 2002 that addressed maternal involvement in premature infant care. Articles reviewed were written in the English language and had been accessed using CINAHL, MEDLINE, and PSYCHLIT computerized databases.

Results of the literature analysis revealed that various phases resulted in major changes in the care of premature infants. In the 19th century, parents cared for premature infants in their homes until the incubator was developed by Tarnier, a French obstetrician, which greatly increased the survival of preterm infants. Because of special care with the incubator and concerns about infections, care of preterm infants quickly became institutionalized. High maternal death rates from home births eventually led to acceptance of women going to the hospital for infant deliveries. Because premature delivery was identified as the major cause of infant mortality after World War II, efforts were made to educate women about the importance of prenatal care. In the 1960s, neonatology became a recognized medical specialty and special problems from life-saving therapies were identified. Studies addressing infant psychological health were performed and benefits of having mothers actively involved in preterm infant care demonstrated improved mother–infant bonding, increased maternal confidence in caring for preterm infants, and increased weight gain. The fear of infectious exposure was dispelled through research studies. Social changes in the late 1960s and early 1970s transformed obstetric care with demands for analgesic-free deliveries, husbands as labor coaches, natural childbirth and breastfeeding. Renewed efforts toward birth as a natural, healthy process and prenatal care importance occurred resulting in the development of family centered maternity care. By the late 1970s, studies pointed to problems of early parent–infant separation especially on child development and socialization. Increased rates of child abuse were found with early parent–child separation. Research in the 1990s demonstrated physiologic and psychological benefits to preterm infants who received close contact with mothers.

This review of historical literature, although limited in scope, reveals the need for parents to be actively involved in the care of preterm infants. Neonatal nurses serve as a major means to help parents spend time with and master the basic care skills for preterm infants even though they may be frightened by the technology, the small size of the infant and an uncertain prognosis.

Despite federal government recognition of unique professional nursing contributions to health care, the American public continued to see mixed pictures of professional nursing. Prime time news programs became popular; *Dateline* featured a story about a nurse who had murdered several patients in a Veterans hospital. The show *ER* debuted with an episode featuring a suicide attempt of an emergency department employee, Nurse Hathaway. In future episodes, Nurse Hathaway became the epitome of the caring nurse who secretly provided health care services to persons without the ability to pay for them. Unlike previous portrayals of oppressed nurses, Nurse Hathaway never let fear get in the way of confronting potential errors or injustices.

## ● NURSING IN THE POSTMODERN ERA (2000–BEYOND)

Scholars debate when the postmodern era actually began. Some acknowledge that the postmodern era began in the 1960s; others claim it began with the introduction of the computer and Internet. Another group of scholars herald the beginning of the postmodern age with questioning of scientific method as the best approach for discoveries to achieve the questions surrounding humanity, the environment and health-related issues. Wilson (1998) introduced the term **consilience,** a term to describe the unity of knowledge. Consilience represents the point where the scientific, artistic, ethical, spiritual, social, environmental and personal knowledge intersect. Recent research has discovered that spirituality plays a key role in health and healing, and qualitative research methods hold the same status as quantitative research methods.

Currently, professional nursing finds itself in a state of flux. Scientific advances promise increased complexity and costs of health care. Limited resources for health care drive its delivery. As the population of the United States grows older and lives longer, nursing services are in high demand. The gap between the rich and poor continues to widen resulting in an increase in governmental funding for health care services. Sources of health care insurance for consumers of health care come from employment, private purchase, or the government. Forty-four million persons have joined the ranks of the uninsured. Twenty-eight million persons participate in Medicaid programs. By virtue of education and practice, nurses are the best-equipped health team members to assume the gatekeeper and advocacy roles required of case managers. Nurse practitioners have demonstrated the ability to deliver high quality health care economically without compromising care quality. Hospitals currently employ 66% of working RNs, and nurses work in extended care facilities, homes, clinics, and community health settings (Institute for the Future, 2000).

Along with different settings for professional nurse employment, nurses find that the complexity of information in any given practice area requires continuous education. Professional nursing organizations provide opportunities for further education in a specialized practice field. An Internet search revealed over 130 professional nurse organizations. Specialty areas include critical care, oncology, neuroscience, holistic, parish, maternal–child, psychiatric, and administration to name only a few. Although certification by a recognized nursing specialty organization attests to knowledge and skill in the special area of practice, few positions require certification and many fail to provide financial rewards for professional certification. However, many individuals consider certification prestigious and view it as a means to improve the image of nursing.

Besides being knowledgeable in a specific practice area, nurses realize the importance of being versed in current consumer health care practices. Many alternative or complimentary health care practices affect current medical therapies. Some complimentary therapies such as aromatherapy, guided imagery, therapeutic touch, and massage ease some adverse effects of conventional medical and surgical therapies.

## ● SUMMARY AND SIGNIFICANCE TO PRACTICE

The development of nursing for recognition as a respected profession is ongoing. In the past 100 years, great strides have been made to standardize the nursing curriculum for professional nursing. However, three entry levels of education serve as a major barrier toward professional status. Societal trends have affected recruitment efforts into the profession of nursing. Advances in science provided opportunity for the nursing profession to establish its own scientific body of knowledge. However, with the merging of the hard science with ethics, spirituality, and philosophy, providing individualized holistic care becomes a key challenge for professional nurses. The trend away from "hard science" provides nursing with an opportunity to capture the essence of nursing as a holistic healing art based on scientific evidence. The development of multiple nursing organizations impedes the ability of professional nurses to speak with a united voice, results in duplication of services and fosters competition for membership (Vance, 1999). In many ways, nursing continues to fight the same battles within the profession repeatedly.

## FROM THEORY TO PRACTICE

Review the vignette at the beginning of the chapter and answer the following questions:
1. What are some current issues in health care that might be solved by looking at nursing history?
2. What are the similarities among current and ancient nursing practice?
3. Why is it important for nurses to have knowledge about nursing history?
4. How does modern nursing compare to nursing in various stages of human history?
5. How could nurses use history to guide current and future nursing practice?

## WWW INTERNET EXERCISE

This chapter has provided you with a broad overview of the history of nursing. Visit http://www.internurse.com. View pictures and read more about the nurses who shaped the profession of nursing. Listen to the voice of Florence Nightingale. Write a paragraph or two describing your thoughts and feelings on visiting the site. Please also include information related to your perception of nursing history since reading and visiting this website. Share with your nursing colleagues in class or at work.

## WWW INTERNET RESOURCES

Internurse: http://internurse.com/history.htm. Listen to voice recording of Florence Nightingale and see many nursing historical photographs.

American Association for the History of Nursing: http://www.aahn.org. Read about organizational membership and view nursing history archives.

The Center for the Study of the History of Nursing: http://www.nursing.upenn.edu/history. Visit the gravesites of historical nursing figures and read about their contributions to the profession.

Men in American Nursing History: http://www.geocities.com/Athens/Forum/6011/. Trace the historical role of men in professional nursing and discover current issues confronting men in nursing.

Women's History: http://womenshistory.about.com/homework/womenshistory/cs/nurses. Read about key historical nursing figures and learn about contributions of minority nurses to the profession.

American Nurses Association(ANA): http://www.nursingworld.org. Read about ANA history, membership services, and current issues affecting professional nursing.

Sigma Theta Tau International: http://www.nursingsociety.org. Read about Sigma Theta Tau history, membership criteria, membership services, efforts to promote nursing scholarship, and visit the Virginia Henderson Library.

National League for Nursing(NLN): http://www.nln.org. Learn about NLN history, membership services, standards for professional and vocational nursing program accreditation, testing services, and research initiatives.

American Association of Colleges of Nursing(AACN): http://www.aacn.nche.edu. Read about AACN history, mission, and get a hyperlink to Commission for Credentialing of Nursing Education for program accreditation standards for baccalaureate and graduate nursing educational programs.

Check out past and current media images of professional nurses by visiting http://www.nursingadvocacy.org.

## REFERENCES

Berens, M. J. (2000). Nursing mistakes kill, injure thousands. *The Chicago Tribune*. Available at: http://www.chicagotribune.com/news/specials/chi-0009101,1,2682439.story?ctrack=1?cset=true/. Accessd June 25, 2005.

Bodenheimer, T., & Grumbach, K. (1995). The reconfiguration of U.S. medicine. *Journal of the American Medical Association, 274,* 85–90.

Bogdanich, W. (1991, November 1). Danger in white: The shadowy world of 'temp' nurses. *The Wall Street Journal*, pp. B1, B4.

Brown, E. L. (1948). *Nursing for the future (Brown report)*. New York: Russell Sage Foundation.

Brooten, D., & Naylor, M. D. (1995). Nurses' effect on changing patient outcomes. *Image, 27,* 95–99.

Buerhaus, P. I. (1995). Economic pressures building in the hospital employed RN labor market. *Nursing Economics, 13,* 137–141.

Burgess, M. A. (1928). *Committee on the grading of nursing schools: Nurses, patients and pocketbooks*. New York: Commonwealth Fund.

Cohen, E. L., & Cesta, T. G. (2001). *Nursing case management from essentials to advanced practice applications* (3rd ed.). St. Louis: Mosby.

Davis, L., Mohay, H., & Edwards, H. (2003). Mothers' involvement in caring for their premature infants: An historical overview. *Journal of Advanced Nursing, 42,* 578–586.

Dock, L. L. (1912). *A history of nursing, Vol. III*. New York: G.P. Putnam.

Flanagan, L. (1976). *One strong voice: The story of the American Nurses Association*. Kansas City, MO: American Nurses Association.

Flexner, A. (1910). *Medical education in the United States and Canada*. The Carnegie Foundation for the Advancement of Teaching. Boston: Merrymount Press.

Ginsberg, E. (1995). A cautionary note on market reforms in health care. *Journal of the American Medical Association, 274,* 1633–1634.

Ginzberg, E. (1949). *A pattern for hospital care*. New York: Columbia University Press.

Goldmark, J. (1923). *Nursing and nursing education in the United States*. New York: Macmillan.

Greenberg, L. (1994). Work redesign: An overview. *Journal of Emergency Nursing, 20,* 28A–32A.

Institute for the Future (2000). *Health and Health Care 2010. The forecast, the challenge*. San Francisco: Jossey-Bass.

Jamieson E. M., & Sewall, M. F. (1954). *Trends in nursing history* (4th ed.). Philadelphia: WB Saunders.

Kalisch, P. A., & Kalisch, B. J. (2004). *The advance of American nursing* (4th ed.). Philadelphia: Lippincott Williams & Wilkins.

Kjervik, D. K., & Martinson, I. J. M. (1979). *Women in stress: A nursing perspective*. New York: Appleton-Century-Crofts.

Meehan, T. C. (2003). Careful nursing: a model for contemporary nursing practice. *Journal of Advanced Nursing, 44,* 99–107.

Montag, M. (1951). *The education of nursing technicians*. New York: Putman.

Muff, J. (1988). Of images and ideals: A look at socialization and sexism in nursing. In A. H. Jones (Ed.), *Images of nurses: Perspectives from history, art, and literature* (pp. 197–220). Philadelphia: University of Pennsylvania Press.

National League for Nursing, (1939). More graduate duty nurses. *American Journal of Nursing, 39,* 898.

Nutting, M. A., & Dock, L. L. (1935a). *A History of Nursing, volume 2, The evolution of nursing systems from the earliest times to the foundation of the first English and American training schools.* New York: Putman.

Nutting, M. A. and Dock, L. L. (1935b). *A History of Nursing, volume 3, The evolution of nursing systems from the earliest times to the foundation of the first English and American training schools.* New York: Putman.

Roberts, M. M. (1954). *American nursing: History and interpretation.* New York: Macmillan.

Spradley, B. W. (1990). *Community health nursing: Concepts and practice.* Glenview, IL: Scott Foresman/Little Brown.

Vance, C. (1999). Nursing the global arena. In E. Sullivan, (Ed.). *Creating nursing's future: Issues, opportunities, and challenges* (pp. 334–344). St. Louis: Mosby.

Wheeler, W. (1999). Florence: Death of an icon? *Nursing Times, 95,* 24–26.

Wilson, E. O. (1998). *Consilience: The unity of knowledge.* New York: Alfred A. Knopf.

# CHAPTER 3

# Contextual, Philosophical, and Ethical Elements of Professional Nursing

## KEY TERMS AND CONCEPTS

Values

Beliefs

Context

Philosophy

Contextual Elements of Nursing Practice

Mission

Morality

Ethics

Principalism

Care

Contextualism

Ethical Decision-Making Process

## LEARNING OUTCOMES

By the end of this chapter, the learner will be able to:

**1** Identify environmental factors that constitute the context for nursing practice.

**2** Outline the essential elements of a nursing philosophy.

**3** Develop a personal nursing philosophy.

**4** Outline key steps for effective analysis of ethical dilemmas.

**5** Use a structured method for making ethical decisions.

**6** Specify fallacies that might occur when making ethical decisions.

**7** Explain how demographic, cultural, economic, environmental, and ethical factors influence professional practice.

**8** Incorporate knowledge, freedom, and choice while using nursing process.

## VIGNETTE

Jane has been in nursing for 15 years. She yearns for the "good old days" when client care was focused on persons rather than on business. Currently, Jane feels detached from her clients and perceives herself as a client-care machine. However, she knows in her heart that she does make a difference in her clients' lives and she derives profound satisfaction from helping others through times of pain and suffering. Jane is considering a career change, but she feels passionate about helping other people.

As a science, nursing focuses on humanity in a highly objective manner using interventions based on scientific evidence. As advances in technology create a more complex world, making sense of the world becomes more important. A well-defined set of **values** (principles or what things are important) and **beliefs** (ideas regarded as truths) provides a firm foundation for nursing practice. Nurses who rely exclusively on thinking and approach nursing using only the hard sciences would appear cold and distant to their clients. However, professional nurses also connect emotionally and spiritually with clients, thereby allowing genuine warmth and authentic compassion to guide clinical practice. Values and beliefs influence perceptions, thoughts, and feelings.

Values and beliefs directly interact with the environment. All environmental and situational conditions create the **context** of nursing practice. One definition states that context refers to "the interrelated conditions in which something exists or occurs" (Mish, 1994, p. 250). Each nurse brings a personal set of beliefs about people, the world, health, and nursing. This set of beliefs constitutes a **philosophy** of nursing. When providing nursing care, nurses interact with the environment which is comprised of contextual factors in which a nurse's philosophy plays a key role. The pragmatic professional self focuses on using nursing for a practical purpose such as solving client health-related problems. The idealistic professional self pays serious attention to the ideal conceptualizations of nursing practice and views nursing as a means for forming authentic and caring relationships with others to help them achieve their maximal health potential. The realistic professional self emphasizes facts and scientific principles during nursing practice. The existentialist professional self shows great regard for individual choice with acceptance of responsibility for choices made as nursing care is delivered. Some degree of congruence with the vastly different worldviews is desirable for authentic, humane, scientific-based, nonpaternalistic nursing practice.

Development of an individual nursing philosophy helps nurses come to terms with diverse worldviews. However, to begin developing a personal nursing philosophy, nurses need to be cognizant of contextual elements of nursing practice. **Contextual elements of nursing practice** are all of the demographic, economic, environmental, and ethical factors that surround a client care situation. Contextual elements surrounding a clinical situation affect the professional roles assumed by nurses and the clinical decisions they make. These elements, along with a personal nursing philosophy, help nurses develop a meaningful and thoughtful practice.

## ✦ CONTEXTUAL BASIS OF NURSING PRACTICE

What is the world of nursing like today? Before that question can be answered, we must look at the world environment, the place where nursing occurs. Professional nursing practice does not occur in isolation; rather, nursing is one piece of the health care delivery systems. When one area of health care experiences a change, all areas of health care delivery experience change. Dramatic changes have occurred in health care over the past two decades that have profoundly affected professional nursing practice. Future changes may occur so quickly that nurses (and other persons) may have difficulty in fully comprehending the effects of change and coping with the implications of nonstop change (Porter-O'Grady & Malloch, 2003). Professional nursing is a complex phenomenon. Many contextual elements affect professional practice, making it impossible to present all of them in a single chapter. To capture an accurate picture of current professional practice, the following discussion focuses on quantum science that requires relational and whole systems thinking, technology and consumerism, the global community, communication, and the desire for equality while maintaining personal identity.

## Quantum Science: Relational and Whole Systems Thinking in Health Care

Because change is constant, no one can avoid it (Hawking, 2002). To survive, humans must learn new ways of thinking. The world is a complex place full of chaos. Everything is interconnected. Structure becomes defined by wholes rather than individual parts (Hawking; Porter-O'Grady & Malloch, 2003). When looking into a hologram, the entire large picture is seen on any size fraction of the entire picture. Such is the nature of overall structure. The smallest structural unit of a system mirrors its entire system in terms of organization pattern and behavior. Systems work continuously to renew and reinvent themselves while maintaining their basic integrity. Systems are composed of multiple interacting feedback loops. Structure has disorder and disorder has structure. Quantum science eliminates dualistic or "either–or" thinking, and envisions new possibilities of combining ideas through the use of synthesis. Synthesis involves putting ideas or things together in a new way. For example, Porter-O'Grady and Malloch define competence as using one's skills to attain a desired outcome rather than just having skills. As caregivers, coordinators, and change agents, nurses are frequently called upon to look for new ways of delivering client care to meet optimal outcomes.

Relational thinking involves recognition of the interconnectedness of all things. All things become interdependent. A complex algorithm (series of steps or events) is required for things to occur or exist (Porter-O'Grady & Malloch, 2003). For example, human health is a complex process that involves a safe environment, intact physical and mental capabilities, meaningful interpersonal relationships, and spiritual dimensions. Recent advances in the field of psychoneuroimmunology emphasize the importance of mental health and finding meaning in one's existence as a determinant of health status (Antonovsky, 1987). As client advocates, caregivers, coordinators, teachers, and counselors, nurses look at the client holistically to determine what resources are required to promote health.

The holistic approach also requires whole systems thinking. Whole systems thinking envisions the "whole." Many smaller interacting systems create the larger (or whole) system (Porter-O'Grady & Malloch, 2003). For example, a hospital consists of many departments (surgery, radiology, laboratory central supply, pharmacy, nursing, dietary, rehabilitation services, etc.). Each department assumes responsibility for an integral part of client care. In the case of nursing departments, client care is delivered 24 hours a day, 7 days a week. Thus, different teams of nursing personnel staff the hospital during the different shifts. Each nursing unit also represents another system. The nursing team on a unit may be broken down even further to represent the professional nurse, a vocational (or practical) nurse, and unlicensed care providers. Each person providing client care is also a complex system with many personal needs. When engaging in whole systems thinking, persons look at the complex nature of all the interacting systems. To further emphasize the nature of whole systems thinking, consider the hospital as being only a smaller system of the health care delivery system. Nurses use whole systems thinking frequently in daily clinical practice. As coordinators, nurses look for ways to use resources optimally to meet client care needs (e.g., staffing nursing units to meet client care needs). When assuming the role of client advocate, nurses frequently refer clients to community agencies for assistance when needed.

Because of the complex nature of practice and health care delivery, nurses consider many factors when providing client care. Quantum science and relational and systems thinking provide nurses with the ability to consider not only the impact of clinical decisions on clients, but also on the institutional, national, and global communities. Because change remains constant, nurses must stay abreast of factors that influence professional practice. The ability to use relational and systems thinking enables the nurse to appraise the entire client care situation before making decisions focused on the client's best interest. The following discussion provides a broad overview of factors that affect professional nursing practice.

## Technology, Communications, and Consumerism in Health Care

Technology has transformed human lives. Increased use of technology in health care has resulted in people surviving illnesses once thought as untreatable, enabled instant access to information, increased the cost of health care, and created more savvy health care consumers. Pharmaceutical companies post new information about medications on the Internet and target consumers with advertising. In the United States, consumers drive the delivery of health care. Frequently, health care consumers rely on information obtained from the Internet. When assessing client knowledge of health-related information, nurses must find out what clients know *and* the source of the information. As educators, professional nurses should assist clients in determining the quality of information accessed from various Internet sites (see Chapter 15, Informatics and Technology in Nursing Practice). Clients sometimes demand the newest (not always the best) health care treatments from providers (Herzlinger, 2004). Because of the array of sources of health information on the Internet, professional nurses must stay abreast of developments in health promotion and disease management to remain effective caregivers and educators.

In some instances, clients may know more about their health problems than health care providers (Herzlinger, 2004). For example, a young woman, newly diagnosed with myasthenia gravis (MG), finds detailed information about her disease from visiting the National Myasthenia Gravis Foundation website. She learns what medications may result in increased muscle weakness. When she needs surgery that requires hospitalization, she brings the long list of medications known to increase muscle weakness in persons with MG to the hospital so that she will not receive them. However, her action may have been unnecessary because nurses and physicians providing her care have access to the same information via the Internet using a desktop or handheld computer.

Constant connections to cellular telephones and pagers serve as distractions to focusing on persons with whom one is interacting and frequently result in ineffective interpersonal communication. Nurses have always valued developing therapeutic relationships with clients. Clients expect nurses to care for them by assuring their safety, being competent in nursing, taking action that is in their best interests, and listening to them. Some health care organizations provide nurses with pagers (or cellular telephones) so nurses can receive instant messages (in case of client emergency or other client needs). These devices can prevent nurses from devoting their entire attention to the client whom they are helping. In addition, some clients become distracted when their own cellular telephones ring while receiving health care and may miss critical information on how to best manage their health (Herzlinger, 2004).

Along with the latest developments in traditional medical care, many clients have knowledge of alternative and complementary health care therapies. Some consumers expect health care professionals, including nurses, to have knowledge of, and provide them with, these therapies or to offer advice about them (Herzlinger, 2004; Ross, Wenzel, & Mytlyng, 2002; Porter-O'Grady & Malloch, 2003). Professional nurses must inquire as to all health care practices used by clients to assure safety of prescribed, traditional medical therapies and to determine if any complementary or alternative therapies may pose client health hazards.

## The Global Community and Health Care

Besides technology, the emergence of a single world economy and the acknowledgment of finite earth resources for all persons have resulted in a changed context for professional practice. Disparities in the quality of life and health care have surfaced. Whereas undeveloped and overpopulated nations are looking for ways to combat malnutrition and infectious diseases, citizens of highly developed nations suffer from health problems related to a life of excess, such as obesity, diabetes mellitus, and cardiovascular disease. Developed nations have well-refined health care delivery systems along with access to sophisticated treatments, while undeveloped nations (especially those in political turmoil) may have no organized systems to meet the health care needs of residents (Fried & Gaydos, 2002).

Along with differences in health problems related to wealth, the nations of the world are connected as a global economic community. Companies looking to reduce labor costs set up manufacturing and service centers in countries where there are fewer regulations to protect workers, and where persons just want income to provide the basics (food, clothing, and shelter) for their families. Outsourcing of jobs decreases the tax revenue that would have been generated to finance governmental health care programs, and newly unemployed workers find themselves without health insurance coverage (Fried & Gaydos, 2002).

Political and social unrest in one nation has the potential to disrupt the economies of many nations. Fried and Gaydos characterize the current global phenomena that threaten the health of the world population:

1. The exacerbation of old infections (multidrug resistant TB, smallpox as a potential biologic weapon)
2. The emergence of new infections (HIV/AIDS pandemic)
3. Environmental devastation (natural or manmade disasters)
4. Lowering of occupational and environmental standards for workers (especially in underprivileged countries)
5. Global drug trafficking
6. War
7. Terrorism
8. Domestic violence
9. Suicide

According to infectious disease experts, their worst nightmare would be the birth of a new, highly contagious lethal flu virus. Because of worldwide air travel, the virus could spread to many areas of the world within 100 days of its emergence. In this scenario, clusters of cases would pop up simultaneously in Sydney, London, Toronto, and Los Angeles, and hundreds of persons would die as their lungs filled with fluid. In actuality, public health officials cooperating globally prevented a pandemic of severe acute respiratory syndrome (SARS) in 2003 (Enserink, 2004).

### Desire for Equality While Maintaining a Personal Cultural Identity

Despite globalization and access to information from around the world, persons strive to maintain ties to their culture. Current geopolitical unrest stems from the perception that democracy, capitalism, and freedom are best for, and wanted by, all persons. Many persons immigrate to developed wealthier nations to escape political persecution or less-than-ideal economic situations. Others may come to developed nations to secure treatment for diseases. Many persons born in developed nations value their cultural heritage. As caregivers, nurses who deliver culturally sensitive nursing care acknowledge the cultural needs of clients. Culturally sensitive health care enables the health care system to accommodate client needs to abide by specific cultural practices. Some health care facilities use computers that permit printing of discharge instructions in more than one language and have interpreters for staff to use when working with clients from diverse cultures. In some cases, folk healers are permitted to practice in inpatient settings (Dossey, Keegan, & Guzzetta, 2005). As client advocates, sometimes nurses have to question specific cultural practices that might be detrimental to client health. (More detailed information on Multicultural Issues in Professional Practice is presented in Chapter 11.)

When questioning client health practices, nurses use personal values and belief systems. Determining if and when a client's health practices are questionable depends on the individual nurse's knowledge and beliefs systems. Part of education involves discovery of things unknown about oneself. The next section offers a discussion about philosophy and its significance for professional nursing practice.

## ⬥ PHILOSOPHY

Philosophy is a conceptual discipline and involves things that cannot be directly touched or observed. The word philosophy is derived from the following Greek words: *philia* (love or friendship) and *sophia* (wisdom). Philosophers strive after wisdom, not necessarily to possess it. "Wisdom is used inclusively to cover the sustained intellectual inquiry in any area, the understanding and practice of morality, and the cultivation of such enlightened opinions and attitudes as lead to a life of happiness and contentment" (Earle, 1992, p. 2). People have been searching for meaning and happiness in their lives for centuries. Development of a personal philosophy requires examination of beliefs and values about life and requires a little time. However, development of a collective philosophy (group philosophy) requires much time and consolidation of individual beliefs and values. Philosophies may change as people gain new knowledge and skills through life journeys.

Anyone can be a philosopher. Tools used by philosophers include analyzing concepts (in terms of necessary and sufficient conditions, specific criteria, and by counterexamples), doubting everything, and describing our inner lives (phenomenology or lived experience). When describing lived experiences, persons capture the essence of the situation (Earle, 1992). Finding meaning in one's life enables persons to survive harsh conditions (Frankl, 1963) and promotes health (Antonovsky, 1987).

## Building the Foundation

The discipline of philosophy consists of eight major areas, each of which is summarized below:

1. Logic: the systematic study of arguments for logical or illogical reasoning. Does this make sense?
2. Epistemology: the study of knowledge. What is knowledge? How do people acquire it?
3. Philosophy of science: the explanation of the successes of science. How is science used? What are the benefits of hard sciences to humans?
4. Metaphysics (ontology): the analysis of issues surrounding the ultimate nature of existence, reality, and experience. What is there? This branch also addresses the reality of abstractions (from mathematical constructs such as numbers, to religious concepts such as God, angels, and the human soul), and the existence of abstractions in the absence of human thought.
5. Philosophy of mind: the study of the nature of the mental dimension of people. What is the mind? How should we understand intentions, desires, beliefs, emotions, pleasure, and pain? How do mental processes explain human behavior?
6. Ethics (moral philosophy): the study of the appropriateness of possible courses of action based on a system of moral principles and values. What is morality? What actions are obligatory, morally permissible, or impermissible?
7. Sociopolitical philosophy: the study of the control and regulation of persons living in a society, and the means to improve their lives. Where do states come from? What does it mean to be a citizen of a state? Must we obey laws, and why? When should laws be changed?
8. Philosophy of religion: the study of the meaning of human life. Is religious language meaningful? Does God exist? Is there good and evil? What other basis can give meaning to life if the religious assumptions were to be proven false?
9. Aesthetics: the study of what constitutes beauty. What is beauty? What makes something a work of art? Why are art and other forms of artistic expression important?

Philosophy focuses on conceptual clarity and requires an individual journey. It provides a foundation for human action (Earle, 1992). For clarity, philosophy of nursing is defined as the intellectual and affective outcomes of the professional nurses' efforts to:

1. Understand the ultimate relationships between humans, environment, and health.
2. Approach nursing as a scientific discipline.
3. Integrate a sense of values into practice.
4. Appreciate aesthetic elements that contribute to health and well-being.

5. Define the mission of nursing.
6. Articulate a personal belief systems about human beings, environment, health, and nursing.

## Significance of Philosophy for Nursing

Achievement of intellectual enlightenment is considered better protection against calamitous mistakes than ignorance. Thus, over time, the study of philosophy has accrued great benefits for individuals, societies, and particularly, specific sciences. Pursuing the objectives of philosophy provides individuals an opportunity to develop an understanding of the world around them and to exercise value judgments. The quest for reason develops understanding. Development of a personal system of values requires making ethical and aesthetic decisions. Science benefits from philosophy essentially because philosophy governs scientific methods through logic and ethics.

The nursing profession needs nursing philosophers who articulate visions for nursing as a scientific discipline, emphasize concern for the ultimate good of humankind, develop belief systems reflecting sound ethics, reflect upon the meaning of nursing, and conduct periodic review of philosophies of nursing. Never carved in stone, a nursing philosophy remains a constant work in progress.

Practitioners of the profession of nursing need personal philosophies that reflect a belief in recasting the health system to benefit all humankind rather than assuring institutional survival. Nursing philosophers analyze current health care systems and conceptualize the bases for nursing practice, research, and education. These nursing philosophers also concern themselves with moral issues surrounding nursing and health care while promoting behavior based on a professional code of ethics.

Rafael (1996) coined the term "empowered caring" to denote leadership as a unity of power and caring that values the characteristics and experiences of women, and a system of ethics that "stems from a heightened awareness of interrelatedness and emerges as a sense of responsibility toward others" (p. 15). Rafael's writing demonstrates the work of a nursing philosopher who provides novel thinking and uses this to shift from a hierarchical approach to nursing to one where nurses and nurse leaders share knowledge and expertise with clients (and each other).

Finally, nurse leaders have identified a system of values to guide the nursing profession. The American Association of Colleges of Nursing (AACN) in 1986 defined values as "beliefs or ideals to which an individual is committed and which guide behavior" (p. 5). According to AACN (1986), values should be "reflected in attitudes, personal qualities, and consistent patterns of behavior" (p. 5). The AACN has identified altruism, equality, aesthetics, freedom, human dignity, justice, and truth as values that underpin the practice of professional nursing.

## Developing a Personal Nursing Philosophy

A nursing philosophy provides a personal perspective for nursing practice, research, and scholarship (Salsberry, 1994). A philosophy combines the way of doing with the way of being (Rew, 1994). Development of a nursing philosophy requires that the nurse embark on a journey of self-discovery. As knowledge and experience in nursing expand, a personal nursing philosophy may change. A personal nursing philosophy is never complete, but always remains a work in progress. Because the profession of nursing concerns itself with human beings, health, nursing, and the environment, most personal philosophies of nursing address these key concepts. Carper (1978) identified four patterns of knowing in nursing: personal knowledge, empirics, aesthetics, and ethics (presented in more detail in Chapter 4, Patterns of Knowing and Nursing Science). A well-developed nursing philosophy represents personal knowledge related to professional nursing.

To construct a personal philosophy of nursing, one must engage in reflective thinking about one's relationship to the universe. Discovery of a personal **mission** or goal within the realm of nursing solidifies the decision to practice professional nursing. Because nursing focuses on individuals and the environment, a beginning nursing philosophy should minimally address these concepts.

From a nursing perspective, to develop a nursing philosophy, the individual nurse should examine and answer the following questions:

1. What is the environment and what is the nature of the relationship between humans and the environment?
2. What is your central belief about the individual person and that person's potential?
3. What is your central belief about the family and its potential?
4. What is your central belief about the community and its potential?
5. What are your central beliefs about the relationship between society and health?
6. What is your view on health? Is it a continuum? A state? A process?
7. How do illness and wellness relate to health?
8. What is the central reason for the existence of nursing?
9. Who is the recipient of nursing care?

From the perspective of a philosophers' concern with knowledge, the individual nurse should look at the following questions that consider essential elements of the scientific discipline:

1. Is nursing a science or art? Or both?
2. From what cognitive base does the professional nurse operate?
3. What is nursing process? How is it implemented?
4. What is necessary to apply nursing knowledge?
5. How is the theory base for nursing derived?
6. What is the theoretical framework for the profession?
7. What are the purposes and processes of nursing research?

From the philosopher's concern with ethics and aesthetics, the professional nurse must attempt to answer the following questions reflecting the valuation elements of nursing:

1. What are the essential rights and responsibilities of the professional nurse?
2. What are the essential rights and responsibilities of recipients of nursing care?
3. What are the governing ethical principles in the delivery of nursing care and the conduct of nursing research?
4. What are your beliefs about the educational requirements for the practice of the profession?
5. What are your beliefs about the teaching–learning process?
6. What is the ultimate goal of professional nursing care?

The greatest opportunity to begin developing answers to the preceding questions begins with the first nursing course. However, as nurses attain higher levels of education, beginning a new course becomes an opportune time to evaluate and modify a professional nursing philosophy. A nurse's professional self-concept is built on the foundation of personal life, and educational and clinical practice experiences. As a nurse progresses on his or her life journey, finding meaning in one's personal and professional existence remains a constant challenge. Articulation of a personal nursing philosophy helps the nurse find purpose, create meaning, and increase commitment to the profession of nursing. A sample and abbreviated nursing philosophy is found in Display 3-1. In the sample philosophy, the author uses an analogy to present her philosophical views about nursing. Analogies are useful to some when presenting deeply held beliefs. However, a nursing philosophy does not require using an analogy; statements about personal beliefs serve just as well. As you develop your philosophy, realize that there is no "right" nursing philosophy. You may also find that your nursing philosophy may change.

---

### A Sample Nursing Philosophy

DISPLAY 3-1 ●

Nursing is like a diamond ring. Special conditions must exist for a diamond ring to be created, and special care must be taken to maximize its luster.

Nurses hold a sacred trust with their clients when clients put their lives in the nurse's hands. The nurse **has a mission** to focus on what is best for the client when making decisions concerning care. When possible, the nurse and clients work as partners to promote health. **Together they carve out a multifaceted** plan of care that integrates the needs of body, mind, and spirit. The nurse always considers client choices for care. However, when the client is no longer able to choose, the nurse abides by information left previously by the client or by the family's wishes. Along with caring for individuals, the nurse cares for families and communities. A diamond ring never shows its luster if left in a box; **a nurse fails to shine when unable to care for others.**

---

Once you have an established nursing philosophy, you can use it in many ways. When seeking employment, ask to see the potential employer's organizational philosophy and see how closely it matches your own. A recent trend in health care is the development of a unit-based philosophy. To engage in the process, all unit staff meet and draft a philosophy. This process is time-consuming and creates some interesting debates among staff members. When organizational and personal philosophies match, people have more commitment to work processes and increased job satisfaction.

## ● MORALITY AND ETHICS IN NURSING PRACTICE

Within any practice context, nurses feel compelled to do what is "right" for their clients. **Morality,** as defined by O'Neill (1995, p. 224), encompasses "the oughts of a given society." **Ethics** is "the philosophical study of morality" (Noddings, 1984, p. 1). Nurses confront many situations in which they rely upon their consciences for decision making. When working with coherent clients, nurses provide information and share decision making with them.

By virtue of being a nurse, individual nurses are expected to care. Caring permeates the profession of nursing. Early Indian and Christian nurses tended to the infirmed as a way to express altruism. Nurses provide holistic health care services in a caring manner. Persons acknowledge that a desire to care for others stimulated them to enter the nursing profession (Boughn, 1994; Boughn, 2001; Okrainec, 1994; Streubert, 1994). The science and art of nursing centers around the concept of caring. Experts in caring theory emphasize that before one can effectively care for others over a lifetime, the person must be able to care for the self (Benner, 1994; Benner & Wrubel, 1989; Watson, 1988). Watson (1988) proclaims that caring is a moral imperative. Nurses enter the nursing profession with an intention to care, and society expects them to care.

Recent changes in health care delivery prevent nurses from having the time to express caring in practice. Some institutions treat nurses as replaceable technicians who have sophisticated skills. Clients become consumers. Instead of individualized care, health care consumers receive care from standardized plans. Nurses feel pressure to streamline care to maximize use of health care resources.

The shift of nursing care to a "trade service" rings true, especially when managed care looks for cost-cutting measures such as increased use of unlicensed care providers. Health insurers limit covered health care services and an individual's right to choose health care providers. Access to and justification for care supersede the more important, close interpersonal relationships that nurses build with clients. Therefore, the main stimulus for entering nursing, caring, becomes less valued by health care providers.

Gilligan (1982) identifies two ways of thinking about moral development. She associates these conceptions of morality with male and female modes of describing relationships betweens others and self (Gilligan, 1982, p. 19):

1. Fairness: connecting moral development to the understanding of rights and rules (male mode).
2. Concern with the activity of care: connecting moral development to the understanding of responsibilities and relationships (female mode).

Traditional views of moral development emphasize "rights" over relationships and responsibilities (Kohlberg, 1981). Noddings (1984) proposes that morality and ethics should be "rooted in receptivity, relatedness and responsiveness" (p. 2). Haegert (2004) adapts Nodding's work on the ethics of caring to professional nursing practice. For Noddings, caring involves two aspects of human nature in the embodied and ethical self. The first encompasses an ideal self that is "synonymous with caring" and the "vision that implied a picture of goodness toward the one caring (the nurse) and the one cared for (the patient)" (Haegert, 2004, p. 434). As nurses practice, much energy is devoted to the development of authentic, therapeutic, and caring relationships with clients. Nurses also consider legal and institutional standards of care, along with client rights for self-determination and the equal access to care. Therefore, nursing presents a unique opportunity for blending different approaches to morality and ethics. However, as long as society values fairness and responsibility over receptivity, relatedness, and responsiveness, contributions made by professional nurses may not be as valued as those made by members of other health professions.

Morality supersedes status when persons entrust their lives, a sacred trust, to others. Therefore, moral principles guide health care providers in practice. Several moral principles central to nursing include beneficence, fidelity, and veracity. According to Flynn

(1987), the principle of beneficence is to do only good. This principle also requires that persons act to prevent harm. Aroskar (1987) views fidelity as undisputed and primary loyalty and faithfulness to the client. Finally, veracity requires absolute truth-telling. Professional nurses use these principles daily when providing care to clients.

Moral and ethical principles create dilemmas for nurses. Disagreements surface regarding what is good for a client, depending upon the situation (Flynn, 1987). Individual members of health care teams may disagree what is best for a terminally ill person. Fidelity specifies that nurses should always remain loyal and faithful to the client and to abide by the client's wishes. Sometimes, nurses encounter situations that require them to deceive or withhold information from clients to protect the institutions in which they work, or physicians with whom they serve. Most institutions require nurses to report errors using some form of incident reporting. However, many institutional policies specify that the nurse should not document completion of an incident report.

When nurses encounter situations in which there is no good outcome, the principle of double-effect (known as choosing the 'lesser evil') guides practice. Keegen (1995, p. 140) outlines that the following four conditions should be met to justify actions:

1. The act itself must be morally good or at least indifferent.
2. The good effect must not be achieved by means of the bad effect.
3. Only the good effect must be intended, although the bad effect is foreseen and known.
4. The good effect intended must be equal to or greater than the bad effect.

As client advocates, nurses must act on behalf of clients. To assess a particular clinical situation, nurses use critical thinking skills to collect and analyze information, and to formulate possible courses of action. As critical thinkers, nurses also anticipate consequences of actions before choosing the best course to take. Professional nurses use values and philosophical beliefs to set priorities and establish action plans in ethically and morally charged situations. For example, Mrs. G. is a 96-year-old woman in a coma from a head injury from an automobile accident in which she was the driver. Before the accident, she lived independently and volunteered at the library teaching adults to read. Mrs. G. has been unresponsive and ventilator-dependent for 3 days. She has shown no improvement, but her son is insisting on a tracheostomy so that his mother can be maintained on the ventilator until she regains consciousness. In this situation, nurses caring for Mrs. G turn to ethics when having to make value-based decisions about how to provide the best care for Mrs. G. and her son.

## ◆ ETHICAL DECISION-MAKING PROCESS

According to Bandman and Bandman (1995), nursing ethics focus on doing good and avoiding harm. Ethical behavior relies on the ability to make choices. The nurse bears responsibility for valuing choices that clients make. Choices may be clearly articulated when persons complete living wills before becoming incapacitated. However, when persons fail to make desires known before they are unable, health care professionals rely on families for treatment-related decisions. In the absence of family, health care professions use moral and ethical tenets to guide actions.

Nurses, like all other scientists and philosophers, base decisions on outcomes of inquiry. Munhall (1988) links nursing inquiry to ethical reflection with the ultimate ethical question being "toward what goal and what end?" (p. 151). Munhall adds that "many of our research endeavors focus on facilitating 'health.' The search for a means to produce a desired health outcome requires critical ethical reflection" (Munhall, 1988, p. 152).

## Three Perspectives

Three perspectives provide a foundation for and influence ethical thinking: principalism, care, and contextualism. Of the three, the most prevalent framework is **principalism,** which is "an orientation incorporating duties, rights, and principles" (O'Neill, 1995, p. 232); this perspective values rationalism. However, O'Neill acknowledges the importance of incorporating analysis of individual situations, sensitivity to the needs of others, and relationship dynamics when principalism guides ethical decision making.

The **care** perspective values dialogue to discover the particular needs of the person(s) involved in the decision. Finally, in **contextualism,** individual situations become the paradigm cases that provide "rules of thumb" to follow. In the contextualist perspective, practical experience in patient care is highly valued (O'Neill, 1995). Nursing based on contextualism supports detailed analysis of individual nursing situations and determines the best approaches to fit each situation.

In a postmodern world, persons tend to discount the simpler, monolithic approach to life and prefer pluralism. However, some persons may experience confusion in how to figure out life and find meaning in it when rules are abandoned. They may desire to find the "right" way to approach a given situation and develop radical, steadfast approaches that fuel political debates and conflict. For years, nursing scholars have debated if nursing is an art or a science. Emphasis on technology, scientific evidence, and quality improvement suggests that nursing is a science. However, considering the beauty of the deep, meaningful, interpersonal relationship among nurses and clients and capturing how they unfold suggest that nursing may really be an art.

### Research Brief 3-1

Appleton, C. (1993). The art of nursing: the experience of patients and nursing. *Journal of Advanced Nursing, 18,* 892–899.

By combining two qualitative research approaches: phenomenology (identifying the lived experience) and hermeneutics (identifying the deep personal meaning), the investigator sought to explicate a view of nursing as an art. The broad research question that was asked during 17 nurse and patient interviews was "What is the experience of the art of nursing for you?" (p. 893).

**Themes that Express the Art of Nursing**

The study identified the following five overriding themes to express the art of nursing:

1. The way of being there in caring.
2. The way of being-with in understanding caring.
3. The way of creating opportunities for fullness of being through caring.
4. A transcendent togetherness.
5. The context of caring (p. 894).

Nurse-identified themes in the nurse's way of being there in caring included centering on the whole person, while valuing the patient's individual dignity and worth. Patient-identified themes related to being there in caring focused on needing care, feeling vulnerable, and personally wanting help in caring. Themes identified for being-with in caring included knowing that caring is the core of practice, describing the essence of caring as establishing mutually shared meaning and "creating situations for caring to flourish" (p. 895). Themes emerging for the way of creating opportunities for nurses feeling more as persons included nurse preparation for personal well-being, responsible decision making, and self-guidance of expression. Finally, the context of caring centered around "nursing as the primary source of caring and valuing the art of nursing" (p. 897).

Because all participants were white women, the patients were child-bearing age, and the nurses had practiced for 10 or more years, results of this study may not reflect perceptions of men and nurses with less clinical experience. Women may value the emotional elements of a nursing encounter more than do men. Seasoned nursing professionals have established clinical competence and may be able to focus more on establishing meaningful relationships with patients.

### Clinical Implications

Clinical implications of this study include that caring may be the essence of the art of nursing and nursing care may mean liberating help. Because nurses synthesize basic, applied, and practical sciences and use personal, aesthetic, ethical, and empirical knowledge to guide practice, nursing may indeed be an art. The art of nursing might explain the science of nursing. Nursing education and clinical practice provide ways that enable nurses to freely attain fullness of being; provide opportunities for reflection on and reflection in action; look for innovative means to promote active partnerships among nurses and patients; and create caring cultures. Because nursing considers the holistic nature of humans, nursing as an art may more effectively describe the essence of nursing than does nursing as a science. Additional research related to capturing the essence of professional nursing is needed to arrive at a more clear and concise definition of nursing.

### Questions for Reflection 3-1

1. What are my beliefs and values about human life?
2. How strong are these beliefs and values?
3. What would I do if I encountered a client care situation in which decisions were made that were against my values and beliefs? Why would I act this way?

## An Ethical Decision-Making Process

Nurses frequently encounter moral and ethical problems in practice, thereby creating a need for a workable method with which to analyze and resolve ethical dilemmas. Fowler (1987, pp. 183–184) proposes a systematic **ethical decision-making process** that incorporates principalism, care, and contextualism to help nurses thoughtfully address moral problems in practice. Fowler's steps are outlined in Table 3-1, and Display 3-2 provides an example of how the process is used. Consistent use of a sequential process for ethical decision making enables nurses to consider all aspects surrounding a situation

**TABLE 3-1**

## Process for Ethical Decision Making

| Step | Thoughts and Actions |
|------|---------------------|
| Identify the problem. | Analyze the situation to clearly identify the problem.<br>Determine the presence of more than one ethical concern.<br>Look for any conflict of duties with personal or professional values.<br>Determine if the ethical conflict rightly belongs to you. |
| Identify the morally relevant facts. | Examine the complete context of the dilemma (how it occurred, likelihood of arising again).<br>Identify the key players and their views and vested interest(s).<br>Identify administrative, political, economic, legal, medical, and aesthetic concerns. |
| Evaluate the ethical problem. | Examine the ethical norms by reviewing the literature, code of ethics for nursing, and moral traditions in the profession.<br>Based on information from the review, identify guides for moral actions that are appropriate for the situation.<br>Consider broader ethical principles, such as justice and autonomy to provide directions for action.<br>Consider aspects that are unique to the dilemma.<br>Examine the dilemma using each ethical principle.<br>Assign priorities to each of the ethical principles (Chapter 1) according to professional and personal values. |
| Identify and analyze action alternatives. | Determine all possible options for action.<br>Create new options not found elsewhere.<br>Analyze each alternative action for potential harms and benefits.<br>Speculate the possible outcomes for each benefit for the key players.<br>Identify which actions will produce subsequent dilemmas.<br>Analyze each alternative according to institutional procedures. |
| Choose and act. | Choose a course of action (preferably in consultation with others).<br>Modify the plan in accordance with legal, institutional, or other values while remaining true to your moral values and norms.<br>Implement the alternative action selected. |
| Evaluate and modify the plan. | Identify the result of action taken.<br>Clarify your moral feelings about your actions.<br>Generate modifications to the plan used if you encounter similar situations in the future.<br>Modify the current plan if the ethical dilemma persists. |

Adapted from Fowler, M. D. M., & Levine-Ariff, J. (Eds.) (1987). *Ethics at the bedside: A source book for the critical care nurse* (pp. 183; 184). Philadelphia: J. B. Lippincott.

before taking action. Once the situation has resolved, engagement in evaluation facilitates the nurse to reflect on actions taken, and to generate ideas for ways to manage a future, similar situation.

---

**An Example Using Fowler's Process**                    **DISPLAY 3-2** ◆

Mary is a nurse who works the night shift on an acute general surgical unit. Because of budget cuts, the hospital has eliminated two night shift professional nursing positions, resulting in a consistent staffing pattern of one professional nurse for 15 patients. Mary has always valued her ability to provide individualized nursing care to postoperative patients. However, since she has been working under the new staffing pattern, Mary knows that patients are receiving substandard care (problem identified). Mary realizes that the hospital has been losing revenue, but she also feels that the staffing pattern is unsafe. Her recent complaints to her nurse manager have been futile. Because of unsafe care situations, Mary knows that she will have to inform her nurse manager's supervisor and possibly, the director of nursing and hospital administration to analyze the entire situation (morally relevant facts identified). Mary reads current literature and identifies serious gaps in the accepted standards of practice and examines the effects of the new staffing practice on each ethical principle (ethical problem evaluated). After sharing her concerns with her coworkers and manager, Mary and her colleagues work as a team to develop three action plans. They discuss the pros and cons of each plan (alternatives identified and analyzed). The nursing team decides to meet with the director of nursing to share their concerns about unsafe patient care (course of action chosen and implemented). The director of nursing thanks the nurses for informing her of the situation and promises action to increase the number of professional nurses for the night shift on the unit. Two months pass and no change in staffing results. The nurses decide to meet with hospital administration to voice their concerns (plan evaluated and modified).

---

Bandman and Bandman (1995, pp. 110) talk about the pitfalls that may occur when nurses use an ethical decision-making process. They label these pitfalls "fallacies" or errors in reasoning. Such errors in reasoning include:

1. Arguing that because something (X) is the case, therefore, something else (Y) ought to be the case.
2. Making someone accept the conclusion of another based on force alone (appealing to force).
3. Abusing the person rather than addressing the person's reasons for making a particular decision.
4. Arguing that because everybody does something, that something must be good.
5. Appealing to inappropriate authority to justify a decision.
6. Assuming that if one exception is made to a rule, then uncontrolled events with unwanted circumstances will occur (called the 'slippery slope fallacy').
7. Refusing to allow evidence to be shared if it contradicts one's personal position.

Bandman and Bandman (1995) offer suggestions for ways to avoid fallacies by using the following principles for ethical decision making:

1. Valuing and respecting the client's self-determination.
2. Serving the client's well-being in practice in a manner that prevents harm and does good.

3. Treating clients fairly and equally by respecting their rights and treatment options and by making them equal partners in shared health care decisions.

Nursing practice, education, and research provide many opportunities for the professional nurse to make ethical decisions and to experience the satisfactions of resolving ethical dilemmas. Situations that generate ethical dilemmas arise from the nurse's efforts to determine what is right. In dealing with each of these ethical issues, the primary responsibility of the professional nurse in caring for the client is always to respect the person as a unified being. Despite variations in the definition of responsibility in nursing, most nursing leaders would probably agree that the structure of the professional nurses' responsibility is to self, to client, and to the profession, always for improving health.

## ● MAJOR CONTEXTUAL ELEMENTS AFFECTING NURSING PRACTICE

To understand the moral or ethical dimension of nursing more fully, the nurse needs to understand the contextual elements of nursing practice that either reinforce or challenge belief and value systems. Display 3-3 briefly summarizes selected demographic, economic, cultural, environmental, and ethical factors that characterize the context of nursing practice which are discussed subsequently. Public policy, another significant contextual element, is discussed in Chapter 16, The Professional Nurse's Role in Public Policy. The following discussion aims to provide a general overview of factors chosen as being most influential to professional nursing practice.

---

### Five Major Contextual Elements Affecting Professional Nursing Practice

DISPLAY 3-3 ●

**Demographic:** These characteristics reflect social and economic conditions. The demographics of a population influence the opportunities an individual has to form or maintain cooperative and interdependent relationships with fellow human beings.

**Economic:** Economics primarily focuses on the considerations of costs and return for provided services. In cultures in which health services are viewed as commodities, providers must be reimbursed for their services. However, when societies view health care as a basic right, governments usually provide a national health insurance plan for all citizens.

**Cultural:** Provides organization and structure for groups of people. Within a culture, people share common values, beliefs, norms, and practices (Giger & Davidhizar, 1999). Culture plays a key role in the development of human behavior patterns.

Sometimes cultural beliefs clash with scientifically based health care practices.

**Environmental:** These elements consist of global health influences. Along with safe food sources, the human species requires clean air and water for survival. Kleffel (1996) presents an ecocentric view of the world by describing that "the environment is considered to be whole, living, and interconnected" (p. 1).

**Ethical:** These elements encompass the moral obligations and duties that emerge from an individual's struggle with good and bad, and right and wrong. Ethical nurses act in accordance with approved standards or codes for professional behavior. Nurses confront ethical issues in daily practice. Ethical dilemmas occur when nurses confront situations in which alternatives for action produce unsatisfactory results. Sometimes, what is ethically right can be legally or morally wrong.

## Demographic Elements

Within the next decade, Americans will be living longer and growing older. By 2010, 40 million Americans will be 65 years old or older. The life expectancy for American women will be 81 years, and for American men, 76 years. By 2030, one in five Americans (70 million persons) will be older than age 65 years (National Center for Health Statistics, 2004). The Institute for the Future (2003) estimates that over 100,000 centenarians will reside in the United States in 2010. The percentage of elderly will also increase in Europe, Asia, and Latin America, with China having close to 290 million persons older than age 60 years in 2030 (Institute for the Future, 2004). Elderly persons use more health care resources and have different care needs than younger persons (Institute for the Future, 2003; National Center for Health Statistics, 2004). Nurses need to consider specific needs of the elderly when providing care to them.

The increased elderly population may strain current health care resources because this age group has an increased risk for chronic illness. Persons older than 65 have higher rates of hospital admittance and may have greater need for assistance with activities of daily living. In 2004, the National Center for Health Statistics reported that 51% of Americans older than the age of 75 years had mobility limitations, and 23% relied on family members for assistance.

According to Horrigan (2004) at the United States Department of Labor Bureau of Labor Statistics, 623,156 new nurses will be needed to meet the demand for registered nurses in 2012 (an increase of 25.2%). The increased numbers stem from nurses needed to care for the aging population and to replace aging nurses who currently practice.

Perhaps the most important health care need for the American population is the need for health promotion and disease prevention services. Nurses need to look for ways to promote healthy aging. Efforts should target persons of all ages, especially adults and adolescents whose current lifestyles and health habits will significantly affect their future wellness (United States Department of Health & Human Services, 2000). Middle-aged adults find themselves torn between meeting career obligations, raising teenagers, and caring for aging parents. In the role of counselor, professional nurses can provide clients (their children or spouses) support by inquiring about the stresses associated with fulfilling multiple role responsibilities.

## Cultural Elements

America's population will continue to become more diverse. Sixty-nine percent of the American population is non-Hispanic white. The distribution of ethnic groups is not equal in all areas of the United States. The western United States enjoys the highest concentration of ethnic and racial minorities, with Hispanics being the largest group (17%). In 2010, the southern United States is projected to have the largest percentage (18%) of the African American population (Institute for the Future, 2003). Increasing diversity increases the complexity of providing effective nursing care.

In locations with large Hispanic populations, nurses may need to communicate with clients who may not be fluent in English. In addition, many immigrant groups tend to settle in a specific community (Institute for the Future, 2003). Nurses need to be aware of culturally diverse population clusters and their usual health practices to provide effective nursing care. Meeting the health care demands of a culturally diverse population means that nurses need to understand biophysiologic variations related to risk for specific health problems, development, and medication metabolism, along with specific cultural values, beliefs, and health practices (See Chapter 11 for more specific information).

## Economic Elements

Along with age and diversity population changes, the population is expected to be better educated by 2005, with 55% of persons over age 25 years having the equivalent of 1 year of college. However, income disparity will increase slightly, with the mean income of an American family projected to be $53,000 (in 1998 dollars). Fortunately, persons with higher income tend to enjoy better health (Institute for the Future, 2003).

Unfortunately, projections for access to health care will be three-tiered, with 38% being empowered, 43% being worried, and 28% being excluded. Consumers excluded from accessing health care will be the poor, uninsured, unemployed, and uneducated, with the poor and uneducated having the poorest access. Currently, 45 million persons (15%) in America do not have health insurance (National Center for Health Statistics, 2004). The newly uninsured are young adults, persons who are self-employed, and employees of small businesses. If no changes are made to either the health care system or insurance regulations, estimates project that up to 16% of the American population will have no health insurance coverage in 2010 (Herzlinger, 2004). The worried consumers include early retirees and persons dependent on employer-provided health insurance. As health expenditures continue to escalate, employers may have to reduce health care benefits or pass on increased costs to employees to afford any form of health insurance coverage. Empowered health care consumers have discretionary income that can be used to cover health care costs. They also tend to be well educated and frequently use technology (especially the Internet) as a source for health care information. Empowered consumers frequently actively participate when making health-related decisions with physicians and other health care professionals (Institute for the Future, 2003).

Health care spending is expected to increase. Health care expenditures accounted for 14.1% of the gross domestic product (GDP) in 2002. By 2012, the Department of Health and Human Services (2004) forecasts that health care expenditures will account for 17.7% of the GDP. Companies providing health care insurance to employees have seen 12% to 15% increases in premiums over the past 3 years. Within the next 5 years, company costs for providing health insurance are expected to double. Increased costs for health insurance will be passed on to employees who then may not be able to afford the increased copayments, thereby increasing the numbers of more uninsured Americans (Herzlinger).

According to the Institute for the Future (2003), the following factors determine personal health status: access to care (10%), genetics (20%), personal health behaviors (50%), and uncontrollable factors (30%). Uninsured Americans have limited access to health care. Personal health-promoting habits require that individuals know what lifestyle behaviors promote health and that they have the resources to obtain them. Persons without health insurance may use free clinics and public health departments for primary health care services. In these settings, an advanced practice nurse assumes the role of caregiver. Other clients may prefer a more holistic approach to health care. These consumers may turn to nurses rather than physicians for primary care services. As educators, professional nurses can teach clients health-promoting strategies. However, if clients do not have the ability to practice them, then nurses can refer them to social or governmental agencies to help them (nurse as client advocate). As change agents, nurses can engage in efforts to change the health care system by actively participating in public policy development (see Chapter 16).

## ● SUMMARY AND SIGNIFICANCE TO PRACTICE

Professional nursing centers on caring for others. When delivering care to individuals, groups, and communities, professional nurses use individual value systems as a basis for some clinical decisions. Many contextual elements affect health care delivery and clinical practice. Sometimes the contextual elements create ethical dilemmas that need to be resolved. Nurses who have examined their beliefs and have developed a personal nursing philosophy have a basis for finding meaning in professional practice and for resolving ethical dilemmas. Nurses assume a variety of professional roles when providing direct care services and when working toward promoting health for all.

### FROM THEORY TO PRACTICE

1. What does it mean to be a professional nurse?
2. How do nurses make differences in the lives of others?
3. After reading this chapter, how would you help Jane, the nurse, in the vignette? Outline a plan for you to help Jane make a decision whether or not to continue in her current job or to be a professional nurse.
4. Stephen is often the only registered nurse on duty during the evenings in a nursing home in which he works. Lately, he has become increasingly concerned about one of his patients. Mrs. Moore is a 77-year-old woman with advanced Parkinson's disease who has to be restrained to keep her from pulling out her feeding tube. Whenever Mrs. Moore speaks, she begs to be allowed to die. Mrs. Moore's son and daughter refuse to let the physician remove the feeding tube. Stephen agonizes about what he should do. Analyze this case using the guidelines for the ethical decision-making process outlined in this chapter and decide what decision should be made about Mrs. Moore.
5. Look at your nursing program and departmental/organizational philosophies where you work. Compare these to your own personal philosophy and outline key similarities and differences.

### WWW INTERNET EXERCISES

1. Search the web for any college- or university-based nursing program and see if they have the philosophy of the school of nursing posted on the home page.
2. Visit the home page of the American Holistic Nurses Association (AHNA) and read this organization's philosophy of nursing at http://www.ahna.org.
3. Select a nursing organization that interests you. Use the search engine of your choice to get the home page of the organization. Visit the site and see whether you can find the organization's values, mission, and philosophy. Based on a review of available information, outline reasons why you might or might not join the organization.

## INTERNET RESOURCES

For an example of an integrated health system: Visit the website of Saint Luke's Health System in Kansas City at http://www.saint-lukes.org. View the mission, vision, and value statements.

For a sample nursing department philosophy, view the nursing department philosophy of Barnes Jewish Hospital in St. Louis, Missouri, at http://www.barnesjewish .org/groups?NavID=636.

Sample nursing organization philosophy: The New Jersey State Nurses Association at http://www.njsna.org/about.htm.

## REFERENCES

American Association of Colleges of Nursing (AACN) (1986). *Final report: Project on the essentials of college and university education for professional nursing.* Washington, DC: Author.

Antonovsky, A. (1987). *Unraveling the mystery of health.* San Francisco: Jossey-Bass.

Appleton, C. (1993). The art of nursing: the experience of patients and nursing. *Journal of Advanced Nursing, 18,* 892–899.

Aroskar, M. A. (1987). Fidelity and veracity: Questions of promise keeping, truth telling, and loyalty. In M. D. M. Fowler & J. Levine-Ariff (Eds.). *Ethics at the bedside: A source for the critical care nurse.* Philadelphia: Lippincott Williams & Wilkins.

Bandman E. L., and Bandman, B. (1995). *Nursing ethics through the lifespan* (3rd ed.). Stamford, CT: Appleton & Lange.

Benner, P. (1984). *From novice to expert: Excellence and power in clinical nursing practice.* Menlo Park, CA: Addison-Wesley.

Benner, P., & Wrubel, J. (1989). *The primacy of caring: Stress and coping in health and illness.* Menlo Park, CA: Addison-Wesley.

Boughn, S. (1994). Why do men choose nursing? *Nursing and Health Care, 15,* 406–411.

Boughn, S. (2001). Why women and men choose nursing. *Nursing and Health Perspectives, 22,* 14–19.

Carper, B. A. (1978). Fundamental patterns of knowing in nursing. *Advances in Nursing Science, 1,* 13–23.

Dossey, B., Keegan, L., Guzzetta, C. (2005). *Holistic nursing: a handbook for practice* (4th ed.). Sudbury, MA: Jones & Bartlett.

Earle, W. J. (1992). *Introduction to Philosophy.* New York: McGraw-Hill.

Enserink, P. M. (2004). Looking the pandemic in the eye. *Science, 306,* 392–394.

Flynn, P. A. R. (1987). Questions of risk, duty, and paternalism: Problems in beneficence. In M. D. M. Fowler & J. Levine-Ariff (Eds.). *Ethics at the bedside: A source for the critical care nurse.* Philadelphia: Lippincott Williams & Wilkins.

Fowler, M. D. M., & Levine-Ariff, J. (Eds.). (1987). *Ethics at the bedside: A source for the critical care nurse.* Philadelphia: Lippincott Williams & Wilkins.

Frankl, V. (1963). *Man's search for meaning.* New York: Washington Square Press.

Fried, B. J., & Gaydos, L. M. (Eds.). (2002). *World health systems, challenges and perspectives.* Chicago: Health Administration Press.

Giger, J. N., & Davidhizar, R. E. (1999) *Transcultural nursing assessment and intervention* (3rd ed.). St. Louis: Mosby.

Gilligan, C. (1982). *In a different voice: Psychological theory and women's development.* Cambridge MA: Harvard University Press.

Haegart, S. (2004). The ethics of self. *Nursing Ethics, 11,* 434–443.

Hawking, S. (2002). *The theory of everything.* Beverly Hills, CA: New Millennium Press.

Herzlinger, R. (2004). *Consumer-driven health care.* San Francisco: Jossey-Bass.

Horrigan, M. (2004). Employment projections to 2012: Concepts and context. *Monthly Labor Review,* (February, 2004), 3–22.

Institute for the Future (2003). *Health & health care 2010* (2nd ed.). San Francisco: Jossey-Bass.

Institute for the Future (2004). *2004 map of the decade.* Menlo Park, CA: Author.

Keegan, L. (1995). Holistic ethics. In B. M. Dossey, L. Keegan, C. E. Guzzetta, & L. G. Kolkmeier (Eds.). *Holistic nursing: A handbook for practice* (2nd ed.). Gaithersburg, MD: Aspen.

Kleffel, D. (1996). Environmental paradigms: Moving toward an eccocentric approach. *Advances in Nursing Science, 18,* 1–10.

Kohlberg, L. (1981). *The philosophy of moral development: Moral stages and the idea of justice.* New York: Harper & Row.

McKay, M. L. (2001). The growth of health care. *American Journal of Nursing, 101,* 24F–24H.

Mish, F. C. (Ed.). (1994). *Merriam Webster's Collegiate Dictionary* (10th ed.). Springfield, MA: Merriam-Webster.

Munhall, P. (1988). Ethical considerations in qualitative research. *Western Journal of Nursing Research, 10,* 150–162.

National Center of Health Statistics (2004). National health care expenditures projections: 2002–2012. Available at: http://www.cms.hhs.gov/statistics/nhe/projections-2002/proj2002.pdf. Accessed June 25, 2005.

Noddings, N. (1984). *Caring: A feminine approach to ethics and moral education.* Berkeley: University of California Press.

O'Neill, J. (1995). Ethical decision making and the role of nursing. In G. L. Deloughery (Ed.). *Issues and trends in nursing* (2nd ed.). St. Louis: Mosby-Year Book.

Okrainec, G. D. (1994). Perception of nursing education held by male nursing students. *Western Journal of Nursing Research, 16,* 94–107.

Porter-O'Grady, T., & Malloch, K. (2003). *Quantum leadership: a textbook of new leadership.* Sudbury, MA: Jones & Bartlett.

Rafael, A. R. (1996). Power and caring: A dialectic in nursing. *Advances in Nursing Science, 19,* 3–17.

Rew, L. (1994). Commentary. In J. F. Kikuchi, & H. Simmons. (Eds.). *Developing a philosophy of nursing* (pp. 20–31). Thousand Oaks, CA: Sage.

Ross, A., Wenzel, F., & Mitlyng, J. (2002). *Leadership for the future: core competencies in healthcare.* Chicago: Health Administration Press.

Salsberry, P. J. (1994). A philosophy of nursing: What is it? What is it not? In J. F. Kikuchi & H. Simmons (Eds.). *Developing a philosophy of nursing* (pp. 11–19). Thousand Oaks, CA: Sage.

Streubert, H. (1994). Male nursing students' perceptions of clinical experience. *Nurse Educator, 19,* 28–32.

Watson, J. (1988). A case study: Curriculum in transition. In National League for Nursing. *Curriculum revolution: Mandate for change* (pp. 1–8). New York: Author

United States Department of Health and Human Services (2000). *Healthy People 2010.* Washington, DC. U.S. Government Printing Office.

United States Department of Health and Human Services (2004). National health care expenditures projections: 2002–2012. Available at: http://www.cms.hhs.gov/statistics/nhe/projections-2002/proj2002.pdf. Accessed June 25, 2005.

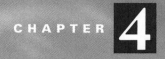

# CHAPTER 4

# Patterns of Knowing and Nursing Science

## KEY TERMS AND CONCEPTS

Certainty
Relativity
Rationalism
Intuition
Empiricism
Historicism
Postmodernism
Empirical Knowing
Empirical Knowledge
Aesthetic Knowing
Aesthetic Knowledge
Personal Knowledge
Personal Knowing
Ethical Knowledge
Ethical Knowing
Nursing Science
Concepts
Theories
Nursing Conceptual Models
Four Central Concepts of Nursing

## LEARNING OUTCOMES

By the end of this chapter, the learner will be able to:

1 Discuss the evolution of three systems of thought about how to organize developing knowledge in science.

2 Describe the differences among logical empiricism, historicism, and postmodernism in their philosophic approaches to the development of knowledge.

3 Explain the differences among the four patterns of nursing knowledge.

4 Know the four central concepts of nursing that identify the focus for scientific inquiry.

5 Appreciate why theory is essential to the practice of nursing.

## VIGNETTE

Paul, a registered nurse (RN) for 7 years, just completed a bachelor of science in nursing (BSN) degree program. He believes that knowledge from "hard science" is the only way nursing can become as respected as other health care professions. He also believes that research is only useful if it directly improves patient care, and he disregards conceptual or explanatory research. He wants to do research because he feels that it looks good on a résumé and is a good way to "get ahead."

Understanding a body of knowledge is essential for competent professional practice. Knowledge can be obtained from a number of sources, including experience, reflection, and values. Science is "a unified body of knowledge about phenomena that is supported by agreed-on evidence" (Meleis, 1997, p. 10). "Since nursing is a learned profession, it is both a science and an art. The practice of nurses, [therefore], is the creative use of [this] knowledge in human service" (Rogers, 1992, pp. 28–29).

The science of nursing incorporates the study of relationships among nurses, clients, and environments within the context of health. It also is the result of interrelationships among theory, practice, research, and education. Theory provides the tools to direct nursing practice. Practice provides the professional individual with the setting to apply and test nursing knowledge and develop theories. Research provides the means to test theories. Education provides the means to shape belief systems and to synthesize and disseminate knowledge.

Nursing science is emerging as an autonomous, distinctive professional discipline that is valued by society. As an emerging science, nursing uses and builds on knowledge developed in many disciplines through centuries of evolution.

**Questions for Reflection 4-1**

1. What are the benefits of establishing a base of nursing science for the profession of nursing?
2. What consequences arise for the nursing profession if it fails to generate a specialized knowledge base?

## ● THE EVOLUTION OF SCIENTIFIC THOUGHT

Human life has greatly changed since prehistoric times and many of the changes have been the result of the advancement of science. To a large degree, science accounts for humankind's progress. This chapter addresses three systems of thought about organizing and developing human knowledge because it is impossible to cover each era of human history and the entire evolution of human knowledge (Spradlin & Porterfield, 1984).

At first, ancient humans knew about the world through magical beliefs and they believed that they were controlled by forces beyond human understanding or control. A second way of trying to know about the world began during the scientific revolution (around 1500) and continued until recently. Science emphasized observations, measurement, and quantification as the means for understanding the world. Since Einstein's discovery of relativity in the early 20th century, humans began to accept uncertainty and focused on processes that have influenced human thought.

### Ancient Humans

Early humans differentiated the world into two parts: me (internal) and not me (external). They viewed the external world as being populated by spirits, demons, and gods, who assumed both good and evil characteristics of humans. Because gods were believed to be irrational and to be moved by whims and passions, humans tried to influence the gods' behavior, instead of trying to figure out rational causes of events.

Through trial and error, humans discovered that some patterns of action led to predictable outcomes, which could be reproduced as long as the procedure was followed exactly (as one would with recipes from a cookbook). Thus, in an elementary way, humans studied and observed phenomena sufficiently to gather many isolated facts. However, the facts remained isolated, rather than being organized into a body of data that could form the basis for scientific conclusions. To the extent that nursing functioned primarily from protocols and procedures for many years, it somewhat followed the methods of science that existed until approximately two centuries ago.

Because disease, aches, and pains were assumed to be caused by gods and evil spirits, early medicine was associated with religion or magical beliefs. However, time and attention to cause and effect led to practical approaches and logical sequencing of steps of treatment. Hippocrates (460–377 BC) was followed by Aristotle (384–322 BC), who emphasized classification of signs and symptoms. Increasingly, attention was paid to exploring the mechanisms of the human body (Spradlin & Porterfield, 1984).

## Questions for Reflection 4-2

1. What current superstitions have I encountered in my professional practice?
2. How do these superstitions affect my practice and the profession?
3. What are the consequences of relying on superstitions to guide professional practice?

## The Search for Certainty

By the 1500s, the development of mathematics coincided with increasing interest in scientific study of humans and nature. The ability to count made relationships appear more logical and the world more predictable. The philosophy of logical positivism drove the search for **certainty.** This was based on a belief that the world was like a simple machine, but only God understood the laws by which it operated. Time and space were absolute. Time flowed smoothly and uniformly. A reductionistic approach was used to identify causes to predict effects.

Scientific scholars became engulfed in a spiral of logic and increasing certainty about quantification of relationships among absolute entities that led to concepts of truths that could be validated. . . . We could, with the use of observation, measurement, and logical reasoning, know the laws of nature. . . . All the entities that composed the whole of nature could be reduced to their smallest parts, studied and understood, and rebuilt (Spradlin & Porterfield, 1984, p. 106).

Reduction of humans into separate psyche and soma (Cartesian dualism), both of which could be measured physically, was advanced by Descartes (1596–1650), who saw the human being as a machine ruled by the same laws as all of nature (Spradlin & Porterfield, 1984, p. 108). The separation of mind from matter (body) and the emphasis on the human being as the sum of minute parts has dominated medical and nursing science ever since.

Four basic assumptions about humans and the universe are inherent in this kind of a mechanistic world view: determinism, quantity, continuity, and impersonality. Leaving no room for uncertainty, the principle of determinism reflects the belief that "nature proceeds by a strict chain of events from cause to effect, the configuration of causes at any instant fully determining the event in the next instant, and so on forever" (Ware, Panikaar, & Romein, 1966, p. 127). The ability to predict comes out of this principle, whereas lack of predictability and the presence of uncertainty represent ignorance.

The quantitative principle expresses the exact nature of science. It reflects the belief that science consists of "measuring things and setting up precise relations between the measurements" (Ware et al., 1966, p. 129). In this view, humans and the universe are described by numbers (e.g., spatial coordinates, time, position, amounts, and locations) that quantify physical properties and by relations among these quantitative characteristics.

Continuity, the third principle, is concerned with the "transitions of nature from one state to another [and] express[es] the sense, deeply engrained in the outlook of the age, that the movements of nature are gradual" (Ware et al., 1966, p. 129). This principle reflects the belief that the processes involving humans and the universe are continuous.

In the fourth principle, impersonality, the scientist is viewed as an instrument, not a person. The scientist uses observation rather than imagination, passively finds order in phenomena rather than creating it, and does not permit personal influence on the phenomena under observation (Ware et al., 1966, p. 129).

Belief in these principles led Galileo (1564–1642) and Sir Isaac Newton (1642–1727) to develop the scientific method, based on a particular method of reasoning: logic. Logic encompasses principles of reasoning applicable to any branch of knowledge. Because logic is based on reason and sound judgment, it can be convincing.

Inquiry is a technique of science. It seeks truth, information, or knowledge to meet the goal of problem solving. A problem is any question or matter involving doubt, uncertainty, or difficulty that needs solution. Solution is the act of solving a problem by finding the answer or explanation. The most extensive investigative process of science is the systematic inquiry of research.

**Questions for Reflection 4-3**

1. How do I use logic, science, and inquiry in my professional practice?
2. What are the consequences of using logic, science, and inquiry in my professional practice and for the profession?

## The Relative World of Process

By the 20th century, scientists realized that the physical world consisted of matter and forces that interact with matter, such as gravity, magnetism, and electricity. By exploring the cell, genetic mechanisms and mechanisms that influenced cellular structure and function were explained. It appeared that "the immutable laws which governed the world" were being discovered.

Then, in the early 20th century, Albert Einstein demonstrated that the world was composed not of events, but of observations, which were relative to the place and velocity of the observer. "Any absolutes or cause and effect sequences [are] illusions. . . testable only in a retrospect organization of events" (Spradlin & Porterfield, 1984, p. vi). Heisenberg's (1971) and Bertalanffy's (1968) work in quantum physics led to postulation that mass, energy, time, and space coordinates are interchangeable. All systems are considered interrelated and interdependent, on a continuum of **relativity** and probability, and thus uncertainty.

The implications of this different conceptual system are enormous. Continuity is replaced by discontinuity, and probability (determined statistically) replaces certainty. Emphasis is placed on patterning, rather than on discrete entities, and on interactions, rather than on isolated events. The scientist is no longer an isolated objective observer of events. "Man came to be seen not as a detached observer but as an irremovable part of his observations" (Ware et al., 1966, p. 148). In addition, awareness of the limitations and biases of individual perception has increased, implying that truth and meaning are not absolute but are relative to history and context.

Nonetheless, "while physicists have become increasingly concerned with . . . a relative world of process, biologists have until recently tended to be even more involved in the reductionistic approach to life" (Spradlin & Porterfield, 1984, p. 189). Because one's belief system is critical to determining sources and methods of discovering knowledge, the following section discusses differing approaches to the philosophy of science that currently influence nursing science.

### Questions for Reflection 4-4

1. How does relativism affect nursing practice?
2. How have I used relativism to justify some nursing actions that I have taken?
3. What are the consequences of use of relativism for patients, myself as a professional nurse, and the nursing profession?

## ● PHILOSOPHY OF KNOWLEDGE

Based on Plato's concepts, knowledge is considered to be belief that has been justified through reason (Stumpf, 1993). What constitutes adequate justification is the concern of the discipline of philosophy. Philosophy considers questions such as whether there is such a thing as truth and how one can be certain that something is true. It is necessary to accept that some things can be true to question the truth or falseness of any particular thing. But must certainty be beyond all possible doubt, or is certainty sufficient if it is beyond logical and reasonable doubt? How does an individual acquire knowledge? What are the roles of intellect, perception, and intuition in the process of knowing?

### Processes of Knowing

The three primary processes of knowing are rationalism, empiricism, and intuition. **Rationalism** involves belief in the possibility of knowing truth by thinking and by use of reason that is a priori, or independent of experience. Empiricism involves belief that the only source of certainty about knowledge is immediate experience. However, because raw experience is subject to individual perception, the emphasis must be on verification and on confirmation or refutation of observations. **Intuition** is sometimes described as "just knowing." The source of the knowing is internal to the individual and often is perceived as occurring independently of experience or reason. It is subjective and personal in origin, although it can be validated through experience and interaction with others.

## Approaches to Knowing

### Logical Empiricism

Logical **empiricism,** a philosophic approach to the development of knowledge accepted since the 16th century, is based on the following assumptions:

1. A body of facts and principles that explain the way the world operates is waiting to be discovered. These include abstract, general, and universal principles. Theories provide alternative explanations of how the body of facts is ordered and systematically unified.
2. Cause-and-effect (linear) relationships can be established by using deductive processes and experimental methodology. The results are context-free generalizations that can be applied to all individuals. Truth is achieved through sensory data and controlled experiments.
3. It is necessary to control values and biases to achieve "objective" knowledge; therefore, the observer must be separated from the observed world. Science is value free. Social relevance is unimportant.
4. Theoretical reduction is an important scientific goal. It is assumed that the ultimate character of reality will be best explained using the logic and simplicity of the fewest possible theoretical concepts and laws.
5. The whole is the sum of its parts. Circumscribing (reducing) observations to small parts of the whole gives better control of the data and stronger explanatory power.

### Historicism

**Historicism,** advanced since the 1930s under the influence of concepts such as relativity and process, is based on the following assumptions:

1. Because "truth" is dynamic and constantly changing, what is important is the effectiveness of a theory for solving problems.
2. The whole is more than the sum of its parts. Reducing the whole to parts is counterproductive. Interrelationships and interactions are part of what must be studied.
3. An individual or a phenomenon must be studied as a whole in a natural setting. The observer is part of the setting, so interactions between the observer and the setting should be described, rather than controlled. Emphasis is on process, rather than fact.

4. Multiple research traditions are desirable (e.g., theories from psychology, physiology, education, and so forth) to explain different dimensions of the same phenomenon. Synthesis and development of multiple theories are encouraged.
5. Knowledge is related to context. Values, subjectivity, intuition, history, and tradition are useful for discovery.

### Postmodernism

**Postmodernism** is a social movement and a philosophy that originated in Europe in the 1960s (Reed, 1995). Postmodern perspectives on knowledge development are based on the following assumptions:

1. There is a focus on understanding multiple meanings and ways of knowing reality, rather than "a single, transcendent meaning of reality" (Reed, 1995, p. 71). As a result, conceptual models and grand theories are considered irrelevant.
2. Because "multiple truths" are accepted, knowledge is considered to be uncertain and provisional (Holmes & Warelow, 2000). Contradictory positions have value for generating alternative meanings.
3. Statements "reflect a concern for context rather than universality, specificity rather than generalization, uniqueness rather than sameness, and relativism rather than absolutism" (Holmes & Warelow, 2000, p. 90).
4. The emphasis of knowledge development shifts "from concern over the truth of one's findings to concern over the practical significance of the findings" (Reed, 1995, p. 72).
5. Problems are not "solved," but rather are "deconstructed," which means that efforts are made to disentangle or separate concerns from underlying values and beliefs. Language is analyzed for the meanings of words and assumed power structures.
6. With lack of concern about generalization is a shift toward lived experience, and toward "creativity, flexibility, uniqueness, and local value" (Holmes & Warelow, 2000, p. 96). Instead of probable "truth," relevance and usefulness for practice and the potential to generate additional study are the criteria for research.

Until recently, nursing research and theory were dominated by empiricism and logical positivistic philosophy. However, beginning with Rogers (1970) and increasing in the 1980s, nurse scientists incorporated principles of historicism and process into theory, research, and practice. In the mid 1990s, principles of postmodernism began to appear in the nursing literature.

Currently, a debate about the appropriate methods for developing nursing knowledge is being waged in the nursing literature. Some authors in support of qualitative methods maintain that "human behaviors cannot be isolated and quantified and that the attempt to do so results in misleading and dehumanizing outcomes rather than in knowledge that is useful for nursing practice" (Campbell & Bunting, 1991, p. 2). Others suggest that quantitative and qualitative methods can be used at different times to serve different purposes. Meleis advocates development of a

world view [Weltanschauung] that includes an integration of norms emanating from different theories of truth. It combines rigor and intuition, sensory data as they exist and as they appear, perceptions of the subject and of the theoretician, and logic with observable clinical data (1997, p. 87).

Such a synthesis of philosophical approaches would encourage various methods for development of nursing science.

The next section discusses patterns (ways) of knowing and methods for their use.

## ⊕ PATTERNS OF NURSING KNOWLEDGE

Chinn and Kramer (1999, pp. 1, 7) describe knowing as "ways of perceiving and understanding the self and the world . . . Nursing's patterns of knowing are interrelated and arise from the whole of experience."

Gender differences have been identified in the ways in which men and women may develop frameworks for the organization of knowledge. Perry (1970) identified four positions through which men make sense of their educational experiences:

1. Basic dualism: Authorities hand down the truth, and the learner is passive. Choices are perceived as either right or wrong, black or white, good or bad, we or they.
2. Multiplicity: The teacher may not have the right answer. A personal opinion is acceptable and may be valid.
3. Relative subordinate position: Evidence is sought for opinions. The emphasis is on analysis and evaluation of information.
4. Full relativism: Truth is relative. The meaning of knowledge depends on its context.

Perry suggested that the positions occurred in a linear sequence, with each position an advance over the previous.

In a study of women's perceptions, Belenky, Clinchy, Goldberger, and Tarule (1986) described five major categories used for the organization of knowledge:

1. Silence: The individual is subject to the whims of an external authority and perceives herself to be mindless and voiceless.
2. Received knowledge: External authority is all-knowing. The individual is capable of receiving and even reproducing knowledge, but not of creating it.
3. Subjective knowledge: Truth and knowledge are personal, private, and subjectively known or intuited.
4. Procedural knowledge: The individual is invested in learning and in applying objective procedures for obtaining and communicating knowledge.
5. Constructed knowledge: The individual experiences herself as a creator of knowledge. She views knowledge as contextual and values both objective and subjective strategies for knowing.

Additional study is needed to identify whether these categories develop sequentially.

Gender has been linked to the distribution of power and privilege in society (Marecek, 1995). Doering (1992, p. 26) states that knowledge reinforces and supports existing power relations that "subtly support male dominance and reinforce female submissiveness."

"When the male model is assumed to be the human model, women are viewed as the 'other,' deviant from the male norm or prototype" (p. 31). However, Doering continues, "since power is always exercised in relation to a resistance" (p. 31), ways of knowing (such as intuitive knowing, and contextual, phenomena-centered knowledge) that are not based on a male world view "may alter the balance of the nursing–medicine power relation" (p. 32).

Carper (1992, p. 73), in "an effort to understand the kinds of knowledge comprising the discipline of nursing," analyzed the nursing literature published between 1964 and 1975. Her results, which were published in a seminal 1978 article, identified four fundamental patterns, or ways, of knowing in nursing: empiricism, aesthetics, personal knowledge, and ethics. These ways of knowing have been extended by Chinn and Kramer (1999) and White (1995).

## Empirical Knowledge

The pattern of **empirical knowing** constitutes the science of nursing. It "encompasses publically verifiable, factual descriptions, explanations, and predictions based on subjective or objective group data" (Fawcett, Watson, Neuman, Walker, & Fitzpatrick, 2001, pp. 115–116). "Empirical data, obtained by either direct or indirect observation and measurement . . . are formulated as scientific principles, generalizations, laws, and theories that provide explanation and prediction" (Carper, 1992, p. 76) or enrich understanding through interpretation or description (White, 1995). **Empirical knowledge** is obtained through the senses, can be verified, is credible, and is used to impart understanding. Processes related to creating empiric knowledge include explaining and structuring (Chinn & Kramer, 1999).

## Aesthetic Knowledge

**Aesthetic knowing** in nursing "is that aspect of knowing that connects with deep meanings of a situation and calls forth inner creative resources that transform experience" (Chinn & Kramer, 1999, p. 183). This knowledge is not universal but is uniquely experienced and expressed and has subjective meaning. Aesthetic knowing involves the creative processes of rehearsing and envisioning (Chinn & Kramer).

"Art begins with the assumption of a common, generalizable human experience . . . and seeks expression of the infinite creative possibilities for experiencing or responding to the human experience" (Chinn, 1994, p. 30). Intuition, defined as "an immediate apprehension, or the power of gaining knowledge without evidence of rational thought" (Mitchell, 1994, p. 2), can be an important component of **aesthetic knowledge** in nursing practice.

Benner and Tanner (1987) discuss six aspects of intuitive judgment previously identified by Dreyfus and Dreyfus (1985). These aspects are not sequential but rather are used in combination by the practitioner.

1. Pattern recognition is the ability to recognize patterns and relationships without prior consideration of the separate components.
2. Similarity recognition is the ability to see similarities and parallels among patient situations, even when there are marked dissimilarities in objective features.

3. Common sense understanding is "a deep grasp of the culture and language, so that flexible understanding in diverse situations is possible. It is the basis for understanding the illness experience, in contrast to knowing the disease" (Benner & Tanner, 1987, p. 25). It is a way of "tuning in" to the patient and grasping the patient's experience.
4. Skilled know-how is based on a combination of knowledge and experience that permits flexibility of actions and judgment.
5. A sense of salience makes it possible to differentiate what is particularly significant in a situation.
6. Deliberative rationality involves the use of analysis and past experience to consider alternative interpretations of a clinical situation.

Carper emphasizes the importance of integrating aesthetic knowledge into the nursing process. The experience of helping and caring "must be perceived and designed as an integral component of its desired result rather than conceived separately as an independent action imposed on an independent subject" (Carper, 1978, p. 17). The result is a richness and appreciation of the practice of nursing as an art as well as a science.

## Personal Knowledge

**Personal knowledge** involves a "person's individualized and subjective ways of learning, storing, and retrieving information about the world" (Rew, 1996, p. 96). "The pattern of **personal knowing** refers to the quality and authenticity of the interpersonal process between each nurse and each [client]" (Fawcett et al., 2001, p. 116). Both the nurse and the client are considered to be "integrated, open system(s) incorporating movement toward growth and fulfillment of human potential" (Carper, 1978, p. 19). In the process of mutually establishing a nurse–client relationship, there must be efforts toward "receptive attending" (Moch, 1990, p. 155) and engagement, rather than detachment and a manipulative impersonal orientation. The result is an authentic knowing of an individual apart from the category of nurse or client. The creative processes of personal knowing include opening and centering (Chinn & Kramer, 1999).

Because personal knowing "concerns the inner experience of becoming a whole, aware, genuine self" (Chinn & Kramer, 1999, p. 5), the individual needs to accept ambiguity, vagueness, and discrepancies in what is essentially a subjective and existential process. There is no specific methodology that can be used consistently. The individual must be open to experience and intuitive feelings, be honest with self, and make efforts to acknowledge the responses of others. This is an ongoing process, because the self is constantly changing.

Belenky and colleagues state that

educators can help women develop their own authentic voices if they emphasize connection over separation, understanding and acceptance over assessment, and collaboration over debate; if they accord respect to and allow time for the knowledge that emerges from firsthand experience; if instead of imposing their own expectations and arbitrary requirements, they encourage students to evolve their own patterns of work based on the problems they are pursuing (1986, p. 229).

Moch (1990, pp. 156–159) describes three overlapping components of personal knowing:

1. Experiential knowing involves becoming aware through participation in which the knower learns through self-observation, by observing others, through feeling, and through sensing.
2. Interpersonal knowing is increased awareness through connectedness or interaction, which can involve intense attending, opening oneself to another, and conveying feelings to another.
3. Intuitive knowing involves the immediate knowing of something without the use of reason. The knower often describes this as a "hunch" or as a "feeling about something."

Moch believes that personal knowing can be viewed only from within a context of wholeness; includes a process of encountering, passion, commitment, and integrity; and entails a shift in connectedness at the conscious or unconscious level (1990, p. 159).

In identifying implications for research and knowledge development, Moch (1990, p. 162) suggests the following assumptions for capturing and transmitting personal knowing:

1. All perceptions are involved in data gathering.
2. The process of the experience may take precedence over the product.
3. The product of knowing is validated by the knower with both internal and external validation criteria.
4. No attempts are made to reproduce the process or the product because each situation is unique.

"The processing may consist of any combination of human and environmental interaction, rational intuiting, appraisal, active comprehension, and personal judgment" (Sweeney, 1994, p. 917).

## Ethical Knowledge

Ethics in nursing focuses on an obligation, or "what ought to be done" (Chinn & Kramer, 1999, p. 5). Sarvimaki (1995) describes four aspects that represent different ways of organizing and expressing moral knowledge. Theoretical/**ethical knowledge** "stands for an intellectual conception of what is good and right. It is organized into concepts and propositions that are formulated into judgments, rules, principles, and theories" (p. 344). Moral action knowledge means "having the skill necessary for performing the act as well as having good judgment. . . . Values and principles are manifested in action" (p. 345). Personal moral knowledge "refers to the way in which morality is organized in the person, that is, in his motives, inclinations, emotions and commitments" (p. 346). Situational knowledge "means being aware of the moral significance of the situation and being able to identify its morally significant traits" (p. 347).

Biomedical ethics are derived from models of patient good, rights-based notions of autonomy, or the social contract of medical practice (Fry, 1989). However, it has been argued (Fry, 1989; Sarvimaki, 1995; White, 1995) that nursing ethics should be based on an ethic of caring and must consider the nature of the nurse–client relationship. A caring orientation is based on the moral ideal of doing what is good, rather than that which is just. Mutuality, not autonomy, is foundational (White, 1995). "Creative processes of **ethical knowing** in nursing include clarifying and valuing" (Chinn & Kramer, 1999).

White (1995) proposes that a fifth way of knowing, sociopolitical knowing, needs to be added to the original patterns identified by Carper. "The pattern of sociopolitical knowing addresses the 'wherein'" (White, p. 83), a broader context that includes the context of nurse and client (including cultural identity), and the context of nursing as a practice profession. White (p. 85) states, "a sociopolitical understanding in which to frame all other patterns of knowing is an essential part of nursing's future in an increasingly economically driven world."

In addition, Munhall (1993) proposes "unknowing" as another pattern of knowing in nursing. She argues that the state of mind of unknowing is a condition of openness, and "a de-centering process from one's own organizing principles of the world" (p. 125). The intent is to "come to know the patient's world" (p. 126), and "lead to a much deeper knowledge of another being, of different meanings, and interpretations of all our various perceptions of experience" (p. 128).

Three different perspectives, each described as reflecting a different point of view (paradigm) of the way to develop nursing knowledge, have been identified (Newman, Sime, & Corcoran-Perry, 1991, p. 4):

1. Particulate–deterministic perspective: Phenomena are viewed as "isolatable, reducible entities having definable properties that can be measured." Knowledge includes facts and universal laws that can be used to predict and control change.
2. Interactive–integrative perspective: Phenomena are viewed as having multiple, interrelated parts. Reality is assumed to be multidimensional and contextual. Relationships may be reciprocal (rather than linear and causal), and knowledge may be context-dependent.
3. Unitary–transformative perspective: Each phenomenon is viewed as a unitary self-organizing field embedded in a larger self-organizing field. It is identified by pattern and by interaction with the larger whole. Change is unpredictable. Knowledge is personal and involves pattern recognition. Both the viewer and the phenomenon are involved in a process of "mutuality and creative unfolding."

Patterns as ways of knowing are not mutually exclusive; rather, they "are interrelated and arise from the whole of experience" (Chinn & Kramer, 1999, p. 7). Different ways of knowing are not judged against one another. Each of the ways of knowing and of creating knowledge are useful. Because each pattern adds only one specific component, none alone is a sufficient source of knowledge for **nursing science.** Comprehensive nursing knowledge must be based on an integration of all the ways of knowing. "Nursing depends on the specific knowledge of human behavior in health and in illness, the aesthetic perception of significant human experience, a personal understanding of the unique individuality of the self and the capacity to make choices within concrete situations involving particular judgments" (Carper, 1978, p. 22).

## ● THE DEVELOPMENT OF NURSING SCIENCE

Because of the complexity of the discipline of nursing and competing worldview perspectives (particular–deterministic, interactive–integrative and unitary–transformative), defining nursing science poses a challenge. However, attaining a clear definition of nursing science would provide a foundation for the profession's unique body of knowledge. Specialized branches of science develop knowledge and theories. First come the ideas and theories. Scientists then test the theories and depending upon the results, the ideas and theories are refined. Nursing contributes uniquely to health care delivery, but failure to articulate exact contributions may place the profession at risk.

## Concepts

For a discipline to have growth of knowledge, the **concepts**—highly abstract and general "word[s] or phrase[s] that summarize the essential characteristics or properties of a phenomenon" (Fawcett, 2000, p. 3)—that are important for the discipline must be identified, and there must be a shared acceptance of conceptual definitions. Four concepts have been commonly accepted as central to the discipline of nursing: the human being (who may be a nurse or client individual, a family, group, or community); the environment (which may be alive or inanimate); health (which may include well-being and illness); and nursing actions (which include all the interactions among nurse, client, and the environment in the pursuit of health).

In addition, there recently has been renewed interest in the concept of caring. Newman and colleagues even assert that "nursing is the study of caring in the human health experience" (1991, p. 3). However, others have expressed concern that "caring is relatively underdeveloped as a concept, has not been clearly explicated and often lacks relevance for nursing practice" (Morse, Bottorff, Neander, & Solberg, 1991, p. 119).

At least five conceptualizations of caring have been identified: a human trait, a moral imperative, an affect, an interpersonal interaction, and a therapeutic intervention (Morse et al., 1991). Caring seems to be part of content and relationship (Knowlden, 1991) and associated with varying outcomes, such as the client's physical response and the client's or the nurse's subjective experience (Morse et al., 1991).

At present, in the absence of consensus on definitions for these concepts, multiple definitions coexist (see Chapter 5, Nursing Models and Theories).

## Theories

**Theories** generally are introduced when scientists have studied a class of phenomena and have found a system of uniformities that can be expressed in the form of laws. A theory is a "creative and rigorous structuring of ideas that project a tentative, purposeful, and systematic view of phenomena" (Chinn & Kramer, 1999, p. 258). All theories include relationships among defined concepts, have a structure that gives them a systematic nature, and are tentative because they are based on assumptions, values, judgments, and empirical observations. Theories help nurses understand how and why the phenomena of nursing are associated with one another.

Higgins and Shirley have described two types of theory (2000, p. 179): explanatory theory "describes concepts and provides understanding of interactions among concepts"; and predictive theory "anticipates a particular set of outcomes."

Effectiveness in practice is directly related to the ability to understand, describe, explain, and anticipate human responses concerning health.

## Theoretical Frameworks

A theoretical or conceptual framework has been defined as "a logical grouping of related concepts or theories" (Chinn & Kramer, 1999, p. 258). A model is composed of abstract and general concepts and propositions that are linked together in a distinctive way. Fawcett states that a conceptual model "provides a unique focus that has a profound influence on individuals' perceptions" (2000, p. 16). Developing theoretical frameworks for nursing ensures practice that is effective in achieving the overall goal of the profession: improving quality of health.

## Models for Nursing

Several nurse scientists have proposed individual and distinctive models about the interrelationships of concepts that form the nature and processes of nursing. Each nurse scholar who has proposed a conceptual model has based the model on empirical observation, intuitive insights, or deductive reasoning "that creatively combine[s] ideas from several fields of inquiry" (Fawcett, 2000, p. 16). Although they may present diverse views of nursing phenomena, each conceptual model is useful for professional nursing because of the organization it provides for thinking, observing, and interpreting in nursing practice. Each provides principles from which guidelines for practice can be derived. See Chapter 5, for a discussion of selected conceptual models. **Nursing conceptual models** identify the interventions that nurses use in practice while explaining the **four central concepts of nursing**: human, environment, health, and nursing (Villarruel, Bishop, Simpson, Jemmott, & Fawcett, 2001).

## ⬥ SUMMARY AND SIGNIFICANCE TO PRACTICE

There is growing agreement on the central concepts of the discipline of nursing. The central concepts that could be used as parameters of the science of nursing are the client or consumer of nursing actions, the nurse and the accompanying nursing actions, the environment, and the processes of health of the consumer and the nurse.

The science of nursing evolves from these four components and their inseparable interrelationships. Indices for observing and understanding the phenomena and their interrelationships are emerging as the true scientific study of nursing evolves.

### FROM THEORY TO PRACTICE

1. How do I use the empirical, aesthetic, personal, and ethical ways of knowing in my professional practice? How do my attitudes about the ways of knowing affect my professional practice? Why are the ways of knowing important for professional nurses?
2. How has reading this chapter affected my views about nursing science and nursing theory?
3. What ideas would I use to debate Paul on his perception that nursing advancements should be based on "hard science" only? How do I think Paul would respond to each of my points? What are the consequences of having a narrowly defined perception of what constitutes nursing knowledge?

## REFERENCES

Belenky, M. F., Clinchy, B. M., Goldberger, N. R., & Tarule, J. M. (1986). *Women's ways of knowing: The development of self, voice and mind*. New York: Basic Books.

Benner, P., & Tanner, C. (1987). Clinical judgment: How expert nurses use intuition. *American Journal of Nursing, 87,* 23–31.

Bertalanffy, L. von. (1968). *General system theory*. New York: Braziller.

Campbell, J. C., & Bunting, S. (1991). Voices and paradigms: Perspectives on critical and feminist theory in nursing. *Advances in Nursing Science, 13,* 1–5.

Carper B. A. (1978). Fundamental patterns of knowing in nursing. *Advances in Nursing Science, 1,* 13–23.

Carper, B. A. (1992). Philosophical inquiry in nursing: An application. In J. F. Kikuchi & H. Simmons (Eds.). *Philosophic inquiry in nursing* (pp. 71–80). Newbury Park, CA: Sage.

Chinn, P. L. (1994). Developing a method for aesthetic knowing in nursing. In P. L. Chinn & J. Watson (Eds.). *Art and aesthetics in nursing* (pp. 19–40). New York: National League for Nursing.

Chinn, P. L., & Kramer, M. K. (1999). *Theory and nursing: Integrated knowledge development* (5th ed.). St. Louis: Mosby-Year Book.

Doering, L. (1992). Power and knowledge in nursing: A feminist poststructuralist view. *Advances in Nursing Science, 14,* 24–33.

Dreyfus, H., & Dreyfus, S. (1985). *Mind over machine: The power of human intuition and expertise in the era of the computer*. New York: Macmillan Free Press.

Fawcett, J. (2000). *Analysis and evaluation of contemporary nursing knowledge: Nursing models and theories*. Philadelphia: F. A. Davis.

Fawcett, J., Watson, J., Neuman, B., Walker, P. H., & Fitzpatrick, J. J. (2001). On nursing theories and evidence. *Journal of Nursing Scholarship, 33,* 115–119.

Fry, S. T. (1989). Toward a theory of nursing ethics. *Advances in Nursing Science, 11,* 9–22.

Heisenberg, W. (1971). *Physics and beyond*. New York: Harper & Row.

Higgins, P. A., & Shirley, M. M. (2000). Levels of theoretical thinking in nursing. *Nursing Outlook, 48,* 179–183.

Holmes, C. A., & Warelow, P. J. (2000). Some implications of postmodernism for nursing theory, research, and practice. *Canadian Journal of Nursing Research, 32,* 89–101.

Knowlden, V. (1991). Nurse caring as constructed knowledge. In R. M. Neil & R. Watts (Eds.), *Caring and nursing: Explorations in feminist perspectives* (pp. 201–208). New York: National League for Nursing.

Marecek, J. (1995). Gender, politics, and psychology's ways of knowing. *American Psychologist, 50,* 162–163.

Meleis, A. (1997). *Theoretical nursing: Development and progress* (3rd ed.). Philadelphia: Lippincott.

Mitchell, G. J. (1994). Intuitive knowing: Exposing a myth in theory development. *Nursing Science Quarterly, 7,* 2–3.

Moch, S. D. (1990). Personal knowing: Evolving research and practice. *Scholarly Inquiry for Nursing Practice, 4,* 155–170.

Morse, J. M., Bottorff, J., Neander, W., & Solberg, S. (1991). Comparative analysis of conceptualizations and theories of caring. *Image, 23,* 119–126.

Munhall, P. L. (1993). 'Unknowing': Toward another pattern of knowing in nursing. *Nursing Outlook, 41,* 125–128.

Newman, M. A., Sime, A. M., & Corcoran-Perry, S. A. (1991). The focus of the discipline of nursing. *Advances in Nursing Science, 14,* 1–6.

Perry, W. G. (1970). Forms of intellectual and ethical development in the college years. New York: Holt, Rinehart and Winston.

Reed, P. G. (1995). A treatise on nursing knowledge development for the 21st century: Beyond postmodernism. *Advances in Nursing Science, 17,* 70–84.

Rew, L. (1996). *Awareness in healing*. Albany, NY: Delmar.

Rogers, M. E. (1970). *An introduction to the theoretical basis of nursing*. Philadelphia: F. A. Davis.

Rogers, M. E. (1992). Nursing science and the space age. *Nursing Science Quarterly, 5,* 27–34.

Sarvimaki, A. (1995). Aspects of moral knowledge in nursing. *Scholarly Inquiry for Nursing Practice, 9,* 343–358.

Spradlin, W. W., & Porterfield, P. B. (1984). *The search for certainty*. New York: Springer-Verlag.

Stumpf, S. E. (1993). *Socrates to Sartre: A history of philosophy* (5th ed.). New York: McGraw-Hill.

Sweeney, N. M. (1994). A concept analysis of personal knowledge: Application to nursing education. *Journal of Advanced Nursing, 20,* 917–924.

Villarruel, A. M., Bishop, T. L., Simpson, E. M., Jemmott, L. S., & Fawcett, J. (2001). Borrowed theories, shared theories, and the advancement of nursing knowledge. *Nursing Science Quarterly, 14,* 158–163.

Ware, C. F., Panikaar, K. M., & Romein, J. M. (1966). *History of mankind, cultural and scientific development: Vol. 6. The twentieth century.* New York: Harper & Row.

White, J. (1995). Patterns of knowing: Review, critique, and update. *Advances in Nursing Science, 17,* 73–86.

# Nursing Models and Theories

## KEY TERMS AND CONCEPTS

Metaparadigm

Conceptual Model

Nursing Models

Theory

Stability Model of Change

Systems Theory

King's Systems Interaction Model (Theory of Goal Attainment)

Neuman's Health Care Systems Model

Roy Adaptation Model

Growth Model of Change

Caring

Orem's Self-Care Deficit Theory

Watson's Human Science and Human Care Theory

Complexity Theory

Rogers' Science of Unitary Human Beings

Parse's Human Becoming Theory

Newman's Theory of Health as Expanding Consciousness

Leddy's Human Energy Model

## LEARNING OUTCOMES

By the end of this chapter, the learner will be able to:

1. Compare and contrast systems, adaptation, caring, and complexity theories.

2. Outline differences in how nursing's meta-paradigm concepts are defined in each of the nursing models presented.

3. Explain the key differences among rote, stereotypical, and theoretically based nursing practice.

4. Identify assumptions in the various nursing models presented in the chapter.

5. Determine the strengths and weaknesses of current nursing models/theories.

6. Apply each of the presented nursing models/theories to a clinical practice situation.

Nancy and Ann are two nurses working the night shift. Tonight, Ms. Green uses the call light every 5 minutes because she cannot sleep. Her nurse, Nancy, asks Ann for help because Ann always seems to know just what to do. After Ann spends 5 minutes with Ms. Green, she goes to sleep. Nancy asks "How do you always know what to do to help the restless patients?" Ann shares her knowledge about Parse's Human Becoming Theory emphasizing being truly present with clients. Ann also summarizes key concepts and approaches presented by other nursing theorists that she learned in her undergraduate nursing program. Ann mentions that although she prefers to use Parse's model, she finds that other nursing models help in different client care situations.

 ## MODELS AND THEORIES FOR PROFESSIONAL NURSING

The discipline of nursing is highly complex. Over the years, most nursing scholars have adopted the following four key concepts to serve as a **metaparadigm**: person (the recipient of nursing care), environment (physical and social), health (a process or state), and nursing (goals, roles, and functions) (Fawcett, 2000). The term *metaparadigm* comes from the Greek prefix "meta," which means more comprehensive or transcending, and the word Greek word "paradigm," which means a philosophical or theoretical framework of a discipline upon which all theories, laws, and generalizations are formulated (*Merriam-Webster's Collegiate Dictionary*, 1994). All existing nursing models and theories address these four concepts. Although nursing models and theories vary according to philosophical world views, all flow from the metaparadigm of nursing.

## NURSING MODELS

Before 1950, the writings of Florence Nightingale served as the primary source of nursing theory and nursing science was derived principally from social, biologic, and medical science theories. Nursing science started to emerge as part of the profession in the 1950s and continues to flourish as nursing theorists develop and refine models of nursing. Some nursing theories and models arose when nurses tried to generate a clear, concise definition of nursing.

A model, as an abstraction of reality, provides a way to visualize reality to simplify thinking. For example, a spaceship model provides a representation of a spaceship. A **conceptual model** gives structure to and shows how various concepts are interrelated. Conceptual models serve as a foundation for theory development or can also apply theories to predict or evaluate consequences of alternative actions. According to Fawcett (2000), a conceptual model "gives direction to the search for relevant questions about the phenomena of central interest to a discipline and suggests solutions to practical problems" (Fawcett, p. 16). **Nursing models** tend to be more abstract than nursing theory.

## Nursing Theory

Chinn and Kramer (1999) define **theory** as "a creative and rigorous structuring of ideas that projects a tentative, purposeful, and systematic view of phenomena" (p. 83). Professional nurses apply concepts, principles, and theories from many disciplines. For example, nurses use physics when placing cardiac monitor electrodes on client chests, pharmacology when monitoring clients receiving medications, psychology when providing emotional support, microbiology when using asepsis, family theory when assessing effective mother–infant bonding, and human development theory when caring for clients of all ages. However, these borrowed theories and principles fail to capture the essence of professional nursing. Theories create a different way of looking at a particular phenomenon by interrelating concepts in a logical manner and provide a framework for describing, explaining, and predicting practice. They also provide a relatively simple, yet generalizable view for testable hypothesis development. Once validated through research, theories expand discipline-specific knowledge while identifying other questions for future investigation.

Many nurses base their practice on intuition, experience, or "how I learned it in nursing school." These methods lead to rote and stereotypical practice. Nurses rely on memorization and habit when engaging in rote practice. Rote practice enables nurses to provide care while in an "autopilot" or robotic mode. When nurses use long-standing traditions and incorporate the expectations of others in practice, they engage in stereotypical practice. In the stereotypical practice mode, nurses try to fulfill expectations others may have of them such as blindly following physician orders or willingly assuming the role of the self-sacrificing angel of mercy.

However, practice based on models or theories allows for hypotheses about practice, which make it possible to derive a rationale for nursing actions. When using a specific nursing model or theory, nurses use key concepts and relationships to direct client assessments and interventions. Testable theories provide a knowledge base for the science of nursing. As the science of nursing develops, nurses will be able to more accurately understand and explain events, and to provide a basis for predicting and controlling future events. In addition, practice based on science fosters the recognition of nursing as a professional discipline. Looking at philosophical differences helps to explain why nursing models and theories vary in approaches to professional practice.

### Questions for Reflection 5-1

1. How do I rely on traditions and personal experience when I practice nursing?
2. What consequences have resulted when I used traditions to guide my nursing practice?
3. What is my personal attitude toward nursing models and theories? Why do I feel this way about them?

## Categories of Nursing Models and Theories

Because many nursing conceptual models and theories exist today, this chapter presents nine models that are commonly used. To distinguish differences among them, the models and theories have been classified according to the following criteria:

1. The world view of change reflected by the model (growth or stability).
2. The major theoretical/conceptual classification with which the model seems most consistent (systems, stress/adaptation, caring, or growth/development).

Providing a structure for grouping the models and theories should provide the reader with a basis for understanding conceptual similarities and differences.

Many nurses fail to appreciate nursing models and theories. By revealing the essence of each model or theory, from original sources as much as possible, the chapter aims to provide concise summaries so that the reader can appreciate similarities and differences among them and identify points of congruence with the world views on which the model/theory is based. Some nurse theorists coin words, define family words in different ways, and develop new concepts. This chapter aims to clarify the models, rather than critique them or to select a single best model or theory for use. The selection of a nursing model or theory to guide practice is an individual decision. Interpretations of the professional nursing processes based on theses models will be presented in Chapter 6, "Professional Nursing Processes."

## Growth and Stability Models of Change

Two basic philosophical world views exist about the nature of change. Change remains constant; however, perceptions of change differ among people. In 1989, Fawcett presented world views according to perceptions of change. One world view recognizes change as continuous, a desired opportunity for growth to attain maximum human potential. The other world view is persistence, which maintains that persons strive for stability and that endurance results from ". . . a synthesis of growth and stability" (p. 12). The persistence world view focuses on continuing and maintaining patterns by emphasizing balance and equilibrium. Although the world views differ, they are not mutually exclusive. However, the selected nursing models in this chapter approach change differently and provides a means to classify them.

## ⬥ THE STABILITY MODEL OF CHANGE

The **stability model of change** proposes that the natural order of things revolves around consistency. Although change is inevitable and may be undesirable, it forces adaptation. Stability means that the organism attains a new and stable equilibrium.

### Questions for Reflection 5-2

1. Which world view seems more compatible with my personal philosophy, the change or persistence world view?
2. Why is this world view more compatible with my philosophy?
3. Is it possible to embrace both world views? Why or why not?

## Systems Theory

**Systems theory** is concerned with elements and interactions among all the factors (variables) in a situation. Interactions between the person and the environment occur continuously, thereby creating a complex, constantly changing situation. Systems theory provides a way to understand the many influences on the whole person and the possible impact of change of any part on the whole. This theory can help nurses to understand, predict, and control the possible effects of nursing care on the client system and the concurrent effects of the interaction on the nurse system and environment.

Auger (1976) defines a system as "a whole with interrelated parts, in which the parts have a function and the system as a totality has a function" (p. 21). Within the systems framework, single systems (subsystems) form more complex systems (suprasystems). Subsystems may be smaller than the tiniest cell of an organism. Suprasystems extend beyond what humans know as the universe.

A person is composed of cells, organs, and physiologic systems—the subsystems of humans. These subsystems are continuously interacting and changing. As a person eats, the blood supply to the gastrointestinal organs increases. Absorption of carbohydrates increases the blood glucose level, which results in increased insulin secretion. Simultaneously, changes in the blood circulation and blood glucose level affect the attention level and the feeling of hunger. The person may feel satisfied and contented.

The whole person is the suprasystem for multiple interacting subsystems. The person's internal environment consists of interacting subsystems that are contained within bodily boundaries.

The person holds membership in a subsystem called family (which is a suprasystem of the person), which is a subsystem of the community system, and so on. Subsystems may be isolated for study, but human beings are more than and different from the sum of their parts (Rogers, 1970). Thus, a person cannot be characterized by describing physiologic, psychological, and sociocultural subsystems. A person's behavior is holistic; a reflection of the person as a whole. The focus of systems theory is on understanding the interaction among the various parts of the system, rather than on describing the function of the parts themselves (Auger, 1976).

As open systems, persons exchange matter, energy, and information across their boundaries with the environment (Sills & Hall, 1977). A person's internal environment interacts constantly with an ever-changing external environment. Changes occurring in one affect the other. For example, walking into a cold room (change in the external environment) affects various physiologic and psychological subsystems of the internal environment, which in turn reduces blood flow to the periphery, the ability to concentrate, and the feeling of comfort. Similarly, a person's angry outburst (change in the internal environment) may have a demonstrable effect on the moods of others. This openness of human systems makes nursing intervention possible. Under general systems theory, nurses interact with clients to help them attain homeostasis defined as the constancy of the internal environment caused by action of regulatory mechanisms. Constancy does not mean that the internal environment is static, but rather constantly changing. This relative equilibrium is maintained by homeodynamics (Cannon, 1932).

Systems analysis assumes that structure and stability can be measured during an arbitrarily frozen period. The system seeks equilibrium, or a steady state, in which a balance exists among the various forces operating within and on the system. Factors from the environment impinge on the system across the system boundary. These factors cause tension, stress, strain, or conflict that may upset system balance. Change is a process of tension reduction and dynamic equilibrium, which restores a new position of system balance after a disturbance (Chin, 1976).

Energy, information, or matter provide system input. The system "transforms, creates, and organizes input in the process known as throughput, which results in a reorganization of the input" (Sills & Hall, 1977, p. 21). Thus, each system modifies its input. Simultaneously, energy, information, or matter is given off into the environment as output. When output is returned to the system as input, the process is known as feedback.

For example, information about a therapeutic diet given to the client by the nurse is system input for the client system. What the client eats would be one type of system output, based on the throughput related to assimilation and acceptance of the information originally given. The nurse, using the client's reported food intake as feedback, can help reinforce or modify the client's future behavior (Figure 5-1).

A person can be viewed as "an interrelated, interdependent, interacting, complex organism, constantly influencing and being influenced by [the] environment" (Sills & Hall, 1977, p. 24). Because the person is in constant interaction with the environment, many interrelated factors, including the nurse, affect the person's health status. The person's response, in turn, results in environmental change. Because of these interactions, a change in any part affects the whole human–environment system.

Using systems theory to guide nursing process directs assessment of the relationships among all variables that affect the client–environment interaction, including the influence of the nurse. While intervening, the nurse must anticipate the system-wide impact from change in any part of the system and appreciate the simultaneous, rather than cause-and-effect, nature of change in open systems.

Systems theory provides one approach for nursing practice. Imogene King and Betty Neuman developed nursing models based on systems theory and are described subsequently.

### Imogene King's Systems Interaction Model (Theory of Goal Attainment)

Imogene King stresses interactions and mutuality in her nursing model known as **King's Systems Interaction Model (Theory of Goal Attainment).** King developed her model when she was trying to outline essential content for a new graduate nursing program (Fawcett, 2001). According to Imogene King's systems interaction model, the purpose of nursing is to help people attain, maintain, or restore health, primarily by mutual goal setting. King describes the nurse–patient interaction as *transaction,* which means the following: Nurse–patient mutual understanding of events, mutually set goals, and agreement on means to achieve the goal.

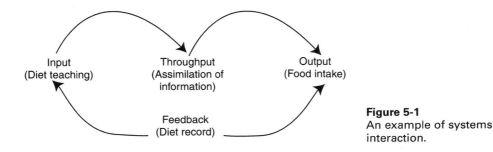

Input
(Diet teaching)

Throughput
(Assimilation of
information)

Output
(Food intake)

Feedback
(Diet record)

**Figure 5-1**
An example of systems interaction.

King's model has its roots in sociology and focuses on "individuals whose interactions in groups within social systems influence behavior within the systems" (King, 1989, p. 152). King defines humans as "open systems interacting with environment" (King, 1981, p. 10) and as "rational, sentient, reacting, social, controlling, purposeful, time-oriented, and action-oriented" (King, 1987, p. 107). The human "perceives the world as a total person" (King, 1981, p. 141) resulting in environmental interactions to which he or she must constantly adjust. King delineates the environment as internal (within the body/person) and external (King, 1981). King proposes that the personal system underlies each person as a whole system who interacts with one or more persons thereby creating interpersonal systems. When interpersonal systems expand to include large groups of persons, social systems are developed. King emphasized that the three systems interact with the other and "represent organized wholes in constant interaction in one's environment" (King, 1999, p. 292). As humans interact with their environment, their perceptions influence their behavior and health. Nurses interact with clients to facilitate achievement of mutually determined health-related goals.

Perception is the comprehensive concept in personal systems. It is "a characteristic of a human process of interaction, and along with communication provides a channel for passage of information from one person to another" (King, 1989, p. 153). Concepts of self, growth and development, learning, body image, time, and space also relate to individuals as personal systems.

Interaction is the comprehensive concept in interpersonal systems. Related concepts include communication, transactions, roles, stress, and all the concepts identified in personal systems. Organization is the comprehensive concept in social systems, with related concepts of power, authority, status, decision making, and control (King, 1989).

Health assumes achievement of maximum potential for daily living and an ability to function in social roles. It is the "dynamic life experiences of a human being, which implies continuous adjustment to stressors in the internal and external environment through optimum use of one's resources to achieve maximum potential for daily living" (King, 1981, p. 5). "Illness is a deviation from normal, that is, an imbalance in a person's biological structure or in his psychological makeup, or a conflict in a person's social relationships" (King, 1989, p. 5).

"The goal of nursing is to help individuals and groups attain, maintain, and restore health" (King, 1981, p. 13). "Nursing's domain involves human beings, families, and communities as a framework within which nurses make transactions in multiple environments with health as a goal" (King, 1996, p. 61). Nursing care is accomplished within goal-oriented nurse–client interactions "whereby each perceives the other and the situation, and through communications, they set goals, explore the means to achieve them, agree to the means, and their actions indicate movement toward goal achievement" (King, 1987, p. 113). The emphasis of health-related goal attainment provides the name of theory of goal attainment.

King, (1987) identifies the following ten relevant concepts to understand the dynamic interacting systems delineated in her model:

1. Interaction: "a process of perception and communication between person and environment and between person and person, represented by verbal and nonverbal behaviors that are goal-directed."
2. Perception: "each person's representation of reality."
3. Communication: "a process whereby information is given from one person to another."

4. Transaction: "an observable behavior of human beings interacting with their environment . . . [in which] valuation is a component of human interaction."
5. Role: "a set of behaviors expected of persons occupying a position in a social system."
6. Stress: "a dynamic state whereby a human being interacts with the environment to maintain balance for growth, development, and performance."
7. Growth and development: "continuous change in individuals at the cellular, molecular, and behavioral levels of activities."
8. Time: "a continuous flow of events in successive order that implies change, a past, and a future."
9. Self: "a personal system defined as a unified, complex whole."
10. Space: "existing in all direction and the same everywhere" (pp. 109–110).

King has proposed the theory of goal attainment in which these concepts are interrelated in a number of propositions and hypotheses that indicate the nature of nurse–client interactions that lead to goal attainment" (King, 1995, p. 27). Decision making is "a shared collaborative process in which client and nurse give information to each other, identify goals, and explore means to attain goals; each moves forward to attain goals. This is identified in the theory as a critical independent variable called mutual goal setting" (King, 1989, p. 155). From the theory, a transaction process model has been designed to lead to goal attainment when practiced (King, 1999). Examples of testable hypotheses generated from King's theory include the following: the process of mutual goal setting with clients, strengths of mutual goal setting, and role conflict between client and nurse in nursing situations (King, 1987).

King's model and the theory of goal attainment provide a "theoretical base for applying the traditional nursing process . . . aimed at maintaining or restoring health" (Magan, 1987, pp. 129, 132). King's model has provided theoretical foundation for international nursing practice, nursing departments, nurse empowerment and client satisfaction (Fawcett, 2001). A recent computerized literature search using the Cumulative Index of Nursing and Allied Health Literature reveals that over 80 research articles have been published that use King's model. Published studies using King's model have been performed internationally and includes the areas of client decision-making processes and effectiveness of client education. Besides research, King's model serves as a foundation for undergraduate and graduate nursing programs and nursing service departments (Fawcett, 2002). The King International Nursing Group formed in 1998 and publishes an annual newsletter. Table 5-1 presents the major concepts of this model.

## Betty Neuman's Health Care Systems Model

Betty Neuman also uses systems theory to provide a foundation for her nursing model known as **Neuman's Health Care Systems Model.** She developed her model while she attempted to help nursing students organize their thinking and look at clients holistically (Neuman, 2002). The Neuman's health care systems model specifies that the purpose of nursing is to facilitate optimal client system stability by reducing the impact of environmental stimuli or stressors.

Neuman describes the person as having a core that is protected by buffering systems. The following four key concepts describe interaction of the person with the environmental stressors that determine health status.

**TABLE 5-1**

## Major Concepts as Defined in King's Model

| Person (human being) | A personal system that interacts with interpersonal and social systems |
| --- | --- |
| Environment | A context "within which human beings grow, develop, and perform daily activities" (King, 1981, p. 18) |
| Health | "dynamic life experiences of a human being, which implies continuous adjustment to stressors in the internal and external environment through optimum use of one's resources to achieve maximum potential for daily living" (King, 1981, p. 5) |
| Nursing | A process of human interaction |

1. Central core: the basic structure and energy reserves of the human that make life possible.
2. Flexible lines of defense: adaptive responses that fluctuate and protect the core from stressor penetration.
3. Normal line of defense: a conscious adaptation response usually used by an individual to protect the core from stressor penetration.
4. Lines of resistance: protection factors activated when stressors have penetrated the normal line of defense that are usually unconscious in nature.

Neuman's model focuses on stress reduction and addresses how stress and individual response to it affects the development, maintenance, and restoration of health. The person is a composite of physiologic, psychological, sociocultural, developmental, and spiritual variables that act harmoniously and simultaneously when encountering stressors from either the internal or external environments. Neuman defines clients as individuals, families, groups, or communities who interact constantly with the environment.

The environment includes "all internal and external factors or influences surrounding the identified client or client system" (Neuman, 2002, p. 18). The internal environment is composed of interacting elements within the human body. The external environment consists of anything outside of the human body. The created environment encompasses individual perceptions of the internal and external environments.

A person constantly encounters stressors from the internal, external, or created environment. Stressors are tension-producing stimuli that have the potential to disturb a person's equilibrium or normal line of defense. This normal line of defense is the person's "usual steady state." It is the way in which an individual usually deals with stressors. Stressors may be positive (eustress) or negative (distress). Stressors may be of three types: intrapersonal (arising from within the person), interpersonal (arising between two or more persons), or extrapersonal (arising from the external environment rather than other persons).

According to Neuman (1982, 2002), the basic structure and energy resources of humans need protection from encountered stressors. Reactions and resistance to stressors are provided by lines of defenses. Neuman calls the outermost line of defense the flexible lines of defense. This dynamic protective buffer consists of physiologic, psychological, sociocultural, developmental, and spiritual variables affecting a person at any given moment. These variables may include a person's current physiologic state, mood, beliefs, cognitive state, nutritional status, spiritual beliefs, developmental state, and cognitive ability. If the flexible line of defense is no longer able to protect the person against a stressor, the normal lines of defense work to buffer the effects produced. The normal lines of defense encompass the usual response used by the person. Examples of normal lines of defense include exercise regimens, health habits (such as basic hygiene), typical methods of relaxation, and conscious coping methods. The final protections for the core are the lines of resistance. Examples of lines of resistance include immunologic responses and unconscious emotional defense mechanisms. Obvious reactions to stress become visible when lines of resistance are penetrated. The reaction to stressors may lead to restoration of balance or to death. Three factors influence the person's reaction and recovery to encountered stressors: the number and strength of the stressors affecting the person, the length of exposure to the stressor(s), and the meaningfulness of the stressor(s) to the person.

Neuman intends for the nurse to "assist clients to retain, attain, or maintain optimal system stability" (Neuman, 1996, p. 69). Thus, health (wellness) seems to be related to dynamic equilibrium of the normal line of defense, where stressors are successfully overcome or avoided by the flexible line of defense. Neuman defines illness as "a state of insufficiency with disrupting needs unsatisfied" (Neuman, 2002, p. 25). Illness appears to be a separate state when a stressor breaks through the normal line of defense and causes a reaction with the person's lines of resistance.

Nurses use primary, secondary, or tertiary prevention to help clients attain optimal wellness. Primary prevention covers interventions to promote health. Secondary prevention occurs once a stressor has penetrated the normal lines of defense or lines of resistance (e.g., pain medication). Tertiary prevention focuses on restoration of balance (e.g., rehabilitation). When restoration is complete, nursing interventions return to primary prevention.

The Neuman systems model has compatibility with the traditional medical model. Over 300 research articles using the Neuman systems model have been published, including research conducted by nurses in the Pacific Rim and Europe. The model serves as the framework for the World Health Organization project "Nest of Love" and for delivery of mental health services in Holland (Fawcett, 2004). The Neuman Trustee Group promotes utilization of the Neuman systems model. Table 5-2 summarizes major concepts as defined in Neuman's model.

**TABLE 5-2**

## Major Concepts as Defined in Neuman's Model

| | |
|---|---|
| Person (client system) | A composite of physiological, psychological, sociocultural, developmental, and spiritual variables in interaction with the internal and external environment |
| Environment | All internal and external factors of influences surrounding the client system |
| Health | A continuum of wellness to illness |
| Nursing | Prevention as intervention |

## Stress/Adaptation Theory as a Framework

In contrast to systems theory, stress and adaptation theories view change in terms of accommodation. People adjust to environmental changes to avoid disturbing a balanced existence. Adaptation theory provides a way to understand both how the balance is maintained and the possible effects of disturbed equilibrium. This theory has been widely applied to explain, predict, and control biologic (physiologic and psychological) responses of persons and serves as traditional medical therapy.

The regulatory systems operate by way of compensation. Any change in the internal environment automatically initiates a response to minimize or counteract the change. For example, when the blood glucose level drops, the endocrine system responds with increased cortisol secretion, which decreases the rate at which cells use glucose and stimulates the conversion of amino acids into glucose. These compensatory actions cause the blood glucose level to increase. If it should increase above acceptable limits, insulin secretion would increase the rate of glucose uptake by cells, tending to reduce the blood glucose level.

Compensation occurs constantly as the body adjusts to stimuli that tend to disturb equilibrium. Stimuli may be anything that creates change in the internal environment and thus places demands on the body to compensate. Examples of stimuli include changes in external environmental temperature or sleep pattern, hunger, joy, and infection. Stimuli, either beneficial or harmful, all require the body to adapt.

A person's ability to adapt to changes in life events may determine the potential for health or disease. One way that a person adapts is through coping mechanisms that aim "to master conditions of harm, threat, or challenge when a routine or automatic response is not readily available" (Monat & Lazarus, 1977, p. 8). Some regard coping methods primarily as psychological barriers when stimuli are perceived as threats. Thus, a person's reaction to stimuli involves cognitive appraisal and psychological coping methods, in addition to physiologic reactions. One of the best-known nursing models that use adaptation theory is the model developed by Sister Callista Roy.

### Callista Roy's Adaptation Model

Roy developed the adaptation model when confronted with the challenge of defining nursing as a graduate nursing student (Fawcett, 2002). The **Roy Adaptation Model** outlines the purpose of nursing as promoting a person's adaptation, the process and outcome by which thinking and feeling persons use conscious awareness and choice to create human and environmental integration. Roy uses the following five key terms in her model:

1. Stimulus: point of interaction of the human system and environment. Stimulus produces a response.
2. Adaptive modes: ways that a person adapts (e.g., through physiologic needs self-concept, role function, or interdependent relations).
3. Classes of stimuli: focal (immediately confronting the person), contextual (all other stimuli present), and residual (nonspecific stimuli, such as beliefs or attitudes).
4. Adaptation level: range of a person's ability to adapt and create changes in the integrated, compensatory, and compromised environments.
5. Coping: ways of responding to the changing environment.

Roy organizes her model around adaptive behaviors that encompass the set of processes by which a person adapts to environmental stimuli. The person as a unified system is viewed as a "set of parts connected to function as a whole" (Roy & Andrews, 1999, p. 36) through homeostatic and homeodynamic systems. The person constantly interacts with an ever-changing environment. The person's ability to respond positively reflects the level of adaptation.

Environmental stimuli affect the person. A focal stimulus is an environmental change that requires an immediate adaptive response from the person. Accompanying the focal stimulus are contextual (all other stimuli present) and residual stimuli (other relevant factors such as nonspecific stimuli), which mediate and contribute to the effect of the focal stimulus.

The pooled effect of the three classes of stimuli establishes the person's adaptation level. The person's adaptation level determines a zone that indicates the range of additional stimulation that will have a positive or adaptive response. If additional stimuli fall outside of the zone, the person cannot respond effectively and compromised adaptation ensues. Effective adaptation results in free energy available for use in subsequent adaptation to stimuli.

According to Roy and Roberts (1981, p. 56), "Coping refers to routine, accustomed patterns of behaviors to deal with daily situations as well as to the production of new ways of behaving when drastic changes defy the familiar responses." The two major coping mechanisms for individuals are the regulator subsystem, comprised mainly of automatic neural, endocrine, and chemical activity, and the cognator subsystem, which includes cognitive–emotive channels and provides for perceptual/information processing, learning, judgment, and emotion (Andrews & Roy, 1986, p. 7).

In 1997, Roy redefined adaptation as the "process and outcome whereby the thinking and feeling person uses conscious awareness and choice to create human and environmental integration" (p. 44). Roy identified four adaptive modes: physiologic–physical, self-concept–group identity, role function, and interdependence. The desired result is a state in which conditions promote the person's goals, including survival, growth, reproduction, mastery, and person and environment transformations.

Health "is viewed in light of human goals and the purposefulness of human existence. The fulfillment of this purpose in life is reflected in becoming integrated and whole" (Roy & Andrews, 1999, p. 54). Thus, health is viewed as both "a state and a process of being and becoming an integrated and whole human being" (p. 54).

The goal of nursing is "to promote adaptation by the use of the nursing process, in each of the adaptive modes, thus contributing to health, quality of life, and dying with dignity" (Roy, 1987, p. 43). Nursing assessment and intervention fosters the goal of adaptation with the client actively participating in the processes. The criteria for goal attainment encompasses generally any positive response by the person that creates free energy that can be used for responding to other stimuli (Riehl & Roy, 1980). The goal of adaptation is fostered through nursing assessment and intervention, with the client as an active participant.

Roy's model provides a classification system for stimuli that may affect adaptation, as well as a system for classifying nursing assessment. The model "has been useful in supporting the traditional concept of nursing practice within the medical model perspective" (Huch, 1987, p. 63). Frederickson (2000) found more than 200 quantitative studies based on the Roy Adaptation Model. According to a literature search done in

TABLE 5-3

## Major Concepts as Defined in Roy's Model

| | |
|---|---|
| Person (human system) | "a whole with parts that function as a unity" (Roy & Andrews, 1999, p. 31) |
| Environment | "the world within and around humans as adaptive systems" (Roy & Andrews, 1999, p. 51) |
| Health | "a state and process of being and becoming an integrated and whole human being" (Roy & Andrews, 1999, p. 54) |
| Nursing | Manipulation of stimuli to foster successful adaptation |

2004, 617 articles have been published, about half of them research articles using Roy's model as a theoretical framework, some in Spanish and Japanese. The Roy Adaptive Association based in Boston offers support to nurses conducting research using the model. Nurses use Roy's model as a framework for nursing education in baccalaureate and higher degree programs, as a foundation for health assessment in clinical practice, and as guidance for application in nursing service departments. Roy also advocates the use of the model by other health care professionals (Fawcett, 2002; 2003). Table 5-3 summarized the major concepts as defined in Roy's model.

## ● THE GROWTH MODEL OF CHANGE

Unlike the previous models, which focus on achievement or restoration of stability, nursing models based on the **growth model of change** tend to focus on helping persons grow to realize and attain their full human potential. The models of nursing that espouse the growth change model tend to use caring theory or complexity theory as an underlying framework.

### Caring Theory as a Framework

Nursing practice focuses on caring for and about others. No single, universally accepted definition exists for caring in the nursing context as it can be used as a verb or noun (The nurse cared for the client. Nursing care was given.). Morse, Solberg, Neander, Bottorff, and Johnson (1990, p. 2) point out that the literature includes references to care or **caring** as actions performed (as in to take care of), as well as concern demonstrated (as in caring about). An analysis of the literature reveals at least five perspectives or categories of caring, including caring as a human trait (Benner & Wrubel, 1989; Gaut & Leininger, 1991), caring as a moral imperative (Watson, 1985, 1999), caring as an interpersonal relationship (Parse, 1987), caring as a therapeutic intervention (Orem, 1980), and caring as an affect (Morse et al., 1990).

Clients perceive as caring "those nursing ministrations that are person-centered, protective, anticipatory, physically comforting, and that go beyond routine care" (Swanson, 1991, p. 161). Kyle (1995, p. 509) concludes that there is a "marked difference between the patients' perceptions of caring and those of nurses, with the nurses focusing on the psychosocial skills and the patient on those skills which demonstrate professional competency." Caring outcomes may be demonstrated in terms of either subjective experiences or objective client outcomes.

Several classifications of the components of caring have been published. Swanson (1991, p. 162) defines caring as "a nurturing way of relating to a valued other toward whom one feels a personal sense of commitment and responsibility." She identifies the five caring processes:

1. Knowing: striving to understand an event as it has meaning in the life of another.
2. Being with: being emotionally present for the other.
3. Doing for: doing for the other as he would do for himself if it were possible.
4. Enabling: facilitating the other's passage through life transitions and unfamiliar events.
5. Maintaining belief: sustaining faith in the other's capacity to get through an event or transition and face a future with meaning.

Koldjeski (1990) also describes the five "essences" of caring as:

1. Interpersonal valuing and involvement.
2. Being there for and experiencing with the other.
3. Instilling faith.
4. Concern and love for the other.
5. Actualization.

Table 5-4 compares Swanson's and Koldjeski's theoretical components of caring.

**TABLE 5-4**

### A Comparison of Components of Caring

| Swanson | Koldjeski |
|---|---|
| Knowing | Interpersonal involvement |
| Being with | Experiencing with concern and love |
| Doing for | Nursing actions |
| Enabling | Actualization |
| Maintaining belief | Instillment of faith |

### Questions for Reflection 5-3

1. What are the characteristics that I identify when I have been the recipient of a caring interaction?
2. What results from a caring interaction between two persons?
3. Why is caring an important aspect of professional nursing?

The concept of caring permeates the nursing literature and appears in many nursing models. **Orem's Self-care Deficit Theory** uses the term "care" primarily as action; whereas Watson uses the term to describe an attitude or display of compassion that is a moral imperative for nurses.

### Dorothea Orem's Self-care Deficit Theory

Orem proposes that the purpose of nursing is to help people meet their self-care needs. She suggests that nurses do for others what they cannot do for themselves. Orem uses the following five key concepts in her Self-care deficit theory:

1. Self-care: learned behaviors that a person performs for self (when able) that contribute to health.
2. Self-care deficit: a relationship between actions a person should take for healthy functioning and the capability for action.
3. Self-care requisites: needs that are universal or associated with development or deviation from health.
4. Self-care demand: therapeutic actions to meet needs.
5. Agency: capability to engage in self-care.

The essence of Orem's three-part nursing theory "focuses on persons in relations. The theory of self-care focuses on the self, the I; the theory of self-care deficit focuses on you and me; and the theory of nursing systems focuses on we, persons in community" (Orem, 1990, p. 49). Orem's general theory, the self-care deficit theory, integrates the theory of self-care, the theory of self-care deficit, and the theory of nursing systems (Orem, 1995).

Orem defines self-care as the "voluntary regulation of one's own human functioning and development that is necessary for individuals to maintain life, health, and well-being" (Orem, 1995, p. 95). People learn self-care activities as they mature. Culture, society, and family customs play key roles in determining individual self-care activities. Age, developmental state, or health status can affect the ability to perform self-care activities. For example, parents or guardians must provide continuous care for infants and toddlers.

Orem (1980) specifies that nursing is concerned with the person's need for self-care action to "sustain life and health, recover from disease or injury, and cope with their effects" ( p. 6). In Orem's view, nursing care may be offered to individuals and groups. However, Orem emphasizes that only persons have self-care requisites. The nurse cares for, assists, or does something for the client to achieve client desired health outcomes (Orem, 1980).

Orem (1985, p. 179) implies that health is "a state of a person that is characterized by soundness or wholeness of developed human structures and of bodily and mental functioning." Orem proposes that individual perception (well-being) affects health.

Orem addresses the physical, psychological, interpersonal, and social aspects of health but indicates that they are inseparable in the person: "Health describes the state of wholeness or integrity of human beings" (Orem, 1995, p. 96). "If there is acceptance of the real unity of individual human beings, there should be no difficulty in recognizing structural and functional differentiation within the unity" (Orem, 1980, p. 180). Orem views individuals as moving "toward maturation and achievement of the individual's human potential" (Orem, 1985, p. 180) rather than organisms seeking a steady state.

Orem suggests that some people may have self-care requisites (needs) associated with development or with health deviations. Self-care requisites are essential enduring needs; whereas other needs may surface because of internal or external conditions that alter the ability to care for oneself. Orem identifies the following universal self-care requisites (Orem, 1980, p. 42):

1. Maintenance of sufficient air, water, and food intake.
2. Provision of care associated with elimination processes and excrements.
3. Maintenance of a balance between activity and rest and between solitude and social interaction.
4. Prevention of hazards to life, functioning, and well-being.
5. Promotion of human functioning and development within social groups in accord with potential, known limitations, and the desire to be normal.

Identified self-care requisites require actions known as "therapeutic self-care demands." Therapeutic self-care demands can be determined by:

1. Identifying existing or potential self-care requisites.
2. Developing methods for meeting self-care requisites by considering basic factors (e.g., developmental state, general health status, living patterns) that "condition the values of patients' self-care agency and therapeutic self-care demands as well as the means that are valid for meeting self-care requisites and in regulating self-care agency at particular times" (Orem, 1985, p. 78).
3. Designing, implementing, and evaluating a plan of action. Orem tends to use nursing process as a way to develop a system of nursing.

The theory of nursing systems involves "an interpersonal unity in a particular time–space localization. This unity is formed by nurses, persons who have entered into an agreement to accept and participate in nursing, and the relatives or persons who are responsible for the individuals who require nursing" (Orem, 1990, p. 54). Thus, candidates for nursing care are clients who have insufficient current or projected capability for providing self-care. "It is the need for compensatory action (to overcome an inability or limited ability to engage in care) or for action to help in the development or regulation of self-care abilities that is the basis for a nursing relationship" (Orem, 1980, p. 58). Other concepts and theories that have been derived from the self-care deficit theory include self-care agency, dependent care, and dependent care agency (Taylor, Geden, Isaramalai, & Wongvatunyu, 2000).

Orem's theory specifies that nurses help clients when the client is unable to provide for his or her own self-care requisites. Nursing interventions may be aimed at maintaining health, preventing illness, or restoring health, and they may involve actions for or with the client. The theory, which is compatible with the traditional medical model, has been widely used in practice and education and recently has been the basis for research. Although more than 440 research-based journal articles have used Orem's theory, most of the research tends to be descriptive in nature. Major concepts as defined in Orem's model are summarized in Table 5-5.

### Jean Watson's Human Science and Human Care Theory

Jean Watson developed **Watson's Human Science and Human Care Theory** while writing a book about a BSN-integrated nursing curriculum (Fawcett, 2002a). Watson proposes that the purpose of nursing is to help persons gain greater harmony within the mind, body, and soul. Key concepts in Watson's model are the phenomenal field, which

**TABLE 5-5**

## Major Concepts as Defined in Orem's Theory

| Person (patient) | A person under the care of a nurse |
| --- | --- |
| Environment | Physical, chemical, biologic, and social contexts within which human beings exist |
| Health | "A state characterized by soundness or wholeness of developed human structures and of bodily and mental functioning" (Orem, 1995, p. 101) |
| Nursing | Actions to overcome or prevent the development of a self-care deficit or provide therapeutic self-care for a patient who is unable to do so |

is the totality of past, present, and future influences on the person, and carative factors, which are interventions that demonstrate caring as a moral ideal of nursing.

Watson's theory blends Eastern philosophy while representing phenomenological, existential, and spiritual orientations. The model arises from her conception of "transpersonal caring" as "a moral ideal of nursing with a concern for preservation of humanity, dignity, and freedom of self" (Watson, 1985, p. 74). Watson wants nursing "to concern itself more with meaning, relationships, context, and patterns" (Watson, p. 2).

"Human life . . . is defined as (spiritual–mental–physical) being-in-the-world which is continuous in time and space" (Watson, 1985, p. 47). Although the soul, mind, and body are explicitly identified as spheres of the human being, they are viewed as integrated and inseparable.

Health is related to "unity and harmony within the mind, body, and soul," and illness is "subjective turmoil or disharmony within a person's inner self or soul at some level or disharmony within the spheres of the person, for example, in the mind, body, and soul, either consciously or unconsciously" (Watson, 1985, p. 48). A distinction is made between the self as perceived and as experienced, with the degree of congruence between these perceptions being related to health.

Watson views humans as being open to the environment, within which interrelationships occur with other humans and nature. She uses the concept of a phenomenal field to describe "the totality of human experience" (Watson, 1985, p. 54). The human being, with a unique life history, "imaged future," and "presenting moment," interacts with others in the environment to create an event, "a focal point in space and time from which experience and perception are taking place" (Watson, 1985, p. 59). An event, as a "moment of coming together," provides an actual caring occasion for human care through nursing. "An actual caring occasion, or transpersonal caring moment, involves action and choice by both the one-caring and the one-being-cared-for" (Watson, 1999, p. 116).

"Nursing consists of transpersonal human-to-human attempts to protect, enhance and preserve humanity by helping a person find meaning in illness, suffering, pain, and existence; to help another gain self-knowledge, control, and self-healing wherein a sense of inner harmony is restored regardless of the external circumstances" (Watson, 1985, p. 54).

Caring is "a moral ideal, rather than an interpersonal technique" (Watson, 1985, p. 58), which can be demonstrated through the carative factors (nursing interventions) that "allow for contact between the subjective world of the experiencing persons"

(Watson, 1985, p. 58). The following carative factors are all presupposed by a knowledge base and clinical competence (Watson, 1989, pp. 227–228).

1. Formation of a humanistic–altruistic system of values.
2. Nurturing of faith and hope.
3. Cultivation of sensitivity to one's self and others.
4. Development of a helping–trusting, human caring relationship.
5. Promotion and acceptance of the expression of positive and negative feelings.
6. Use of creative problem-solving caring processes.
7. Promotion of transpersonal teaching–learning.
8. Provision for a supportive, protective, or corrective mental, physical, socio-cultural, and spiritual environment.
9. Assistance with gratification of human needs.
10. Allowance for existential–phenomenologic–spiritual forces.

During the human care process (nursing), both the nurse and the client are in a process of "being and becoming." "The agent of change . . . is viewed as the individual patient, but the nurse can be a coparticipant in change" (Watson, 1985, p. 74). Each person has human freedom, choice, and responsibility, with the moral ideal being the "protection, enhancement, and preservation of human dignity . . . Human caring involves values, a will and a commitment to care, knowledge, caring actions, and consequences" (Watson, 1985, p. 29). "Emphasis is on helping other(s), through advanced nursing caring-healing modalities, to gain more self-knowledge, self-control, and even self-healing potential" (Watson, 1996, p. 148).

"Connectedness with other, and yet beyond self and other, keeps alive our common humanity" (Watson, 1999, p. 117).

Watson's theory provides one framework for the study of caring that has served as foundation for many nursing research studies across the world. A current literature search revealed 687 articles using Watson's framework. Smith (2004) outlined four categories addressed by nurse researchers using Watson's theory: the nature of nurse caring, client and nurse perceptions of the nurse caring experience, human experiences, and human caring needs. Nurses use Watson's theory to measure caring behaviors, attitudes, and efficacy; in practice across various specialty areas and in nursing education research (Smith, 2004). The University of Colorado hosts the Center for Human Caring, where nurses study and practice the human science and human care theory. Table 5-6 summarizes the key concepts as defined in Watson's theory.

**TABLE 5-6**

## Major Concepts as Defined in Watson's Theory

| | |
|---|---|
| Person (human) | A "unity of mindbodyspirit/nature" (Watson, 1996, p. 147) |
| Environment | A "field of connectedness" at all levels (Watson, 1996, p. 147) |
| Health (healing) | Manifested by harmony, wholeness, and comfort |
| Nursing | Reciprocal transpersonal relationship in caring moments guided by carative factors |

## Complexity Theory as a Framework

Like stability theory, **complexity theory** assumes that reality continuously changes. However, change occurs with irregularity and cannot be predicted. Complexity theory "emphasizes change over time, long-term unpredictability, and openness to the environment with mutual simultaneous interactions . . . The complexity perspective seeks to understand patterns of phenomena as wholes within their contexts" (Maliski & Holditch-Davis, 1995, p. 25). Unlike systems theory, interacting systems cannot be separated because they are one.

Complexity theory replaces the metaphors of separation and interaction (reductionistic) with the metaphor of participation (holistic) (Porter, 1995). The whole cannot be known from the sum of the parts, nor can the sum of the parts be more than the whole because everything is unitary.

Assumptions of complexity theory include:

- Nonlinear change over time.
- Long-term unpredictability.
- Openness to the environment.
- Mutual, simultaneous interactions.
- Continual fluctuations that reveal patterns.
- Variable patterns appear at critical points.

Because the theory assumes mutual change of human being and environment, which provides potential for restructuring in new patterns, linear cause and effect is difficult to infer. The theory suggests that multiple, dynamic, mutual relationships, rather than enduring "causes," influence change. Thus, change of an individual, because it is related to initial conditions, is not generalizable.

Nursing models/theories with complexity theory as foundation emphasize becoming of the human being in terms of potential for change. Some nurses find models based on complexity theories difficult to understand because complexity theory challenges them to think in multiple dimensions.

### Martha Rogers' Science of Unitary Human Beings

Martha Rogers developed **Rogers' Science of Unitary Human Beings** while searching for a specific and unique body of knowledge for nursing during the late 1970s (Fawcett, 2003a). In Rogers' science of unitary human beings, the purpose of nursing is to foster health potential. Rogers incorporates the following three key concepts in her model:

1. Unitary human being: an irreducible, indivisible, pandimensional energy field identified by pattern.
2. Unified energy field: a pandimensional nonlinear domain without spatial or temporal attributes.
3. Mutual process: changes within the human and environmental fields that occur simultaneously.

Rogers' model builds on an assumption of the person as a unified energy field that continuously exchanges energy with an environmental energy field. Rogers proposes that "man is a unified whole possessing his own integrity and manifesting characteristics that are more than and different from the sum of his parts" (Rogers, 1970, p. 47). Physical, biologic, psychological, social, cultural, and spiritual attributes are merged into behavior that reflects the total person as an indivisible whole. Rogers believes that it is impossible to describe humans by combining attributes of each of the parts. Only as the parts lose their particular identity is it possible to describe the person.

The person is an organized energy field that has a unique pattern. The continuous mutual process of energy field with environmental energy field results in continuous pattern manifestation changes in both the person and the environment (Rogers, 1970). This results in increasing complexity and innovativeness of the person. Rogers believes that this life process "evolves irreversibly and unidirectionally along the space–time continuum" (Rogers, 1970, p. 59). She conceptualizes this unidirectionality as a spiral, with self-regulation "directed toward achieving increasing complexity of organization— not toward achieving equilibrium and stability" (Rogers, 1970, p. 64). The person also is characterized by "the capacity for abstraction and imagery, language and thought, sensation and emotion" (Rogers, 1970, p. 73).

Rogers believes that health serves as an "index of field patterning" (Maliski & Holditch-Davis, 1995, p. 27). Health and illness are not separate states, good or bad, nor in a linear relationship. "Ease and disease are dichotomous notions that cannot be used to account for the dynamic complexity and uncertain fulfillment of man's unfolding" (Rogers, 1970, p. 42). Thus, observable manifestations are all "manifestations of patterning (that) emerge out of the human/environmental field mutual process and are continuously innovative" (Rogers, 1990, p. 8).

Nursing intervention is aimed toward promoting the betterment of humans wherever they may be (Rogers, 1992). Rogers also specifies that nurses must address health promotion with consumers because disease and pathology may always be a potential manifestation of human patterns. Rogers (1992) views caring in nursing as "simply a way of using knowledge" (p. 46).

Rogers (1990 p. 333) has described three principles that explain change: integrality, helicy, and resonancy. The principle of integrality emphasizes that the human energy field and the environmental energy field are continuous and must be perceived simultaneously. The relationship is one of constant interaction and mutual simultaneous change. In other words, "they are reciprocal systems in which molding and being molded are taking place at the same time" (Rogers, 1970, p. 97).

The principle of helicy predicts that change occurs as a "continuous innovative, unpredictable, increasing diversity of human and environmental field patterns" (Rogers, 1990, p. 8). The human field becomes increasingly diverse with time. As the person ages, behavior is not repeated but may recur at ever more complex levels. The principle of resonancy indicates that change in pattern and organization toward increased complexity of the field occurs by way of waves, "manifesting continuous change from lower-frequency, longer wave patterns to higher-frequency, shorter wave patterns" (Rogers, 1980, p. 333).

Rogers believes that an understanding of the mechanisms that affect the life process in humans makes it possible for the nurse to purposefully intervene to affect client pattern manifestations in a desired direction. In the process, the nurse also is changed. She sees the future as "one of growing diversity, of accelerating evolution, and of nonrepeating rhythmicities" (Rogers, 1992, p. 33). Rogers' emphasis on holism and on the simultaneous and mutuality of humans and the environment are concepts that have been widely accepted in nursing. Rogers proposed that the science of unitary human beings would serve as a foundation for future theory development to make this abstract science applicable to practice (Fawcett, 2003). Parse (1987), Newman (1986), and Leddy (2004)

TABLE 5-7

## Major Concepts as Defined in Rogers' Theory

| | |
|---|---|
| Person (human being) | A unitary energy field with a unique pattern |
| Environment | An energy field in mutual process with the human being |
| Health | An indication of the complexity and innovativeness of patterning of the energy field that is the person |
| Nursing | Intervening to improve pattern manifestations and the environment to achieve maximum health potentials |

use the science of unitary human beings as foundation for practice. Barrett developed a theory of power using the science that nurses use to guide nursing service departments (Fawcett, 2003b). Over 600 nursing articles have been published addressing Rogerian science. Nurse researchers use Rogers' theory as a foundation in validating effectiveness of complementary and alternative health practice (e.g., therapeutic touch, guided imagery, and other energy therapies). Table 5-7 presents major concepts as defined in Rogers' model.

### Rosemarie Parse's Human Becoming Theory

Like Rogers, Parse suggests that the purpose of nursing is to improve the quality of life for both the client and nurse in **Parse's Human Becoming Theory.** Parse coins words to describe the essence of nursing and the following three key concepts in her model:

1. Coconstitution: development of patterning through person–environment interaction.
2. Coexistence: dynamic mutual processes between the person and the environment.
3. Situated freedom: freedom of choice in a situation.

Parse's model incorporates a combination of Rogers' principles and building blocks "with the tenets of human subjectivity and intentionality and the concepts of coconstitution, coexistence, and situated freedom from existential phenomenological thought" (Parse, 1987, p. 161). The emphasis is on the meaning and values that influence a person's active choices of behavior. "The person constructs his or her own meaning" (Parse, 1996, p. 57).

Parse defines the person as "an open being, more than and different from the sum of parts in mutual simultaneous interchange with the environment who chooses from options and bears responsibility for choices" (Parse, 1987, p. 160). As a person interacts with the environment, patterns of relating are established that provide insight into his or her patterning and values at that moment. Health is viewed as a "nonlinear entity," a constantly changing process of becoming that incorporates values. Because it is not a state, health cannot be contrasted with disease. "The human becoming nurse's goal is to be truly present with people as they enhance their quality of life" (Parse, 1998, p. 69).

Parse (1987, pp. 164–165) defines nine key concepts in her model.

1. Imaging: "picturing or making real of events, ideas, and people."
2. Valuing: "living of cherished beliefs."

3. Languaging: "speaking and moving . . . the way one represents the structure of personal reality."
4. Connecting–separating: " the rhythmical process of distancing and relating."
5. Powering: "the pushing–resisting of inter-human encounters that originates in the uniqueness in the process of transforming."
6. Transforming: "the changing of change."
7. Originating: "generating unique ways of living."
8. Revealing–concealing: "rhythmical patterns of relating with others."
9. Enabling–limiting: "infinite number of possibilities within choice."

Parse (1987, p. 163) has combined these concepts into three principles. Meaning is structured multidimensionally as humans and the environment together create (cocreate) reality through "the languaging of valuing and imaging." In other words, the meaning of human beliefs and values is developed and demonstrated through words and movement. Rhythmicity of patterns of relating is cocreated through "living the paradoxical unity of revealing–concealing, enabling–limiting, and connecting–separating." In other words, human patterns in relating to others are derived from multiple choices and involve rhythmical processes of moving closer to and away from others. Cotranscendence with possibilities is "powering unique ways of originating in the process of transforming." In other words, it involves the processes of distancing and moving closer in interrelationships that provide the force for change and creativity. "The unitary human freely chooses meaning in situation, bears responsibility for the choices, and transcends with possibles" (Parse, 1998, p. 31).

From these concepts and principles, Parse (1987, pp. 168–169) has derived three implications for practice:

1. Illuminating meaning by explicating what is appearing through language.
2. Synchronizing rhythms by dwelling with the flow of connecting–separating.
3. Mobilizing transcendence by moving toward possibles in transforming.

Parse states that, "the way of living the belief system is through true presence" (Parse, 1996, p. 57), "which is a non-routinized, unconditional loving way of being within which the nurse witnesses the blossoming of others" (p. 57). Practicing within this model, the nurse would provide an empathic sounding board for clients and families to express and therefore uncover the meaning of thoughts and feelings, values, and changing views. In the process of expression through language and movement, and in "dwelling with" the rhythm of the client and family, new possibilities for change in the quality of life would become apparent. "The new insights shift the rhythm and all participants move beyond the moment toward what is not-yet. This is mobilizing transcendence" (Parse, 1989, p. 257). In this model, the nurse connects with clients through focused interactions rather than doing things for them (Phillips, 1987). Therefore, Parse blends caring with Rogers' science of unitary human being.

Parse (1998) also has developed a phenomenological–hermeneutic research methodology to test relationships suggested by the model. The methodology uses "dialogical engagement," a researcher–participant encounter, to uncover the meaning of the live experience being studied (Parse, 1989, p. 256), and serves as the research methodology for many qualitative nursing studies. To date, over 200 published nursing research studies use Parse's human becoming theory as a conceptual framework. The following list presents some of the research topics addressed in published studies based on Parse's theory: client-lived experiences of tiredness; spiritual perspectives of nurses; use of therapeutic touch, quiet, and dialogue in cancer patients; client perceptions of being cared for; and concerns of family caregivers. In the human becoming practice methodology, the "goal is to be truly present with people" (Parse, 1998, p. 69), who are the experts about what will enhance quality of life.

Parse's theory emphasizes the importance of the meaning that underlies behavior and provides a structure for the identification and clarification of "manifestations of whole people as they interrelate with the environment" (Phillips, 1987, p. 188). Hansen-Ketchum (2004) specifies that outcomes for nursing practice using Parse's theory include opportunities for multidimensional client healing, enhanced personal growth (for client and nurse), and continued professional growth (for the nurse). Table 5-8 summarizes the major concepts as defined in Parse's theory.

### Margaret Newman's Theory of Health as Expanding Consciousness

Like Parse, Newman uses principles from Rogers's Science of Unitary Beings in **Newman's Theory of Health as Expanding Consciousness.** Margaret Newman states that the purpose of nursing in this theory is to promote a higher level of consciousness in both client and nurse. Newman uses the concept of consciousness as the capacity of the system (person) to interact with its environment; the informational capacity of the system in her nursing model.

Newman's theory incorporates Rogers' concept of a unitary person as a center of energy in constant interaction with the environment. Persons are characterized by patterning that is constantly changing. According to Newman, "the focus of nursing is the pattern of the whole, health as pattern of the evolving whole, with caring as a moral imperative" (Newman, 1994, p. xix).

"The total pattern of the person-environment can be viewed as a network of consciousness (Newman, 1986, p. 33) that is expanding toward higher levels: the patterns of interaction of person-environment constitute health. . . . Health is the expansion of consciousness" (Newman, 1986, pp. 3, 18), and "health and the evolving pattern of consciousness are the same" (Newman, 1990, p. 38). "Consciousness is defined as the information of the system: the capacity of the system to interact with the environment" (Newman, 1994, p. 38).

Health is viewed as a process that encompasses both disease and "non-disease." Instead of the familiar linear relationship between health as good and disease (or illness) as bad, Newman conceptualizes disease as a meaningful component of the whole and a possible facilitator of health. "Sickness can provide a kind of shock that reorganizes the

**TABLE 5-8**

| Major Concepts as Defined in Parse's Theory | |
|---|---|
| Person | An open being, more than and different from the sum of parts |
| Environment | In mutual process with the person |
| Health | Continuously changing process of becoming |
| Nursing | Use of true presence to facilitate the becoming of the participant |

relationships of the person's pattern in a more harmonious way" (Newman, 1994, p. 11). As the person interacts with the environment, "the fluctuating patterns of harmony–disharmony can be regarded as peaks and troughs of the rhythmic life process" (Newman, 1986, p. 21).

Newman posits four major ways in which person–environment patterning is manifest: movement, time, space, and consciousness. Consciousness is expressed in patterns of rhythmic movement toward higher levels that can be described in time and space. Manifestations of these patterns include exchanging, communicating, relating, valuing, choosing, moving, perceiving, feeling, and knowing (Newman, 1986, p. 74). The task for nursing intervention is to recognize patterning and relate to it in an "authentic" (genuine, sincere) way.

The new paradigm is relational. The professional enters into a partnership with the client with the mutual goal of participating in an authentic relationship, trusting that in the process of its evolving, both will grow and become healthier in the sense of higher levels of consciousness (Newman, 1986, p. 68).

Nursing facilitates the process of evolving to higher levels of consciousness by "rhythmic connecting of the nurse with the client in an authentic way for the purpose of illuminating the pattern and discovering the new rules of a higher level of organization" (Newman, 1990, p. 40).

Newman's theory contributes to the development of a body of knowledge about manifestations of healthy patterning of unitary human beings. Newman has described a methodology for using practice as the basis for research within the model, and recently, over 100 research studies based on the theory have been reported in the literature. Areas for research based on Newman's theory include nurses as cancer survivors, use of nursing spiritual interventions, empowerment of cancer patients, nurse–family relationships with medically fragile children, family caring, and perceived health of men with human immunodeficiency virus. Table 5-9 lists major concepts as defined in Newman's theory.

### Susan Leddy's Human Energy Model

**Leddy's Human Energy Model** was influenced by Rogers' science of unitary human beings, Eastern philosophy, and quantum physics and complexity theories. This model identifies three aspects of universal essence: matter, information, and energy, which constitute an undivided whole. In the human energy model, Leddy (2004) proposes that the purpose of nursing is to facilitate the harmonious pattern of the essence fields of both client and nurse. Leddy (2004) uses five key concepts in her model.

**TABLE 5-9**

| Major Concepts as Defined in Newman's Theory | |
|---|---|
| Person (human being) | "unitary and continuous with the undivided wholeness of the universe" (Newman, 1994, p. 83) |
| Environment | "undivided wholeness of the universe" (Newman, 1994, p. 83) |
| Health | Expansion of consciousness |
| Nursing | Facilitating repatterning of the client to higher levels of consciousness |

1. Self-organization: the structure of the human being demonstrated by pattern and its manifestations.
2. Energy field: a dynamic web of energy interactions.
3. Awareness: an energy that links humans with the environment.
4. Energy: manifested by movement and change.
5. Pattern: a web of relationships.

Leddy views the human being (person) as "a unitary energy field that is open to and continuously interacting with an environmental universal essence field" that can only be understood as a whole. Sensitivity to complementary facets and vantage points for observation provides a view of the whole from different perspectives" (Leddy, 1998, p. 192; 2003, p. 68). "Self-organization distinguishes the human energy field from the environmental field with which it is inseparable and intermingled" (Leddy, 2003, p. 68). "Self-organization is a synthesis of continuity and change that provides identity while the human evolves toward a sense of integrity, meaning, and purpose in living" (Leddy, 1998, p. 192). Humans also have awareness that enables the development of self-identity, construction of meaning, and the capability to influence change by making choices (Leddy, 2004).

Leddy (2004) views the environment as the context in which the human is embedded. People are one with the environment. Change can be partially predicted and partially unpredictable. She explains that the universal essence environment is ordered, and has a rhythmic pattern while constantly changing "through continuous transformation of matter and information" (Leddy, 2004, p. 14). However, change ". . . is also influenced by the inherent order of the universe" (Leddy, 2003, p. 68). Along with the order of the universe, history, pattern, and choice also shape change.

Leddy (2003) defines health as being "the pattern of the whole" (p. 68). This pattern is rhythmic, varying in quality and intensity over time. Health is characterized by a changing pattern of harmony/dissonance.

Knowledge-based consciousness in a goal-directed relationship with the client is the basis for nursing. "A nurse–client relationship is a commitment characterized by intentionality, authenticity, trust, respect, and genuine sense of connection. The nurse is a knowledgeable, concerned facilitator. The client is responsible for choices that influence health and healing" (Leddy, 1998, pp. 192–193). The facilitation of harmonious health patterning for both client and nurse is identified as the purpose of nursing.

Leddy (2004) has derived three theories from the model: the theory of healthiness, theory of participation, and the theory of energetic patterning. In the theory of healthiness, healthiness is defined as a manifestation of a health pattern. Healthiness is defined as a process characterized by purpose, connections, and power to attain goals. The theory proposes that healthiness acts as a resource that influences the ongoing patterning that is reflected in health (Leddy & Fawcett, 1997).

The Leddy Healthiness Scale (LHS) (1996) includes items that measure meaningfulness, connections, ends, capability, control, choice, challenge, capacity, and confidence. In studies with the LHS (Leddy, 1996; Leddy & Fawcett, 1997), healthiness has been found to be moderately and negatively related to fatigue and symptom experience in women with breast cancer; and moderately and positively related to mental health, health status, and satisfaction with life in a sample of healthy people.

In the theory of participation, participation is defined as the experience of continuous human–environment mutual process. Leddy (2004) defines participation as the experience of expansiveness (fullness and activity) and ease (smoothness and calmness of the

**TABLE 5-10**

## Major Concepts as Defined in Leddy's Theory

| | |
|---|---|
| Person (human being) | A unitary, self-organized field of matter, energy and information that constantly interacts with an environmental universal essence field |
| Environment | A dynamic, ordered, connected web in continuous transformation of energy, matter, and information with the human being (environmental universal essence) |
| Health | The rhythmic pattern of harmony/dissonance of the whole |
| Nursing | Knowledge-based consciousness involved in a mutual, connected, and goal-directed relationship with clients |

mutual process of the human and environmental fields). The Person–Environment Participation Scale (PEPS) (Leddy, 1995) measures expansiveness and the ease of participation. In studies with the PEPS to date, participation has been found to be moderately and positively correlated with healthiness, sense of coherence (Antonovsky, 1987), and power (Barrett, 1990), and moderately and negatively correlated with fatigue and symptom experience in healthy people.

The theory of energetic patterning proposes that nursing interventions to facilitate the harmonious pattern of both client and nurse are accomplished through health pattern appraisal, recognition of patterns, and energy-based nursing interventions (Leddy, 2004). Nursing healing interventions promote healing by surrounding, supporting, or penetrating the human body. The six domains of energetic patterning are:

1. Coursing: to reestablish free flow of energy.
2. Conveying: to foster redirection of energy away from areas of excess to depleted areas.
3. Converting: to augment energy resources.
4. Collecting: to reduce energy depletion.
5. Clearing: to facilitate the release of energy tied to old patterns.
6. Connecting: to promote harmony within the human field and with the environmental field.

A number of types of interventions are consistent with this theory, including nutrition, exercise, touch modalities, bodywork, light therapy, music, imagery, relaxation, and stress reduction (Leddy, 2003; 2004).

Leddy's conceptual model offers a unique and modern perspective for nursing; however, because it is a newer model, its usefulness for practice and research remains to be demonstrated. Table 5-10 presents major concepts as defined in Leddy's model.

## ● NURSING MODELS IN RESEARCH AND PRACTICE

### Model Use in Nursing Research

Most published nursing research studies fail to use conceptual nursing models as study foundations. Currently, three kinds of research related to models of nursing are being conducted: testing the relationships predicted by a model, using a model as a framework for descriptive analysis, and attempting to modify nursing care through use of a model.

For example, Leddy and Fawcett (1997) interpreted the results of a study to explain relationships among theoretical variables (participation, change, energy, and healthiness) derived from the human energy model, as being supportive of the model. In another example, Hart (1995), in a study of pregnant women, derived research variables from Orem's general theory and tested the relationships between the variables. The results were interpreted as supporting Orem's model.

Models also have been used as a framework for descriptive analysis. For example, concepts from Watson's science of human caring and Newman's health as expanding consciousness were used to describe personal (DeMarco, Picard, & Agretelis, 2004) and professional (Picard, Argretelis, & DeMarco, 2004) experiences of nurses who survived cancer. Picard and colleagues' (2004) study demonstrates how nursing models may be used to guide clinical research. Scura, Budin, and Garfing (2004) used the Roy Adaptation Model to organize and categorize data in a pilot study using telephone social support and education to promote adaptation in men with prostate cancer. Roy's Adaptation Model was also used to organize study variables in a study looking at change in exercise tolerance, activity and sleep patterns and quality of life in cancer patients who participated in a structured exercise program (Young-McCaughan, et al., 2003). Bauer (2001) demonstrated how Newman's theory may be helpful in establishing patterns common to persons with similar health problems.

## Research Brief 5-1

Picard, C., Agretelis, J., & DeMarco, R. (2004). Nurse experiences as cancer survivors: Part II-Professional. *Oncology Nursing Forum, 31*, 537–542.

The investigators employed a descriptive phenomenological research design based on Watson's caring theory and Newman's health as expanding consciousness theory to discover the professional experiences of nurses who have survived cancer. Twenty-five registered nurses were interviewed by the investigators on two occasions. The first interview asked about the experiences of being a professional nurse who had survived cancer; in the second interview, the participant verified written researcher understanding, and reflected on a researcher-generated piece of artwork. VanManen's approach was used to capture key dimensions of professional aspects of nurse cancer survivor experiences. Five key professional experiences emerged from the data from at least 20 of the participants: "(a) role ambiguity, (b) deepening of compassion for patients and others, (c) self-disclosure as a therapeutic intervention, (d) becoming an advocate for change, and (e) volunteerism" (p. 538). The nurses participating in this study also mentioned that their experiences of being health care consumers had caused professional practice changes. Increased compassion for others resulted in personal changes. They felt a moral obligation to volunteer in cancer care organizations, work to increase client voices in cancer care treatment decisions, and improve their work environments. Although considered taboo, the nurses felt that self-disclosure about their cancer survivorship provided hope for persons undergoing cancer treatments. Finally, the nurses had difficulty separating professional needs and obligations from personal ones.

The clinical significance of this study is that when nurses are consumers of health care, they experience problems with role ambiguity and may need additional support to confront this issue. Talking about their experiences resulted in heightened self-awareness about the experience, which in turn led to renewed and deeper compassion for clients. Also, nurses like many clients confronting cancer, undergo a process of remoralization that results in increased professional commitments to clients. Because of the small sample size (25 breast cancer cases) and self-selection for participation in the study, results of this study may not be applicable for all nurse cancer survivors. More research is needed to address the personal and professional experiences of nurses who survive potentially terminal illnesses.

A few studies attempt to modify nursing care through use of a model. For example, Kelly, Sullivan, Fawcett, and Samarel (2004) tested the effects of therapeutic touch, quiet time, and dialogue on women's perceptions of breast cancer using Rogerian science. They found that only women receiving therapeutic touch experience bodily sensations of tingling, magnetic pull, or being touched. Experimental and control groups both found quiet time and dialogue with the nurse as calming and relaxing. Therefore, nurses should not overlook therapeutic results from just spending time with clients.

## Model Use in Practice

As more nurses receive baccalaureate degrees and graduate nursing education, model use in practice may become more prevalent. Nursing models and theories provide guidance to nurses engaged in practice for holistic assessments, rationale for various nursing interventions, and delineation of professional nursing roles in health care delivery. Some hospitals identify a particular theory as a basis for use of nursing process. For example, nurses at St. Luke's Hospital of Kansas City use Orem's Self-Care Deficit Theory as a foundation and guide for nursing practice. The American Nurses Association requests that nursing departments specify nursing model and theory use by the organization as part of the Magnet Hospital application process.

However, nursing model use in professional practice seems irrelevant to some nurses. Do models make real differences in nursing care delivered to clients? Does it matter if the client need is called a "noxious influence" affecting a behavioral subsystem, a "self-care deficit" leading to a "self-care demand," or a "focal stimulus" that is a stressor? How is the care given any different if its purpose is labeled to "limit self-care deficits," "reduce stressors," or "foster coping"? Why does the profession need specific nursing models and theories?

Although nursing science remains in an early stage of development, nursing scholars agree on categories of concepts (person, environment, health, and nursing) that are central to nursing knowledge. Nursing science must attain distinction from medical science. Much discussion about whether there should be one model for nursing has occurred, but the popularity of a growing number of models within different paradigms and frameworks indicates that disagreement still exists about how professional nursing should be described and how its goals can best be achieved. Perhaps multiple approaches and definitions of nursing would be advantageous due to the complex nature of nursing.

However, the profession continues to progress in defining nursing, identifying the unique nursing contributions to health care, developing nursing theory, and using nursing models and theories in practice. As health care evolves, nursing must demonstrate an ability to articulate its important and unique contribution to client care and perhaps, new models and theories may be needed.

> **Questions for Reflection 5-4**
>
> 1. What is my personal attitude toward nursing models and theories?
> 2. Has my attitude changed since reading this chapter?
> 3. Why do I feel this way about them?
> 4. What are the consequences of my attitudes toward nursing models and theories?

## ● SUMMARY AND SIGNIFICANCE TO PRACTICE

The nursing models discussed in this chapter use the metaparadigm concepts of person, environment, health, and nursing. Philosophical differences between the change as stability paradigm and the change as growth paradigm are pronounced. Professional nurses have the freedom to select which models to use in clinical practice based on personal philosophy and world views. Sometimes, a particular nursing model may fit a clinical situation better than others. Nursing models do not compete with each other but provide a variety of approaches and explanations for the phenomena associated with professional nursing practice.

A comparison of concepts in selected theories is presented in Table 5-11. The major differences and similarities among models can be seen by comparing Table 5-12 with Table 5-13. More research is needed to see if the models provide an effective description of nursing and make differences in client care outcomes.

**TABLE 5-11**

### Comparison of Concepts in Selected Theories

| Theory | Human | Human–Environment Interaction | Health | Examples of Nursing Implication |
|---|---|---|---|---|
| Systems | Multiple interacting subsystems that form the human system | Simultaneous change in both systems | Tendency toward increased complexity | Nurse system and client system are mutually affected |
| Stress and adaptation | Multiple subsystems that share an internal environment | Humans cope and compensate for environmental change | Constancy of the internal environment within normal parameters | Support coping mechanisms of client |
| Complexity | Unitary whole | Mutual simultaneous interaction; nonlinear | Pattern of the whole | Stimulate repatterning |

## TABLE 5-12

# Similarities and Differences of Conceptualization in Nursing Models Within the Change as Stability Paradigm

| Model | Person | | Health | Environment | Nursing | |
|-------|--------|--|--------|-------------|---------|--|
| | Goal | Composition | | | Nature | Purpose |
| King | Functioning in social roles | Open system | Dynamic state of well-being | Internal and external stressors | Goal-oriented interaction | Attainment maintenance, or restoration of health |
| Orem | Constancy | Whole with physical, psychological, interpersonal, social aspects | Meeting self-care needs | External forces | Systems that address self-care requisites | Help people to meet self-care needs |
| Roy | Become integrated and whole | System with biopsychosocial components | Adaptation | External conditions | Manipulation of stimuli to foster coping | Promotion of adaptation |
| Neuman | Balance | Composite of physiologic, psychological, sociocultural, developmental of spiritual variables | Equilibrium | Internal and external stressors | Stress-reducing activities | Promotion of equilibrium |

# TABLE 5-13

## Similarities and Differences of Conceptualization in Nursing Models Within the Change as Growth Paradigm

| Model | Person | | | Environment | Nursing | |
|---|---|---|---|---|---|---|
| | Goal | Composition | Health | | Nature | Purpose |
| Peplau | Equilibrium | System with physiologic, psychological, and social components | Foreward movement of the personality | Significant others | Therapeutic interpersonal process | Helping people to meet needs and to develop |
| Watson | Sense of inner harmony | Integrated and inseparable spiritual, mental, and physical spheres | Unity and harmony | Energy field external to the person | Transpersonal caring | Promoting harmony |
| Rogers | Increased complexity of pattern | Indivisible energy field | Increasing innovativeness of patterning | Contiguous, continuously interacting energy field | Promotion of repatterning | Facilitating health potential |
| Newman | Expansion of consciousness | Center of energy | Patterns of person–environment interaction expanding toward higher levels | Energy field in continuous interaction with the person | Repatterning partnership | Promoting higher level of consciousness |
| Parse | Process of becoming | Open being | Process of becoming | Energy field in continuous interaction with the person | Interpersonal processes | Improving quality of life |
| Leddy | Harmony, integrity, meaning, and purpose | Unitary energy field | Pattern of the whole | Energy field and person are one | Goal-directed relationship | Facilitation of harmonious health patterning |

## FROM THEORY TO PRACTICE

Reread the vignette at the beginning of the chapter and answer the following questions:

1. Do you believe that because Ann uses theory to guide her nursing practice, she is a better nurse than Nancy? Why or why not?
2. Which of the nursing models or theories presented in this chapter appeals to you the most?
3. How would you incorporate the theory identified in question 2 into your professional practice?
4. What are the consequences of using a nursing model or theory to guide clinical practice?

## WWW INTERNET EXERCISE

1. Visit one of the nursing theory websites listed below or found on the Clayton College and State University Nursing Theory websites and answer the following questions:
   a. Can you contact the nursing theorist?
   b. Who maintains the nursing theory website?
   c. What materials are available on the website to explain the nursing theory?
   d. Where can you go to find additional information about the nursing theory?
   e. Would you recommend the website to a colleague interested in the selected nursing theory? Why or why not?

## WWW INTERNET RESOURCES

Clayton College and State University Department of Nursing's Nursing Theory: http://www.healthsci.clayton.edu/eichelberger/nursing.htm.
Neuman's health system model: http://www.neumansystemsmodel.com.
Newman's health as expanding consciousness: http://www.healthasexpandingconsciousness.org.
Orem's self-care deficit nursing theory: http://www.muhealth.org/~nursing/scdnt/scdnt.html.
Parse's human becoming theory: http://www.humanbecoming.org.
Roy's adaptation model: http://www2.bc.edu/~royca/.
Rogers's science of unitary human beings: http://medweb.uwcm.ac.uk/martha.
Watson's theory of caring and the Colorado Center for Human Caring: http://www2.uchsc.edu/son/caring/content.

## REFERENCES

Andrews, H. A., & Roy, C. (1986). *Essentials of the Roy adaptation model*. Norwalk, CT: Appleton-Century-Crofts.
Antonovsky, A. (1987). *Unraveling the mystery of health*. San Francisco: Jossey-Bass.
Auger, J. R. (1976). *Behavioral systems and nursing*. Englewood Cliffs, NJ: Prentice-Hall.
Barrett, E. A. M. (1990). A measure of power as knowing participation in change. In O. L. Strickland & C. F. Waltz (Eds.). *Measurement of nursing outcomes* (pp. 159–180). New York: Springer.

Bauer, D. J. (2001). Common patterns of person-environment interaction in persons with rheumatoid arthristis. *Western Journal of Nursing Research, 23*(4), 414–430.

Benner, P., & Wrubel, J. (1989). *The primacy of caring. Stress and coping in health and illness.* Menlo Park, CA: Addison-Wesley.

Cannon, W. B. (1932). *The wisdom of the body* (rev. ed.). New York: Norton.

Chin, R. (1976). The utility of systems models and developmental models for practitioners. In W. G. Bennis, K. D. Benne, K. E. Corey, & R. Chin (Eds.). *The planning of change* (3rd ed., pp. 90–122). New York: Holt, Rinehart and Winston.

Chinn, P. L., & Kramer, M. K. (1999). *Theory and nursing: Integrated knowledge development* (5th ed.). St. Louis: Mosby-Year Book.

DeMarco, R., Picard, C. & Agretelis, J. (2004). Nurse experiences as cancer survivors: Part 1-Personal. *Oncology Nursing Forum, 31*, 523–530.

Fawcett, J. (1989). *Analysis and evaluation of conceptual models of nursing* (2nd ed.). Philadelphia: F. A. Davis.

Fawcett, J. (2000). *Analysis and evaluation of contemporary nursing knowledge: Nursing models and theories*. Philadelphia: F. A. Davis.

Fawcett, J. (2001). The nurse theorists: 21st-century updates—Imogene M. King. *Nursing Science Quarterly, 14*, 311–315.

Fawcett, J. (2002). The nurse theorists: 21st-century updates—Callista Roy. *Nursing Science Quarterly, 15*, 308–310.

Fawcett, J. (2002a). The nurse theorists: 21st-century updates—Jean Watson. *Nursing Science Quarterly, 15*, 214–219.

Fawcett, J. (2003). Conceptual models of nursing: International in scope and substance? The case of the Roy adaptation model. *Nursing Science Quarterly, 16*, 315–318.

Fawcett, J. (2003a). The nurse theorists: 21st-century updates—Martha E. Rogers. *Nursing Science Quarterly, 16*, 44–51.

Fawcett, J. (2003b). Conceptuual models of nursing: International in scope and substance. The case of the Roy Adaptation Model. *Nursing Science Quarterly, 16,* 315–318.

Fawcett, J. (2004). Conceptual models of nursing: International in scope and substance? The case of the Neuman Systems model. *Nursing Science Quarterly, 17*, 50–54.

Frederickson, K. (2000). Nursing knowledge development through research: Using the Roy adaptation model. *Nursing Science Quarterly, 13,* 12–17.

Gaut, D., & Leininger, M. (1991). *Caring: The compassionate healer.* New York: NLN Press.

Hansen-Ketchum, P. (2004). Parse's theory in practice. *Journal of Holistic Nursing, 22*, 57–72.

Hart, M. A. (1995). Orem's self-care deficit theory: Research with pregnant women. *Nursing Science Quarterly, 8,* 120–126.

Huch, M. H. (1987). A critique of the Roy adaptation model. In R. R. Parse (Ed.), *Nursing science: Major paradigms, theories, and critiques* (pp. 47–66). Philadelphia: WB Saunders.

Kelly, A., Sullivan, P., Fawcett, J., & Samarel, N. (2004). Therapeutic touch, quiet time, and dialogue: Perceptions of women with breast cancer. *Oncology Nursing Forum, 31*, 625–631.

King, I. M. (1981). *A theory for nursing: Systems, concepts, process.* New York: Wiley.

King, I. M. (1987). King's theory of goal attainment. In R. R. Parse (Ed.), *Nursing science: Major paradigms, theories, and critiques* (pp. 107–113). Philadelphia: WB Saunders.

King, I. M. (1989). King's general systems framework and theory. In J. P. Riehl-Sisca (Ed.), *Conceptual models for nursing practice* (pp. 149–158). Norwalk, CT: Appleton & Lange.

King, I. M. (1995). The theory of goal attainment. In M. A. Frey & C. L. Sieloff (Eds.), *Advancing King's systems framework and theory of nursing* (pp. 23–32). Thousand Oaks, CA: Sage.

King, I. M. (1996). The theory of goal attainment in research and practice. *Nursing Science Quarterly, 9*, 61–66.

King, I. M. (1999). A theory of goal attainment: Philosophical and ethical implications. *Nursing Science Quarterly, 12,* 292–296.

Koldjeski, D. (1990). Toward a theory of professional nursing caring: A unifying perspective. In M. Leininger & J. Watson (Eds.), *The caring imperative in education* (pp. 45–57). New York: National League for Nursing.

Kyle, T. V. (1995). The concept of caring: A review of the literature. *Journal of Advanced Nursing, 21,* 506–514.

Leddy, S. K. (1995). Measuring mutual process: Development and psychometric testing of the person-environment participation scale. *Visions: The Journal of Rogerian Nursing Science, 3,* 20–31.

Leddy, S. K. (1996). Incentives and barriers to exercise in women with a history of breast cancer. *Oncology Nursing Forum, 24,* 885–890.

Leddy, S. K. (1998). *Leddy & Pepper's conceptual bases for professional nursing,* (4th ed.). Philadelphia: Lippincott.

Leddy, S. K. (2003). *Integrative health promotion.* Thorofare, NJ: Slack.

Leddy, S. K. (2004). Human Energy: A conceptual model of unitary nursing science. *Visions: The Journal of Rogerian Scholarship, 12,* 14–27.

Leddy, S. K., & Fawcett, J. (1997). Testing the theory of healthiness: Conceptual and methodological issues. In M. Madrid (Ed.), *Patterns of Rogerian knowing* (pp. 75–86). New York: National League for Nursing.

Magan, S. J. (1987). A critique of King's theory. In R. R. Parse (Ed.), *Nursing science: Major paradigms, theories and critiques* (pp. 115–133). Philadelphia: WB Saunders.

Maliski, S. L., & Holditch-Davis, D. (1995). Linking biology and biography: Complex nonlinear dynamical systems as a framework for nursing inquiry. *Complexity and Chaos in Nursing, 2,* 25–35.

Monat, A., & Lazarus, R. (Eds.). (1977). *Stress and coping: An anthology.* New York: Columbia University Press.

*Merriam-Webster's collegiate dictionary* (10th ed.). (1994). Springfield, MA: Merriam-Webster.

Morse, J. M., Solberg, S. M., Neander, W. L., Bottorff, J. L., & Johnson, J. L. (1990). Concepts of caring and caring as a concept. *Advances in Nursing Science, 13,* 1–14.

Neuman, B. (1982). *The Neuman systems model: Application to nursing education and practice.* Norwalk, CT: Appleton-Century-Crofts.

Neuman, B. (1996). The Neuman systems model in research and practice. *Nursing Science Quarterly, 9,* 67–70.

Neuman, B. (2002). The Neuman systems model. In B. Neuman & J. Fawcett (Eds.), *The Neuman systems model* (4th ed.). Upper Saddle River, NJ: Prentice-Hall.

Newman, M. A. (1986). *Health as expanding consciousness.* St. Louis: Mosby.

Newman, M. A. (1990). Toward an integrative model of professional practice. *Journal of Professional Nursing, 6,* 167–173.

Newman, M. A. (1994). *Health as expanding consciousness* (2nd ed.). New York: National League for Nursing.

Orem, D. E. (1980). *Nursing: Concepts of practice* (2nd ed.). New York: McGraw-Hill.

Orem, D. E. (1985). *Nursing: Concepts of practice* (3rd ed.). New York: McGraw-Hill.

Orem, D. E. (1990). A nursing practice theory in three parts, 1956–1989. In M. E. Parker (Ed.), *Nursing theories in practice* (pp. 47–60). New York: National League for Nursing.

Orem, D. E. (1995). *Nursing: Concepts of practice* (5th ed.). St. Louis: Mosby.

Parse, R. R. (1987). *Nursing science: Major paradigms, theories, and critiques.* Philadelphia: WB Saunders.

Parse, R. R. (1989). Man-living-health: A theory of nursing. In J. P. Riehl-Sisca (Ed.), *Conceptual models for nursing practice* (pp. 253–257). Norwalk, CT: Appleton & Lange.

Parse, R. R. (1996). The human becoming theory: Challenges in practice and research. *Nursing Science Quarterly, 9,* 55–60.

Parse, R. R. (1998). *The human becoming school of thought.* Thousand Oaks, CA: Sage.

Phillips, J. R. (1987). A critique of Parse's man-living-health theory. In R. R. Parse (Ed.), *Nursing science: Major paradigms, theories, and critiques* (pp. 181–202). Philadelphia: WB Saunders.

Picard, C., Agretelis, J., & DeMarco, R. (2004). Nurse experiences as cancer survivors: Part II-Professional. *Oncology Nursing Forum, 31,* 537–542.

Porter, E. J. (1995). Non-equilibrium systems theory: Some applications for gerontological nursing practice. *Journal of Gerontological Nursing, 21,* 24–31.

Riehl, J. P., & Roy, C. (1980). *Conceptual models for nursing practice.* New York: Appleton-Century-Crofts.

Rogers, M. E. (1970). *An introduction to the theoretical basis of nursing.* Philadelphia: F. A. Davis.

Rogers, M. E. (1980). Nursing: A science of unitary man. In J. P. Riehl & C. Roy (Eds.), *Conceptual models for nursing practice* (pp. 329–337). New York: Appleton-Century-Crofts.

Rogers, M. E. (1990). Nursing: Science of unitary, irreducible human beings: Update 1990. In E. A. M. Barrett (Ed.), *Visions of Rogers' science-based nursing* (pp. 5–11). New York: National League for Nursing.

Rogers, M. E. (1992). Nursing science and the space age. *Nursing Science Quarterly, 5,* 27–34.

Roy, C. (1987). Roy's adaptation model. In R. R. Parse (Ed.), *Nursing science: Major paradigms, theories, and critiques* (pp. 35–45). Philadelphia: WB Saunders.

Roy, C., & Andrews, H. A. (1999). *The Roy Adaptation Model* (2nd ed.). Stamford, CT: Appleton & Lange.

Roy, C., & Roberts, S. L. (1981). *Theory construction in nursing: An adaptation model.* Englewood Cliffs, NJ: Prentice-Hall.

Scura, K., Budin, W., & Garfing, E. (2004). Telephone social support and education for adaptation to prostate cancer: A pilot study. *Oncology Nursing Forum, 32,* 335–338.

Sills, G. M., & Hall, J. E. (1977). A general systems perspective for nursing. In J. E. Hall & B. R. Weaver (Eds.), *Distributive nursing practice: A systems approach to community health* (pp. 22–43). Philadelphia: Lippincott.

Smith, M. (2004). Review of research related to Watson's theory of caring. *Nursing Science Quarterly, 17*(1), 13–25.

Swanson, K. M. (1991). Empirical development of a middle range theory of caring. *Nursing Research, 40,* 161–166.

Taylor, S. G., Geden, E., Isaramalai, S., & Wongvatunyu, S. (2000). Orem's self-care deficit nursing theory: Its philosophic foundation and the state of the science. *Nursing Science Quarterly, 13,* 104–110.

Watson, J. (1985). *Nursing: Human science and human care.* Norwalk, CT: Appleton-Century-Crofts.

Watson, J. (1989). Watson's philosophy and theory of human caring in nursing. In J. P. Riehl-Sisca (Ed.), *Conceptual models for nursing practice* (pp. 219–235). Norwalk, CT: Appleton & Lange.

Watson, J. (1996). Watson's theory of transpersonal caring. In P. H. Walker & B. Neuman (Eds.), *A blueprint for use of nursing models: Education, research, practice and administration* (pp. 141–184). New York: National League for Nursing.

Watson, J. (1999). *Postmodern nursing and beyond.* Edinburgh: Churchill Livingstone.

Young-McCaughan, S., Mays, M., Arzola, S., Yoder, L., Dramiga, S., Leclerc, K., Caton, J., Sheffler, R., & Nowlin, M. (2003). Research and Commentary: Change in exercise tolerance, activity and sleep patterns, and quality of life in patients with cancer participating in a structured exercise program. *Oncology Nursing Forum, 30,* 441–454.

# Professional Nursing Processes

## KEY TERMS AND CONCEPTS

Critical Thinking

Nursing Process

Assessment

Diagnosis

Planning

Implementation

Evaluation

Nursing Diagnosis

Goals

Outcomes

Nursing Outcomes Classification (NOC)

Nursing Interventions

Nursing Interventions Classification (NIC)

Intuition

Reflection

Reflection-in-action

Reflection-on-action

Interpersonal Processes

Psychomotor Processes

Patterning Nursing Processes

## LEARNING OUTCOMES

By the end of this chapter, the learner will be able to:

1 Outline cognitive processes nurses use in clinical practice.

2 Specify the steps of nursing processes.

3 Appraise the strengths and weaknesses of using nursing process in practice.

4 Discuss variances in the use of nursing process when practice is based upon a selected nursing model.

5 Compare and contrast critical thinking, reflection, and intuition.

6 Differentiate among the stages of the novice-to-expert model of clinical practice.

7 Distinguish between linear and integrated cognitive nursing processes.

8 Discuss interpersonal nursing processes consistent with selected nursing conceptual models.

9 Outline psychomotor processes for patterning of health.

Carol, a nurse employed in a university-based health clinic, serves as a preceptor for community health nursing students from a local baccalaureate nursing program. Today is her first day working with Jane, a senior nursing student. Carol receives a telephone call from the University Campus Police informing her that they are bringing an obese student who fell and has a very swollen ankle. Before the student arrives, Carol asks Jane, "What is the first thing we should do when the injured student arrives?" Jane replies, "I think we should find out her name and how the accident happened." Carol responds "OK. What other information do we need?" Jane begins to shake and answers, "I never had a client with an orthopedic problem, so I really don't know where to begin. It seems like I always get confused in the clinical setting what I should do first. Maybe I should not be a nurse." Knowing the frustration she experienced as a nursing student, Carol replies, "Once I understood nursing process, it seemed as though what to do in the clinical setting fell into place for me when I was a nursing student. Can you tell me the steps of nursing process and what nursing theorist you use?" "I get the steps of nursing process confused all of the time, and the program has us use Rogers' nursing theory," replies Jane. Carol sighs and thinks to herself, "How can a nursing student get this far in her education without understanding how to use nursing process? What can I do to help Jane master nursing process quickly?" Carol instructs Jane just to observe while she handles the injured student and tells Jane that the two of them will talk about nursing process and Rogers' nursing theory later.

### Questions for Reflection 6-1

1. How would I explain nursing process to someone else?
2. Why is nursing process important to practice?

Beliefs about nursing shape the way nurses practice. Consider the nature of nursing when nurses practice using the medical model. Much of nursing, as taught and practiced, is standardized according to medical diagnoses and supports medical intervention. The physician does the assessment needed for the medical diagnosis, and this information serves as the basis for the medical orders. Nursing focuses on human responses to health status and the medical plan of care. When so-called nursing knowledge is actually borrowed from medicine, nurses focus on detailed knowledge of pathophysiology, symptoms of disease, standard medical interventions, and a single "best" way to perform treatments and procedures.

In contrast, nursing practice differs greatly when the nature of nursing is based on a model of autonomous professional practice. In an autonomous nursing model, nurses focus on supporting the client to improve well-being status and develop human potential. Nursing knowledge includes detailed understanding of the client as a whole person, health and the factors that promote health, the environment and the mutual and ongoing interaction between environment and humans, and the purpose and functions of nursing. Nurses perform their own client assessments, gathering information about each client's well-being status, including client:

1. Strengths and weaknesses.
2. Whole responses to health concerns.

3. Analysis of circumstances associated with well-being status.
4. Knowledge related to health and well-being.
5. Beliefs and values about health.
6. Lifestyle.
7. Health-related goals.
8. Support systems.

Because nurses view clients as whole persons and consider themselves key partners in an interdisciplinary health care team, they also have knowledge about the care regimens of the other providers, such as physicians, pharmacists, and physical therapists. Understanding care regimens outlined by other health team members helps nurses to appreciate the global health care plan and acknowledge its impact on the whole client. By sharing knowledge about the plan, nurses help clients assume mutual and equal responsibility for setting health-related goals and participating as equal members of the health care team.

The knowledge projected by the model of nursing, accepted by the nurse, provides the basis for all nursing processes. Skill in the integrated use of cognitive, interpersonal, and psychomotor processes in client care is basic to the practice of professional nursing. This chapter emphasizes the relationship between nursing processes and the practice of professional nursing according to the nursing models discussed in Chapter 5.

## ● CRITICAL THINKING

Many different definitions of critical thinking appear in the nursing and higher education literature. Table 6-1 outlines some of the more common definitions of critical thinking used in nursing and higher education. Although they vary somewhat, elements that consistently appear in the definitions include that **critical thinking** appears to be a highly complex thinking pattern that requires higher-order thinking. Persons who critically think take time to examine situations in terms of content and context, instead of jumping into action to make personal judgments and clinical decisions or to solve problems. Critical thinkers also take time to examine consequences of anticipated actions. Finally, critical thinking also demands that persons have solid, logical reasons for judgments and actions.

Critical thinking scholars debate whether the critical thinking process is a general skill that applies to all areas of life. If viewed as a general life skill, critical thinking must be learned by everyone to survive in a rapidly changing world (Paul, 1993). Fortunately, skills can be taught. However, basic elements of critical thinking may have to be altered to "fit" the context of the situation (Paul). When a nurse encounters a person without a pulse and respirations, spending time critically thinking about the situation would cause great harm; immediate action is warranted. However, after the emergency has been handled, the professional nurse could spend some time engaged in critical reflection about why the arrest occurred, how it could have been avoided, and the effectiveness of professional actions.

Other authors, such as Facione, Facione, and Sanchez (1994), propose that critical thinking may be a personal quality and relies on attitude in addition to cognitive skills. Before persons can engage in regular critical thinking, they must value truth seeking,

TABLE 6-1

## Some Commonly Used Definitions of Critical Thinking

| Author(s) | Definition |
| --- | --- |
| Bandman & Bandman (1995) | "The rational examination of ideas, inferences, assumptions, principles, arguments, conclusions, ideas, statement, beliefs and action" (p. 7) |
| Brookfield (1987) | "Reflecting on the assumptions underlying our and others' ideas and action and contemplative alternative ways of thinking and living." Four components of critical thinking:<br><br>• Identifying and challenging assumptions<br><br>• Acknowledging the importance of context<br><br>• Exploring and imagining alternatives<br><br>• Reflective skepticism (Boychuk-Duchscher, 1999) |
| Dauer (1989) | "The art of assessing truth claims according to certain general principles or canons" (p. 3) |
| Kennedy, Fisher, & Ennis (1991) | "Reasonable and reflective thinking that is focused upon deciding what to believe or do" (p. 46) |
| Facione, Facione, & Sanchez (1994) | The "ideal critical thinker is one who is habitually inquisitive, well-informed, trustful of reason, open-minded, flexible, fair-minded in evaluation, honest in facing personal biases, prudent in making judgments, willing to reconsider, clear about issues, orderly in complex matters, diligent in seeking relevant information, reasonable in the selection of criteria, focused in inquiry and persistent in seeking results which are as precise as the subject and circumstances of inquiry permit" (p. 345). |
| Kataoka-Yahiro & Saylor (1994) | "Reflective and reasonable thinking about nursing problems" (p. 352) |
| Kurfiss (1988) | "An investigation whose purpose is to explore a situation, phenomenon, question, or problem to arrive at a hypothesis or conclusion about it that integrates all available information and that, therefore, can be convincingly justified" (p. 37) |
| McPeck (1981) | "The propensity and skill to engage in an activity with reflective skepticism" (p. 8) |
| National League for Nursing Accrediting Commission (2000) | "The deliberative nonlinear process of collecting, interpreting, analyzing, drawing conclusions about, presenting and evaluating information that is both factual and belief based" (p. 8) |
| Paul (1983) | "A unique kind of purposeful thinking in which the thinker systematically and habitually imposes criteria and intellectual standards upon the thinking, taking charge of the construction of thinking, guiding the construction of the thinking according to the standards, and assessing the effectiveness of the thinking according to the purpose, the criteria and the standards" (p. 21) |
| Scheffer & Rubenfeld (2000) | "Inquiry type thinking" (p. 94) |
| Watson & Glaser (1990) | Problem definition<br>Decision making about pertinent information for problem solving<br>Identifying and recognizing overt and covert assumptions<br>Hypothesis formation and selection<br>Drawing valid conclusions and judging validity of inferences (p. 1) |

open-mindedness, analyticity (recognizing potential problems, anticipating results, prizing the use of reason), systematicity (the orderly, focused approach to inquiry), and inquisitiveness (natural curiosity) while having the maturity to make honest, reflective judgments and self-confidence in reasoning processes (Facione, Facione, & Giancarlo, 1996). This view of critical thinking fits well with Benner's novice-to-expert model, which illustrates the idea that experts develop certain characteristics related to practice (confidence, competence, and maturity) that enable them to quickly make correct clinical judgments that seem to simultaneously spring into action. Critical thinking is integrated throughout the cognitive nursing processes.

## ● COGNITIVE NURSING PROCESSES

### The Nursing Process

Clients rely on nurses to make effective clinical decisions. Kataoka-Yahiro and Saylor (1994) suggested that the **nursing process,** as a method for problem solving and decision making in nursing practice, represents a discipline-specific version of critical thinking. Nursing process consists of the following five steps:

1. **Assessment:** comprehensive data collection of factors related to client health status.
2. **Diagnosis:** a judgment that identifies actual or potential client health strengths and weaknesses.
3. **Planning:** a two-phase step that determines health-related goals (or outcomes) and specifies a series of actions to be taken to attain them.
4. **Implementation:** execution of the action plan outlined in step 3.
5. **Evaluation:** determining the effectiveness of the implemented action plan either to make needed revisions or restart nursing process with step 1.

Nursing process has been compared with the scientific method and problem solving. Effective problem solving relies on extensive data collection for proper problem identification. Nurses assess clients holistically to determine actual and potential health-related problems or strengths (nursing diagnoses). Problem solving, the scientific method, and nursing process incorporate planning as a key step. When determining ways to solve the problem, test hypotheses, or deliver individualized nursing care, people generate action plans consisting of a desired goal and steps for attainment. After execution of action plans, problem solving, scientific method, and nursing process evaluate the effectiveness of predetermined action plans in meeting the desired outcome.

The nursing process "provides a systematic guide or method to assist students and novices develop a style of thinking that leads to appropriate clinical judgments" (Christensen & Kenney, 1995, pp. 8–9). The nursing process provides a logical and rational way for the nurse to solve problems and make decisions so that the care given is appropriate and effective. Nurses use critical thinking skills while using all steps of the nursing process. Critical thinking enables nurses to collect relevant data from a variety of sources, sift out irrelevant pieces of data, determine what data are important, and validate meaning of data with others if uncertain. Nurses use critical thinking to organize data into meaningful patterns, determine if more data are required, compare data patterns with norms and known theories, examine assumptions about client situation, and identify the major client health concerns to arrive at a nursing diagnosis. Critical thinking helps nurses to set safe care priorities, set realistic care outcomes, determine appropriate nursing interventions, and generate rationale for interventions while considering client needs and concerns. Nurses use critical thinking while applying knowledge for intervention performance, test the efficacy of interventions, update and revise care plans as needed, noting changes in client status, and determining when to consult other health team members. Finally, critical thinking is used by nurses to evaluate the effectiveness of the care plan, determine alternative approaches and interventions, monitor the quality of care delivered, track client progress toward desired outcomes, and revise the plan as needed. Although nursing process has its roots from the scientific process, nurses execute it in a sensitive and caring manner when working with human beings. Nurses consider client individual needs and preferences when providing client care. Nurses use creativity to individualize nursing care for clients. Thus, the nursing process is an artistic and scientific process.

Invariably, the nursing process is presented as a series of four or five phases, with a number of steps within each phase. The net effect is a procedure that appears linear (or at best overlapping or circular) and cumbersome. However, all parts of the process are interrelated and influence the whole. The parts or phases of the nursing process occur sequentially, but they are not linear. Planning may lead to intervention, or evaluation during planning may result in more assessment. Figure 6-1 depicts the nursing process viewed from an interactional perspective. The following discussion presents an overview of each phase of the nursing process.

### The Assessment Step

During assessment, the nurses collect subjective and objective data about the client's health status. Subjective data consist of information that the client or significant other shares with the nurse. Objective data consist of information that can be directly measured or observed. For example, a client's report of right flank pain (particularly the presence of pain, its location, intensity, and aggravating and alleviating factors) represents subjective data. Increased blood pressure, pulse, and respiratory rates represent objective data. Other forms of objective data include diagnostic test results. Nurses collect data systematically and verify its accuracy with clients. If unable to collect desired data, nurses use critical thinking to determine reasons for obstacles and devise alternative approaches to collect it. When working with clients, nurses continuously collect data and analyze it to make nursing decisions. Nurses document data collected so that other members of the health care team have access to it.

Before nurses can begin collecting data, clients must trust them. Usually, nurses initiate client relationships. When possible, nurses and clients work together as partners

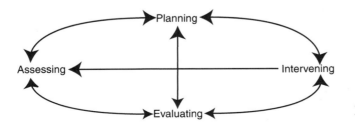

**Figure 6-1**
An interactional approach to the nursing process.

to outline specific care goals and specify responsibilities and ways to tailor nursing care to meet individual client needs. Nurses use critical thinking to evaluate client responses and determine ways to facilitate communication.

Most nurses use an organized process for data collection. They decide which data are desirable and significant to collect in a particular situation and determine what sources and methods would be best to obtain these data. Data provide evidence for determining nursing diagnoses and planning nursing care. Nurse-collected data should supplement, rather than duplicate, data collected by other health professionals (e.g., history) and should focus on information needed for nursing care. During data collection, nurses review all data to determine if more needs to be collected. When data collection is complete, nurses organize and begin planning nursing care.

First, the nurse must know who the client is, why the client needs nursing care, and what factors currently influence the client's health status. Therefore, the nurse must collect key data, such as the client's name, age, gender, marital status, occupation, education, economic status, existing knowledge about health–illness status, and family (and significant other) attitudes toward health care. Second, to individualize care, the nurse collects data regarding the client's personal habits, communication styles, cultural influences, growth and development status, learning capacity, supports and resources, previous experience with the health care system, medical diagnosis and regimen, coping patterns, personal values, and desired changes. Finally, the nurse uses a preferred conceptual nursing model to guide and organize data collection using suggestions outlined in Table 6-2.

As data are collected, the nurse validates the findings with the client and other sources. If discrepancies are noted, they should be clarified, and those data should not be used as the basis for inferences or judgments. Evaluation of the data should consider accuracy and whether all relevant factors have been included. As data collection continues, the organization and analysis of patterns within the data proceed concurrently, which may identify additional data collection needs. When all of this is completed, the nurse moves to the second phase of the nursing process.

## The Diagnosis Step

Nurses derive nursing diagnoses from client data. Using all the data collected during the assessment, nurses organize data into clusters and interpret what they reveal about the client. Effective data analysis and synthesis require that nurses remain objective, engage in thoughtful deliberation, make sound judgments, and discriminate relevant from irrelevant pieces of information.

The North American Nursing Diagnosis Association (NANDA) defines **nursing diagnosis** as:

a clinical judgment about the individual, family or community response to actual or potential health problems/life processes. Nursing diagnosis provides the bases for selection of nursing interventions to achieve outcomes for which the nurse is accountable (Carpenito, 2002, p. 8).

NANDA identifies five types of nursing diagnoses: actual, risk, possible, wellness, and syndrome. Nursing diagnoses exclusively address care situations for which the professional nurse has responsibility. Although nursing practice may vary across state and national boundaries, nurses make independent judgments when clustering data to

TABLE 6-2

## Implications for Data Collection in Selected Nursing Models Organized by Theoretical Frameworks

| Nursing Models | Implications for Data Collection |
| --- | --- |
| **Systems Theory** | |
| King | Perceptions of self, level of growth and development, level of stress, abilities to function in usual role, decision-making abilities, and abilities to communicate |
| Neuman | Stressors, indications of disruption of the lines of defense, resistance factors |
| **Stress/Adaptation** | |
| Roy | Adaptation level (related to three classes of stimuli), coping in relation to modes of adaptation, position on the health-illness continuum |
| **Caring** | |
| Orem | Therapeutic self-care demand, presence of self-care deficits, ability of clients to meet self-care requisites |
| Watson | Phenomenal field (self within life space and motivational factors for health), values, needs for information, problem-solving abilities, developmental conflicts, losses, feelings about the human predicament |
| **Complexity** | |
| Peplau | Physiologic and personality needs, illness symptoms, relationships with significant others, influences on establishment and maintenance of the nurse–client relationship |
| Rogers | Characteristics of patterning, health potential, rhythms of life, simultaneous states of the individual and environment |
| Parse | Thoughts and feelings about the situation, the synchronizing rhythms in human relationships, personal meanings, ways of being alike and different, and values |
| Newman | Person-environment interactions, patterns of energy exchange, client's responses to symptoms, transforming potential, client's feelings and what he does because of those feelings, patterns of life |
| Leddy | Characteristics of human universal essence field and enviornmental essence field |

formulate nursing diagnoses. Professional nursing responsibility means that the nurse has the legal qualifications and accountability to take action. Nursing diagnoses may apply to individuals, families, or communities (Carpenito, 2002).

When defining characteristics of a nursing diagnosis are present, nurses work with an actual nursing diagnosis. Actual nursing diagnoses are written using a three-phrase clause: the client problem, followed by the words "related to," then the etiology. Proper formatting of actual nursing diagnoses forbids the use of the name of a disease or surgical procedure as the related-to clause. NANDA has other classifications of nursing diagnoses to fit a variety of clinical situations. Wellness diagnoses occur when a person, family, or community experiences a transition to a higher level of wellness. When persons or groups are at risk to develop a specific human response, but the signs and symptoms (diagnostic cues) are absent, nurses formulate at-risk nursing diagnoses. Nurses use a syndrome diagnosis when a particular clinical situation results in a predictable cluster of commonly encountered actual or at-risk nursing diagnoses. Finally, nurses may encounter a clinical situation in which insufficient data are present to designate an actual, at-risk, wellness, or syndrome diagnosis. The possible nursing diagnosis presents a nurse with an option to address the human response despite insufficient data. Finally, when nurses monitor for possible complications from medications or an invasive procedure, nurses use collaborative problem statements (Carpenito, 2002). The number of clauses in a nursing diagnosis varies according to its classification. Table 6-3 offers definitions, specific formats, and examples of the various classifications of nursing diagnoses.

Although nurses develop nursing diagnoses, they need to validate the data on which they are based with clients. When nurses involve clients in the generation of nursing diagnoses, clients become more aware of the goals, and have opportunity to determine desired outcomes of nursing care. Human response patterns and functional health patterns of health perception provide different ways for nurses to collect and organize data to compile nursing diagnosis. NANDA developed nine human response patterns in efforts to define and classify nursing diagnoses. The patterns identified by NANDA are: exchanging, communicating, relating, valuing, choosing, moving, perceiving, knowing, and feeling. Gordon (1995) outlines the following 11 functional health patterns that apply to all persons:

1. Health perception–health management.
2. Nutritional–metabolic.
3. Elimination.
4. Activity–exercise.
5. Sleep–rest.
6. Cognitive–perceptual.
7. Self-perception–self-concept.
8. Role–relationship.
9. Sexuality–reproduction.
10. Coping–stress tolerance.
11. Value–belief.

NANDA advocates the use of human response patterns for classifying and defining nursing diagnoses and Gordon's functional health patterns as a means for client data collection (Carpenito, 2002). However, human response patterns tend toward a more Western thought process, whereas Gordon's functional health patterns tend to be understood by all nurses.

Although the more commonly used nursing diagnoses tend to be problem oriented only, nurses help clients to enhance their health and address potential health concerns. Nursing diagnoses focusing on enhancing wellness and preventing potential health problems enable nurses to focus on client strengths and use them to improve client health.

## The Planning Step

Once a comprehensive list of nursing diagnoses has been generated, professional nurses develop a plan of care to communicate specific client care needs to nursing personnel so that desired outcomes are attained. Care plans guide and direct client care efforts to assure continuity of care when different nurses assume client care responsibilities. In addition, care plans designate specific interventions to meet client care goals. Finally, nursing care plans outline contributions nurses make to client health care delivery.

Nurses follow certain guidelines to generate effective nursing care plans. When planning client care, nurses establish a set of nursing diagnoses in priority order, designate desired nursing goals and client outcomes, and prescribe specific nursing interventions.

TABLE 6-3

## Definition, Format, and Examples of Nursing and Collaborative Diagnoses

| Nursing Diagnosis Classification | Definition | Format | Examples |
|---|---|---|---|
| Actual | A clinical judgment identifying a problem with major defining characteristics being present with identified contributing factors influencing the health status change. | Three clauses: 1. The human response 2. Etiology (or contributing factors) 3. Clinical signs and symptoms | Altered nutrition less than body requires (1) related to persistent nausea and vomiting (2) as evidenced by no food intake for 1 week, refusal to eat, weight loss of 10 pounds within 2 weeks, (3) prealbumin of 14.8 mg/dl and c/o "feel tired all the time" and statement "I am afraid to eat because I will throw up." |
| Risk | A clinical judgment identifying a potential problem because of increased vulnerability to developing it. | Two clause statement designating the potential human response and the etiology | Risk for infection related to compromised host defenses from the potentially immunosuppressive effects of chemotherapy and presence of Groshong central venous catheter |
| Syndrome | A clinical judgment identifying health-altering situation resulting in the likely presence of multiple nursing diagnoses | One clause statement designating the type of altered health | Battered child syndrome |
| Wellness | A clinical judgment identifying a transition from a current wellness level to a higher one | One clause statement designating a human response with the possibility of moving toward greater wellness | Potential for enhanced spiritual well-being |
| Possible | A clinical judgment describing a suspected problem not validated by available data | Two clause statement designating the human response and possible etiology | Possible death anxiety related to recent cancer diagnosis |
| Collaborative problems and diagnostic statements | Potential complications arising from a disease process or medical interventions | Two-part phrase including the words: *Potential complication* | Potential complication: hemorrhage Potential complications of cardiac catheterization |

Adapted from Carpenito, L. J. (2002). *Nursing diagnosis application to clinical practice* (9th ed.). Philadelphia: Lippincott Williams & Wilkins.

Nurses set priorities based on preserving client functional status (except in the terminally ill), promoting client comfort, and meeting mutually agreed-on client goals.

Because of the need to streamline care and improve client outcomes, some nurses rely on standardized care plans. Standardized nursing care plans provide less variance in care delivered to clients with similar health problems. They address all critical assessments and customary interventions for medical therapies, invasive procedures, and diagnostic tests. When nurses follow standardized care plans, they may forget to include clients in care decisions or neglect client preferences.

The nursing care plan includes the priorities and the prescribed nursing interventions to achieve desired **goals** (the global desired state) derived from the nursing diagnoses. Ideally, nurses and clients work together to develop desired goals and outcomes of nursing care. Once goals are defined, specific outcomes can be generated. **Outcomes** are end results that, when measured, determine client progress toward resolution of the nursing diagnosis. These expected outcomes must be realistic and stated clearly and concisely as they provide the basis for evaluating nursing care plan effectiveness. Broad guidelines for goal setting in selected nursing models are presented in Table 6-4. Because the nursing models vary, the foci of nursing goals differ.

### Nursing Outcomes Classification

The **Nursing Outcomes Classification (NOC)** provides an alternative approach to delineating client outcomes. Since the 1990s, increased importance has been placed on

**TABLE 6-4**

### Broad Guidelines for Goal Setting in Selected Nursing Models Organized by Theoretical Frameworks

| Nursing Models | Broad Guidelines for Goal Setting |
|---|---|
| **Systems Theory** | |
| King | Achievement of goals and solution of problems related to personal, interpersonal, and social systems |
| Newman | Maintenance or restoration of dynamic equilibrium by reducing stressor penetration or strengthening the normal line of defense |
| **Stress/Adaptation** | |
| Roy | Promotion of adaptation from successful coping |
| **Caring** | |
| Orem | Restoration of external and internal constancy |
| Watson | Meeting human needs and solving problems in a caring interpersonal relationship |
| **Complexity** | |
| Rogers | Help people design ways to attain optimal rhythmic patterns |
| Parse | Illuminating meaning, synchronizing rhythms, and mobilizing transcendence |
| Newman | Transformation of patterns of life and facilitation of evolving consciousness |
| Leddy | Mutual process to define meaningful goals to attain an optimal pattern of the whole |

determining the effectiveness of nursing care. To meet this challenge of developing measurable client outcomes, nurse researchers at the University of Iowa developed NOC, a research-based classification of nursing care outcomes. Currently, NOC provides nurses with more than 200 scales to measure outcomes of holistic nursing care. For example, NOC has a scale to measure personal safety behaviors. Nurses can use this scale to identify client risk for injury. After client education about personal safety or correction of metabolic disorders, nurses can re-assess the client using the scale to determine if improvement in behavior has occurred. NOC facilitates the development of computerized information systems for tracking nursing care outcomes across health care settings. NOC also facilitates comparable data collection, substantiates nursing care contributions, creates uniform nursing data sets, provides nurses with outcome measurement tools, facilitates electronic documentation of client care, improves reimbursement for nursing services, enables creation of uniform nursing data sets, facilitates electronic documentation of client care, and standardizes ways nurses can evaluate nursing care innovations. Through the process of determining measurable, standardized outcomes, professional nurses clearly articulate the contributions they make to client care while developing a unique body of nursing knowledge (Johnson, Maas, & Moorhead, 2000).

Not all nurses use the NOC in clinical practice. However, the planning phase requires that goals, objectives, or outcomes are determined within the client plan of care. After the goals and outcomes for care have been established, priorities must be set among them. When survival is threatened, physical needs must take precedence. Cost, available personnel and resources, and time may influence priorities. For example, for the overweight student who has a broken leg, weight loss may be considered an important goal, but because of the time needed to accomplish substantial weight loss, it may be assigned a lower priority than learning how to use crutches, which is needed immediately for mobility. The theory or model being used to organize care also can influence determination of priorities. For example, use of Maslow's theory would assign higher priority to physiologic, safety, and security needs, and lower priority to love, self-esteem, and self-actualization needs. In addition, as always, the client must be closely involved in priority setting.

Once the priorities among goals and outcomes have been determined, alternative options for care can be generated and their probability for success predicted. The possible solutions or approaches are heavily influenced by availability of resources and by factors in the client's lifestyle and cultural background. For example, the student's weight loss could be achieved by 2 weeks' residence at a health spa, or a self-monitored weight reduction program consisting of weighing portions of food and following a prescribed exercise program. However, financial constraints may make the spa trip unfeasible, and time and lifestyle constraints may influence the desirability of the exercise or food-weighing approaches. With NOC, nurses working with the client would look at adherence to the outlined dietary regimen, compliance, knowledge and use of health-promoting behaviors, knowledge about prescribed diet, and specific weight control behaviors along with weight reduction measurements. The NOC provides a standardized method to track client progress toward care objectives across inpatient, community, and home settings (Johnson et al., 2000).

Unfortunately, nurses sometimes neglect the process of choosing approaches from among a number of alternatives, especially when they are pressed for time. As a result, the first solution thought of becomes the one implemented, with limited assessment of its likelihood of success or its appropriateness in the particular situation. Time constraints, an instilled belief in a single best way for goal attainment, and the need for rapid closure results in a tendency for nurses to avoid collaborative brainstorming.

Nurses must make conscious efforts to avoid choosing a prescribed "cookbook recipe" approach to delineating care outcomes. To preserve nursing as a collaborative partnership with clients, the nurse and client together must select from alternative goals that have the best likelihood of success within a specific nursing situation. The individualized and collaborative approach then can be translated into specific actions, the desired frequency of the actions, who will be assigned to carry them out (e.g., nurse, client, other health team members), and the timetable for expected achievements.

Along with the establishment of goals, outcomes (or objectives) for nursing care, the nursing care plan outlines specific nursing interventions. **Nursing interventions** are actions nurses take to attain care goals and outcomes. Frequently, nursing students find written nursing care plans challenging and complex. Because of its rigorous nature, students sometimes dread the assignment. Unlike practicing nurses, student care plans usually require written rationale for proposed nursing interventions. Nursing care plans may consist of multiple nursing diagnoses. For each nursing diagnosis, nurses develop priority lists for each nursing diagnosis, expected outcomes and goals, and prescribe specific interventions (establish frequencies and time for each action).

As part of the care plan, the nurse can prescribe independent interventions (those not requiring a physician order such as using a pillow under a client's foot to keep the heels off the mattress), designate collaborative interventions (those requiring a physician order, such as administration of prescription medications), and outline specific interventions to screen for potential complications associated with medical or surgical treatments. Ideally, another nurse should be able to follow the care plan exactly as written by the nurse who developed it. Nurses can find published care plans in books, journal articles, computer programs, and on the Internet.

### Nursing Interventions Classification

In 1987, the University of Iowa developed the **Nursing Interventions Classification (NIC)** system as a means to standardize all possible nursing interventions. NIC contains over 486 standard nursing interventions and outlines 12,000 nursing activities. Most interventions contain 10 to 30 specific activities that include information related to assessing and assisting clients in managing health-related issues, maintaining safe care environments, providing client and family education, offering psychosocial and spiritual support, engaging in consultation with professionals, and referring clients to community support services. NIC facilitates nursing professionalism by standardizing nursing treatment nomenclature; strengthening links between nursing knowledge, diagnoses, interventions, and outcomes; facilitates electronic documentation of nursing care; assists in determining costs and resources needed for nursing interventions; provides a theoretical foundation to help beginning nurses learn clinical decision making; and increasing nursing-specific knowledge (McCloskey & Bulechek, 2000).

To explicate the use of NIC and compare it to traditional nursing process, the example of a client on a weight reduction plan continues. The NIC contains two interventions related to weight reduction and management. The NIC uses the label "weight reduction assistance" for the nursing intervention for the following nursing diagnosis: Alteration in nutrition: more than body requires, related to reduced activity secondary to nonbearing weight status for fractured leg. Nursing activities for the intervention include assessment of eating patterns, reasons for overconsumption, and weekly weight determinations. Development of weight-loss goals, an exercise program, and a daily eating plan with the client appears as a nursing activity. Teaching activities include appropriate energy-expending activities, nutritional needs to promote fracture healing without increasing caloric intake, and calculation of fat content in food. Food selections to stay within predetermined daily caloric limit when eating out or participating in social gatherings also appears as a desired client outcome. The NIC suggests other tips, such as posting weekly weight-loss goals in a strategic location (such as the refrigerator), charting weight loss weekly, referring to community weight reduction support groups, and rewarding the client for meeting goals. Because NIC designates a framework for nursing interventions that can be computer coded (and clients can be charged for them), NIC use in clinical practice has become standard practice in some health care organizations. Evaluation of the care plan occurs by using NOC (McCloskey & Bulechek, 2000).

### Client Care Paths

Since the 1990s, many acute care and outpatient centers have developed client care paths. The nursing care plan for commonly encountered human responses to a specific illness, surgery, or procedure and potential complications are outlined on the client care path. Client care paths have reduced variation of nursing care received by clients with the same clinical problem; streamlined care to reduce costs; reduced care errors and oversights (health team members become specialists in care protocols); and decreased the time nurses spend in documentation (paths frequently contain checklists, instead of requiring nurses to write detailed narrative notes). Clients receive a copy of the care path so they can track progress toward health restoration. In addition, care paths outline specific instructions to follow when they assume self-care responsibilities. Most care paths have methods to accommodate instances when care delivery fails to follow the path exactly because of an unexpected client response. Criticisms of care paths include reduced individualization of client care plans and decreased critical thinking by nurses because of feeling the need to follow the path exactly as outlined.

## The Implementation Step

During implementation, nurses execute proposed nursing care plans. Nursing actions support and compliment the medical plan of care. Ideally, professional nurses use interventions based on scientific evidence. Successful care plan implementation requires that nurses have many diverse skills including the ability to teach and manage others, group process, conflict resolution, competently perform technical skills, and above all, effective communication.

All client–nurse interactions should be goal directed and purposeful. As nursing actions are performed, nurses collaborate with the clients and their significant others while striving to involve them appropriately in the care. Nurses perform interventions with sensitivity to the client's feelings and individual preferences in mind. Conceptual models play a role in the organization of nursing care. Table 6-5 outlines how conceptual models may be used to organize care along with possible implications for nursing interventions.

An important part of implementation is the documentation of results of nursing interventions. Documentation provides a means to track client progress toward desired outcomes while providing a key method for communication among all health team members. When interventions are determined to be ineffective, the nurse revises the nursing

TABLE 6-5

## Implications for Nursing Interventions in Selected Nursing Models Organized by Theoretical Frameworks

| Nursing Models | Implications for Nursing Interventions |
|---|---|
| **Systems Theory** | |
| King | Emphasis is on exploration of the situation, shared information, mutually set goals, and explored means to resolve problems, achieve goals, and move forward. |
| Neuman | Emphasis is on primary, secondary, or tertiary prevention to reduce stressors or strengthen the lines of defense. |
| **Stress/Adaptation** | |
| Roy | Emphasis is on increasing, decreasing, or maintaining focal contextual, or residual stimuli. |
| **Caring** | |
| Orem | Emphasis is on self-care actions for or with the client if he is unable to perform them for himself. |
| Watson | Emphasis is on caring that reflects interpersonal teaching–learning, mutual formulation of the problem, joint appraisals, shared need for problem-solving, joint planning, provision of cognitive information, and evaluation of helpfulness for learning and coping. |
| **Complexity** | |
| Rogers | Emphasis is on mobilization of the client's resources and repatterning of the human–environment interaction. |
| Parse | Emphasis is on guidance to relate the meaning of the client's situation, to share thoughts and feelings with one another, and to change the meaning of the situation by making it more explicit. |
| Newman | Emphasis is on the process of growth in which the nurse focuses on the client's evolving capacities, diversity, and complexity in the process of expanding consciousness. |
| Leddy | Emphasis is on the mutual process of transforming energy to create change. |

care plan. Changes in client condition may mean an alteration in the frequency of prescribed interventions, modification of the current one, or prescription of new ones. The process of intervention is integrally involved with the final phase of nursing process, evaluation.

### The Evaluation Step

During evaluation, nurses and clients collaborate to determine if progress is being made toward the attainment of the health-related goal in ideal client care situations. Processes included in the evaluation of care include reassessment, review and reordering (if necessary) care priorities, establishing new goals, and revision of the care plan. Evaluation occurs continuously throughout each phase of the nursing process. However, during evaluation, the main purpose is to compare changes in client behavior or health status with the determined goals or expected outcomes specified in the nursing care plan. Results of evaluation may reveal one or a combination of the following:

1. Goals and outcomes were fully met and future client contacts are needed to reaffirm that the health status change remains permanent.
2. Goals and outcomes were partially met, revealing that the health problem or desired health status change has not been resolved. However, progress continues. Continued monitoring is warranted; more time may be needed with the current plan before considering modification.
3. Goals and outcomes were not met. The client has little or no evidence in change in health status or health problem since the initial assessment. The care plan needs revision.
4. New problems have emerged and the entire care plan needs to be revised to address them.

Because not all client-related health goals are amenable to quantification, nurses sometimes have difficulty finding valid and reliable tools to objectively measure progress toward some goals. It may be helpful to consider whether there are appropriate tools to measure progress toward goals when the goals are established. For example, weight loss and blood pressure reduction are easily validated. However, it is difficult to assess improved self-concept or attitudes toward a more healthful lifestyle. Sources for instruments to measure progress may be found in NOC, journal articles, websites, and instrument handbooks. However, not all goals may be effectively quantified.

Because the nursing process is systematic, logical, and goal directed, it is assumed that adherence to the process will result in desired attainment of goals. When evaluation of progress indicates that the problem is not resolved, it is necessary to consider possible reasons, which may involve the client, the nurse, the client's significant others, or health care team members.

Depending on the outcome of evaluation, the nurse and client may need to modify the goals or interventions, continue the planned strategies with a modified timetable, or, if the goals have been met and no new ones have emerged, terminate the relationship. Both the client and the nurse may have difficulty terminating the relationship. Clients may be unsure of their ability to maintain the changes in health behavior or well-being status on their own. The nurse may have ambivalence about not being needed any longer. Awareness and an open sharing of these feelings can lead to satisfaction in having accomplished the desired goals and acceptance of the need to end the relationship.

Despite the extensive attention given to nursing process, many nurses continue to intervene using standardized procedures based on medical diagnoses. Perhaps, nursing process may not be how experienced nurses practice. Efforts to standardize client care have resulted in the development of client care paths. In many institutions, professional nurses helped develop client care paths that incorporate nursing assessments and interventions to address commonly encountered nursing diagnoses for specific health problems. These nurses tend to engage in rote practice.

However, when nurses use nursing models to guide care, they engage in critical thinking because models provide solid reasoning behind clinical practice. In the following section, two brief examples illustrate that nurses can approach the nursing process differently when they use conceptual nursing models to guide practice.

**Questions for Reflection 6-2**

1. How does my clinical practice setting promote/discourage the use of nursing process in clinical practice?
2. What are the barriers to developing individualized nursing care plans for clients in my current practice setting?
3. Why do I perceive these as barriers?
4. How could I change the practice setting to facilitate individualization of client care?
5. What are the consequences of not individualizing client care in practice?

## Conceptual Models Emphasizing the Nursing Process

Roy and Neuman address nursing process specifically in their nursing models. Instead of keeping with the five-step process, they refined it. Roy keeps nursing process focused on nursing practice, whereas Neuman (2002) proposes use of nursing process for all health care professionals because it is based on the scientific method.

### The Roy Adaptation Model

In the Roy adaptation model, the goal of nursing is to promote adaptation. The nurse manipulates stimuli to move the client in the desired direction of change toward adaptation. The process of nursing is described as a six-step problem-solving method (Roy & Andrews, 1999).

1. First-level assessment: Examine client behaviors in the adaptation modes and make a judgment about whether behaviors in the four modes are adaptive or ineffective.
2. Second-level assessment: Analyze stimuli that influence ineffective behaviors and determine nursing care priorities.
3. State problem areas as nursing diagnoses.
4. Determine specific goals.
5. Determine interventions.
6. Evaluate as behavior changes, and modify as needed.

### The Neuman Systems Model

In the Neuman systems model, the purpose of nursing action is "to best retain, attain and maintain optimal client health or wellness using the three preventions as intervention to keep the system stable" (Neuman, 2002, p. 25). Client stability depends upon the depth of stressor penetration. Nurses assess for actual and potential effects of environmental stressors before making judgments of taking action. Neuman proposed a modification of the nursing process to incorporate the following three steps:

a. Determine a nursing diagnosis.
b. Establish nursing goals.
c. Determine nursing outcomes with interventions classified as primary (wellness retention), secondary (attainment of health), or tertiary (maintenance of health) prevention (Neuman, 2002).

### Benefits and Criticisms of the Nursing Process

The American Nurses Association (ANA) *Standards of Clinical Practice* (1997) states that professional nurses use all five phases of the nursing process when engaging in professional practice. Many professional nurses use nursing process daily in clinical practice and many organizations have documentation forms based on the steps of nursing process. Research has demonstrated that nurses hold a relatively positive attitude toward the nursing process (Martin et al., 1994). In addition, nursing process provides an organized way of thinking about client care and fosters deliberate nursing actions.

However, some nurses express concerns about using nursing process solely as the template for thinking when delivering client care. They perceive that nursing process is too time-consuming to be practical and dislike the emphasis on "nurse-centered power" by overlooking essential rights of health care consumers and collaboration with other health team members (Varcoe, 1996). Henderson (1987), Lindsey and Hartrick (1996), Rew (1996), and Varcoe (1996) offer the following concerns that the nursing process is:

1. Inconsistent with real-world practice because it is a linear, rational problem-solving process.
2. Focused on problems rather than client strengths and potential.
3. Time-consuming and requires elaborate nursing jargon for its use.
4. Preferential to rules over interaction.
5. Antithetical to a holistic approach to client care.
6. Labeling clients by nursing diagnoses.
7. Minimizing disallowance of nursing intuition.
8. A questionable approach for expert nursing practice.

The formulaic structure of the nursing process has been useful to teach rules to novice learners. However, many nurses treat the nursing process as if it were *the only process* in nursing practice. Research has demonstrated that the nursing process is inadequate "when sensory data are changing rapidly or are ambiguous, uncertain, or conflicting" (Rew). Interestingly, a relationship between critical thinking ability and professional competence has not been demonstrated (Maynard, 1996). In addition, Benner, Tanner, and Chesla (1996) found that clinically proficient and expert nurses use intuitive cognitive processes, rather than rule-based thinking, to make clinical judgments. In the research brief, Bucknall (2003) outlines how these processes and other factors are used by professional nurses as they make clinical decisions. The following section highlights these integrative processes.

### Research Brief 6-1

Bucknall, T. (2003). The clinical landscape of critical care: nurses' decision-making. *Journal of Advanced Nursing, 43,* (3), 310–319.

By observing 18 critical care nurses in private, public, and rural hospitals, the investigator sought to identify environmental influences on nursing decisions made in critical care settings. The nurses were observed during clinical practice for 2 hours and then participated in a semistructured interview within 24 hours that addressed nurse perceptions of the recorded clinical practice session.

With use of content analysis, the following key concepts and themes emerged as key to nursing care decisions made by the nurse participants: the patient situation, clinical resources (physical and personnel), interpersonal relationships (between the nurse and client, family and other health team members), time, and risk. Results reveal that clinical decision making relies on a multitude of contextual factors rather than the nurse to follow the steps of nursing process.

This study demonstrates how complex clinical decision making is for professional nurses. Because of the small sample and sharp clinical focus (critical care settings), results from this study must be exercised with caution. More research is needed to explicate more fully the thought processes and actions nurses use to make clinical decisions.

## Integrated Models for Clinical Judgment

Along with nursing process, nurses use other models to make clinical judgments. Benner and colleagues (1996) suggest that "the clinical judgment of experienced nurses resembles much more [the] engaged, practical reasoning . . . than the disengaged, scientific, or theoretical reasoning . . . represented in the nursing process" (p. 1). Experienced nurses tend to bypass some steps of nursing process, whereas novice nurses comply with each of the five steps.

### Intuition

Studies of expert clinical practice have identified intuition, knowing the patient, and reflection as important characteristics. **Intuition** has been described as "another way of knowing wherein facts or truths are known or felt directly rather than arrived at through a linear process of rational analysis" (Rew, 1996, p. 149), or as "an instantaneous, direct grasping of reality" (Mishlove, 1994, p. 32). In a study that supported the novice-to-expert model, Polge (1995, p. 8) found that "as the level of nursing proficiency increases from advanced beginner to expert, there is a significant increase in the use of intuitive critical thinking to make clinical nursing judgments." Young (1987) proposed that intuition is multidimensional. The functional dimension of intuition is comprised of cues and judgment, in which actions do not have a logical link with data. Intuition as a personal way of knowing relies on direct patient contact, self-receptivity, experience, energy, and self-confidence. Many nurses have saved lives by acting on intuitive feelings. In some cases, physicians have been known to come and see hospitalized clients because the nurse identified intuition as the reason for contacting the physician.

### Questions for Reflection 6-3

1. How have I used intuition to guide personal or professional actions?
2. What were the consequences of using intuition in the situation(s) identified above?
3. What advice would I give to someone about using intuition to guide action?
4. Would the advice I give be different for a professional colleague than if I were giving it to a friend? Why or why not?

### Reflection

**Reflection** is a process of thinking about concerns associated with an experience. Reflection develops the affective domain of learning and allows nurses to relate to the aspects of their experience that are the most profound at the time. Consequently, reflection has the potential to provide for personal growth. Reflective learning is multidimensional and may be triggered by a sense of inner discomfort. When things do not go according to plan, nurses engage in reflection to identify and clarify concerns surrounding a clinical situation. Effective reflection requires that the nurse be open to new information that may arise from nonempirical sources. Sometimes reflection results in the resolution (or "aha moment") in confounding situations, or with the feeling that one has learned something that is personally significant. Reflection may result in profound changes in attitudes or behaviors.

The Pew Health Professions Commission (1998) identifies reflection as one essential skill that health professionals must be able to perform along with critical thinking and rational problem solving. Health care professionals need to develop skills in reflective and critical thinking to identify and respond to new situations and practice dilemmas. Professionals also use reflection during practice and afterward to evaluate professional performance. Schon (1987) identifies two ways in which professionals use reflection: **reflection-in-action,** and **reflection-on-action.** During reflection-in-action, health care practitioners think about the purposes and reasons behind actions being performed. Reflection-on-action thinking is a self-evaluative process in which practitioners analyze personal performance in a given clinical situation, think of what could have been done better, and determine plans to improve performance the next time a similar clinical situation is encountered.

Brookfield (1995, p. 8) proposes that reflection becomes critical reflection when it "questions assumptions and practices" as well as seeking to understand power forces behind current practice. Reflection also provides opportunities for professionals to find meaning in practice (Brookfield; Schon, 1987). Reflection takes time to master, especially in today's fast-paced society. A variety of means help persons to develop skills in reflection, including writing one's autobiography, keeping professional logs, auditing self-performance, constructing criteria for role model profiles, developing survival advice memos, videotaping oneself in professional action, having peer evaluations, identifying critical incidents, and engaging in meaningful dialogues with others (Brookfield, 1995).

## Knowing the Patient

Tanner, Benner, Chesla, and Gordon (1993) argue that when nurses are constrained from knowing their clients by organizational factors and economic constraints, the groundwork "for safe and astute nursing care is undermined . . . and nursing is reduced to a technology" (p. 23). Knowing the client involves knowing the client as a person and knowing the client's typical pattern of responses. To know patients, nurses must spend time with them.

Radwin (1995) identifies familiarity and intimacy as the properties of knowing the client. Radwin identifies the following four strategies for nurses for knowing the client:

1. Empathizing: "The nurse imagines what her feelings and perceptions might be if she were in the patient's situation" (p. 367).
2. Matching a pattern: The nurse matches knowledge about the patient being cared for with "a pattern or configuration comprising the experiences, behaviors, feelings, and/or perceptions of previously cared for patients in similar situations" (p. 367).

3. Developing a bigger picture: "The nurse combines understanding of the patient within and outside the acute care setting to produce a broader perspective" (p. 367).
4. Balancing preferences with difficulties: "The nurse has an understanding of patient experiences, behaviors, feelings, and/or perceptions . . . and preferences" (p. 368).

Intuition and reflection are professional nursing processes that integrate experience with cognition. Knowing the client integrates experience and cognition and also adds the dimension of interpersonal processes. Cognitive processes receive more attention during discussions related to nursing process, intuition, and reflection. Without attention to interpersonal processes, nursing practice may become impersonal, dominated by technology and self-serving. Therefore, the next section showcases interpersonal processes as guided by selected nursing conceptual models/theories.

## ✦ INTERPERSONAL PROCESSES

The nurse–client relationship requires that nurses use interpersonal processes. **Interpersonal processes** can be defined as interactions between two or more persons. Many nursing conceptual models and theories differ in descriptions of interpersonal processes. The following content provides brief examples of different approaches used by selected nursing conceptual models and theories.

### King's Theory of Goal Attainment

In King's (1995) theory, the goal of nursing is to help individuals maintain their health so they can function in their roles. Nursing is a process of action, reaction, and interaction that results in goal attainment. Although the process proposed by this theory is classified according to the steps in the nursing process, the emphasis is on interpersonal processes within the steps. Assessment incorporates perception, communication, and interaction of the nurse and the client. Planning includes mutual determination of goals and agreement on means to attain them. Implementation is the process in which transactions are made. Finally, evaluation is the process in which nurses ask, "Was the goal attained?"

### Peplau's Interpersonal Relations Model

In Peplau's model (Reed, 1996), nursing is a therapeutic, interpersonal process. Nurses use the interpersonal process as an educative instrument, a maturing force that aims to promote forward movement of the personality. The interpersonal process is the method by which nurses facilitate useful transformation of the client's energy or anxiety. The interpersonal process is based on a participatory relationship between the nurse and client, in which the nurse governs the purpose for and the process in the relationship and the client controls the content. The process consists of the following four phases.

1. Orientation: Clients become aware of the availability of and trust in the nurse's abilities.
2. Identification: The nurse facilitates expression of feelings without rejection.

3. Exploitation: The client derives the full value from the relationship.
4. Resolution: The client is gradually freed from identification with the helping professional. The client's ability to meet his or her needs is strengthened.

## Paterson and Zderad's Humanistic Theory

In the humanistic nursing practice theory, nursing is perceived as a lived experience between human beings. "Nursing is a response to the human situation. One human being needs a kind of help and another gives it" (Paterson & Zderad, 1988, p. 11). The humanistic nursing effort is directed toward increasing the possibilities of making responsible choices. The process, which is labeled the phenomenologic method of nursology (science of nursing), consists of five phases.

Phase I: The nurse knower prepares for coming to know.
Phase II: The nurse intuitively knows the "other."
Phase III: The nurse scientifically knows the other by:

- Analyzing the situation
- Considering relationships between components
- Synthesizing themes or patterns
- Conceptualizing or symbolically interpreting a sequential view of this post-lived reality

Phase IV: The nurse complementarily synthesizes known others by:

- Comparing similarities and differences
- Synthesizing the similarities and differences to create an increased knowing

Phase V: Succession occurs within the nurse from the many to the paradoxical one—"a conception or abstraction that is inclusive of and beyond the multiplicities and contradictions" (Paterson & Zderad, 1988, p. 74).

## Parse's Human Becoming Theory

In Parse's (1996) theory, the goal of practice is quality of life from the client's perspective, with the focus on the meaning constructed by the client. The nurse is present in a nonroutine, unconditional, loving way of being with the client. The full attention of the nurse is with the client "as they move beyond the moment." The methodology in this theory consists of three processes:

1. Explicating (illuminating meaning): making clear what is appearing now through languaging.
2. Dwelling with (synchronizing rhythms): giving of self over to the flow of the struggle in connecting–separating.
3. Moving beyond (mobilizing transcendence): propelling with visioned possibles in transforming.

## Newman's Theory of Health as Expanding Consciousness

Newman describes nursing as "caring in the human health experience" (Newman, 1994, p. 139). "The responsibility of the nurse is not to make people well, or to prevent their getting sick, but to assist people to recognize the power that is within them to move to higher levels of consciousness" (Newman, 1994, p. xv). The focus of nursing in this theory is the pattern of the whole that is clarified through a praxis (practice) method. The method starts with the establishment of a partnership with the client with a mutual goal of participating in an authentic relationship that requires meeting and forming connections. The nurse and client then form a shared consciousness that serves as the basis for increasing awareness. When client and nurse goals are met, they move apart. Each participant in the nursing encounter tells his or her story in his or her way.

The nurse is free to be authentic and fully present. "Awareness of being, rather than doing, is the primary mechanism of helping" (Newman, 1994, p. 104). To develop a sequential pattern over time, the nurse organizes data in chronological order as a narrative.

## ⊕ PSYCHOMOTOR PROCESSES

In addition to cognitive and interpersonal processes, nursing care includes psychomotor processes. **Psychomotor processes** are defined as the manual dexterity, coordination, and ability to use equipment effectively while performing nursing procedures. Skill in the performance of physician-ordered, often invasive, disease or problem-related interventions is a major emphasis in much of nursing clinical practice. Associate degree programs emphasize these technical aspects of nursing, whereas baccalaureate and higher degree programs focus on cognitive and interpersonal processes. Health care consumers and organizations expect nurses to have the ability to carry out complex procedures smoothly and efficiently.

## ⊕ PATTERNING NURSING PROCESSES

**Patterning nursing processes** use energy to enhance health and well being. Patterning processes are more compatible with a unitary approach to nursing practice. Some complementary and alternative health care interventions incorporate manipulation of human–environmental energy fields. Table 6-6 presents some noninvasive nursing interventions to promote self-patterning.

### Rogers' Science of Unitary Human Beings

Nursing from an interaction perspective delineates structure in qualities and persons in the environments. Rogers' Science of Unitary Human Beings proposes that separations do not exist, but rather all things form a single constellation. Rogers (1988, 1992) specified that the purpose of nursing is to create optimal health and well-being for all persons. The science of unitary human beings defines health not as a separate state or as the result of lifestyle choices or an encounter with illness. Instead, health is viewed as "an index of field patterning" (Malinski, 1986, p. 27). "Pattern is concerned with qualities and is expressed by the map of the configuration of relationships" (Bartol & Courts, 2005, p. 114). Only manifestations of patterns can be accessed by humans (Leddy, 2004).

In Rogerian science, behavior patterns are viewed as manifestations of the human–environment field. Field manifestations may include lifestyle parameters, such

TABLE 6-6

## Noninvasive Nursing Interventions to Promote Self-Patterning

| Intervention | Example(s) |
|---|---|
| Imagery | Guided imagery in which client visualizes healing occurring |
| Relaxation | Progressive relaxation exercises or warm bath |
| Affirmations | Positive self-talk |
| Sound | Listening to 60 beats/second cycle music |
| Exercise | Yoga or Tai Chi |
| Wave modulation | Color or light therapy |
| Nutrition | Special diet or herbal, vitamin, or mineral supplements |
| Meaningful presence | Being with another |
| Humor | Clowning, sharing appropriate jokes |
| Authentic dialogue | Guided reminiscence |
| Wellness counseling | Health education |
| Therapeutic touch | Centering and altering energy fields |
| Movement therapy | Dance or imposed motions |
| Journaling | Diary writing or critical incident written records |
| Balancing | Finding balances between activity rest, work, and fun |
| Bibliotherapy | Reading self-help or inspirational literature |
| Body therapy | Acupressure, massage, or healing touch |

as nutrition, work, and play; exercise; sleep–wake cycles; safety; interpersonal network; and decelerated–accelerated field rhythms.

Examples of field-rhythm manifestations might include diversity (from greater to lesser), motion (from slower to seeming continuous), time (from slower to timelessness), and creativity (from pragmatic to visionary). The client is a knowing participant in change in this model. Through being aware, having choices and the freedom to act intentionally, and being involved in creating changes, the client is a mutual participant with the nurse in the patterning process. A healing relationship is characterized by certain principles.

1. The focus is on strengths and skills.
2. Nurse and client are involved in creating changes and influencing outcomes.
3. Nurse and client are equal partners, but the client has the major responsibility for change decisions.
4. A balance of exchange or reciprocity occurs.
5. Presence and involvement or connectedness emerge.
6. Flow and harmony exist.

The patterning process has two phases, appraisal and deliberative patterning. The elements of appraisal in Phase 1 include:

1. Using multiple modes of awareness, including recognizing, being aware, and being sensitive.

2. Tuning into a person's unique patterns.
3. Appreciating manifestations of the human field in the form of experience, perception, and expressions.
4. Constructing pattern knowing through synthesis.
5. Verifying with the client.

Phase 2 involves the mutual deliberative patterning of behavior, which is possible because of the integral connectedness of the person–environment. Although diversity is considered a norm, patterning of each individual is unique. Each individual has an intrinsic potential for growth, which can be identified through exploring the meaning of experiences for the individual. The client and nurse are viewed as connected, and the healing milieu is as important as the particular modality selected as a treatment. Because change is viewed as inevitable, the challenge is to reframe problems into opportunities for positive becoming. By tuning in to the client's rhythms, the nurse can help the client to free energy for self-patterning through a number of possible noninvasive interventions.

- Imagery
- Relaxation
- Affirmation
- Sound (music)
- Exercise
- Color/light (wave modalities)
- Nutrition (diet, vitamins, minerals, herbs)
- Meaningful presence
- Humor
- Authentic dialogue (guided reminiscence)
- Wellness counseling (health education)
- Therapeutic touch (centering)
- Movement (dance, imposed motion)
- Journal keeping
- Balance between activity and rest
- Bibliotherapy
- Acupressure
- Bodywork (massage, touch for health)

**Questions for Reflection 6-4**

1. How do I feel about using energy to promote healing and health?
2. Which of the patterning process would I like to try to enhance my health? Why would I like to try this one?

The science of the unitary human being seems highly compatible with traditional and integrative approaches to health care. As clients become more aware of complementary and alternative health care treatments, professional nurses need the knowledge to help them make wise choices for health enhancement.

## ● SUMMARY AND SIGNIFICANCE TO PRACTICE

Cognitive, interpersonal, and patterning nursing processes provide methods by which the nurse sensitively and systematically approaches practice to achieve mutually determined health goals with the client. Although nursing process arises out of scientific foundations, nurses can be artistic when developing individualized client care plans. In addition to nurse cognitive processes, the nurse–patient relationship facilitates data collection and goal setting for nursing care plans. Recent efforts to standardize nursing diagnoses, outcomes, and interventions may interfere with the ability to provide individualized client care developed in partnership with clients. Critical thinking enables nurses to effectively use nursing cognitive processes in clinical practice. The use of interactive processes may provide enriching relationships for the client and the nurse because authenticity provides the basis for therapeutic partnerships. Patterning processes provide a complex holographic approach to nursing care, in which nurses focus on maximizing client human potential. The various nursing models and theories presented in the chapter guide nursing practice. However, the individual nurse decides the approaches and processes used to meet desired outcomes determined by the nurse and client.

### FROM THEORY TO PRACTICE

1. Why is it important for professional nurses to use cognitive, interactive, and patterning processes when engaging in clinical practice?
2. Which of the professional nursing processes do you use most frequently in clinical practice? Why? What assumptions underlie your most frequently used professional nursing process?
3. Based on the vignette, how would you respond to the nursing student having difficulty using nursing process? Why is it so important that beginning nurses understand nursing process?

### WWW INTERNET EXERCISE

Read Phillipa O'Reilly's on-line article, "Barriers to Clinical Decision Making in Nursing." To access the article quickly, perform a Google search using the terms "Barriers to Clinical Decision Making in Nursing" and hit the "I Feel Lucky" tab, or do a basic Internet search using the search engine of your choice. The article is housed in a New South Wales Australian government website that does not permit a hyperlink. The article appears in the hospital policy section of the St. Vincent's Hospital in Sydney, Australia.

1. What did you think of the article?
2. List the factors for effective decision making that you commonly use in your clinical practice.
3. List the factors that impede your decision making in your clinical practice.
4. Outline a plan to improve your clinical decision-making process.
5. Would you forward this article to a colleague? Why or why not?

## 🖱️ INTERNET RESOURCES

Critical Thinking Consortium: http://www.criticalthinking.org.
California Academic Press: http://www.insightassessment.com.
North American Nursing Diagnosis Association (NANDA): http://www.nanda.org.
Center for Nursing Classification and Clinical Effectiveness:
    http://www.nursing.uiowa.edu/cncce.

## REFERENCES

American Nurses Association (ANA). (1997). *Scope and standards of college health nursing practice.* Washington, DC: American Nurses Publishing.

Bandman, E. L., & Bandman, B. (1995). *Critical thinking in nursing* (2nd ed.). East Norwalk, CT: Appleton & Lange.

Bartol, G., & Courts, N. (2005). The psychophysiology of body mind healing. In B. Dossey, L. Keegan, & C. Guzzetta (Eds.), *Holistic nursing, a handbook for practice,* (4th ed., pp. 111–133). Sudbury, MA: Jones & Bartlett.

Benner, P., Tanner, C. A., & Chesla, C. A., (Eds.). (1996). *Expertise in nursing practice: Caring, clinical judgment, and ethics.* New York: Springer.

Brookfield, S. D. (1987). *Developing critical thinkers: Challenging adults to explore alternative ways of thinking and acting.* San Francisco: Jossey-Bass.

Brookfield, S. D. (1995). *Becoming a critically reflective teacher.* San Francisco: Jossey-Bass.

Bucknall, T. (2003). The clinical landscape of critical care: nurses' decision-making. *Journal of Advanced Nursing, 43,* 310–319.

Carpenito, L. (2002). *Nursing diagnosis application to clinical practice,* (9th ed.). Philadelphia: Lippincott Williams & Wilkins.

Christensen, P. J., & Kenney, J. W. (1995). *Nursing process: Application of conceptual models* (4th ed.). St. Louis: Mosby-Year Book.

Dauer, E. W. (1989). *Critical thinking: An introduction to reasoning.* New York: Barnes & Noble Books and Noble Books in cooperation with Oxford University Press.

Facione, N. C., Facione, P. A., & Sanchez, C. A. (1994). Critical thinking disposition as a measure of competent clinical judgment: The development of the California Critical Thinking Disposition Inventory. *Journal of Nursing Education, 33,* 345–350.

Facione, P. A., Facione, N. C., & Giancarlo, C. A. (1996). *The California Critical Thinking Disposition Inventory test manual.* Millbrae, CA: California Academic Press.

Gordon, M. (1995). *Manual of nursing diagnosis, 1995–1996.* St. Louis: Mosby-Year Book.

Henderson, V. (1987). Nursing process: A critique. *Holistic Nursing Practice, 1,* 7–18.

Johnson, M., Maas, M., & Moorhead, S. (2000). *Nursing outcomes classification* (NOC) (2nd ed.). St. Louis: Mosby.

Kataoka-Yahiro, M., & Saylor, C. (1994). A critical thinking model for nursing judgment. *Journal of Nursing Education, 33,* 351–356.

Kennedy, M., Fisher, M. B., & Ennis, R. H. (1991). Critical thinking: Literature review and needed research. In L. Idol & B. F. Jones (Eds.), *Educational values and cognitive instruction: Implications for reform.* Hinsdale, NJ: Lawrence Erlbaum.

King, I. M. (1995). The theory of goal attainment. In M. A. Frey & C. L. Sieloff (Eds.), *Advancing King's systems framework and theory of nursing* (pp. 23–32). Thousand Oaks, CA: Sage.

Kurfiss, J. (1988). *Critical thinking theory, research, practice and possibilities.* Washington, DC: Association for the Study of Higher Education.

Leddy, S. (2004). Human energy: a conceptual model of unitary nursing science. *Visions: The Journal of Rogerian Scholarship, 12,* 14–28.

Lindsey, E., & Hartrick, G. (1996). Health-promoting nursing practice: The demise of the nursing process? *Journal of Advanced Nursing, 23,* 106–112.

Malinski, V. M. (1986). *Explorations on Martha Rogers' science of unitary human beings.* Norwalk, CT: Appleton-Century-Crofts.

Martin, P. A., Dugan, J., Freundl, M., Miller, S. E., Phillips, R., & Sharritts, L. (1994). Nurses' attitudes toward nursing process as measured by the Dayton Attitude Scale. *Journal of Continuing Education for Nurses, 25,* 35–40.

Maynard, C. A. (1996). Relationship of critical thinking ability to professional nursing competence. *Journal of Nursing Education, 35,* 12–18.

McCloskey, J., & Bulechek, G. (2000). *Nursing interventions classification (NIC)* (3rd ed.). St. Louis: Mosby.

McPeck, J. E. (1981). *Critical thining and education.* New York: St. Martin's Press.

Mishlove, J. (1994). Intuition: The source of true knowing. *Noetic Sciences Review, 29,* 31–36.

National League for Nursing Accrediting Commission. (2000). *Standards for the accreditation of baccalaureate and higher degree nursing programs.* New York: Author.

Neuman, B., & Fawcett, J. (2002). *The Neuman systems model,* (4th ed.). Upper Saddle River, NJ: Prentice-Hall.

Newman, M. A. (1994). *Health as expanding consciousness* (2nd ed.). St. Louis: Mosby.

Parse, R. R. (1996). The human becoming theory: Challenges in practice and research. *Nursing Science Quarterly, 9,* 55–60.

Paterson, J. G., & Zderad, L. T. (1988). *Humanistic nursing.* New York: National League for Nursing.

Paul, R. (1983). *Critical thinking: What every person needs to survive in a rapidly changing world* (3rd ed.). Santa Rosa, CA: Foundation for Critical Thinking.

PEW Health Professions Commission (1998). *Recreating health professional practice for a new century.* San Francisco: University of California, San Francisco Center for the Health Professions.

Polge, J. (1995). Critical thinking: The use of intuition in making clinical nursing judgments. *Journal of the New York State Nurses Association, 26,* 4–9.

Radwin, L. E. (1995). Knowing the patient: A process model for individualized interventions. *Nursing Research, 44,* 364–370.

Reed, P. G. (1996). Peplau's interpersonal relations model. In J. J. Fitzpatrick & A. L. Whall (Eds.), *Conceptual models of nursing: Analysis and application* (3rd ed., pp. 55–76). Stamford, CT: Appleton & Lange.

Rew, L. (1996). *Awareness in healing.* Albany, NY: Delmar.

Rogers, M. E. (1988). Nursing science and art: A prospective. *Nursing Science Quarterly, 1,* 99–102.

Rogers, M. E. (1992). Nursing science and the space age. *Nursing Science Quarterly, 5,* 27–34.

Roy, C., & Andrews, H. A. (1999). *The Roy adaptation model* (2nd ed.). Stamford, CT: Appleton & Lange.

Scheffer, B. K., & Rubenfeld, M. G. (2000). A consensus statement on critical thinking in nursing. *Journal of Nursing Education, 39,* 352–359.

Schon, D. A. (1987). *Educating the reflective practitioner: Toward a new design for teaching and learning in the professions.* San Francisco: Jossey-Bass.

Tanner, C. A., Benner, P., Chesla, C., & Gordon, D. R. (1993). The phenomenology of knowing the patient. *Image, 25,* 273–280.

Varcoe, C. (1996). Disparagement of the nursing process: The new dogma? *Journal of Advanced Nursing, 23,* 120–125.

Watson, J. M., & Glaser, E. M. (1990). *The Watson-Glaser Critical Thinking Appraisal Manual.* San Antonio, TX: The Psychological Corp., Harcourt, Brace Jovanovich, Inc.

Young, C. E. (1987). Intuition and nursing process. *Holistic Nursing Practice, 1,* 52–62.

# Professional Communication to Establish Helping and Healing Relationships

## KEY TERMS AND CONCEPTS

Helping Relationships
Communication
Metacommunication
Verbal Communication
Nonverbal Communication
Interpretation
Perception
Collaborative Relationships
Principles of Communication
Nurses as Helpers
Stages of the Nurse–Client Relationship
Mutuality
Anxiety
Caring Interaction
Noncaring Behaviors
Healing Relationships
Professional Partnerships

## LEARNING OUTCOMES

By the end of this chapter, the learner will be able to:

1 Explain why communication is an essential element of professional nursing.
2 Outline major purposes of communication.
3 Discuss principles to establish helpfulness in nurse–client communication.
4 Outline the stages of nurse–client relationship development.
5 Outline outcomes of mutuality in helping relationships.
6 Differentiate therapeutic from nontherapeutic relationships.
7 Discuss how nurses use relationships to promote client healing.
8 Explain how health team members can develop meaningful professional partnerships.

## VIGNETTE

Margie, an emergency department nurse, has just arrived at work. As she finishes receiving reports and her assignment to be the triage nurse, a middle-aged man with severe chest pain and dyspnea arrives with his family. Margie gets immediate help for the man, who is rushed to the cardiac catheterization laboratory. Margie notices that the family members seem very anxious and distressed. When she asks them if they would like anything, they reply "no", but the wife tries to hold back tears as she wrings her hands, the daughter's hands shake, and the son paces. Margie notes that the nonverbal behavior of the family is incongruent with the verbal message and wonders what would be the best course of action to help this distressed family.

The long-supported axiom of the helping professions—that behavioral change occurs by way of emotional experience—serves as the basis for emphasizing communication in nursing practice. The human need for relatedness binds people together, and communication serves as the exchange medium in these relationships. The verbal and nonverbal messages exchanged during human relationships determine the structure and function of feelings. Indeed, the whole existence and the health status of human beings depend on communication because the affective dimension of life cannot be separated from the biologic or spiritual dimensions.

## ● COMMUNICATION AS INTERACTION

Nurses and clients rely on communication during nurse–client interactions. Without communication, nurses cannot effectively use nursing process to provide safe, effective client care.

### The Interpersonal Component of Professional Nursing

Effective use of nursing process requires that nurses and clients communicate with each other. When nurses and clients interact, they experience emotions as they communicate. Nurses strive to maximize the client's potential for optimal health. To live out this commitment, nurses must clearly understand the power of communication in shaping professional relationships. Without well-refined communication skills, nurses cannot establish therapeutic relationships with clients. Thus, the quality of communication between the nurse and the client is an essential determinant of the success of the professional relationship. Mutual goals cannot be defined or achieved in the relationship without effective communication that positively influences the emotions of both the client and the nurse. This chapter focuses on communication as the interpersonal component of the nursing process and the essential component of **helping relationships.**

Assuming that humans possess all the characteristics of an open system, the nurse concludes that people are influenced by and influence all human beings with whom they are associated. Indeed, this reciprocal process suggests that the most important human attributes are not only openness to interpersonal experiences but also power to influence self and others. Sullivan (1953, p. 32) assumes that "everyone is more simply human than otherwise."

Human beings influence others primarily through communication. **Communication** is described as the "exchange of meanings between and among individuals through a shared system of symbols that have the same meaning for both the sender and the receiver of the message" (Vestal, 1995, p. 51). Through communication during nursing interactions with a client, the nurse hopes to create new client attitudes and situations that will influence the client to live in a healthier manner. This goal can be achieved only if the nurse is knowledgeable about the content and process of the nurse–client relationship.

To understand content in nursing situations, the nurse must have knowledge of the person as a human system interacting with the environment and striving for health, and of specific factors that promote positive change in human systems. To understand the process in the nurse–client relationship, the nurse must have knowledge of communication and experience in developing helping relationships. Thus, to participate effectively in nurse–client relationships, intradisciplinary or interdisciplinary relationships, and personal relationships, the nurse must understand the structure and the functions of communication.

Nursing, as an organized body of professionals, has not always been successful in portraying an image of being an autonomous professional discipline. Disagreement among nursing theorists, practitioners, and educators about the purpose and meaning of nursing and key concepts such as nursing diagnosis has led to multiple, and sometimes conflicting, images of nursing. Currently, nurses generally agree that contemporary nursing practice addresses the client holistically to address the full range of human responses and illness. Nurses also agree that assessment of objective and subjective factors related to client health is essential. They concur that that evidence (scientific, intuitive, or mystical) may be used to guide practice. Finally, most nurses in practice acknowledge that the importance in establishing authentic, caring relationships with clients is essential to promote health and healing.

Nursing's unique service to society consists of dealing with human responses in health and illness. These responses are the substance of communication. Thus, professional nursing's business is communication and the purposeful use of communication in nurse–client relationships. The relationship should be "characterized by compassion, continuity, and respect for the client's choice. The focus is on the process: the process of the client–environment interaction and the process of the nurse–client relationship" (Newman, Lamb, & Michaels, 1991, p. 406).

## The Structure of Communication

Human communication not only conveys information and influences another throughout a relationship, but "communication is the relationship" (Sundeen, Stuart, Rankin, & Cohen, 1994, p. 94). It is the dynamic interaction between two or more persons in which ideas, goals, beliefs and values, feelings, and feelings about feelings are exchanged. Experiencing even a minute communication exchange affects change in all parties in the communication process.

Communication is defined only in the context of process. Because human beings are continually and irrevocably exchanging energy with the environment, and life is continually being repatterned, it can be assumed that the individual human being reflects only dynamic actions. Each person is always affected by others and is always affecting others. One constantly communicates, thereby generating change in others and experiencing change in self.

Although communication is a dynamic process, it is possible to identify components and to analyze the interrelationships among the components. Berlo (1960), a noted authority on communications, traced the various models of communication from Aristotle to the 1960s. Aristotle identified the related components as the speaker, the speech, and the audience. After analyzing behavioral science research and several points of view, Berlo (pp. 30–32) postulated a communication model that is generally accepted today.

1. An (interpersonal) source: some person(s) with ideas, needs, intentions, information, and a reason for communicating.
2. A message: a coded, systematic set of symbols representing ideas, purposes, intentions, and feelings.

3. An encoder: the mechanism for expressing or translating the purpose of the communication into the message (in human beings, these are the motor mechanisms—the vocal mechanism for oral messages, the muscles of the hands for written messages, and the muscle systems elsewhere in the body for gestures).
4. A channel: the medium for carrying the message.
5. A decoder: the mechanism for translating the message into a form that the recipient can use (in human beings, the sensory receptor mechanisms).
6. A receiver: the target or recipient of the message.

In this model, the transmission of meaning occurs via a dynamic process in which

1. A person has an intention or purpose (the communication source).
2. The purpose is translated into a communicable form by the person's set of motor mechanisms and skills (encoder).
3. The message is transmitted through a channel.
4. The message is translated into receivable form by the recipient's sensory mechanisms and skills (decoder).
5. The recipient receives the message (the communication receiver).

Since this model was postulated, system theorists have further explained the reciprocal relationship between the participants in the communication process. At any time, the individual person is both an active initiator and a recipient of meanings in an interpersonal situation. Thus, it is important for nurses to understand that they are simultaneously acting and reacting by using nursing processes and that clients' meanings have an equal effect on the outcome of purposeful relationships. The process just described has been labeled "transactional."

The dynamic nature of the communication process dictates the need for the nurse to evaluate his or her actions and reactions when using the nursing process with a client. Without such awareness and evaluation, the professional will be less likely to experience successful communication with the feeling of satisfaction associated with transmitting clear meanings and the validation that the message intended was the message received. Validation of meanings is essential to achieving any therapeutic goals in helping relationships.

## Functions and Types of Communication

Synthesizing from several communication models, Ceccio and Ceccio (1982) propose four major purposes of communication: to inquire, inform, persuade, and entertain. The nurse may attempt to achieve any of these purposes with clients, the health care delivery system, peers, interdisciplinary team members, and even the self. In attempts to achieve one or more of these purposes, the nurse transmits messages.

People transmit messages verbally and nonverbally. In addition, implicit in all models of communication is the concept that communication has two interacting components:

1. The content value of the message.
2. The interactional or perceptual value of the message and its participants.

The informational aspect of the message, the content value, is expressed in verbal or nonverbal forms. The interactional or perceptual value of the message (referred to as

**"metacommunication"**) identifies how the participants interpret content and how they perceive the interpersonal relationship. Metacommunication may be expressed in verbal and nonverbal forms.

## Verbal Communication

**Verbal communication** consists of the spoken word. Verbal communication requires functional physiologic and cognitive mechanisms that produce, recognize, and receive speech. Although a major influence, specific words are not the greatest influences on communication. Nonverbal communication may override verbal communication. Language comprises an elaborate system of symbols. Words symbolize actual objects or concepts. Lack of congruence in language between the nurse and the client usually interferes with initiating relationships and creates obstacles to validation of meanings—the essential characteristic of an effective message.

Two primary influences on verbal communications are developmental age and cultural heritage. Developmental age affects verbal abilities through the person's physiologic ability to change sounds into words and the cognitive ability to symbolize through language. Through the process of acculturation, the person develops culture-based variations from others in defining meanings for words. Although denotative meanings are equal among different persons (i.e., the concrete representations of words are the same), connotative meanings often vary among persons of different cultures and their accompanying acculturation.

Three types of problems with which the nurse needs to be concerned are associated with words being symbols of communication (Ceccio & Ceccio, 1982):

1. The technical problem: How accurately can one transmit the symbols of communication?
2. The semantic problem: How precise are the symbols in transmitting the intended message?
3. The influential problem: How effectively does the received meaning affect conduct?

The verbal content of communication can be used to evaluate the content theme of the communication process. If one evaluates the seemingly varied topics of discussion, the words that underlie or link together several ideas will reflect the "what" (or content) of the communication.

## Nonverbal Communication

Nonverbal communication usually exerts more influence on communication than the words said. **Nonverbal communication** consists of all forms of communication that do not involve the spoken or written word. Perception of nonverbal communication involves all the senses, especially hearing, that are used for the perception of verbal messages. Kinesics (facial expressions, gaze, gestures, and all body movements that are not specific signs), objects (all intentional and unintentional display of material things), and proxemics (the use of space) are powerful nonverbal messages perceived by the senses (Northouse & Northouse, 1998).

Besides receiving verbal messages, Sundeen and colleagues (1994) identify the additional purposes of nonverbal communication: expressing emotion and interpersonal attitudes; establishing, developing, and maintaining social relationships; presenting the self; engaging in rituals; and supporting verbal communication (p. 99).

The tactile senses represent the most primitive sensory process developed by humans. Bonding between the infant and the parent figure (important to infant development) occurs largely through nonverbal tactile communication. Touch remains a powerful communication tool throughout life.

Deprivation of tactile stimulation in infancy may impair the achievement of some developmental tasks. The young child orients himself or herself to space through touch. As the child develops into the adult, touch as nonverbal communication takes on specific cultural meanings.

Nurses must understand taboos concerning touch and distance if they desire to be purposeful in nonverbal and verbal communication. For example, to one person, a touch on the knee might mean concern, whereas to another it may be interpreted as seduction. Used sensitively at the proper time and within the context of the client's culture, touch is a powerful nonverbal tool for the nurse.

All the sensory processes become powerful components of the communication process as human beings exchange nonverbal and verbal messages with others throughout life. For example, the olfactory (smell) and gustatory (taste) senses make it possible for the person to distinguish pleasant from not-so-pleasant odors and tastes. When persons have adequate smelling and tasting capacities, odor and taste become significant nonverbal messages in the communication process. The nurse needs to manipulate the health care environment to control odors.

The sense of hearing the spoken word also has a nonverbal component: that of interpreting the qualities of the voice. Hunsaker and Alessandra (1980) identify the following voice qualities as strong determinants of effective communication: resonance, the intensity with which the voice fills the environmental space; rhythm, the flow, pace, and movement of the voice; speed, how fast the voice is used; pitch, the highness or lowness of the voice that relates to the tightening of the vocal cords; volume or loudness; inflection, the change in pitch or volume of voice; and clarity, the articulation and enunciation capacity of the voice.

People move during communication and these motor or kinesic actions are perhaps most often performed with little or no awareness. Body movements are largely determined through socialization. Developed in a particular psychosocial and cultural setting, motor actions vary according to gender, socioeconomic status, age, and ethnic background. Misinterpretations of culturally variable kinesic behaviors produce barriers to effective communication. For example, eye motions involved with eye contact communicate culturally specific messages. If the nurse and client assign different meanings to this nonverbal communication, the effectiveness of the nurse–client relationship is likely to be reduced.

Hunsaker and Alessandra (1980) suggest that 90% of meaning comes from nonverbal communication; thus, nonverbal behavior has a significant impact on the recipient of the communicated message. Therefore, nonverbal behavior has great significance for nurses as they engage in all professional nursing roles, especially leadership roles. It conveys the greatest meaning to persons involved in leadership processes. For example, the following motor actions (which are commonly observed) may be highly influential in the communication process (Hunsaker & Alessandra):

1. Gently rubbing behind the ear with the index finger—interpreted as doubt.
2. Casually rubbing the eye with one finger—interpreted as the recipient in the communication process does not understand what is being communicated.

3. Cupping hands over the mouth—interpreted that the gesturer is trying to hide something.
4. Leaning back with both hands supporting the head—interpreted as confidence or superiority.
5. Pinching the bridge of the nose with eyes closed—interpreted as thoughtful evaluation.
6. Moving eyeglasses to the lower bridge of the nose and peering over them—interpreted as a powerful negative evaluation.

Kinesics, the meaning of motor actions, and proxemics, or the function of space in nonverbal communication, also play important roles in all aspects of life. Space is a constant. It may be perceived either as surrounding persons or as existing between them. Nurses must strive purposefully for congruence among their own nonverbal behaviors and the verbal communications they intend to convey. In addition, nurses must recognize that culture affects all aspects of nonverbal communication (Leininger & McFarland, 2002). For example:

- Proximity/spacing. Persons from various cultures define appropriate personal space differently. For example, Americans prefer more personal space (6 inches to 4 feet) than Latin Americans. Nurses must abide by client preferences for personal space to facilitate effective communication.
- Touching. Any physical contact or touching that is part of an individual's communication style can create problems or discomfort for people from many cultures. Nurses need not abandon hands on a shoulder or arm to show support and caring. Rather, clients should feel empowered to tell the nurse if such touching makes them feel uncomfortable.
- Gestures. People from some cultures may be more animated than others, using gestures and body language to communicate their message. In addition, gestures that have a positive meaning in one culture may be insulting and rude in another.
- Eye contact. Traditionally, Americans have valued direct eye contact as a sign of confidence and respect, whereas not making eye contact has negative connotations. However, in many cultures, making eye contact with an authority figure is considered an insult.
- Use of silence. People from some cultures prefer active verbal interaction and are uncomfortable with silence. Other cultures may value periods of contemplative silence, leading to the potential for misunderstanding of communication style and motivation.
- Body language. The body is one of the more subtle ways people communicate meaning and sincerity. The nurse may say all the right things but communicate tension through body language.

With an awareness of what a client perceives as acceptable use of space and how body position and direction affect the meaning of the relationship, the nurse can manipulate personal and environmental space for the benefit of the client during clinical practice.

### Metacommunication
Occurring on both verbal and nonverbal levels, metacommunication represents an integrative level that defines the "what," the "who," and the relationship between the "what" and the "who" of the communication process. Because this level of communication is

influential in determining the effectiveness of relationships, the nurse must evaluate communication in terms of its context and the relationships among its parts. Understanding themes of the relationship helps the nurse evaluate the metacommunication occurring in the nursing process. The nurse searches for the content theme (the central underlying idea or links), the mood theme (the emotion communicated—the how of the message), and the interaction theme (the dynamics between the communicating participants).

Knowing that change occurs more readily and more effectively if congruence exists between the verbal and nonverbal components of communication, the nurse must be alert to indicators of the degree of agreement on the meaning of the content and on the process of the relationship. When a discrepancy arises between verbal and nonverbal components, the nonverbal component usually is the more accurate indicator. However, nonverbal behavior is more open to subjective meaning and variations; thus, it must be verbally validated. This validation process plays an important part in effectively using metacommunication in the nursing process.

## Interpretation and Perception

The capacity for **interpretation** makes communication between humans possible. When engaged in interpretation, persons assign meaning to the interpersonal interaction. Interpretation involves perception, symbolization, memory, and thinking. Perhaps the most important of these is perception, the basic component after which the others follow. Taylor (1977) defines **perception** as the selection and organization of sensations so that they are meaningful. Taylor proposes that humans learn perceptions and that what they learn depends on socialization experiences. Perceptual expectations are influenced by emotions, language, and attitude, and vary widely from one individual to another. Thus, one's interpretation ability highly depends on individual perceptual ability.

Factors affecting perception in the nurse–client relationship are the capacity for attention (reception of sensations) by both the nurse and client, the perspective each brings to the relationship, and the physical condition of the receptors. Anxiety (the actual or anticipated negative appraisal by the other) in the nurse or the client limits the ability to be attentive in the communication process, interferes with the validation of individual perspectives, and decreases physical capacities. Therefore, anxiety must be controlled in the nurse–client relationship. Validated perceptions between nurse and client are essential to goal setting and achievement. The nurse must constantly be aware of the power and influence of perception on the outcomes of a communication, regardless of its form.

## Self-Concept and Interpersonal Relationships

The relationships among participants greatly affect communication. The self-concept of each participant largely determines the nurse–client relationship. Clients receiving care from a nurse with low self-esteem will question the nurse's competence and actions more frequently. Whereas, clients will feel more comfortable when receiving care from a confident, self-assured nurse.

According to Brill (1990, p. vii), "In dealing with people it is essential that workers possess awareness of themselves, their own needs, the ways in which they satisfy these needs, the ways in which they use themselves in relationship with others." In addition to self-awareness, other factors involved in the self-concept are essential to effective communication:

- Ability to share with individuals (a function of achievement of interpersonal developmental tasks).
- Ability to establish, maintain, and terminate the kind of relationship in which one is comfortable (a function of the human need to perpetuate a personal self-concept).
- Ability to share power (a reflection of the person's view of self and others).

If the major reason for nurses' communication with clients is to influence clients toward better health, nurses must develop concepts of self that are most effective in facilitating the potential of the client for growth. These concepts include an awareness of one's perceptions of and feelings about self; the ability to derive satisfaction by sharing with the client the responsibility for the nurse–client relationship; the ability to view the self as the therapeutic tool for implementing the nursing process; and an appreciation of the value of shared power in activities directed toward change.

### Questions for Reflection 7-1

1. When I see nonverbal behavior not matching verbal messages of clients, what do I do? Why is it important to act when I see this incongruence?
2. How do I come across as a professional nurse? (you may have to ask a colleague for the answer to this one; it may surprise you) Why is it important to know how others perceive me as a professional nurse?

## Principles of Communication in Collaborative Relationships

When engaged in communication with clients, nurses empathize with, demonstrate respect for, and respond genuinely to them. When nurses and clients equally share the responsibility and authority for steps of the nursing process, they enter into **collaborative relationships.** Collaborative relationships promote client sharing of essential information as the nurse performs a health assessment. During diagnosis, the nurse must verify conclusions with the client so that accurate conclusions based on client data related to human response have been drawn. The nurse and client work together to plan and implement nursing care. Finally, the client reports success or failure of nursing interventions or proposes alternative courses of action during evaluation. Collaboration of this magnitude cannot occur without presence, empathy, respect, and genuineness. Presence, empathy, and respect are **principles of communication** that facilitate collaboration.

### Presence

Presence is an important part of several nursing conceptual models, including those of Parse (1996), Paterson and Zderad (1988), and Watson (1996). "The core element in presence is 'being there'. . . . It is described as a gift of self and is equated with a use of self that is conveyed through open and giving behaviors of the nurse" (Osterman & Schwartz-Barcott, 1996, p. 24). Characteristics of four ways of "being there" are described in Table 7-1. These ways "reflect degrees of intensity in the context of another" (Osterman & Schwartz-Barcott, p. 29).

TABLE 7-1

## Presence: Characteristics of Four Ways of Being There

| Characteristics of Presence | Presence | Partial Presence | Full Presence | Transcendent Presence |
|---|---|---|---|---|
| Quality of being there | Physically present in context of another | Physically present in context of another | Physically present (there) (physical attending behavior —eye contact, leaning toward) Psychologically (present with) (attentive listening behavior) | Physically present Psychologically present (metaphysical beliefs) Holistic |
| Focus of energy | Self-absorbed<br><br>Personal, subjective reality | Objects or tasks in environment, relevant to the other individual but none of the energy is directed at the other<br>Mechanical/ technical reality | Self/Other (focusing on another influences response—reciprocal)<br><br>Present oriented (here and now)—anchoring in present reality | Centered (drawing from universal energy) Subject/subject— leads to oneness<br>Transcending and oriented beyond here and now—sustaining while transforming reality |
| Nature of interaction | No interaction; self-absorbed, intra-personal encounter | Interaction with part of other encounter | Interactive; essential communication; boundaries— role constraints; professional relationship; dyad caring | Relationship; high degree of skilled communi-cation; role free; human intimacy/love; humanistic caring, no boundaries, monad relationship; |
| Positive outcomes | Reduces stress; reassurance that someone is there; may be quieting and restorative; facilitates creative thinking | Reduces stress; solving a mech-anical problem; reduces amount of stimuli in an encounter | Solving of a human problem; relief of a here-and-now distress | Transformations decreased loneliness expansion of con-sciousness; spiritual peace, hope and meaning in one's existence (love/ connectedness); nice feeling generated in the environment; transpersonal (oneness) |
| Negative outcomes | No interpersonal engagement— missed communi-cation; isolation, withdrawn, increased anxiety | Not interpersonal connectedness | May be too much energy for recipient or feel negative to a recipient; energy not always available for full presence; increased anxiety | Fusion and possible loss of objective reality; danger of taking on recipient's problems |

*Source:* Osterman, P., & Schwartz-Barcott, D. (1996). Presence: Four ways of being there. *Nursing Forum, 31,* 25. Used with permission of the publisher.

By synthesizing these theoretical conceptions of presence, the nurse focuses all her energy on a client when being with the client. The nurse can be present without speaking. Clients and nurses engaged in true presence during an encounter describe an experience that cannot be effectively captured with words. In my experience, presence with a client results in a deep, personal connection for both participants with possible resultant personal transformations. Presence is integrally related to genuineness and a necessary antecedent to empathy.

## Questions for Reflection 7-2

1. Why is it important for me to be truly present with clients?
2. What factors in my clinical practice setting prevent me from being truly present with clients?
3. How could I proceed with changing the clinical practice setting?

### Empathy

Empathy, the ability to understand, sense, share, and accept the feelings of another enables the nurse to develop helping relationships with clients. Therapeutic helping relationships focus on change. Understanding the potential impact of change on clients enables the nurse to identify obstacles for clients to change behaviors and attitudes. When using an empathetic approach, the nurse becomes more tolerant of behaviors, attitudes, and values that differ and could impede progress toward goal attainment. Empathy is defined as "the art of communicating to others that we have understanding [of] how they are feeling and what makes them feel that way" (Keegan, 1994, p. 127). Wiseman (1996, p. 1165) identifies four defining attributes of empathy: seeing the world as others see it, being nonjudgmental, understanding another's feelings, and communicating the understanding.

Nurses possessing empathy show awareness of the uniqueness and individuality of clients. They listen and respond as clients share feelings and concerns. They care about clients as sentient beings like themselves. If clients perceive that nurses care about them and how they feel, the benefits include (Keegan, 1994):

- More trusting relationships with open communication.
- Increased feelings of being connected to another.
- Enhanced client and nurse self-esteem.
- Genuine acceptance of others just as they are.
- Increased self-awareness for both the nurse and the client.
- Increased self-caring and less self-criticism on the part of the client.

To be truly empathic, **nurses as helpers** have to listen so carefully so that they can act as intended, perceive and accept the inner feelings and experiences of clients as the clients experience them, and paraphrase feelings, ideas, and intentions accurately. Two essential actions are necessary for a nurse to develop empathy:

1. Awareness and acceptance of self as a feeling person open to one's experiences.
2. Ability to listen to each message of the client, to identify the client's feelings associated with it, and to respond to those feelings.

Thus, empathy involves far more than the cognitive or thinking part of the self. It involves the acceptance that we are feeling beings, commonly experiencing multiple emotions simultaneously. In effective communication, the nurse and the client know that the nurse perceives and accepts the client's feelings.

## Respect

Respect is feeling or showing deferential regard or esteem (*American Heritage Dictionary of the English Language*, 1992, p. 1536). Respect is the nonpossessive caring for and affirmation of another's personhood as a separate individual. Respect builds self-esteem and positive self-image. In the nurse–client relationship, respect is demonstrated by equality, mutuality, and shared thinking

Certain behaviors display respect toward others. Nurses act respectfully toward clients when they look directly at them when providing care; give them full undivided attention; maintain eye contact if culturally appropriate, smile appropriately, determine how each client wants to be addressed, call clients by name, introduce themselves to clients, and make physical contact such as a handshake or gentle touch. Clients who are members of a cultural group unlike that of the nurse may have special needs for respect and sometimes the aforementioned actions should be avoided because they conflict with cultural norms and values (Leininger & McFarland, 2002).

According to Bradley and Edinberg (1990, p. 226), nurses may be "viewed as being powerful, one-up, and, if from a different racial group, nonempathic. . . . In addition, it can be the nurses who view the clients as powerless, one-down, and different." Respecting the client's dignity is critical to therapeutic communication, "even when the client is in dire social, economic, or health circumstances" (Bradley & Edinberg, p. 226). Respect toward the client facilitates the development of effective helping relationships.

## Genuineness

Genuineness is the state of being real, honest, and sincere. Clients readily detect dishonesty and insincerity when interacting with health care providers. Frequently, genuineness is used synonymously with authenticity.

When defining authenticity, phrases such as "being actually and precisely what is claimed," "genuine," "good faith," and "sincere" are used. Genuine nurses display their real selves to clients. They do not let themselves become distorted or different because of thought or emotions. Genuine nurses act from their hearts and do not need to rehearse or contrive actions. In previous times, nurses were expected to be neutral to attain and maintain a helping relationship (Rogers, 1951). However, neutral behavior often seems depersonalized and sends messages of ambiguity. Ambiguous messages may cause client anxiety because clients may not understand their roles or positions in a relationship.

Nurses take risks to be genuine because it frequently involves expressing negative thoughts and confronting others. However, there may be even more risk when incongruence surfaces between nurse intentions and behaviors. When clients detect incongruence in the nurse–client relationship, feelings of distrust, confusion, and suspicion may arise. Clients may begin to question the credibility of the nurse and the value of the health information being shared. They may only believe the nonverbal messages sent and discount the verbal ones. Finally, therapeutic rapport erodes if clients believe that the nurse is attempting to impress them rather than connect with them.

When a nurse is genuine, action occurs spontaneously. "Being real does not mean being overly familiar"; what the client wants "is an emotionally available, calm, caring proficient resource that can protect, care about, and above all, listen to him or her" (Arnold & Boggs, 1989, p. 439).

Internalizing the principles of empathy, respect, and genuineness makes it possible for the nurse to demonstrate these behaviors and experience satisfaction in professional nursing practice. These principles also help nurses to establish healthy, helping relationships with clients and their significant others.

## ⬤ HELPING RELATIONSHIPS: THE NURSE AS HELPER

The nurse–client relationship is a special helping relationship. Nurses tailor this private, platonic relationship to fit the needs of individual clients. The nurse–client relationship has the power to transform the lives of both the client and the nurse. Because the nurse has specialized knowledge and expertise to serve humanity, the nurse assumes the role as helper.

Rogers (1958) set the following essential conditions of a helping relationship, which are applicable to professional nursing.

1. The individual is capable of and expected to be responsible for himself.
2. Each individual (nurse and client) has a strong drive to become mature and to be socially responsible.
3. The climate of the helping relationship is warm and permits the expression of both positive and negative feelings.
4. Limits, mutually agreed on, are set on behavior only, not on attitudes.
5. The helper communicates understanding and acceptance.

The characteristics of helping as developed by Rogers have positively influenced many health professionals and serve as criteria for nurses as they develop effective helping relationships.

The nurse bears the responsibility to fulfill a helper role, regardless of the specific parameters and purposes of each relationship. The nurse must validate that the client knows why help was sought. The nurse also assumes that both the client and nurse will share the responsibility for the outcomes of the nursing encounter. The helping role is viewed as a facilitative one, in which the nurse uses self and expertise as therapeutic tools to assist the client to overcome threats to health and well-being or obtain optimal health.

The nurse and client bring unique talents, skills, and characteristics that affect the development of a helping relationship. The nurse uses client strengths to facilitate the helping relationship. Table 7-2 displays what the client and the nurse bring to their relationship (Benner, 1984; Northouse & Northouse, 1998; Riley, 2000). When the client is confused or unresponsive, the client's significant others (such as family members, close friends, or those having durable power of attorney) bring these attributes into the therapeutic relationship. At times, as the nurse delivers physical care to the client, efforts are made to fulfill the psychosocial and spiritual needs of the client's significant others.

TABLE 7-2

## Interchange of Knowledge, Attitudes, and Skills Between Client and Nurse in the Helping Relationship

| What the Client Brings to the Client–Nurse Relationship | What the Nurse Brings to the Client–Nurse Relationship |
| --- | --- |
| **Cognitive** | **Cognitive** |
| • Individual ways of perceiving the world | • Individual ways of perceiving the world |
| • Preferred ways of making judgments | • Preferred ways of making judgments |
| • Knowledge and beliefs about health and illness in general | • Knowledge and beliefs about health and illness in general |
| • Specific knowledge related to current health status of illness in general and of the current illness in particular | • Knowledge about his/her clinical specialty |
| • Knowledge and beliefs about health promotion and maintenance in general and information about own health care routines and activities | • Knowledge about what should help this particular client |
| • Ability to solve problems and knowledge of preferred methods of doing so | • Knowledge and beliefs about health behaviors that prevent illness and promote, regain, and maintain health |
| • Ability to learn | • Ability to solve problems and knowledge of preferred methods of doing so while using nursing cognitive and clinical skills |
| • Preferred ways to learn based on individualized learning style | • Knowledge about factors that increase client compliance with treatment regimens |
| • Preferred communication patterns | • Expectations of client based on previous encounters with other clients |
| • Knowledge of how current health affects role responsibilities | • Knowledge of available resources to assist client with this particular health problem |
| • Expectations of encounter with this nurse based on previous encounters with nurses | • Ability to perceive if help is needed for effective nursing management of client health problem |
| **Affective** | **Affective** |
| • Cultural and spiritual values | • Cultural and spiritual values |
| • Self-perceptions | • Professional nursing values |
| • Feelings about seeking help from a nurse | • Self-perceptions |
| • Attitudes toward nurses in general | • Feelings about being a nurse–helper |
| • Attitudes related to previous encounters with nurses | • Attitudes toward clients in general |
| • Attitudes toward previous and currently prescribed treatment regimens | • Attitudes toward this particular client system |
| • Values regarding illness prevention | • Intuitive feelings about the client system |
| • Attitude of either being willing to or fighting actions to take the required measures to improve health status at this time with this particular nurse | • Biases about nursing treatment regimens |
| | • Values placed on being healthy |
| | • Values placed on people actively preventing illness or enhancing well-being |
| | • Willingness to help client take positive action to improve his/her well-being |
| • Personal meaning of current health status and encounter with this nurse | • Personal meaning of current client encounter |

*(continued)*

## Interchange of Knowledge, Attitudes, and Skills Between Client and Nurse in the Helping Relationship (Continued)

| What the Client Brings to the Client–Nurse Relationship | What the Nurse Brings to the Client–Nurse Relationship |
|---|---|
| **Psychomotor[a]** | **Psychomotor** |
| • Ability to relate and communicate with others<br>• Ability to carry out own health care management<br>• Ability to learn new methods of self-care | • Ability to relate and communicate with others using therapeutic communication techniques<br>• Proficiency in administering general and specialized nursing interventions (in some cases the nurse has developed expertise)<br>• Ability to teach nursing interventions to client |

[a]Client may not always be capable of these if health problem has impaired cognitive or motor abilities.
Adapted from Riley, J. B. (2000). *Communications in nursing* (4th ed., p. 28). St. Louis: C.V. Mosby. Used with permission of the publisher. Additional information gathered from Benner (1984) and Northouse & Northouse (1998).

## Nature of Helping in Progressive Stages of the Nurse–Client Relationship

The nurse–client relationship evolves over time. The purposes and functions of the nurse–client relationship vary as the relationship proceeds through predictable sequential stages. Although the nurse in a helping relationship always assumes the roles of facilitator, advocate, and coordinator, specific functions and purposes evolve throughout the relationship. **Stages of the nurse–client relationship** vary according to the purpose of the helping relationship. For example, the facilitator helps the client move toward improved health. The advocate protects the client from stress inherent in the petitioner role and acts on behalf of the client in promoting access to and use of health care delivery services. The coordinator attempts to organize and articulate all the services related to meeting the client's health care needs.

The knowledge base needed to act as a helper in professional nursing was largely developed and shared by Dr. Hildegard Peplau over 50 years ago. Her book, *Interpersonal Relations in Nursing* (Peplau, 1952), presented a thorough analysis of Harry Stack Sullivan's interpersonal theory in psychiatry and gave nursing a sound conceptual model for practice. Although other nurse scholars have developed other models and changed forms of the interpersonal model, Peplau's phases of the nurse–client relationship remain applicable. Following is a brief summary of the phases and their purposes, with associated functions of the nurse in each phase.

### Peplau's Phases of the Relationship
#### Orientation Phase
The purposes of the orientation phase include:

- Introduction of nurse and client.
- Elaboration of the client's need to recognize and understand his or her difficulty and the extent of a need for help.
- Acceptance of the client's need for assistance in recognizing and planning to use services that professional personnel can offer.

- Agreement that the client will direct energies toward the mutual responsibility for defining, understanding, and meeting productively the problem at hand.
- Clarification of limitations and responsibilities in the delivery system environment.

When the nurse and the client validate understanding of the client's need for help and acceptance of resources to meet those needs, and they do so with feelings of shared responsibility and a sense of trust, they move into a new phase of the relationship.

### Identification Phase

The purposes of the identification phase include:

- Provision of the opportunity for the client to respond to the helper's offer to assist.
- Encouragement for the client to express feelings, reorient those feelings, and strengthen positive forces.
- Provision of the opportunity for the nurse and the client to clearly understand each other's preconceptions and expectations.

When the client and nurse articulate agreement that the nurse may help the client, the relationship moves to a different level. The nurse assumes responsibility and accountability to act in a helping manner. The nurse asks the client questions related to how to best help the client meet health-related goals.

### Exploitation Phase

The purposes of the exploitation phase include:

- Full utilization of the nurse–client relationship to mutually work on the solution to problems and the changes needed to improve health.
- Provision of opportunities for the client to explore earlier experiences and behaviors and to have emerging needs met.

This phase represents the working stage of the therapeutic relationship. In an ideal therapeutic relationship, the nurse and client connect and work together to help the client transcend his or her current health status (in growth models of nursing) or attain a stable state (in stability models of nursing). Nurses use a variety of resources, including client referrals to others during this stage.

### Resolution Phase

The purposes of the resolution phase include:

- Provision of opportunity to formulate new goals.
- Encouragement of gradual freeing of the client from identifying with the nurse.
- Promotion of the client's ability to act more independently.

## Other Approaches to Therapeutic Relationship Development

Since Peplau, other persons have established phases of the development of a helping therapeutic relationship. Travelbee (1966, 1971) designates five phases of the client–nurse relationship, starting with the phase of original encounter. During the original encounter, the client and nurse work to view each other as individual human beings, rather than "nurse" and "client." Once the nurse and client transcend their respective roles, they enter the phase of emerging identities, in which both perceive the other's uniqueness, value each other, and decide to make an emotional investment to begin the therapeutic relationship. Once the client and nurse have established their identities in the relationship, they enter the phase of empathy, during which they predict the behavior of each other but fail to genuinely share feelings. Travelbee proposes that after the phase of empathy, the nurse and client enter the phase of sympathy, when the nurse translates sympathy into helpful nursing actions. After the phase of sympathy is complete, the nurse and client enter the phase of rapport, in which the nurse and client enter into a personal, meaningful relationship in which they genuinely communicate deeply with each other (Travelbee, 1964, 1966, 1971). Unlike Peplau, Travelbee never addresses the need to end a helping relationship with the client.

Hames and Joseph (1980) outline the following four stages in the development of a professional helping relationship that is not specific to nursing:

Stage 1: Trust formation, in which the client trusts the nurse because of being the recipient of honesty, respect, positive regard, and empathy as the nurse displays consistent behavior.

Stage 2: Resistance, in which the client pulls away from the relationship, but the nurse continues to show concern.

Stage 3: Working, in which the client and nurse become actively involved in working together to help the client achieve health-related goals.

Stage 4: Termination, in which the client and nurse end the relationship by engaging in closure activities, such as saying good-bye, shaking hands, and extending good wishes for the future.

Northouse and Northouse (1998) designate four phases of the nurse–client relationship that differ slightly from those of Peplau and Hames and Joseph. They also propose that each phase may overlap, depending upon various contextual factors. The following summarizes the phases of the professional helping relationship as viewed by Northouse and Northouse.

1. Preparation: Before the client and nurse can establish a therapeutic relationship, both undergo a preparation phase. For the nurse, this phase involves preparing the setting and oneself for client interactions. The client prepares by making plans to actively seek assistance from a health care provider, such as making an appointment or arranging for a hospital stay.
2. Initiation: During this phase, the nurse uses a variety of therapeutic communication techniques and demonstrates genuine concern, compassion, and respect for the client. The nurse and client also clarify client needs and establish mutual agreement on expected outcomes for the professional encounter.
3. Exploration: During this phase, the client and nurse examine and work on client needs and concerns. The nurse creates an environment to foster client sharing of needs and concerns. The nurse also helps the client to manage anxiety resulting from discussion of sometimes potentially embarrassing personal issues. The nurse and client work together to outline a plan to help the client. Finally, the nurse helps the client develop new skills to learn how to live with or resolve the concern (or need) for which the client sought assistance.
4. Termination: The nurse assesses the client's ability to independently manage and cope with the health-related issue. During this phase, the nurse summarizes client issues and accomplishments. The client and nurse mutually agree upon ending the relationship.

Most of the approaches to developing a helping relationship address the need for the nurse to establish trust with clients by demonstrating the utmost respect for them. The nurse also works with the client so that a mutual plan can be established. Finally, terminating the relationship with adequate closure ends the therapeutic relationships.

Sometimes, the therapeutic relationship has permanent life-changing effects on clients. Occasionally, the nurse may encounter a former client in a social setting (shopping mall, church, or community event) or the client may return to the health care setting for a brief visit. When this happens, memories of previous encounters may surface, resulting in an affirmation of the benefits of the helping relationship.

## The Roles of the Nurse in Therapeutic Relationships

The nurse assumes various roles, depending upon the stage of therapeutic relationship development. Because the stages of therapeutic relationship overlap, the roles assumed by the nurse vary. Table 7-3 outlines roles assumed by the nurse throughout the various phases of therapeutic relationship behavior. Success of the therapeutic relationships relies on nurse consistency in demonstrating deep respect, listening intently, and affirming client thoughts, concerns, and needs throughout all phases. As the relationship unfolds, client dependence on the nurse decreases, and the professional nurse role changes primarily to one of offering support. The relationship ends when the client assumes independence, responsibility, and accountability for meeting his or her own health care needs.

During the various therapeutic relationship phases, the nurse moves back and forth in some of these roles, depending on the client's needs. The nurse uses client responses as a guide to determine which role to assume at a particular time. Role selection requires that the nurse analyze the client response, weigh the pros and cons of the best role to assume, and anticipate consequences of nursing actions. Thus, the nurse constantly assumes the role of critical thinker. However, as the client's needs are met, the nurse essentially assumes the roles that promote client independence. The following discussion outlines characteristics of the helping roles assumed by the nurse.

In the role of stranger, the client perceives the nurse as an unknown individual who may or may not be trustworthy and competent. Peplau points out how it is essential for the nurse in this role to accord the client respect and positive interest to promote open communication. A surrogate is a substitute figure who, in the client's mind, reactivates the feeling generated in earlier relationships. The nurse's responsibility in this role is to help the client to become aware of likenesses and differences and to differentiate the nurse as a person. By permitting clients to re-experience old feelings, the nurse who is acting as surrogate sets up the opportunity for growth experiences.

The resource person role involves the nurse in providing specific information, usually formulated in relation to larger problems. When clients cannot perform activities of daily living or complex care procedures independently, the nurse assumes the role of caregiver. The teacher role involves the nurse sharing information and promoting the client's learning through experience and requires the development of novel alternatives with open-ended outcomes in the nurse–client relationship. The leader role involves the nurse facilitating the client's work on the solution of problems and coaching the client to continue when obstacles are encountered. (The nurse also assumes the leader role

TABLE 7-3

## Various Roles Assumed by the Professional Nurse During the Therapeutic Relationship

| Therapeutic Stage or Phase | Professional Nursing Roles |
| --- | --- |
| **Peplau (1952)** | |
| 1. Orientation stage | 1. Stranger (someone who may or may not be trusted) |
| 2. Identification stage | 2. Unconditional mother surrogate, resource person, teacher, counselor, and surrogate |
| 3. Exploration stage | 3. The above roles and those of support person or coach |
| 4. Resolution stage | 4. Primarily a support person as client has attained independence in managing own health |
| **Travelbee (1971)** | |
| 1. Original encounter phase | 1. Stranger |
| 2. Emerging identities phase | 2. Listener and information giver |
| 3. Empathy phase | 3. Physical caregiver, but client remains uncomfortable sharing deep personal concerns with nurse, early counselor |
| 4. Sympathy phase | 4. Caregiver, counselor, facilitator, coach, support person, client advocate |
| 5. Rapport phase | 5. All professional nursing roles include that of change agent |
| **Hames & Joseph (1980)** | |
| 1. Trust formation stage | 1. Stranger |
| 2. Resistance stage | 2. Counselor (especially in offering self continuously despite rejection) |
| 3. Working stage | 3. Caregiver, counselor, facilitator, leader, resource person, coach, support person, client advocate, change agent |
| 4. Termination | 4. Counselor and support person |
| **Northouse & Northouse (1998)** | |
| 1. Preparation | 1. Critical thinker in deciding how to prepare self and setting for client |
| 2. Initiation | 2. Stranger and counselor |
| 3. Exploration | 3. Caregiver, counselor, resource person, coach, client advocate, change agent, support person, teacher |
| 4. Termination | 4. Counselor and support person |

when working with other members of the nursing and interdisciplinary health care teams.) For clients to become independent in meeting health care needs, they experience change in behavior or attitude. When the nurse facilitates change, the professional role of change agent emerges.

The counselor role incorporates all of the activities associated with promoting experiences leading to health. The counselor helps the client to become aware of health behaviors, to evaluate them, and to plan how to improve them. Counseling focuses primarily on how the client feels about himself and what is happening to him (Peplau, 1952). Throughout the entire relationship, nurses frequently assume the counselor and critical thinker roles.

## Mutuality in Responsibility and Decision Making

Every person involved in a communication process affects and is affected by every other person involved in the communication field. Rogers (1970, p. 97) calls this phenomenon "reciprocity." Reciprocal relationships are the basis of the nursing process. The nurse having the potential to affect the client and to be affected by the client offers the nurse the potential to assist the client to change behaviors in the direction of improved health. Such nurse–client exchanges can be powerful in problem-solving and decision-making situations that determine the nature and direction of change.

Reciprocity is a concept that is similar to the concept of mutuality. Reciprocity "is characterized as an interpersonal exchange, customarily expected to be symmetrical or equivalent" (Mendias, 1997, p. 435). The state of being mutual serves as a lexicon definition of **mutuality.** Merriam-Webster (1994) defines mutual as "a. directed by each other toward the other or others, b. having the same feelings, one for the other . . . c. shared in common" (p. 768). Mutuality appears as a concept in Peplau's (1952), Watson's (1996), and Leddy's (2004) conceptual models in terms of mutual gain in a client–nurse relationship. Leddy (2004) expands the use of the term mutual in terms of shared and connected processes humans have with environments.

Developing these ideas of mutual exchange and gain, Marck (1990) discusses the concept of therapeutic reciprocity as

one phenomenon of caring, [that] allows both the nurse and the client to benefit from their relationship in a mutually empowering manner. . . . Therapeutic reciprocity is a mutual, collaborative, probabilistic, instructive, and empowering exchange of feelings, thought, and behaviors between the nurse and client for the purpose of enhancing the human outcomes of the relationship for all parties concerned (pp. 49, 57).

All of the previously specified roles represent elements of presence, empathy, respect, and genuineness. Communication in these role relationships evolves from diagnostic interactions to therapeutic interactions including educative and supportive interactions as the client moves toward achievement of optimal health. The absolute element of all of these roles is mutuality in responsibility and decision making if both the nurse and the client are expected to grow and experience satisfaction from the nursing process.

## Communication and the Phenomenon of Anxiety

Nursing process results in change. The nature of change includes alternatives of cognitive repatterning (using new information to increase understanding), affective adjustment (using the relationship to become aware of, accept, and express feelings), and synthesis of cognitions and feelings in interpersonal repatterning (using the relationship to learn to interact with others in the social system). The direction of change can be toward health enhancement or deterioration. Obviously, the nurse wants to direct change toward enhanced health.

Every social system has role behaviors for constituents to follow. The way a person communicates is greatly affected by his or her perceived role in the system. Roles "are structures that are imposed on behavior" (Berlo, 1960, p. 153). Three aspects of role must be understood in trying to positively affect the other person in a relationship: role prescription, role description, and role expectations. Berlo defines these aspects as follows.

1. Role prescription: the formal, explicit statement of what behaviors should be performed by persons in a given role.
2. Role description: a report of the behaviors that are performed by persons in a given role.

3. Role expectations: the images that persons have about the behaviors that are performed by persons in a given role (Berlo, p. 153; enumeration added).

In the ideal nurse–client relationship, there is congruence among these three aspects. Together, the nurse and the client agree on the structure and dynamics of their purposeful communication. When there are differences regarding the prescriptions, descriptions, and expectations of role behavior between the nurse and the client, communication breakdowns occur and create uncertainty.

Uncertainty and ambiguity create increased tension and discomfort in the system. Such tension in human systems leads to dissipation of energy and less ability to use the energy to improve. In interpersonal systems, such tension often is called anxiety.

**Anxiety** is the tension state resulting from the actual or anticipated negative appraisal of the significant other in the communication process. Prolonged or intensive anxiety ties up available energy that could be better used for decision making or problem solving aimed to change behavior and attitudes toward enhanced health.

The tension state of anxiety in one person is readily communicated, thus engendering anxiety in the other person(s). Sullivan (1953) attributes great power to the tension of anxiety in a person's interpersonal growth, development, and ability in all stages of life. The actual or anticipated negative appraisals by others that lead to anxiety are perceived as threats to one's self-image. If the anxiety is limited in amount and duration, it simply leads to an increased state of alertness, mediated through physiologic reactions and behavior to reduce the tension. However, if the state of anxiety is unduly prolonged or intense, the level of alertness and successful tension-reducing behaviors are decreased.

Sullivan (1953) postulates that learning occurs through an anxiety gradient extending from mild to severe. A client with mild anxiety can focus energy on most of what is really occurring. A client with moderate anxiety has limited ability to focus on what is really occurring and tends to distort reality. A client with severe anxiety cannot focus energy on what is really happening and thus cannot participate effectively in problem solving or decision making. Because the effective nursing process requires that both the nurse and the client focus on what is really happening, it is essential to control anxiety in the communication process.

The nurse has two primary responsibilities in controlling anxiety:

1. To be aware of his or her own feelings of anxiety and to structure interactions in such a way that limited anxiety is transferred to the client.
2. To use effective strategies for intervening in the client's anxiety. Therapeutic intervention for anxiety relies on the ability of the nurse to recognize client anxiety as well as monitoring and relieving his or her own.

Clinical practice settings often place nurses in stressful situations. Clients find themselves on unfamiliar turf when they enter the health care system. Nurses realize the importance of learning stress-reduction strategies for themselves that they can share with clients. Techniques to help clients (and nurses) recognize, gain insight into, and cope with threats of anxiety are discussed in the following section.

## Communication Strategies That Reflect Caring

Many nurses identify caring as the essence of nursing. Because of its abstract nature, the concept of caring is difficult to define. However, certain behaviors used by others demonstrate caring. The following actions are frequently used by nurses to show that they care: prescencing (being physically, emotionally, and spiritually with another to enter the world of the other), sharing (giving of one's skills, thoughts, and knowledge to help another), supporting (providing fortifying help, displaying concern, trusting others, and affirming persons in their actions), and competence (education and clinical skill). Caring creates the uplifting effects for persons involved in a **caring interaction**: feelings of being respected, feelings of belonging, personal growth, personal transformation, wanting to learn to care, and desire to care (Beck, 2001).

Listening is the most important therapeutic technique in the process of effective communication and in demonstrating caring. Sundeen and colleagues (1994) state that it is devastating to the formation of a helpful relationship if the nurse fails to listen. Listening transmits the messages "You are of value to me," and "I am interested in you." A variety of techniques may be used to develop effective listening skills. However, all include strategies of learning how to ignore internal and external environmental distractions. Guidelines for engaging in effective listening include the following:

1. Give the other person your *full* attention, by facing them directly.
2. Resist external distractions and letting your mind stray.
3. Listen for central ideas and validate them with the client.
4. Ignore gut-feeling traps that confirm prejudices and/or produce biases.
5. Do not become defensive.
6. Watch for nonverbal as well as verbal messages.
7. Do not prejudge worth based on appearance or delivery of the speaker.
8. Listen for ideas and underlying feelings.
9. Do not interrupt the person as he or she speaks or when brief pauses in the conversation occur.
10. Try to see the situation from the other person's point of view.
11. Do not try to have the last word.

To listen effectively and to get clients to share thoughts and feelings, the nurse must use verbal communication techniques that facilitate the client's verbal and nonverbal expressiveness. Such techniques generally are referred to as "therapeutic communication techniques" (Table 7-4). Nurses spend time learning these techniques very early in their nursing careers because people rarely use them on a daily basis. Some nursing students find some of the techniques artificial and phony at first. They need time to refine the use of each technique so that it becomes natural and genuine.

To be helpful, the nurse must respond empathetically, attempt to understand the meaning of health and illness for clients, and respond with respect and authenticity. What does a nurse do to show empathy? The empathetic nurse attends carefully, listens intensely, responds reciprocally to verbal and nonverbal messages, uses appropriate language, times responses appropriately, clarifies and confirms ideas, explores the world from the client's viewpoint, and paces verbal and nonverbal behavior to the client's abilities.

What does a nurse do to show caring? The caring nurse spends time with clients, identifies relationships, and makes connections based on knowledge; states implicit assumptions; conceptualizes trends and patterns; verbalizes implied feelings, thoughts, goals, and attitudes; summarizes appropriately; explains purposes of activities; identifies nonverbal meanings; and assumes responsibility in the nursing process.

**TABLE 7-4**

## Summary of Therapeutic Communication Techniques

| Technique | Definition | Therapeutic Value |
|---|---|---|
| Listening | An active process of receiving information and examining one's reaction to the messages received | Nonverbally communicates to client nurse's interest in client |
| Silence | Periods of no verbal communication among participants | Nonverbally communicates nurse's acceptance of client |
| Establishing guidelines | Statements regarding roles, purpose, and limitations for a particular interaction | Helps client to know what is expected of him |
| Open-ended comments | General comments asking the client to determine the direction the interaction should take | Allows client to decide what material is most relevant and encourages him to continue |
| Reducing distance | Diminishing physical space between the nurse and client | Nonverbally communicates that nurse wants to be involved with client |
| Acknowledgment | Recognition given to a client for contribution to an interaction | Demonstrates the importance of the client's role within the relationship |
| Restating | Repeating to the client what the nurse believes is the main thought or idea expressed | Asks for validation of nurse's interpretation of the message |
| Reflecting | Directing back to the client his ideas, feelings, questions, or content | Attempts to show client the importance of his own ideas, feelings, and interpretations |
| Seeking clarification | Asking for additional inputs to understand the message received | Demonstrates nurse's desire to understand client's communication |
| Seeking consensual validation | Attempts to reach a mutual denotative and connotative meaning of specific words | Demonstrates nurse's desire to understand client's communication |
| Focusing | Questions or statements to help the client develop or expand an idea | Directs conversation toward topics of importance |
| Summarizing | Statement of main areas discussed during interaction | Helps client to separate relevant from irrelevant material; serves as a review and closing for the interaction |
| Planning | Mutual decision making regarding the goals and direction of future interactions | Reiterates client's role within relationship |

*Source:* Sundeen, S. J., Stuart, G. W., Rankin, E. A. D., & Cohen, S. A. (1994). *Nurse-client interaction* (5th ed., p. 124). St. Louis: Mosby. Used with permission of the publisher.

What does a nurse do to show respect? The respectful nurse verbalizes a clear commitment to understand, conveys acceptance, clearly affirms the client's worth as a unique person, and affirms the client's strengths and ability to assume responsibility for self. Such a nurse will help the client to strengthen self-identity. Strengthening self-identity is heard in phrases such as "You have . . ." and "You do . . ."

How does the nurse respond with authenticity? The authentic nurse consistently responds with real thoughts and feelings and resists all urges to play-act; assumes ownership of ideas and feelings; and freely shares emotions with clients. The nurse who is authentic will say, "I feel," "I think," or "I believe."

All of the preceding therapeutic professional nursing activities require the ability to listen. Listening demonstrates genuine concern and prioritizes client needs over the nurse's needs. Nurses frequently overlook the nursing intervention of therapeutic listening and communication techniques in client care documentation. The use of therapeutic techniques facilitates the client's efforts at problem solving, self-expression, and health improvement. Therapeutic communication distinguishes professional nurses from health care technicians.

### Questions for Reflection 7-3

1. As a health care consumer, what caring behaviors have I experienced?
2. What caring behaviors have I seen in a clinical practice setting?
3. What caring behaviors do I display as a nurse?
4. Why are caring behaviors important in professional nursing practice?

## Communication Strategies That Reflect Noncaring

Unfortunately at times, nurses may demonstrate **noncaring behaviors.** Noncaring behaviors communicate the following attitudes: "You have no value," "I am not interested—actually, I'm bored," or "I have more important things to do than to spend time listening to you." Failing to listen to clients is perhaps the most noncaring behavior a nurse can exhibit. Other nurse behaviors that are not helpful to clients include being judgmental (i.e., putting personal values, beliefs, or expectations above the client's); making stereotyped responses (i.e., negating the uniqueness of the client by using platitudes or clichés as responses); and changing the subject (verbally directing the interaction to a new topic of importance to the nurse or by nonverbally signaling that the topic being discussed is not important). Blocks to therapeutic communication are summarized in Table 7-5.

Nurses display noncaring behaviors for several reasons. Generally, one can assume that some of these nurses have some need for regressive behavior. This need, accompanied by increasing anxiety, sometimes leads nurses to adopt an attitude of superiority that is expressed in negative actions, such as moralizing, rejecting, or reacting with hostility.

Defensive behavior commonly occurs in regressive states. For example, a person might demonstrate denial, unconsciously evading or negating the real factors in a situation. Regressive states also may be marked by distortions, rote habitual actions, dogmatic responses, loss of control, invalidated assumptions (jumping to conclusions), parroting, inappropriate timing, and poor judgment. These behaviors represent important components of noncaring and nontherapeutic nursing strategies.

Because therapeutic communication is essential for effective professional nursing practice, nurses should periodically evaluate their communication techniques. If a pattern of nontherapeutic behaviors is identified, the nurse should seek help from a colleague or

TABLE 7-5

## Summary of Nontherapeutic Communication Techniques

| Technique | Definition | Therapeutic Value |
|---|---|---|
| Failure to listen | Not receiving client's intended message | Places needs of nurse above those of client |
| Failure to probe | Inadequate data collection represented by eliciting vague descriptions, getting inadequate answers, following standard forms too closely, and not exploring client's interpretation | Inadequate data base on which to make decisions; client care not individualized |
| Parroting | Continual repetition of client's phrases | The metacommunication is "I am not listening" or "I am not a competent communicator" |
| Being judgmental | Approving or disapproving statements | Implies that nurse has the right to pass judgment; promotes a dependent relationship |
| Reassuring | Attempts to do magic with words | Negates fears, feelings, and other communications of client |
| Rejecting | Refusing to discuss topics with client | Client may feel that not only communication but also the self was rejected |
| Defending | Attempts to protect someone or something from negative feedback | Negates client's right to express an opinion |
| Giving advice | Telling client what nurse thinks should be done | Negates the worth of client as a mutual partner in decision making |
| Stereotyped responses | Use of trite, meaningless verbal expressions | Negates the significance of client's communication |
| Changing topics | Nurse directing the interaction into areas of self-interest, rather than following lead of client | Nonverbally communicates that the nurse is in charge of deciding what will be discussed; possible to miss important topics for individual client |
| Patronizing | Style of communication that displays a condescending attitude toward the client | Implies that the nurse-client relationship is not based on equality; places the nurse in a "superior" position |

Source: Sundeen S. J., Stuart, G. W., Rankin, E. A. D., & Cohen, S. A. (1994). *Nurse-client interaction* (5th ed., p. 132). St. Louis: Mosby. Used with permission of the publisher.

counselor or attend classes or workshops to improve communication techniques. Nurses should let their own feelings be a guide to evaluate effectiveness of communication during nurse–client interactions. The persistent feeling of anxiety or tension is perhaps the best cue that the nurse may be unwittingly communicating in a noncaring and unhelpful way.

Although there are different views on the advantages and disadvantages of nurses (as professionals) being characterized as caring persons, the fact is that nurses do care about their fellow humans. One dilemma for nurses is that they are not always permitted to care for clients to the best of their knowledge or ability. Many factors in clinical environments (such as short staffing, increased focus on cost reduction, and ineffective working relationships with other health team members) impede the ability of nurses to care for clients, as they would like. This results in feelings of frustration. However, when nurses have the opportunity to share their specialized knowledge and compassion, all involved in health care delivery become enriched as desired outcomes are attained.

### Questions for Reflection 7-4

1. As a health care consumer, what noncaring behaviors have I experienced?
2. What noncaring behaviors have I seen in a clinical practice setting?
3. What noncaring behaviors have I displayed as a nurse? What were the factors that contributed to my noncaring behaviors?
4. How could I go about changing characteristics of my practice setting to keep me from displaying noncaring behaviors to clients and families?

## Outcomes of Helping Relationships

The nurse-client relationship has three major desired outcomes:

1. Increased client understanding of how better personal responsibility and accountability for health can be achieved (learning).
2. Attainment of optimal health.
3. Perceived satisfaction in the relationships.

In terms of nurse outcomes, knowing that clients have adequate knowledge and skills to solve problems or take steps to adopt a healthy lifestyle is the desired outcome. When clients have adequate preparation, they can make educated choices, expend the required energy, and assume greater responsibility for their own health.

In the nurse–client relationship, change occurs in two ways: as an outcome of learning in terms of the information gained and understood, and as an outcome of learning in terms of the interpersonal experience in the nursing process. The quality of communication plays the paramount role in change. When change and its effects are not communicated clearly, the change cannot be understood. Lack of understanding leads to resistance.

Hunsaker and Alessandra have proposed a schema for self-evaluation of communication patterns of persons in management positions that apply to nurses when working with clients. They propose several questions that are clearly applicable to the evaluation of communication in the nursing process (Hunsaker & Alessandra, 1980, pp. 140–141, enumeration added).

1. Did I comprehend each point made?
2. Did I make judgments of the words before the speaker was through speaking?
3. Did I make decisions in my own mind while he or she was still speaking?
4. Did I hunt for evidence that would prove the speaker right? Wrong?
5. Did I hunt for evidence that would prove myself right? Wrong?
6. Did I become upset while listening?
7. Did I generally jump to conclusions while listening?
8. Did I let the client speak at least 50% of the time?

9. Did I understand the words in terms of their intended meanings?
10. Did I restate ideas and feelings accurately?
11. Did I study voice, posture, actions, and facial expressions as the client talked?
12. Did I listen between the lines for unspoken meanings behind the words?
13. Did I really try to listen to the client?
14. Did I really want to listen to the client?
15. Did I really show the client I was, in fact, motivated and interested in listening to him?

Nurses should continually evaluate their own communication behaviors. In addition to self-evaluations such as the preceding questions, the nurse should consistently evaluate the effectiveness of communication with the client. Feedback should be sought from the client about what has been said and about how the client feels the relationship is going. The value of the nurse–client interactions should be explored at intervals to promote mutual benefits to nurse and client. A focus on asking the client "How are we doing?" states to the client that the nurse values him or her and cares how the communication affects him or her.

Along with individual evaluations of nurse–patient relationships, much work needs to be done to validate the benefits of helping relationships built by nurses. Therapeutic communication is an independent nursing intervention. However, nurses frequently fail to make entries on client records such as "therapeutic listening" or "explored feelings about the meaning of (client health concern)" when documenting delivered care. Most nursing research studies addressing caring are qualitative or descriptive in nature. Client satisfaction data offer potential to identify the benefits of caring communications and helping relationships from only recipients of nursing care. Nursing job satisfaction studies have potential to explore provider benefits of being a helper. Perhaps, a nursing research program exploring the positive outcomes of helping relationships needs to be established.

## ● HEALING RELATIONSHIPS: THE NURSE'S ROLE IN HEALING

A **healing relationship** might be considered a special type of helping relationship. Because "to heal is the activity of becoming whole" (Kritek, 1997, p. 11), healing has been defined as "a process of bringing parts of one's self together at deep levels of inner knowing, leading to an integration and balance, with each part having equal importance and value" (Dossey, Keegan, & Guzzetta, 2005, p. 6), and as "an inner process through which a person becomes whole" (Lerner, 1994, p. 13). Healing occurs within the person, and external interventions mobilize the client's inner healing resources (Micozzi, 1996). Healing is not synonymous with curing, because persons with terminal illness can become whole in the process of dying (Dossey, Keegan, & Guzzetta, 2005).

Healing encompasses the improvement of the whole person (body, mind, and spirit). Dossey, Keegan, and Guzzetta (2005) identify many healing modalities used by nurses in practice, including the following:

- Body-mind healing (cognitive therapy, self-reflection, relaxation techniques).
- Nutritional healing (healthy diets, dietary restrictions, herbs, vitamin and mineral supplements).

- Exercise and movement therapy (tai chi, walking, dance, yoga).
- Spiritual healing (faith healing, miracles, play, humor, and use of fine arts).
- Energetic healing (meridians, chakras, aura, smells, sounds, colors, magnets, therapeutic touch, and healing touch).
- Environmental healing (reducing toxins, recycling, feng shui).

Along with these integrative healing modalities, nurses engage in healing activities based on traditional scientific medicine when administering medications to clients and following pre- and postprocedure protocols.

Lerner (1994) differentiates among universal, common, and unique conditions of healing. Examples of universal conditions are inner peace and a deep experience of love. Attention and care from friends and family, deeply enjoyed work, laughter, moving music, and great art are examples of common conditions. However, Lerner indicates that the unique conditions of healing are some of the most important. Unique conditions are those that apply only to a single individual and may be the result of life experiences or personal relationships. As a healer, the nurse must assess clients as individuals to identify the particular needs that are most meaningful for each client.

Given that healing occurs within the client, the nurse healer's role is to facilitate another person's growth and life processes toward wholeness or to assist with illness recovery, a more healthy lifestyle, or with transition to peaceful death (Dossey et al., 2005). The nurse assists and responds to the client who is the central force in the healing process. "Nurses assume that their actions, as professionals, aim to facilitate wholeness in others through an interaction based on a mutuality of purpose" (Kritek, 1997, p. 14). Kritek (p. 21) states that four fundamental elements are always present in the healing encounter:

1. Nurse and client interact within a given context.
2. The encounter is in response to a health experience.
3. The nurse works in a pattern of mutuality with the client.
4. Healing is facilitated in response to a client's elicitation of nursing involvement and expertise.

Healing is facilitated within a helping relationship, which is characterized by principles such as presence (being, rather than doing), intention and purpose, empathy, guiding, creativity, imagery, and spirituality (Dossey et al., 2005; Keegan, 1994; Lerner, 1994).

As a healer, the nurse must assess all life dimensions for potential positive and negative forces that might influence the energy available to use when healing another. Effective healers have heightened sensitivity and awareness as they act with conscious intent. Nurses not only must recognize that healing is a unique life gift, but also it must be nurtured. Before healing another, some nurse healers practice preparation rituals. Healing fosters personal growth and the ability to live life to its fullest for both client and nurse (Conti-O'Hare, 2002; McKivergin, 2005).

Healing relationships with clients produce interpersonal connections. Nurses often display intensity and unconditional love when acting as instruments of healing. Nurse healers usually perceive "that healing does not come *from* them, but *through* them" (McKivergin, 2005, p. 243). The potential healing does not come from the healer, but rather it is a mysterious phenomenon involving a higher power and energy within the environment. McKivergin offers the following factors to increase the nurse's capacity as "as instrument of healing" (p. 245):

- Self-care in all of life's dimensions to assure a personal flow of energy and healing.
- Personal interpretations of life's lessons and meanings.
- Rootedness and expansiveness: balancing grounded approaches with intuitive inspirations.
- Understanding of the complex dynamics of holographic nature, the systems metaphor, and the essential nature of life, health, and healing.
- Expansion of consciousness: broaden one's thinking, shift perspectives, and embrace new approaches to life.
- Growth in love.
- Courage.
- Alignment with the Divine.
- Openness to being an instrument of the Creator's healing grace.
- Ability to detach self from the outcomes.
- Groundedness and reliability.
- Patience.
- Authenticity.
- Mindfulness.
- Integrity.

The healing process requires exchange of energy and truth during authentic communication to create an environment of support while helping others become attuned to their own healing capabilities. Outcomes of healing include deep relaxation, and the profound change of becoming more whole.

### Questions for Reflection 7-5

1. Which of Keegan's types of healing have I used in my clinical practice?
2. What would be the consequences for me if I used one of Keegan's healing techniques with clients that were not compatible with the traditional medical model?

## ● HELPING AND HEALING RELATIONSHIPS WITH COLLEAGUES AND OTHER HEALTH TEAM MEMBERS

Professional nurses and other health team members work together to achieve the common mission of providing the absolute best care possible for clients. Each member of the interdisciplinary team brings a unique perspective to and skill set for providing health care to clients. Since the beginning of health care delivery, various conflicts among health team members have surfaced. Physicians have exerted power over nurses. Professional nurses have competed with other health team members, such as pharmacists, laboratory technologists, radiology technicians, and dietitians, for scarce resources. Unlicensed personnel have experienced a lack of respect from professional nurses. As health care professionals find fewer resources for client care, they sometimes turn against each other, instead of working effectively together to provide the best possible care for clients.

With the increasing complexity of client health care needs, members of the health team need to establish professional partnerships to meet client needs and concerns. Currently, many health care organizations do not have healthy working environments for health care providers. Health team members tend to blame each other for shortcomings in client care. The needs of the clients, physicians, and organizational administrators frequently supersede the needs of the nursing staff. In today's fast-paced environment, persons communicate with each other just to get jobs done. Civility and politeness have become icons of the past. The profession of nursing fails to attract young bright persons, and many practicing nurses leave the profession because of intense frustration with practice settings.

Members of the health care team need to establish professional partnerships to dispel competition, exploitation, and frustration in the delivery of health care in the ever-changing health care system. A **professional partnership** is a relationship based on mutual respect to achieve a common mission while each participant lives out his or her life's purpose. "Partnerships join hearts and minds around a common purpose" (Wesorick, Shiparski, Troseth, & Wyngarden, 1997). In health care, the common mission is client care. For a physician, a life purpose may be curing illness in the sick. For a professional nurse, a life purpose may be to care for and help persons as they respond to health alterations. For an unlicensed nursing staff member, a life purpose may be helping persons incapable of caring for themselves. All of these life purposes play essential parts in a common mission: client care.

Theoretical foundations and concepts presented related to the development of healthy helping relationships with clients also apply to interdisciplinary health team members. Healthy working relationships among health care providers require meaningful conversations. Wesorick and Shiparski (1997 [paraphrased from page 40]) say meaningful conversations result when persons use the following principles for communication.

- Intention: creation of a safe place to foster collaborative learning and to share and listen to the thinking of others to connect at a deeply human level (body/mind/spirit).
- Listening: truly hearing oneself and others using physical, mental, and spiritual connections to learn exclusively.
- Advocacy: willingness to share spontaneous personal thinking along with reasons behind the thinking, with the intention only to disclose thoughts, not to defend them.
- Inquiry: willingness to ask others questions to discover new insights and learn by connecting diverse ideas and feelings.
- Silence: time of quiet reflection to learn lessons from unspoken words, personal awareness of "the quiet of the Soul" (p. 40).

### Questions for Reflection 7-6

1. How could I develop professional partnerships with health team members in my clinical practice setting?
2. What personal behaviors/attitudes would I have to change to develop these professional partnerships?

Taking time to abide by these principles could foster the development of more respectful and healthy working relationships among health team members. Development of professional partnerships might facilitate team members to help each other, bolster team member esteem, and heal wounds.

## Research Brief 7-1

McKenna, B., Smith, N., Poole, S., & Coverdale, J. (2003). Horizontal violence: Experiences of registered nurses in their first year of practice. *Journal of Advanced Nursing, 42*, 90–96.

The investigators sought to discover the incidence and effects of horizontal violence on newly registered nurses in their first year of practice. Horizontal violence (aka, bullying) takes the following forms: "verbal abuse, threats, intimidation, humiliation, excessive criticism, innuendo, exclusion, denial of access to opportunity, disinterest, discouragement and withholding of information" (p. 91). Five-hundred eighty-four New Zealand nurses working across a variety of clinical practice settings and with less than 1 year of clinical experience responded to a mailed questionnaire that contained a checklist of horizontal violence incidences, the impact-of-event scale for the various incidences, and open-ended questions about the consequences of the incident.

Results revealed that over half of the respondents reported having felt being undervalued and over a third of them reported that they felt they had experienced blocked access to learning opportunities, neglect, distress from interpersonal conflicts, and situations where they had inadequate supervision for the amount of responsibility they were assuming. More than 15% of respondents indicated that these problems had occurred on more than one occasion. No differences across clinical practice areas were discovered. Rude, abusive, or humiliating comments were the most frequent incidents of horizontal violence reported (58%), followed by feelings of inadequate supervision for the amount of responsibility being assumed (46%). Both of these incidents caused moderate-to-severe distress according to 112 respondents. Horizontally violent incidents most commonly occurred in inpatient wards and were received from experienced female nurses aged 30 to 49 years. Less than half of the respondents reported incidences and only 20 respondents reported receiving counseling or debriefing after the incident. Fourteen percent of the respondents reported being so distressed that they took days off work and 34% of the respondents reported that the incident(s) made them think about leaving the profession. Only seven respondents reported resolution of the incidents because of another staff member and 17 reported changing practice areas.

Implications for clinical practice suggested by the investigators include the following: (1) education of experienced nurses helping new graduates on the behaviors associated with horizontal violence, its prevention, and effective management; (2) nursing programs should cover this content in nursing curriculums; and (3) employers should provide confidential support systems for new graduates who may fall victim to horizontal violence. Even though this study was conducted in New Zealand and nurses from the Pacific Islands and Asian countries were underrepresented, this study provides support that new nurses encounter incidents that reduce self-confidence. The study also supports the need for nurses to develop healthy, helping, healing relationships with each other. More research is needed to determine how best experienced nurses can help new nurses with the transition to independent professional practice and the scope of horizontal violence among experienced nurses.

# ● SUMMARY AND SIGNIFICANCE TO PRACTICE

Professional nurses develop helping and healing relationships with clients. All people have visions of what they would like to accomplish and noble intentions about acting on their dreams. Mastery of communication is necessary for carrying out the agendas of life and promoting health and healing of clients and members of the interdisciplinary health team, including professional nurses.

## FROM THEORY TO PRACTICE

1. Reread the vignette at the beginning of the chapter. What would you do if you were Margie? What would be the consequences of your proposed actions? Are there other actions that you could take?
2. Think about encounters you have had with health care providers as a consumer. Make a list of positive ones and negative ones. Compare the lists. What are characteristics of caring encounters? What are characteristics of noncaring encounters? Has this exercise changed you as a professional nurse? Why or why not?

## WWW INTERNET RESOURCES

The Clinical Practice Model Resource Center: http://www.cpmrc.com.
American Holistic Nurses Association: http://www.ahna.org.
American Psychiatric Nurses Association: http://www.apna.org.
American Psychiatric Association Help Center: http://helping.apa.org.
Healing Touch International: http://www.healingtouch.net.
Therapeutic Touch: http://therapeutictouch.com.

## REFERENCES

*The American heritage dictionary of the English language* (3rd ed.). (1992). Boston: Houghton Mifflin.

Arnold, E., & Boggs, K. (1989). *Interpersonal relationships: Professional communication skills for nurses.* Philadelphia: WB Saunders.

Beck, C. T. (2001). Caring within nursing education: A metasynthesis. *Journal of Nursing Education, 40,* 101–109.

Benner, P. (1984). *From novice to expert.* Menlo Park, CA: Addison-Wesley.

Berlo, D. K. (1960). *The process of communication.* New York: Holt, Rinehart & Winston.

Bradley, J. C., & Edinberg, M. A. (1990). *Communication in the nursing context* (3rd ed.). East Norwalk, CT: Appleton & Lange.

Brill, N. I. (1990). *Working with people: The helping process* (4th ed.). New York: Longman.

Ceccio, J. F., & Ceccio, C. M. (1982). *Effective communication in nursing theory and practice.* New York: Wiley.

Conti-O-Hare, M. (2002). *The nurse as wounded healer from trauma to transcendence.* Sudbury, MA: Jones & Bartlett.

Dossey, B., Keegan, L. & Guzzetta, C. (2005). *Holistic nursing: A handbook for practice.* Sudbury, MA: Jones & Bartlett.

Hames, C. C., & Joseph, D. H. (1980). *Basic concepts of helping—a holistic approach.* New York: Appleton-Century-Crofts.

Hunsaker, P. L., & Alessandra, A. J. (1980). *Art of managing people.* Englewood Cliffs, NJ: Prentice-Hall.

Keegan, L. (1994). *The nurse as healer.* Albany, NY: Delmar.

Kritek, P. B. (1997). Healing: A central nursing construct—reflections on meaning. In P. B. Kritek (Ed.), *Reflections on healing: A central nursing construct* (pp. 11–27). New York: National League for Nursing.

Leddy, S. K. (2004). Human energy: A conceptual model of unitary nursing science. *Visions: The Journal of Rogerian Scholarship, 12,* 14–27.

Leininger, M. & McFarland, M. (2002). *Transcultural nursing: Concepts, theories, research & practice,* (3rd ed.). New York: McGraw-Hill.

Lerner, M. (1994). *Choices in healing.* Cambridge, MA: MIT Press.

Marck, P. (1990). Therapeutic reciprocity: A caring phenomenon. *Advances in Nursing Science, 13,* 49–59.

McKenna, B., Smith, N., Poole, S., & Coverdale, J. (2003). Horizontal violence: Experiences of registered nurses in their first year of practice. *Journal of Advanced Nursing, 42,* 90–96.

McKivergin, M. (2005). The nurse as an instrument of healing. In Dossey, B., Keegan, L., & Guzzetta, C. (Eds.), *Holistic nursing: A handbook for practice* (pp. 233–254). Sudbury. MA: Jones & Bartlett.

Mendias, E. P. (1997). Reciprocity in the healing relationship between nurse and patient. In P. B. Kritek (Ed.), *Reflections on healing: A central nursing construct* (pp. 435–451). New York: National League for Nursing.

*Merriam-Webster's collegiate dictionary* (10th ed.). (1994). Springfield, MA: Merriam-Webster.

Micozzi, M. S. (Ed.). (1996). *Fundamentals of complementary and alternative medicine.* New York: Churchill Livingstone.

Newman, M., Lamb, G. S., & Michaels, C. (1991). Nurse case management: The coming together of theory and practice. *Nursing & Health Care, 12,* 404–408.

Northouse, L. L., & Northouse, P. G. (1998). *Health communication: Strategies for health professionals* (3rd ed.). Stamford, CT: Appleton & Lange.

Osterman, P., & Schwartz-Barcott, D. (1996). Presence: Four ways of being there. *Nursing Forum, 31,* 23–30.

Parse, R. R. (1996). The human becoming theory: Challenges in practice and research. *Nursing Science Quarterly, 9,* 55–60.

Paterson, J. G., & Zderad, L. T. (1988). *Humanistic nursing.* New York: National League for Nursing.

Peplau, H. (1952). *Interpersonal relations in nursing.* New York: G. P. Putnam's Sons.

Riley, J. B. (2000). *Communications in nursing* (4th ed.). St. Louis: Mosby.

Rogers, C. R. (1951). *Client-centered therapy: Its current practice, implications, and theory.* Boston: Houghton Mifflin.

Rogers, C. R. (1958). Characteristics of a helping relationship. *Personnel and Guidance Journal, 37,* 6–16.

Rogers, M. E. (1970). *An introduction to the theoretical basis of nursing.* Philadelphia: F. A. Davis.

Sullivan, H. S. (1953). *The interpersonal theory of psychiatry.* New York: Norton.

Sundeen, S. J., Stuart, G. W., Rankin, E. A. D., & Cohen, S. A. (1994). *Nurse–client interaction* (5th ed.). St. Louis: Mosby.

Taylor, A. (1977). *Communicating.* Englewood Cliffs, NJ: Prentice-Hall.

Travelbee, J. (1966). *Interpersonal aspects of nursing.* Philadelphia: F. A. Davis.

Travelbee, J. (1971). *Interpersonal aspects of nursing* (2nd ed.). Philadelphia: F. A. Davis.

Vestal, K. W. (1995). *Nursing management: Concepts and issues* (2nd ed.). Philadelphia: J. B. Lippincott.

Watson, J. (1996). Watson's theory of transpersonal caring. In P. H. Walker & B. Neuman (Eds.), *Blueprint for use of nursing models: Education, research, practice and administration* (pp. 141–184). New York: National League for Nursing.

Wesorick, B., & Shiparski, L. (1997). *Can the human being thrive in the work place? Dialogue as a strategy of hope.* Grand Rapids, MI: Practice Field Publishing.

Wesorick, B., Shiparski, L., Troseth, M., & Wyngarden, K. (1997). *Partnership Council field book.* Grand Rapids, MI: Practice Field Publishing.

Wiseman, T. A. (1996). A concept analysis of empathy. *Journal of Advanced Nursing, 23,* 1162–1167.

# CHAPTER 8

# The Health Process and Self-Care of the Nurse

## KEY TERMS AND CONCEPTS

Interaction World View
Disease
Illness
Sickness
Well-Being
Wellness
Integration World View
Health Protection
Health Promotion
Alternative Health Practices
Complementary Health Practices
Lifestyle Behavior Change
Health Patterning
Burnout
Health-Enhancing Techniques

## LEARNING OUTCOMES

By the end of this chapter, the learner will be able to:

1 Differentiate wellness from health.

2 Distinguish illness from disease.

3 Compare and contrast the interaction and integration world views of health.

4 Identify factors that contribute to individual variability in wellness.

5 Describe how health/illness can be explained as a unitary concept.

6 Differentiate health protection from health promotion.

7 Outline strategies for changing lifestyle behaviors and health patterning.

8 Identify signs and symptoms of work-related stress, role underload, role overload, and burnout.

9 Describe strategies for managing work-related stress and enhancing personal wellness.

## VIGNETTE

After an exhausting shift, two nurses, Michael and Jane, discuss how ironic it seems that they have worked all day to help others get better at the expense of their own health. Michael states, "The hospital doesn't seem to care about the health and well-being of the staff. We never have time to eat or even take bathroom breaks. Within a few months we will all be ready to occupy one of the beds." Jane continues the discussion, "You know, I have never thought about the toll this job is taking on my health. I wonder what we could do to make this place a more healthful place in which to work?"

Many nurses enter the nursing profession "to help people." Most persons have the perception that nurses help sick people. Because nurses are linked to the discipline of medicine, most people define health using the medical definition, "the absence of disease." Throughout history, persons outside of the medical field have characterized the nurse as the physician's handmaiden.

Curing diseases remains the major focus of medicine despite high costs and sometimes futile efforts. Recently, the public has become aware of the importance of disease prevention and health promotion. Reports on the role of nutrition and exercise in preventing debilitating and fatal illness permeate the airways, Internet, and printed media. Through roles designed to (1) promote health, (2) capitalize on the healthy outlook of people, and (3) reinforce their strengths, the nursing profession has the potential to change societal beliefs about health and health care delivery. Health promotion and patterning are essential nursing activities in all (including acute care) settings for nursing care.

This chapter presents the interaction and the integration world views of health, organizing frameworks for alternate views of the concepts of health, well-being, wellness, disease, illness, and sickness. Later sections of the chapter consider models and nursing interventions for the protection, promotion, and patterning of health. Finally, strategies for nurses to attain optimal health are presented.

# ✦ WORLD VIEWS OF HEALTH

Basic philosophic assumptions about the nature of reality, including human beings and the human–environment relationship, are referred to as paradigms or world views. World views that have been described by nursing scholars include change/persistence (Hall, 1981), totality/simultaneity (Parse, 1987), particulate–deterministic/interactive–integrative/unitary–transformative (Newman, 1992), and reaction/reciprocal interaction/simultaneous action (Fawcett, 1993). Elements of these classifications have been synthesized into the interaction/integration world views of health, which are summarized in this chapter.

## The Interaction World View

In the **interaction world view,** as in the totality world view (Parse, 1987), the human being usually is conceptualized as a whole comprised of parts who interacts with a physically separate environment. The environment exerts stressors on persons to which they must react. The interaction world view supports a belief in linear, predictable, and quantifiable cause-and-effect relationships.

In this world view, persons strive to maintain a balance or state of stability. Whenever the environment changes, persons must change. Environmental changes may pose threats for persons. Effective reactions to environmental changes result in personal changes without negative effects to well-being, wellness, or health.

However, ineffective reactions to environmental changes may result in disease, illness, or sickness that affects personal well-being, wellness, or health.

### Disease

Disease is a medical term consistent with the interaction world view. Benner, Tanner, and Chesla (1996) define **disease** as a "dysfunction of the body" (p. 45). The objective of the physician is to classify observable changes in the body structure or function (signs) into a recognizable clinical syndrome. A correct label, or diagnosis, implies disease course and duration, communicability, prognosis, and appropriate treatment. Medical intervention is aimed at curing the disease. Many nursing interventions support and promote the medical regimen as nurses administer medications, perform treatments, encourage rest, and evaluate the effects of medical and nursing interventions.

Historically, diseases were believed to be attributable to one agent that in a sufficient dose caused certain predictable signs and symptoms. However, a variety of factors related to the person (host), agent, and environment, increasingly are viewed as being interrelated in the cause and effective treatment of disease. All these interactions must be considered in determining a plan for care.

### Illness

**Illness** is a subjective feeling of being unhealthy that may or may not be related to disease. A person may have a disease without feeling ill and may feel ill in the absence of disease. For example, a person may have hypertension (a disease), controlled with medication, diet, and exercise, and be symptom-free (no illness). Another person may have pain and feel ill but may not have an identifiable disease. What is important is how the person feels and what he or she does because of those feelings.

Nursing intervention focuses on the human response to illness, identification of reasons for symptoms, and efforts to decrease symptoms, if possible. In contrast, medical interventions focus on efforts to label and treat the symptoms and cure disease. When a person's illness is accepted by society and thus given legitimacy, it is considered "sickness."

### Sickness

According to Twaddle and Hessler (1977), in a classic reference, **sickness** is "a status, a social entity usually associated with disease or illness, although it may occur independently of them" (p. 97). Once the person fulfills criteria for being sick, others condone various dependent behaviors that otherwise might be considered unacceptable. When working with persons who are sick, nursing roles focus upon assisting the persons until they can reassume responsibility for decision making or independent functioning.

### Well-Being

**Well-being** is a subjective perception of vitality and feeling well that is a component of health within the interaction world view. Although well-being is a variable subjective trait, it can be described objectively, experienced, and measured. Experienced at the lowest degrees, a person might feel ill. Experienced at the highest levels, a person would perceive maximum satisfaction with life, understand what it means to be in harmony with the universe, and feel as though he/she has made a significant contribution to humanity. Thus, well-being status can be plotted on a continuum, as shown in Figure 8-1.

### Health as Wellness

Health is difficult to define. Health is described in various sources as a value judgment, a subjective state, a relative concept, a spectrum, a cycle, a process, and an abstraction that cannot be measured objectively. In many definitions, physiologic and psychological components of health are dichotomized. Other subconcepts that might be included in definitions of health include environmental and social influences, freedom from pain or

**Figure 8-1**
The well-being continuum. (Modified from Terris, M. (1975). Approaches to an epidemiology of health. *American Journal of Public Health*, 65, 1039. Used with permission from the publisher.)

disease, optimum capability, ability to adapt, purposeful direction and meaning in life, and sense of well-being.

In the interaction world view, health indicates the absence of disease and the presence of normal functioning in roles or tasks. In this book, health has been defined as a state or condition of integrity of functioning (functional capacity and ability) and perceived well-being (feeling well). As a result, a person is able to:

- Function adequately (can be observed objectively).
- Adapt adequately to the environment.
- Feel well (as assessed subjectively).

Wellness, as defined in the literature, is similar to the open-ended and eudaimonistic models of health described in this chapter, and in this book will be considered synonymous. Dunn (1977, p. 9), in his classic work on high-level wellness, describes **wellness** as "an integrated method of functioning which is oriented toward maximizing the potential of which the individual is capable, within the environment where he is functioning." Others have characterized wellness–illness as "the human experience of actual or perceived function–dysfunction" (Jensen & Allen, 1994, p. 349). Indications of wellness (health) might include:

- A person's capacity to perform to the best of his or her ability.
- The ability to adjust and adapt to varying situations.
- A reported feeling of well-being.
- A feeling that "everything is together."

Smith (1981, p. 47), in a seminal publication, presents four models of health consistent with the interaction world view that "can be viewed as forming a scale—a progressive expansion of the idea of health": the clinical model, the role performance model, the adaptive model, and the eudaimonistic model.

The clinical model is the narrowest view. People are seen as physiologic systems with interrelated functions. Health is identified as the absence of signs and symptoms of disease or disability, as identified by medical science. Thus, health might be defined as a "state of not being sick" (Ardell, 1979, p. 18) or as a "relatively passive state of freedom from illness . . . a condition of relative homeostasis" (Dunn, 1977, p. 7). Much of the current health care delivery system, which is based on this model of health, is designed to deal with disease and illness after they occur. In the clinical model of health, the opposite end of the continuum from health is disease.

Next on the scale is the idea of health as role performance. This view adds social and psychological standards to the concept of health. The critical criterion of health is that the person has the ability to fulfill societal roles effectively. If a person becomes unable to perform expected roles, this inability can mean illness, even if the individual appears clinically healthy. For example, "Somatic health is . . . the state of optimum capacity for the elective performance of valued tasks" (Parsons, 1958, p. 168). In the role performance model of health, the opposite end of the continuum from health is sickness.

The adaptive model combines the clinical and role performance health models. In the adaptive model, health is perceived as a condition in which the person can engage in effective interaction with the physical and social environment. This model addresses continuous and simultaneous growth and change in persons and the environment. For example, McWilliam, Stewart, Brown, Desai, and Coderre (1996) define health as "the individual's ability to realize aspirations, satisfy needs, and respond positively to the challenges of the environment" (p. 1). The adaptive mode suggests that health may be a process rather than a state of being. In the adaptive model of health, the opposite end of the continuum from health is illness.

The eudaimonistic model provides an even more comprehensive conception of health than the previously presented views. In this viewpoint, health is a condition of actualization or realization of the person's potential. For example, human health is "the actualization of inherent and acquired human potential" (Pender, 2002, p. 22). Health "transcends biological fitness. It is primarily a measure of each person's ability to do what he wants to do and become what he wants to become" (Dubos, 1978, p. 74). In the eudaimonistic model, health is consistent with high-level wellness and at the opposite end of the continuum from disabling illness.

Examples of nursing conceptual models that are consistent with the interaction world view are King's systems interaction model, Neuman's health care systems model, Roy's adaptation model, and Orem's self-care deficit model (see Chapter 5).

## The Integration World View

In the **integration world view,** as in the simultaneity world view (Parse, 1987), the human being is considered to be a unitary, indivisible whole. The human, although distinct, is embedded in and inseparable from environment. Because the person is in mutual process, multiple "causes" and "effects," and nonlinear changes make prediction probabilistic and sometimes imprecise.

In this world view, the goal for a person is to develop his or her potential toward increased diversity. Change is inevitable and provides an opportunity for growth. Health is viewed as a unitary pattern, with manifestations of health reflecting the whole of the human.

### Disease and Illness as Manifestations of Health

In the integration world view, health is viewed as encompassing both disease and "nondisease" (Newman, 1994). Disease can be considered to be "a manifestation of health . . . a meaningful aspect of health" (Newman, p. 5) and "a meaningful aspect of the whole" (p. 7). Illness and health are viewed as a single process of ups and downs that are manifestations of varying degrees of organization and disorganization. Disputing that death is the antithesis of health, Newman (p. 11) proposes that disease and nondisease are not opposites, but rather complementary, to determine health, a unitary process. Illness, like health, simply represents a pattern of life at a particular moment. The tension characteristic of disease throws one off balance, which promotes growth toward a new level of evolving capacities, diversity, and complexity. The person may transform into a new pattern of being.

Therefore, health can be conceptualized as an actively continuing process that involves initiative, ability to assume responsibility for health, value judgments, and integration of the total person. It is a goal, a fluid process, rather than an actual state. Thus, health is difficult to quantify for objective evaluation. In clinical practice, nurses collaborate with clients while trying to help them attain optimal health. Nurses help clients by focusing on client strengths while getting them to acknowledge factors impeding growth toward maximal health potential. Client goals and feelings direct nursing interventions.

Nursing models and theories that are consistent with the integration world view include Rogers' science of unitary human beings, Parse's theory of human becoming, Neuman's theory of health as expanding consciousness, and Leddy's human energy model (see Chapter 5). These models and theories describe health as an evolving or emerging process, a forward movement with mutual person–environment patterns.

### Questions for Reflection 8-1

1. Which of the following world views on health appeal to me the most?
2. Do I view health as a state or a process?
3. How do my views about health affect my professional practice?

## ● HEALTH PROTECTION AND PROMOTION

Health promotion has been defined as "activities directed toward increasing the level of well-being and actualizing the health potential of people, families, community, and society" (Hravnak, 1998, p. 284). Pender (2002) distinguishes health promotion from disease prevention. According to Pender, health promotion is the process of increasing well-being and actualizing an individual's maximal health potential. Individual motivation plays an important role in health promotion. Whereas, **health protection** focuses on efforts for active disease or injury avoidance, and early detection or optimal functioning within the confines of an illness, **health promotion** expands potential for health.

### Goals for Health Promotion and Protection

The United States health care system remains disease oriented, despite increased efforts toward health promotion and fitness. The United States spends more on health care than all other nations with the goal of curing and controlling illness. Health promotion, disease prevention, and health education receive less funding. Efforts for health education mainly address illness prevention. For example, children are taught to brush their teeth to avoid cavities (not because the mouth will feel, look, taste, and smell better) and to eat properly and exercise to prevent diabetes (rather than that they will feel better).

In 2000, the U.S. Department of Health and Human Services published *Healthy People 2010*. This report described national objectives for health promotion and disease prevention, including the following two major goals: "increase quality and years of healthy life" (p. 8) and "eliminate health disparities" (p. 11). The government report specified the following 28 focus areas for improvement in the health of American citizens:

1. Access to quality health services.
2. Arthritis, osteoporosis, and chronic back conditions.
3. Cancer.
4. Chronic kidney disease.
5. Diabetes.
6. Disability and secondary conditions.
7. Educational and community-based programs.
8. Environmental health.
9. Family planning.
10. Food safety.
11. Health communication.
12. Heart disease and stroke.
13. Human immunodeficiency virus.
14. Immunization and infectious diseases.
15. Injury and violence prevention.
16. Maternal, infant, and child health.
17. Medical product safety.
18. Mental health and mental disorders.
19. Nutrition and overweight.
20. Occupational safety and health.
21. Oral health.
22. Physical activity and fitness.
23. Public health infrastructure.
24. Respiratory diseases.
25. Sexually transmitted diseases.
26. Substance abuse.
27. Tobacco use.
28. Vision and hearing (p. 17).

Because all these objectives specify illnesses or injuries to be avoided, the plan represents an extensive program of health protection rather than health promotion.

The concepts of health protection and promotion are consistent with the interaction world view. To guide nurses in interventions targeted for health promotion and protection, the next section discusses various models and strategies for use in clinical practice.

### Questions for Reflection 8-2

1. Think about the last time you engaged in clinical practice. Write down examples of when your practice focused on health protection. Write down examples of when your practice focused on health promotion. Why is it important for professional nurses to engage in client health protection and promotion?
2. Do I have any of the unhealthy conditions or habits outlined in *Healthy People 2010* initiatives? How can I work to become a role model of health for my clients?

## Models for Changing Lifestyle Behavior

### Health Belief Model

Why do people behave in certain ways in certain situations? What kinds of nursing intervention would be most effective in modifying a person's behavior to reduce risk of disease? Rosenstock (1966), in his "health belief" model, which still applies in today's health care situations, includes the following factors:

1. Perceived susceptibility: the client's perception of the likelihood of experiencing a particular illness.
2. Perceived severity: the client's perception of the seriousness of the illness and its potential impact on his or her life.
3. Benefits of action: the client's assessment of the potential of the health action to reduce susceptibility or severity.
4. Perceived threat of disease.
5. Costs of action: the client's estimate of financial costs, time and effort, inconvenience, and possible side effects, such as pain or discomfort.
6. Cues that trigger health-seeking behaviors, such as information in newspapers or on television; internal signals, such as symptoms; and interpersonal relationships with the health care provider and significant others.

The health belief model, called a "rational model," explains how persons work toward improving their general well-being and health. The model assumes that all persons value well-being and that differences vary according to differing perceptions in interactions and motivation. Kasl and Cobb (1966) extended the basic model by specifying a relatively positive variable, the "perceived importance of health matters," in addition to perceived value and perceived threat. Becker and Maiman (1975) expanded the model further by including positive health motivation. In 1988, Rosenstock, Strecher, and Becker urged incorporation of self-efficacy into the model. In a review of 10 years of studies related to the model, Janz and Becker (1984) concluded that only two of the model components, perceived barriers and perceived susceptibility, explained or predicted preventive behaviors. Perceived susceptibility has been found to be strongly related to compliance with medical advice (Vincent & Furnham, 1997).

### Revised Pender Health Promotion Model

The health promotion model (HPM) (Pender, 2002) was developed in the early 1980s and has undergone several revisions based on research findings. The HPM provides a framework for combining professional nursing and behavioral science outlooks on various determinants of health behaviors. Pender categorizes the determinants of health-promoting behavior into cognitive–perceptual factors (individual perceptions), modifying factors, and variables affecting the likelihood of action. Pender distinguishes the HPM from other models explaining health action because it eliminates the "fear" and "threat" perceptions for health action.

Based on extensive research, the HPM was revised in 1996 (Figure 8-2) (Pender, 1996) and has not undergone subsequent revisions. The revised model proposes that health-promoting behavior is related to direct and indirect influences among the 10 determinants of individual characteristics and experiences (e.g., previous related behavior and personal factors); behavior-specific cognitions and affect (e.g., perceived benefits

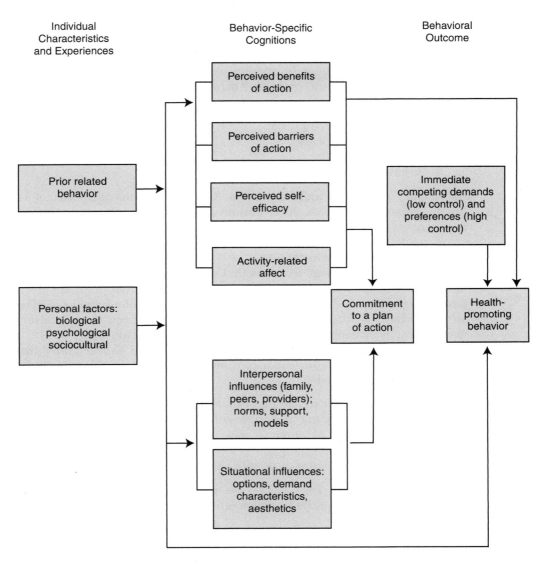

**Figure 8-2**
Health promotion model. (From Pender, N. J., Murdaugh, C. L., & Parsons, M. A. (2002). *Health promotion in nursing practice*, 4th ed. Reprinted with permission of Pearson Education, Inc. Upper Saddle River, NJ.)

of action, perceived barriers to action, perceived self-efficacy, activity-related affect, interpersonal influences, and situational influences); commitment to a plan of action; and immediate competing demands. Pender (1996) considers the behavior-specific cognitions and affect category of variables "to be of major motivational significance . . . (and) constitute a critical 'core' for intervention, because they are subject to modification through nursing actions" (p. 68).

Research has supported the predictive validity of some of the constructs in the revised HPM, such as perceived benefits of action, perceived barriers to action, perceived self-efficacy, interpersonal influences, and situational influences. A review of studies testing the HPM by Pender, Murdaugh, and Parsons (2002) reveals that the following factors contribute to health-promoting behaviors:

1. Perceived benefits of action.
2. Perceived barriers to action.
3. Perceived self-efficacy.
4. Interpersonal influences.
5. Situational influences.

Additional research is needed to validate the contributions of the role of affect during health-promoting activities, the commitment to action, and the competing demands and preferences (Pender, Murdaugh & Parsons, 2002).

## The Transtheoretical Model

The transtheoretical model assumes that change requires movement through discrete motivational stages over time, with the active use of different processes of change at different stages. The model has been supported in studies of a number of lifestyle behaviors, including smoking cessation, weight control, sunscreen use, exercise acquisition, mammography screening, and condom use (Prochaska et al., 1994).

According to Prochaska, Redding, Harlow, Rossi, and Velicer (1994), the stages of change in this model represent a continuum of motivational readiness for behavior change. The stages include:

- Precontemplation: not intending to change.
- Contemplation: intending to change within 6 months.
- Preparation: actively planning change.
- Action: overtly making changes.
- Maintenance: taking steps to sustain change and resist temptation to relapse.

Westberg and Jason (1996, p. 147) describe steps of successful change that are consistent with the stages of the transtheoretical model. The steps are:

1. Acknowledging that something is not right in one's life.
2. Deciding that a change is wanted.
3. Setting a goal or goals.
4. Exploring options for the achievement of goals.
5. Deciding on and trying to implement a plan.
6. Assessing progress.
7. Guarding against backsliding.

Also included in the transtheoretical model is the concept of decisional balance. The model proposes that part of the decision to move toward the action stage of change is based on the relative weight given to the pros and cons of changing behavior to reduce risk. "The pros represent the advantages or positive aspects of changing behavior, and may be thought of as facilitators of change. The cons represent the disadvantages or negative aspects of changing behavior, and may be thought of as barriers to change" (Prochaska et al., 1994, pp. 478–479).

This model provides a rationale for individualizing interventions based on a client's readiness for change. It remains to be demonstrated whether stage-appropriate interventions are effective not only in encouraging behavior change progress, but also in promoting maintenance of the desired change.

## Lifestyle Behavior Change

### Lifestyles and Health

Lifestyle has been described as a "general way of living based on the interplay between living conditions in the wide sense and individual patterns of behavior as determined by sociocultural factors and personal characteristics" (World Health Organization, 1986, p. 118). Some persons elect to incorporate habits that fall outside of traditional scientific-based medicine. When these health practices are used exclusively, they are known as **alternative health practices.** However, when they are used in combination with tradition scientific-based medicine, they become **complementary health practices.** Recent evidence reports that modifying simple lifestyle habits can increase the length of life.

Pender suggests that a healthy lifestyle incorporates both health-protecting behavior and health-promoting behaviors. Health-protecting behavior includes activities such as:

1. Getting adequate sleep (7–8 hours a night).
2. Eating regular meals (not eating between meals); reducing dietary cholesterol and salt intake; and eating a diet with sufficient vitamins, calcium, and fiber.
3. Participating in recreational activity (e.g., long walks, gardening, swimming).
4. Consuming moderate or no alcohol.
5. Never smoking tobacco.
6. Maintaining near-average weight.
7. Establishing the habit of eating breakfast (Belloc & Breslow, 1972).

In contrast, health promotion "is motivated by the desire to increase well-being and actualize human health potential" (Pender, 1996, p. 7). Thus, health-promoting lifestyle activities might promote feelings of vitality, vigor, improved mood and affect, flexibility, relaxation, confidence, and harmony.

Why does a person make healthy lifestyle choices? What factors are important in promoting and sustaining positive changes in lifestyle habits? The answers to these questions are not clear, but some of the variables believed significant include:

- Motivation for change.
- Perceived self-efficacy.
- Supportive relationships.
- Knowledge of benefits.
- Perceived control.
- Definition of health.
- Lack of significant barriers.
- Modifying demographic, interpersonal, and situational variables.
- Positive reinforcement.

People select their lifestyles. Many assume responsibility for their own lifestyle choices; however, some persons may refuse to accept the consequences of personal actions that contribute to a perceived less than optimal lifestyle. The nurse can help facilitate behavioral change for persons who believe that personal actions determine lifestyle and who exhibit sufficient motivation. Thus, the nurse must understand the meaning of health promotion to the client and the client's expectations of outcomes of health promotion interventions. The nurse must shift thinking from using professional expertise to overcome client weaknesses, to empowering clients to help themselves by building on their strengths.

### Health Strengths

A large body of literature associates stress with illness. Stress is assumed to arise when a situation is appraised as threatening or otherwise demanding and an appropriate coping response is not immediately available (Lazarus & Folkman, 1984). When an event is appraised as stressful, emotionally linked responses occur that result in vulnerability to illness.

Certain characteristics, including social support, self-efficacy, and internal locus of control, seem to decrease the relationship between stress and illness. Two models explain the process by which these characteristics might influence well-being. One model suggests that the person is protected, or buffered, from the potentially pathogenic influence of stressful events. In this case, these characteristics would be related to well-being only (or primarily) for persons under stress (Cohen & Wills, 1985, p. 310). The alternative model suggests that health strengths have a beneficial effect, regardless of whether the person is under stress.

Some research suggests that certain personality characteristics reduce the perception of stress or increase resistance to stress and thus may be considered health strengths. In her theory of hardiness, Kobasa (1979) assumes that life is always changing and thus is inevitably stressful. However, people who have a sense of commitment (an overall sense of purpose), control (a belief that one can influence the course of events), and challenge (a view of change as opportunity and incentive for personal growth) are thought to be more resistant to stress. In the sense of coherence theory, Antonovsky (1987) proposes that confidence in comprehensibility (a cognitive sense that information is consistent, clear, and ordered), manageability (a belief that resources are adequate to meet demands), and meaningfulness (a motivational commitment and engagement), provide generalized resistance resources and promotes health. These two theories are compared in Table 8-1.

**TABLE 8-1**

## Comparison of the Subconcepts of the Sense of Coherence and Hardiness Models

| Antonovsky | Kobasa |
| --- | --- |
| Sense of coherence | Hardiness |
| Comprehensibility: cognitive sense | Challenge: change is normative |
| Manageability: adequate resources | Control: internal locus of control |
| Meaningfulness: motivation | Commitment: self-involvement |

### Strategies for Lifestyle Behavior Change

A **lifestyle behavior change** means that a person assumes different activities in multiple aspects of his/her life. The idea of changing health behavior is uncomfortable for many people. Deeply ingrained habits, even harmful ones, can be difficult to change, and most people have difficulty making even minor changes. According to Westberg and Jason (1996, pp. 147–148), people tend to resist change because change of behavior may:

- Require giving up pleasure (e.g., eating high-fat ice cream).
- Be unpleasant (e.g., doing certain exercises).
- Be overtly painful (e.g., discontinuing addictive substances).
- Be stressful (e.g., facing social situations without alcohol).
- Jeopardize social relationships (e.g., engaging in unprotected adolescent sex).
- Not seem important anymore (e.g., in the case of older individuals).
- Require alteration in self-image (e.g., in the case of a hard-working executive learning how to play).

As a result, giving up long-standing habits and attitudes is not easy for most people.

Given that health behavior change is difficult for most people, Westberg and Jason (1996, pp. 148–150) suggest that, to promote "what it takes" to make meaningful, lasting changes in lifestyle, the individual should:

- Endorse the need for change.
- Have "ownership" of the need for change.
- Feel that there is more to gain than to lose.
- Develop an enhanced sense of self-worth.
- Identify realistic goals and workable plans.
- Seek gradual change, rather than a "quick fix."
- Have patience.
- Address starting new behaviors, instead of just focusing on what behaviors should be stopped.
- Practice new behaviors.
- Seek the support of family, friends, colleagues, or health professionals.
- Gain positive reinforcement for the desired behavior.
- Have a strategy for monitoring progress and making needed changes.
- Seek constructive feedback.
- Have a mechanism for follow-up to reduce backsliding.

Learning how to help people adopt and sustain healthy attitudes and habits is a challenge for health professionals. "There are no miracle drugs available for helping people change long-standing patterns of living. Simply telling people to stop smoking, eat less fat, have safe sex, exercise more, discontinue their abusive practices, or reduce their life stresses seldom works" (Westberg & Jason, 1996, p. 146). Clients often do not follow the advice of nurses or physicians, particularly when authoritarian "orders" are given. Clients must be actively involved as collaborative partners who assess their current health, develop a health promotion plan, and monitor plan effectiveness. Rewards facilitate adherence to health promotion plans. The nurse can best assist in promoting and changing health behaviors by providing education (e.g., hazards of the latest health fad), facilitating changes (e.g., positive reinforcement for adhering to a plan), and sustaining positive health behaviors (e.g., reminding clients of how they were before they started the health promotion plan).

According to Prochaska, Redding, and colleagues (1994), some of the most frequently replicated strategies and techniques to help clients modify their behavior include:

- Consciousness raising.
- Self-reevaluation.
- Environmental reevaluation.
- Self-liberation.
- Social liberation.
- Helping relationships.
- Stimulus control.
- Counterconditioning.
- Reinforcement management.

During the contemplation stage of behavior change, consciousness raising occurs as the individual seeks information. The nurse can provide potential information resources so that the individual can be actively involved. The client's perceived incentives and barriers to change can be clarified, and the nurse can help explain and interpret often conflicting or unclear information. In addition, the knowledge and interest of family members can be assessed. It may be helpful for the individual to talk with others who have successfully made the contemplated changes.

As movement occurs toward the preparation and action stages of change, the individual engages in self- and environmental reevaluation. The individual considers how the current problem behavior (or lack of positive behavior) affects the physical and social environment and personal standards and values. Questions that might be asked include: Will I like myself better as a (thinner, nonsmoking, less-stressed) person? Is my environment supportive of the proposed changes? Do I believe that I am able to make and continue the changes needed? The assumption is that changes will not occur unless they are congruent with a person's self-concept.

A strategy that can assist with self- and social liberation is cognitive restructuring. "Cognitive restructuring focuses on client's thinking, imagery, and attitudes toward the self and self-competencies as they affect the change process" (Pender, 1996, p. 171). The nurse can help clients clarify the messages they give themselves about their health and health-related behaviors. Certain beliefs can be irrational. Positive affirmations and imagery, repeated several times daily, can help clients to believe that they have the power to think positively and make desired lifestyle changes.

Helping relationships with family members, friends, colleagues, or health care professionals can be critical in helping to move the individual through the preparation, action, and maintenance stages of change. A self-help group is a strategy that has been found to be helpful for modeling, support, and reinforcement of desired behavior.

Stimulus control, emphasizing activities that precede the desired behavior, can be helpful during the action and maintenance stages of change. The activities, which must be personally relevant for the individual client, might include a postcard reminder for mammography screening, a personal call from the nurse to encourage continued exercise, or a scheduled group meeting to practice relaxation. To encourage the development of a desirable behavior habit it may be helpful to promote the behavior in the same setting or context and time on a daily basis. For example, the client can be encouraged to exercise in a consistent place, early each morning before other activities intervene.

Counterconditioning to break an undesirable association between a stimulus and a response can be desirable during the latter part of the action stage and during the maintenance stage. Undesirable associations can occur that create a negative emotional response to the behavior. For example, many people indicate that exercising can become boring. The nurse can encourage a varied routine, walking outside when the weather permits, and at least occasional exercise with a partner to counteract boredom.

Reinforcement management is an effective strategy, especially during the preparation and action stages of change. "It is based on the premise that all behaviors are determined by their consequences. If positive consequences occur, the probability is high that the behavior will occur again. If negative consequences occur, the probability is low for the behavior's being repeated" (Pender, 1996, p. 172). Immediate reinforcement of the desired behavior is important, especially in the early phases of change. Personalized attention and positive verbal feedback are helpful. Eventually, a desirable consequence of the behavior can become an intrinsic reward. For example, a weekly scale reading indicating decreasing weight can be a reward in itself for continuing a weight reduction diet.

The object of these strategies is to decrease barriers and increase incentives to change behavior. Barriers to change include lack of:

- Knowledge.
- Skills.
- Perception of control.
- Facilities.
- Materials.
- Clear goals.
- Social support.
- Time.
- Motivation.

Incentives to change behavior include:

- Expectation of benefit.
- Sense of personal responsibility.
- Enjoyment of the activity.
- Previous experience.
- Guilt.
- Support from family, peers, or professionals (Leddy & Fawcett, 1997).

The nurse and the client should base the choice of appropriate strategies to foster incentives and reduce barriers and thereby promote behavior change.

The previous section addresses models and strategies for health promotion consistent with the interaction world view of health. In the next section, models and strategies for health patterning consistent with the integration world view for health are discussed.

## ● HEALTH PATTERNING

### Models for Health Patterning

For centuries, the concept of vital life energy, or chi, has been a part of Eastern religion and culture. For example, the ancient Chinese originated the belief that chi circulates through invisible channels called meridians that can be blocked by stressors or by living excesses. A blockage in energy flow results in energy imbalances and areas of the body with energy deficits, producing symptoms or disease.

Leddy's (2004) practice theory of energy (see Chapter 5) proposes that consciousness or focused attention by the nurse can pattern client–nurse energy by clearing (transforming), conveying (carrying), coursing (re-establishing free flow), conserving (decreasing disorder), converting (amplifying resonance), or connecting energy (promoting synchronization to promote harmony).

Martha Rogers introduced the concept of the person as an energy field interacting with an environmental energy field to nursing (see Chapter 5). She conceptualizes that **health patterning** of the human energy field occurs simultaneously and mutually with changes in the environmental energy field. The nurse (part of the environmental energy field) can influence the client's health by redistributing energy and thus repatterning the client's energy field. Nurses work with manifestations of health patterns (Leddy, 2003). Viewing persons as energy fields provides rationale for nontraditional healing modalities that enhance health patterns.

## Health Patterning Modalities

Leddy (2003) identifies integrative nursing interventions to promote health and healing. The following interventions act on the human energy field and can be used by nurses in clinical practice:

1. To relinquish bound energy: herbal preparations and aromatherapy.
2. To re-establish energy flow: physical activity, Tai Chi, Qigong (ChiGung), aerobic and strengthening exercises.
3. To release blocked energy: touch, massage, acupressure, reflexology, applied kinesiology (touch for health), Jin Shin Do, self-massage, Alexander technique, Feldenkrais method, Trager psychophysical integration, Structural Integration (Rolfing).
4. To reduce energy depletion: meditation, autogenic training to elicit the relaxation response, progressive muscle relaxation, deep breathing exercises, yoga, biofeedback, and guided imagery.
5. To regenerate agent optimal nutrition from: foodstuffs, vitamin and mineral supplements, high fiber diet, ingestion of phytonutrients (soy, garlic, onions, and deep-colored fruits and vegetables), antioxidants (vitamins A, C, and E; selenium, coenzyme Q 10, beta carotene).
6. To restore energy field harmony: centering, chromatherapy (color therapy), music therapy, polarity therapy, prayer, Reiki, therapeutic touch.

The literature contains increasing evidence that these kinds of therapies, most of which are noninvasive and involve the client as an active participant in the process, have tangible and highly desirable outcomes for health and healing. Nursing licensing examinations in Europe contain information about the safe use of herbs and essential oils. Before using complementary interventions with clients, the nurse must be educated about how each may affect physiology and potential adverse effects (Dossey, Keegan, & Guzzetta, 2005). In the future, nurses will be increasingly expected to incorporate patterning methods as an integral part of clinical practice.

## ● IMPLICATIONS OF THE NURSE'S VIEW OF HEALTH FOR ROLE PERFORMANCE

"In a positive model of health, emphasis is placed on strengths, resiliencies, resources, potentials, and capabilities rather than on existing pathology" (Pender, 1996, p. 16). The integrative world view supports the beliefs that nurses work with persons who display areas of strength and weakness in health pattern manifestations at a specific time. The effects of the nurse on client manifestations of patterns are complex and nonlinear. Persons entrenched in reductionism or who espouse to an interaction world view may find this approach confusing, and perhaps even nonscientific. However, recent studies have shown that even thinking about or praying for clients may enhance health and healing (Burkhardt & Nagai-Jacobson, 2005).

In trying to improve the quality of health of clients and self, the nurse is obligated to fulfill roles that incorporate promoting health, systematically and strategically planning changes, and using the strengths displayed by the client. Note that the terms "promotion and maintenance of health" were missing. "Maintenance" is an obsolete concept because wellness (health) is an active process in which life moves forward, and the client is always evolving. The nurse may promote well-being and may restore perceptions of well-being, but the process of health does not permit the status quo that maintenance implies.

If health is a process, and if nurses believe that nursing focuses on the person's responses, as a whole, to the environment and to a perception of well-being, then nurses have a basis for a variety of professional roles when clients perceive a sense of harmony, vitality and ability; when they can learn most effectively how to enhance their personal strength and gain greater control of their lives; and when they perceive a lack of harmony, feel consumed by weakness, and feel vulnerable (the illness state).

In this first section, the chapter described strategies the nurse can use to help promote or protect the health of the client. In the next section, the emphasis is on self-care strategies the nurse can use to promote her or his own health.

## ● SELF-CARE OF THE NURSE

### The Stressful Work Environment

A stressful work environment refers to the pressure that is put on nurses by the external organizational forces that determine work conditions. The health care system contributes to nurse burnout through multiple regulations, lack of adequate staffing, mandatory overtime, reimbursement issues, lack of perceived support for quality nursing care at the bedside, and failure to seek nurse input into clinical practice issues. At times, a nurse's work environment could be compared to assembly line work with the goal of moving clients in and out of the system as quickly as possible to reduce costs. Client-care protocols that streamline care and reduce chances for error leave little room for individualization of nursing care. Little time is available to develop therapeutic client relationships and do the small things for clients that make big differences. With reduced client contact, nurses usually cannot see evidence of how their interventions positively affect client outcomes. Being put in the position of having to lower standards to accommodate the employers' financial agenda (especially in for-profit institutions) creates distress for some professional nurses. If left alone, the distress becomes a state of emotional exhaustion known as **burnout.**

The more conscientious nurses, who have a need to give their very best, are most vulnerable to burnout. Cullen (1995) suggests that one of two things happens when nurses work in a system in which they are never able to give their best. Either the nurses lower their standards and work apathetically or they may continue trying to give their best, while constantly bucking a system that fails to have excellence in nursing as a top priority, until they finally experience burnout.

### Questions for Reflection 8-3

1. What current factors in my professional practice setting cause me to feel stressed?
2. How do I currently handle stress?

## Stress and Burnout

A person becomes overstressed when demands exceed perceived resources. Some stress is inevitable and even positive in energizing the person. However, more stress than can be managed may be associated with physical, mental, emotional, and behavioral symptoms in health care providers. According to Mitchell and Cormack (1998), some of the more common symptoms of stress in nurses and other practitioners include:

- Sleep disturbance and fatigue.
- Appetite loss.
- Decreased ability to concentrate.
- Frequent lateness.
- Overeating or increased smoking.
- Sudden mood swings.
- Deep resentment of clients.

If a nurse is constantly exposed to a situation in which demands exceed resources, the nurse's energies gradually will deplete, culminating in the state of emotional and physical apathy and exhaustion known as burnout. Stressful events may be perceived as either challenges that lead to positive growth or threats that can lead to negative consequences (Wells-Federman, 1996). Escalating and continual emotional overload is a common factor in burnout (Kahn & Saulo, 1994). However, job problems alone do not cause burnout. Rather, "it is the worker's lack of control over his job situation that leads to uncertainty, frustration, reduced motivation, and eventually burnout" (Davis, Eshelman, & McKay, 1996, p. 167). The symptoms of stress underload are quite similar to those of stress overload: reduced efficiency, irritability, a sense of time pressure, diminished motivation, poor judgment, and accidents.

The best time to think about burnout is before it happens. Answers to questions such as: "Do I feel little enthusiasm for doing my job," "Do I feel tired even with adequate sleep," and "Do I have too much to do and too little time in which to do it" can help the nurse to identify symptoms and sources of job stress and signs of impending burnout (Davis et al., 1988).

Selected suggestions for ways to manage nursing job stress are listed in Display 8-1. Many of the strategies require that the nurse take time to evaluate current working conditions and require attitudinal and behavioral changes.

---

## Managing Job Stress

**DISPLAY 8-1**

- Identify sources of job stress
- Set realistic goals and priorities to respond effectively to job stress and demands
- Avoid procrastination
- Say no when offered special projects or opportunities
- Toss out clutter in your work environment
- Develop and maintain trusting, mutual, and meaningful collegial relationships with coworkers (and persons outside of the work setting)
- Adopt an attitude that change is a challenge rather than an inconvenience
- Cast off the perception of the nurse being victimized by more powerful members of the health care team
- Inject fun and humor in the work setting
- Create a positive environment by looking at the bright side of adversity
- Take control over nursing work processes
- Participate in decision making
- Schedule time to eat a healthy meal or snacks each day while at work

- Consume a healthy diet (a balanced diet with moderation in refined sugars)
- Take responsibility for successes and failures
- Take a 15–20 minute mini-vacation daily while on the job. Go to a quiet place in the work setting to relax (progressive relaxation, deep breathing exercises, meditation or prayer with your beeper and/or cell phone turned off)
- Confront work issues directly with persons involved
- Engage in a daily regimen of physical exercise that you find enjoyable (stretching, strength building, and aerobic exercises)
- Take vacations and personal days when needed
- Get an adequate amount of sleep (for most persons this is 7–8 hours)
- Balance your work and personal life

*Sources*: Bost, 2005; Boucher, 2004; Cherewatenko & Perry, 2003; Covey, 2004; Davis, Eshelman, & McKay, 2000; Dossey, Keegan, & Guzzetta, 2005; Ellis & Harper, 1961; Kendall-Reed & Reed, 2004; McGraw, 2004; Neuharth, 2004; Sachs, 2001; Schaffner & Ludwig-Beymer, 2003.

---

The following section presents a number of techniques for managing job stress, preventing burnout, and promoting well-being.

## Techniques to Enhance Well-Being

This section emphasizes positive techniques that can be used to avoid burnout, promote health, and reframe stressors into challenges. **Health-enhancing techniques** promote personal well-being. Techniques such as stress management, affirmations, refuting irrational ideas, social support, values clarification, and taking care of oneself are presented.

### Stress Management

"The role of the practitioner needs to be clarified and untangled from notions about being perfectly strong, healthy, in control and omnipotent" (Mitchell & Cormack, 1998, p. 145). However, given that stressors are an inevitable part of personal and professional interactions, a number of techniques have been proposed in the literature as positive ways to build strengths, avoid burnout, and promote well-being. First, it is necessary to identify sources of stress and be aware of tension build-up and situations that are likely to prove stressful. The nurse should try to get in touch with her body, and learn her body's reaction

---

**Organizing Time to Achieve Goals**                          DISPLAY 8-2   ●

- Control situations as much as possible; schedule to avoid too many changes or events happening at the same time.
- Organize your time to accomplish the most important goals; identify values and goals and goal priorities as a framework for time management.
- Set limits; be assertive.
- Say no to demands that are unrealistic or of low priority; imagine yourself protected inside of a bubble.

- Reduce tasks into smaller parts to allow mastery and feelings of competence.
- Delegate responsibilities to others and enlist their assistance; use the skills of others; you don't have to be "all things to all people"; differentiate between time urgencies that are valid and others that are needlessly created; overinvolvement leaves little time for fulfillment of personal needs and often leads to resentment and blame (Wells-Federman, 1996).

---

to and manifestations of stress (sweaty palms, tightening of back and neck muscles, dry mouth). If signs of stress are recognized early, it is possible to start stress-relieving exercises that can keep the effects of stress from increasing (Eliopoulos, 1999).

It is important for the nurse to take care of herself or himself first before attempting to meet someone else's needs (Elder, 1999). Organization of time is one way to focus on the most important goals. Suggestions for ways to organize time are provided in Display 8-2. Goal achievement requires setting time aside to set realistic goals, determining an action plan, using personal values to determine priority goals, and delegating tasks to others.

Enhancement of self-esteem is another way to avoid burnout and promote well-being. Increasing self-awareness of one's positive characteristics can enhance self-esteem. In addition, the nurse should assertively express her thoughts and feelings; share feelings, troubles, and opinions with others; accept shortcomings and imperfections; and maintain a positive and tolerant attitude toward others and the world at large. One way to do this is to change the way a stressor is viewed by putting it in proper perspective to help make the stressor manageable.

To help avoid worrying, it may be helpful to practice the serenity prayer, authored by a medieval monk, St. Francis of Assisi: "God grant me the serenity to accept the things I cannot change, the courage to change the things I can, and the wisdom to know the difference" (Mauk & Schmidt, 2004). In addition, it is helpful for the nurse to try to reduce the "shoulds" and "should nots." "It is reasonable, legitimate, and healthy for clients to express their needs and do what is best for themselves; why do nurses perceive themselves as being different?

. . . . "I should take care of my own needs and I should not worry about what others may think" (Eliopoulos, 1999, p. 311). Display 8-3 lists selected stress reduction or supportive noninvasive modalities. Many of these strategies fall within the realm of health-promoting behaviors.

Additional strategies that might be helpful in achieving a balance between threatening and challenging stress are listed in Display 8-4. Like the other display strategies, these also may require that the nurse ask for help from others.

### Affirmations

Another strategy that can contribute to healthful self-care is to promote affirmations, "a positive thought that you consciously choose to immerse in your consciousness to

| Selected Stress Reduction and Supportive Noninvasive Modalities | DISPLAY 8-3 ● |
| --- | --- |

- Make the environment conducive to relaxation, rather than overstimulating, by adjusting the noise, room temperature, and lighting.
- Follow good health practices by eating a sound diet, avoiding caffeine, avoiding simple carbohydrates ("junk food") and food additives, and supplementing vitamins A, C, E, and the B-complex group.
- Have regular physical activity (exercise).
- Get ample and regular rest and sleep.
- Instead of coffee and cigarette breaks, enjoy short relaxation exercises, recline in a quiet area, or listen to relaxing music.
- Have a pet.
- Practice mindfulness and relaxation.
- Get in touch with nature.

- Build leisure activities into the day; develop a hobby.
- Take vacations and breaks from routine work.
- Use alternative therapies, such as therapeutic massage, guided imagery, progressive relaxation, meditation, yoga, herbs, or aromatherapy.
- Use herbs (e.g., Echinacea or ginseng) to protect the immune system if subjected to chronic or high levels of stress.
- Learn how to center. "The skill of relaxing in the face of stress, taking a deep breath, loosening some of the tension in your neck and shoulders, and quieting your mind for a few moments is called centering. Centering is simply regaining your physical, mental, and emotional balance in order to proceed with the task at hand" (Achterberg, Dossey, & Kolkmeier, 1994, p. 62).

| Additional Strategies to Balance Threatening and Challenging Stress | DISPLAY 8-4 ● |
| --- | --- |

- Develop a sense of balance among physical, mental, and spiritual dimensions.
- Get personal and social support during times of stress and distress; develop personal support systems at work.
- Find ways to maintain interest, enthusiasm, and knowledge at work by remaining alert to new ideas; avoid isolation by attending conferences and discussing your practice with other people; hear and accept the praise from clients and colleagues.

- Leave work behind when you go home.
- Set limits and have priorities other than work.
- Be interested. "Everyone wants to be interesting, but the vitalizing thing is to be interested. . . . Keep a sense of curiosity. . . . Discover new things" (Gardner, 1996, p. 11).
- Avoid unfulfilling or burdensome relationships; minimize contact with people who add more stress, rather than joy, to your life.
- Risk failure.

produce a desired result" (Clark, 1996a, p. 39). Affirmations are positive self-statements that become healthy alternatives to negative self-talk. An affirmation is simply a positive thought, a short phrase, or a saying that has meaning for the person. It can help change assumptions and beliefs that have negative consequences. Affirmations are important in reinforcing new ways of thinking and behaving from moment to moment. They are statements that can be selected to reaffirm new intentions, and they can help to increase the clarity of goals and help the nurse assume responsibility for actions. When starting to feel upset, anxious, frustrated, sad, or overwhelmed, the nurse can stop and examine her or his internal monologue and simply challenge that monologue with language that is more affirming, such as:

- I can ask for what I need.
- I can take care of myself.
- I'm doing the best I can.

- I can find alternatives to problems.
- I can meet my needs.
- I care for myself, and I care for others.

Initially this may seem superficial and uncomfortable, but as the internal monologue is changed, the nurse will begin to notice changes in behavior and in the environment (Wells-Federman, 1996). Do not allow the negative thought patterns of others to distract you from your mission. The guidelines in Display 8-5 are suggestions for the use of affirmations.

### Refuting Irrational Ideas

In a system called rational emotive therapy, Ellis and Harper (1961) proposed that emotions are not caused by actual events. In between the event and the emotion, they said, is realistic or unrealistic self-talk that produces the emotions. Accordingly, the person's own thoughts, directed and controlled by the individual, are what create anxiety, anger, and depression. But irrational self-talk can be changed and the stressful emotions changed with it (Davis et al., 1996).

At the root of all irrational thinking is the assumption that things are done to someone. Statements that interpret experience as catastrophic (e.g., a momentary chest pain is a heart attack) or absolute (e.g., I should, must, ought, always, or never) are examples of irrational thinking. Other examples of irrational ideas are listed in Display 8-6.

Irrational ideas can be disputed and eliminated through a process of rational thinking that includes (Davis et al., 1996; Ellis & Harper, 1961):

1. Writing down the objective facts of the event.
2. Writing down your self-talk, rational and irrational.
3. Focusing on your emotional response.
4. Questioning the rational support (e.g., evidence) for and against an irrational idea.
5. Identifying the worst and best things that could happen.
6. Substituting alternative self-talk.

---

## Guidelines for the Use of Affirmations

**DISPLAY 8-5** ●

- Find a relaxing, sharing atmosphere. Consider using a relaxation exercise before the affirmation process.
- What health issues are you concerned about?
- Is the affirmation best stated in the attitude, feeling, or action mode? Are you ready for action?
- State the affirmation in your own words. Affirmations are best stated in the becoming mode ("It's getting easier," "I'm becoming more comfortable").
- Once you have selected an affirmation, write or say the affirmation 10 to 20 times each day while listening to your inner, gut response to hearing it said or writing it.

- Carry your chosen affirmation with you on an index card and place it in a briefcase, purse, or car dashboard where it will be read throughout the day. Hearing oneself on tape, viewing oneself saying the affirmation, or writing and reading it back provides two kinds of feedback and thus is more powerful than simply saying the affirmation to oneself.
- Provide an ongoing method of reinforcement for continuing the affirmation.
- Try not to become frustrated or expect too much.

*Source*: Clark, 1996b.

---

## Examples of Irrational Ideas

- It is possible to please all persons all of the time.
- Complete competence and perfection is possible in everything.
- Things can always be as I want them to be.
- Misery is created from external factors.
- The unknown, uncertain, and potential dangers instill great fear in me.
- I need to rely upon others at all times.
- Avoiding life's difficulties and responsibilities is easier than facing them.
- The past directs the present and the future.
- Constant relaxation and leisure leads to happiness.
- I am the only one capable to do the job properly.

- Life situations and other persons are the source of pressure.
- It is possible to have it all, all of the time.
- I am responsible for everything that happens.
- Genetics dictate my reactions and life outcomes.
- It is impossible to control my emotions.
- Just getting over things is easy.
- Contributions I make to the world are unimportant.
- All my problems are my fault.
- There is one single best approach to life.

*Sources*: Bost, 2005; Davis, Eshelman, & McKay, 2000; Dossey, Keegan, & Guzzetta, 2005; Ellis & Harper, 1961; McGraw, 2004; Neuharth, 2004.

---

### Social Support

Fellow colleagues can provide the insights and perspectives necessary to cope with commonly shared experiences. "Acknowledging the pain and seeking support from others are the most enduring long-term coping strategies. Practicing collegiality is a way of fostering this social support network. It is a way of building an atmosphere at work where you can support your colleagues and they you" (Wells-Federman, 1996, p. 15).

Building a supportive work environment requires conscious awareness of and action toward valuing yourself and your colleagues. The following are some suggestions (Wells-Federman, 1996) for shaping the quality of the atmosphere in which you work and developing a stronger support network.

- Find someone doing something right, and acknowledge him or her.
- Expect the best from yourself and those with whom you work.
- Model the values you believe. Take responsibility for your health and well-being, and encourage others to do the same.
- Establish a mentoring or buddy system.
- Make decisions based on nursing's ethical values.
- Establish a support group to help deal with the feelings that can arise from professional practice.
- Be supportive, but refer colleagues to professional support when needed.

### Research Brief 8-1

Yip, V. Y. B. (2004). New low back pain in nurses: work activities, work stress and sedentary lifestyle. *Journal of Advanced Nursing, 46,* 430–440.

The investigator sought to identify and predict factors that contributed to the new onset of low back pain in professional nurses. One hundred forty-four nurses who work in six Hong Kong hospitals were interviewed face-to-face and were observed over 12 months using surveys. Fifty-six nurses reported having a new onset of lower back pain during the study. Stepwise logistic regression revealed statistical significant links of the following factors to the new onset of back pain:

1. Being a new nurse on the unit.
2. Working with the back bent.
3. Ineffective working relationships with colleagues.

The findings from this study supported results from other studies in that ineffective collegial relationships with coworkers and bending positions contributed to low back pain in nurses. Social support appears to be an important factor in reducing stress in the workplace. However, this study failed to show support for sedentary leisure activities for nurses as being a predictor of new onset of back pain. Avoiding back bending and effective relationships with coworkers may be factors that promote health in practicing professional nurses.

Implications for practice from this study include the need for nurses not to assume a bending position when working with clients, giving new nurses on a unit extra collegial support, and the importance of building effective nursing teams to protect the physical health of nurses. In addition, the stress of ineffective collegial relationships among staff nurses needs to be addressed. Because the study had a small sample and used nurses in Hong Kong, the findings of this study may not apply to all nurses. Further research addressing potential factors resulting in low back pain in nurses needs to be performed so that nurses can develop ways to protect their physical health.

## Values Clarification

It may be helpful to consider why, despite the drawbacks, nursing can be so rewarding. Editors at *Nursing 2000* magazine ("Nursing top ten rewards," 2000) compiled the following list of 10 values, "qualities that make nursing great," based on interviews with 20 seasoned nurses. Some of these values may be helpful in considering personal strengths of practicing nursing.

- A way to make a difference.
- The human connection.
- Flexibility.
- The chance to use all of yourself.
- Long-term security.
- The chance to mentor.
- A connection between technology and humanity.
- Respect.
- Personal growth and rewards.

There is a procedure known as values clarification that can be used to try to identify values that are most significant for an individual. This process also can be helpful in focusing self-care priorities for the nurse. Clark (1996b, p. 19) describes three steps in a values clarification process.

1. Prizing
   a. Prizing and cherishing. Learn to set priorities, become aware of what the nurse is for or against, begin to trust inner experiences and feelings, and examine why she feels as she does.

    b. Clearly communicate personal values and actively listen to others as they share theirs.

  2. Choosing

    a. Choosing freely by examining values others have imposed on the nurse.

    b. Choosing thoughtfully between alternatives by examining the process by which the nurse chooses and considering the possible consequences of each choice.

  3. Acting

    a. Trying out the value choice by developing a plan of action and trying it out.

    b. Evaluating what happened when action was taken and making plans to reinforce actions that support the values.

## Taking Care of Oneself

As nurses, we have a responsibility to take care of ourselves because we can be in a position to give only when our own needs have, at least to some extent, been acknowledged and satisfied. Mitchell and Cormack (1998, p. 142) suggest ways for the nurse to protect herself or himself from burnout, including:

- Do some honest soul searching to determine whether you're the kind of nurse who needs to express creativity and excellence, who values and displays originality and enthusiasm in your work.
- Objectively evaluate your workplace and respond proactively to achieve a more positive outcome for yourself.
- Don't assume responsibility where you have none.
- Be honest about what you can and can't do in your role, given the constraints on your time and resources.
- Remember you're not on duty 24 hours a day and that nursing is one part of the whole of your life.
- Remember that a good job doesn't love you back, and get your priorities straight.
- Find your own outlets for creativity.
- Don't stay in a situation that consistently fails to meet your needs; give yourself permission to leave.
- Give yourself a break.
- Create support for yourself.
- Love yourself; heal your wounds.
- If the problem is a feeling of helplessness, the solution is to develop personal power.
- Try approaching each task as a challenge.
- Remember that you are here to serve, not to rescue.

    Focusing on the positive sides of giving care to others can be helpful. Helping others as professional nurses provides great rewards. The work is challenging and fulfilling especially when nurses can see the effects of interventions. Some nurses find problem solving thrilling, especially when they have success with creative methods never used. Some nurses derive a deep intrinsic pleasure just by knowing that they helped another person. The personal pleasure becomes enhanced when clients express gratitude, and nurses see the results of efforts to reduce human suffering (Mitchell & Cormack, 1998).

    In summary, nurses need to care for themselves to provide effective care to others. Lifestyle patterns and behaviors of nurses affect the ability to extend themselves to help others. Because nurses are people, they must assume responsibility for **personal health promotion.**

### Barriers to Self-Care

One example of a barrier to self-care is the belief that "it can't happen to me," in which a nurse may feel that she or he will not be in danger of burnout because she or he is too smart or too aware to let negative feelings progress to burnout. Another issue may be rooted in the altruistic nature of many nurses, in which the client or the job may take precedence to considering the nurse's health. So, for example, the nurse may feel that "I don't deserve to be cared for in the same way as others," or "I can't get sick because others depend on me," or "My job is to take care of others, not to look after myself." The essence of this section has been the message that the nurse must take care of herself or himself first. Then, the nurse will be better able to continue to deal with the stresses of the work environment, and advocate for the needs of clients.

## ⊕ SUMMARY AND SIGNIFICANCE TO PRACTICE

In our society, responsibility for illness has been delegated to health professionals who have been prepared and are rewarded for delivering care to the sick. Short-term incentives and rewards to maintain health do not exist for the recipient; in addition, the health care system is not organized to reward providers for keeping clients well.

Clients must be encouraged to assume an increased concern and responsibility for their health potential. Nurses can support, facilitate, and encourage those positive skills, qualities, and plans that will promote health. The client and the nurse, based on goals and a timetable determined by the client, can then devise interventions collaboratively.

In addition, nurses need to take responsibility for self-care. Approaches to managing job stress and techniques such as stress management, affirmations, refuting irrational ideas, social support, values clarification, and taking care of oneself are positive techniques that can be used to avoid burnout, reframe stressors into challenges, and enhance well-being.

### FROM THEORY TO PRACTICE

1. Identify factors within your current lifestyle that fall into the categories of health promotion and health protection. What are the consequences of a lifestyle focused on health protection rather than health promotion?
2. Thinking about Jane and Michael in the vignette, identify factors in their (or your) work environment that are not health promoting. Why is having a colleague to share common experiences important for promoting health?
3. Did you find some of the tips for caring for yourself helpful? If so which ones do you plan to use? If not, why not?

### WWW INTERNET EXERCISES

1. Visit the American Holistic Nurses Association at http://www.ahna.org. Click on the icon, "About AHNA." Read the information. Would you be interested in joining the AHNA ? Why or why not?

2. Using the search engine of your choice, type in one of the nursing interventions for the human energy field identified by Leddy (2003). Come prepared to participate in a class discussion about the information you find. Do you think other health team members would agree that the identified intervention would be beneficial to clients? Why or why not?

## INTERNET RESOURCES

American Association of Retired Persons: http://www.aarp.org. Access information related to healthy living and aging and a wide array of information addressing the special sociocultural concerns of the elderly.

Center for Disease Control and the National Center for Chronic Disease Prevention and Health Promotion: http://www.cdc.gov. Learn the latest information related to prevention of communicable diseases along with health promotion information to reduce the incidence of chronic diseases.

American Institute for Cancer Research: http://www.aicr.org. Consult this site for the research-based information for the prevention of cancer and healthy lifestyle information.

National Institutes of Health: http://www.nih.gov. Read information about the latest government-sponsored health research along with opportunities for funding health promotion research. Read about the National Center for Complementary and Alternative Medicine. www.nccam.nih.gov.

Alternative Medicine Home Page: http://www.pitt.edu/~cbwaltm.html. Jump to a variety of alternative and complementary health care websites from this website maintained by the Falk Library for the Health Sciences at the University of Pittsburgh.

Association for Applied and Therapeutic Humor: http://www.aath.org. Tickle your funny bone by visiting this website and jump to other health care humor sites to lift your spirits.

National Health Information Center: http://health.gov/nhic. Obtain educational materials for clients and yourself using this website.

American Heart Association: http://www.americanheart/org. Visit this site to learn the latest on cardiovascular disease. Because this is a client-oriented site, refer clients and their families to this site.

The American Holistic Nurses Association: http://www.ahna.org.

## REFERENCES

Achterburg, J., Dossey, B., & Kolkmeirer, L. (1994). *Rituals of healing: using imagery for health and wellness*. New York: Bantam.

Antonovsky, A. (1987). *Unraveling the mystery of health*. San Francisco: Jossey-Bass.

Ardell, D. B. (1979). The nature and implications of high level wellness or why 'normal health' is in a rather sorry state of existence. *Health Values, 3,* 17–24.

Becker, M. H., & Maiman, L. A. (1975). Sociobehavioral determinants of compliance with health and medical care recommendations. *Medical Care, 13,* 10–24.

Belloc, N. B., & Breslow, L. (1972). Relationship of physical health status and health practices. *Preventive Medicine, 1,* 409–421.

Benner, P., Tanner, C. A., & Chesla, C. A. (Eds.). (1996). *Expertise in nursing practice: Caring, clinical judgement, and ethics*. New York: Springer.

Bost, B. W. (2005). *The hurried woman syndrome: A seven-step program to conquer fatigue, control weight, and restore passion to your relationship*. New York: McGraw-Hill.

Boucher, J. (2004). *How to love the job you hate: Job satisfaction for the 21st century*. Reno, NV: Beagle Bay Books.

Burkhardt, M. A., & Nagai-Jacobson, M. G. (2005). Spirituality and Health. Chapter 7 (pp. 137-172) in Dossey, B., Keegan, L., & Guzzetta, C. (Eds.). (2005). *Holistic nursing: A handbook for practice*, (4th ed.). Sudbury, MA: Jones and Bartlett.

Cherewatenko, V., & Perry, P. (2003). *The stress cure*. New York: HarperResource.

Clark, C. (1996a). Career fitness guide. Stress management. *Nursing Spectrum, 5,* 65–68.

Clark, C. (1996b). *Wellness practitioner: Concepts, research and strategies* (2nd ed.). New York. Springer.

Cohen, S., & Wills, T. A. (1985). Stress, social support and the buffering hypothesis. *Psychological Bulletin, 98,* 310–357.

Covey, S. R. (2004). *The 8th habit: From effectiveness to greatness*. New York: Free Press.

Cullen, A. (1995). Burnout: Why do we blame the nurse? *American Journal of Nursing, 95,* 22–28.

Davis, M., Eshelman, E. R., & McKay, M. (2000). *The relaxation and stress reduction workbook* (5th ed.). Oakland, CA: New Harbinger.

Dossey, B. M., Keegan, L., & Guzzetta, C. (2005). *Holistic nursing: a handbook for practice* (4th ed.). Sudbury, MA: Jones and Bartlett.

Dubos, R. (1978). Health and creative adaptation. *Human Nature, 1,* 74–82.

Dunn, H. H. (1977). What high-level wellness means. *Health Values, 1,* 9–16.

Elder, A. (1999). Nurturning the caregiver in today's health care arena. *Advance for Nurses,* March 1, 1999, page 7.

Ellis, A., & Harper, R. (1961). *A guide to rational living*. North Hollywood, CA: Wilshire Books.

Eliopoulos, C. (1999). *Integrating conventional and alternative therapies: Holistic care for chronic conditions*. St. Louis: Mosby.

Fawcett, J. (1993). *Conceptual models of nursing* (3rd ed.). Philadelphia: F. A. Davis.

Hall, B. A. (1981). The change paradigm in nursing: Growth versus persistence. *Advances in Nursing Science, 3,* 1–6.

Hravnak, M. (1998). Is there a health promotion and protection foundation to the practice of acute care nurse practitioners? *AACN Clinical Issues, 9,* 283–289.

Janz, N. K., & Becker, M. H. (1984). The health belief model: A decade later. *Health Education Quarterly, 11,* 1–47.

Jensen, L. A., & Allen, M. N. (1994). A synthesis of qualitative research on wellness-illness. *Qualitative Health Research, 4,* 349–369.

Kahn, S., & Saulo, M. (1994). *Healing yourself: A nurse's guide to self-care and renewal*. Albany, NY: Delmar.

Kasl, S., & Cobb, S. (1966). Health behavior, illness behavior and sick role behavior. *Archives of Environmental Health, 12,* 246–266.

Kendall-Reed, P., & Reed, S. (2004). *The complete doctor's stress solution: Understanding, treating and preventing stress and stress-related illnesses*. Toronto: Robert Rose.

Kobasa, S. C. (1979). Stressful life events, personality and health: An inquiry into hardiness. *Journal of Personality and Social Psychology, 37,* 1–11.

Lazarus, R. S., & Folkman, J. (1984). *Stress appraisal and coping*. New York: Springer.

Leddy, S. K. (2003). *Integrative health promotion: Conceptual bases for nursing practice*. Thorofare, NJ: Slack.

Leddy, S. K. (2004). Human energy: A conceptual model of unitary nursing science. *Visions: The Journal of Rogerian Nursing Science, 12,* 14-27.

Leddy, S. K., & Fawcett, J. (1997). Testing the theory of healthiness: Conceptual and methodological issues. In M. Madrid (Ed.), *Patterns of Rogerian knowing* (pp. 75–86). New York: National League for Nursing.

Mauk, K., & Schmidt, N. (2004). *Spiritual care in nursing practice*. Philadelphia: Lippincott Williams & Wilkins.

McGraw, P. R. (2004). *It's not your fault: How healing relationships change your brain and can help you overcome a painful past*. Wilmette, IL: Baha'i Publishing Trust.

McWilliam, C. L., Stewart, M., Brown, J. B., Desai, K., & Coderre, P. (1996). Creating health with chronic illness. *Advances in Nursing Science, 18,* 1–15.

Mitchell, A., & Cormack, M. (1998). *The therapeutic relationship in complementary health care*. Edinburgh: Churchill Livingstone.

Neuharth, D. (2004). *Secrets you keep from yourself: How to stop sabotaging your happiness*. New York: St. Martin's Press.

Newman, M. A. (1992). Prevailing paradigms in nursing. *Nursing Outlook, 40,* 10–13, 32.

Newman, M. A. (1994). *Health as expanding consciousness* (2nd ed.). St. Louis: Mosby.

"Nursing top ten rewards." (2000). *Nursing 2000*, 30, (5), 42–43.

Parse, R. R. (1987). *Nursing science: Major paradigms, theories, and critiques.* Philadelphia: WB Saunders.

Parsons, T. (1958). Definitions of health and illness in the light of American values and social structure. In E. G. Jaco (Ed.), *Patients, physicians, and illness* (pp. 165–187). Glencoe, IL: The Free Press.

Pender, N. J. (1996). *Health promotion in nursing practice* (3rd ed.). Stamford, CT: Appleton & Lange.

Pender, N. J., Murdaugh, C. L., & Parsons, M. (2002). *Health promotion in nursing practice* (4th ed.). Upper Saddle River, NJ: Prentice-Hall.

Prochaska, J. O., Redding, C. A., Harlow, L. L., Rossi, J. S., & Velicer, W. F. (1994a). The transtheoretical model of change and HIV prevention: A review. *Health Education Quarterly, 21,* 471–486.

Prochaska, J. O., Velicer, W. F., Rossi, J. S., Goldstein, M. G., Marcus, B. H., Rakowski, W., Fiore, C., Harlow, L. L., Redding, C. A., Rosenbloom, D., & Rossi, S. R. (1994b). Stages of change and decisional balance for 12 problem behaviors. *Health Psychology, 13,* 39–46.

Rosenstock, I. M. (1966). Why people use health services. *Milbank Memorial Fund Quarterly, 44,* 94–127.

Rosenstock, I. M., Strecher, V. J., & Becker, N. H. (1988). Societal learning theory and the health belief model. *Health Education Quarterly, 25,* 175–183.

Sachs, J. (2001). *20-minute vacations*. Lincolnwood, IL: Contemporary Books.

Schaffner, J. W., & Ludwig-Beymer, P. (2003). *Rx for the nursing shortage: A guidebook*. Chicago: Health Administration Press.

Smith, J. A. (1981). The idea of health: A philosophical inquiry. *Advances in Nursing Science, 3,* 43–50.

Terris, M. (1975). Approaches to an epidemiology of health, *American Journal of Public Health, 65,* 1039.

Twaddle, A. C., & Hessler, R. M., (1977). *A sociology of health*. St. Louis: Mosby.

United States Department of Health and Human Services. (2000). *Healthy people 2010*. Boston: Jones & Bartlett.

Vincent, C., & Furnham, A. (1997). *Complementary medicine: A research perspective*. Chichester: John Wiley & Sons.

Wells-Federman, C. L. (1996). Awakening the nurse healer within. *Holistic Nursing Practice, 10,* 13–29.

Westberg, J., & Jason, H. (1996). Fostering healthy behavior: The process. In S. H. Woolf, S. Jonas, & R. S. Lawrence (Eds.). *Health promotion and disease prevention in clinical practice* (pp. 145–162). Baltimore: Williams & Wilkins.

World Health Organization Health Education Unit. (1986). Lifestyles and health. *Social Science and Medicine, 22,* 117–124.

Yip, V. Y. B. (2004). New low back pain in nurses: work activities, work stress and sedentary lifestyle. *Journal of Advanced Nursing, 46,* 430–440.

Providing access to health care for all persons, delivering nursing care based on strong science and evidence, addressing specific cultural preferences when providing care, balancing accountability to clients in the era of cost containment, creating healthy environments, caring for communities, using technology effectively, and influencing public policy are challenges for today's professional nurses. In addition, spiraling health care costs have led to increased consumer discontent with the health care system, which places health care providers at risk for litigation. This section provides an overview of these challenges while reinforcing professional nursing's goal of doing what is best for clients.

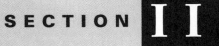

SECTION II

# The Changing Health Care Context

# CHAPTER 9

# Health Care Delivery Systems

## KEY TERMS AND CONCEPTS

Medicare

Medicaid

Prospective Payment

Interdisciplinary Health Care Team

Mandated Insurance Model

Nursing Shortage

Surplus of Physicians

Integrated Health Care Delivery System

## LEARNING OUTCOMES

By the end of this chapter, the learner will be able to:

1 Identify how the historic development of the health care delivery system led to current issues and concerns.

2 Compare and contrast selected health care delivery systems.

3 Explain the major forces that influence change in the health care system.

4 State the gaps in health care delivery between client needs and services offered.

5 Outline the various components of the current American health care system.

6 Identify the impact of changes in the health system on nurses.

7 Specify strategies professional nurses could use to thrive in the current and future health care delivery systems.

8 Explore the ethical issues surrounding current changes in health care delivery.

## VIGNETTE

Jane, a professional nurse, has an elderly father who is hospitalized after falling at home and breaking his hip. Her parents become distraught because of plans being made to transfer Jane's father to an extended care facility 3 days after his surgery. They do not know if their health insurance company is a PPO or HMO when asked by the case manager. Jane's parents express great concern, because the couple had a mutual agreement that one would never put the other in a nursing home.

Health care delivery has undergone radical transformation within the past decade. In the past, the American system was a collection of fragmented services provided on a fee-for-service basis by numerous organizations and providers. Changes in society have resulted in the attitude that health care should be provided to all, regardless of ability to pay. Physicians dominated health care delivery and focused efforts on curing illnesses. Some American health care consumers believe that health care services should be provided to all citizens free of charge. If the consumer does not pay for health care services directly, then either the government or a health insurance plan must cover the costs. Other consumers believe that Americans need to assume responsibility for their own health and pay for services directly. Because health care in America is a big business, some Americans believe that if the government controls the system, then the quality of health care services most certainly will decline. Nurses play an important role in health care delivery. Changes in demography, the economy, technology, attitudes toward health care, and the available labor force have resulted in unprecedented changes in the delivery of health care, with significant implications for nursing as a critical component of the system.

## ✦ HISTORICAL DEVELOPMENT OF CURRENT HEALTH CARE DELIVERY SYSTEMS

Health care delivery systems arose as people identified a need to care for those who are infirm or injured. Societal beliefs about the nature of the world provided foundation for early health care practices. When science offered improved care outcomes, people embraced the new technology and methods. Although medical practice is still largely experientially based, efforts are being made to identify best practices based on solid scientific evidence.

### Health Care, 1492 to 1775

Early expeditions to the New World provided health care services to sailors and passengers. Christopher Columbus staffed his initial expedition with a physician because naval voyagers frequently became afflicted with scurvy and other illnesses contracted before setting sail. The Spaniards sent Dominican, Jesuit, and Franciscan priests with health care expertise on missions to the New World. These religious men strove to protect public health as Europeans penetrated the wilderness and lived with Native Americans. The Jesuits kept detailed records of everyday occurrences, including health-related information obtained from the Native Americans. In the absence of monasteries, religious orders established missions to set up a place for worship, trade, and agriculture. When overwhelming epidemics of diseases originating from Europe occurred, the friars organized disease treatment efforts (Jamieson & Sewall, 1954).

The Franciscans built the first American hospital in 1531. The hospital was named Santa Fe ("holy faith") and served over 30,000 North American Indians. Inclusion of a hospital in the mission resulted in the formation of the first monastery that offered the comprehensive services that were hallmarks of European monasteries. Mission establishment became the general schema for Spanish colonization in the New World. A Franciscan friar, Junipero Serra, bore the responsibility of establishing missions along the California coastline. The missions provided education and training centers for Native

Americans. When outbreaks of European diseases occurred, Native Americans sought care within the confines of the missions (Jamieson & Sewall, 1954).

As the Spanish concentrated on colonization of the West Coast, the French established colonies in Canada. In 1693, the Jesuits built the first hospital in Canada using the support of the wealthy Duchess d'Aiguillon, who was the niece of Cardinal Richelieu. She obtained a land grant and permission to establish a hospital. Three nuns from the Augustinian order were dispatched to run the hospital, which served the city of 250 persons, primarily Native Americans.

Because of epidemics, many Indian and French children became orphans. In response to the dilemma, a rich woman, Mme de la Peltrie was determined to establish an orphanage and school for these children. In May 1639, Mme de la Peltrie, along with Augustinian and Ursuline sisters, established an infirmary at the trading post of Tadoussac, located at the mouth of the St. Lawrence River. The Augustinian sisters established the Hotel Dieu, the first Canadian hospital in Quebec. The Augustinian sisters dispensed medications and offered cheerful encouragement to persons who remained ill but preferred to stay at home. In 1644, Mlle Mance established the Hotel Dieu of Montreal in a building 60 feet long by 24 foot wide. The hospital cared for wounded French and British soldiers during the Seven Years' War (Jamieson & Sewall, 1954).

The British were less successful in establishing health care delivery to settlers. Half of the Mayflower colonists perished. Samuel Fuller, a church deacon on the Mayflower, served as the physician to the colonists. Prayer and various forms of quackery became the mainstay of health care provided to persons in British colonies, where any educated man could assume physician responsibilities (Jamieson & Sewall, 1954).

## Health Care Moves Forward

At the same time, the European health care system continued to evolve. The Church lost control of hospitals. Secular directors were appointed by King Louis XII to run the hospitals, thereby paving the way for government influence in the delivery of health care (Jamieson & Sewall, 1954).

Similar degeneration of religious life occurred in England. The control of hospitals became the responsibility of the cities. Philanthropy and state aid emerged as major funding sources. Physicians learned medicine primarily through an apprenticeship system. Until the germ theory was discovered, surgeons considered wearing blood-stained clothes as an honor and handwashing was nonexistent. In addition, care was delivered by disenfranchised members of society (prisoners or persons from debtors' prisons) with little knowledge of how to care for patients. Hospitalization meant almost certain death (Jamieson & Sewall, 1954).

## Health Care in the Late 19th Century

Until the middle of the 19th century, most American physicians had less than a high school education and a minimal apprenticeship with a European-trained physician. Because physicians had few therapeutic tools, the focus was on nursing care through environmental manipulation provided by family members within the home. Formal education for nursing began in 1873. Epidemics of acute infectious diseases were the predominant health problems. Most diseases were the result of impure food, contaminated water supplies, inadequate sewage disposal, or the poor condition of urban housing. No organized health programs existed because the predominant ethic of the time said that "each person should care for himself, should be self-sufficient, and, should he become dependent, should take advantage of the various charities . . . established for that specific purpose and be grateful for the charity" (Torrens, 1978, p. 12).

The hospital was an almshouse and pesthouse used almost exclusively by socially marginal, overwhelmingly poor people without roots in the community (Vogel, 1979). Because hospitals were supported by the philanthropy of the wealthy, class distinctions were considered to be justified, and hospital patients were stigmatized as dependent and somehow unworthy of societal membership. By 1873, the United States had 178 established hospitals (Jonas, 1998).

However, in Canada, the Fathers of Confederation laid out terms of the British North America Act of 1867 that specified responsibilities of the Canadian government. Within this act, government responsibilities were to take a census, collect vital statistics, determine quarantine regulations, provide hospitals for persons in quarantine, and care for native persons of Canada. Along with these basic responsibilities, a section of the act provided for the establishment of provincial hospitals, asylums, and charities (McIntryre & Thomlinson, 2003).

### Scientific Advancements

In the mid-to-late 1800s, health care delivery was revolutionized by scientific discoveries. Anesthesia was administered by 1847 and antisepsis by 1865, leading to the need for centralized facilities to support expensive equipment for surgery. The typhoid bacillus was isolated in 1880 (with vaccination available in 1896) and the cause of diphtheria was discovered in 1883, which reduced the epidemic spread of those diseases. By 1860, the thermometer, ophthalmoscope, and laryngoscope were in use, joined by the gastroscope, cystoscope, hypodermic needle, and sphygmomanometer by 1883. X-rays were discovered in 1895. Improved hygiene in hospitals and advances in medical diagnostics and therapeutics increasingly led to the referral of middle class and even wealthy clients to hospitals for treatment.

### Health Care Becomes a Flourishing Industry

As immigration and industrialization propelled population increases and urbanization, hospitals flourished. By increasing the number of students in the "schools" of nursing, hospitals could inexpensively meet the demand for care. The medical community became aware of the rich learning resource that hospitalized patients provided for nursing students, and regular hospital affiliations as part of a four-year university medical education slowly became established, following the lead of Johns Hopkins University in 1893. During the same time, medical students also received education in university and clinical settings. An apprenticeship approach dominated nursing and medical education. While medicine developed its independent prestige based on a body of continually increasing scientific knowledge, nursing became associated with a medically dependent scope of practice, with an apprenticeship type of education totally dominated by hospitals.

## Health Care in the Early 20th Century

As the private patients of a greatly expanded class of hospital physicians increasingly provided the money that made hospitals profitable, "the poor and penniless, whom the institution had originally been meant to serve, became a liability" (Vogel, 1979, p. 115). A growing system of public institutions developed to meet the needs of poor patients; private hospitals were owned and controlled largely by physicians. Industrialization and urbanization led to increased specialization of workers, separation of the home from the workplace, and transformation of the social structure. The nuclear family was separated from extended kin, and the streetcar and the telephone became important communication links, especially for the middle classes. Whereas health care had been home oriented and family centered, it now became a stratified and localized system closely attuned to the city.

### The American Medical Association Is Restructured

In 1901, the American Medical Association was restructured, and "doctors sought to assure their financial security and power through their own organization and reform of medical education" (Markowitz & Rosner, 1979, p. 186), as well as by restriction of competition. Foundations added their resources to the centralization of power and decision making in medicine and medical education. There was an effort to replace the rather haphazard art of medical practice with the new scientific medicine, which increasingly involved hospital treatment. As technology developed, it tended to be concentrated in hospitals. The primary causes of death were pneumonia and tuberculosis, with heart disease, nephritis, and accidents close behind. By 1910, the number of hospitals in the United States expanded to 4,400 (Jonas, 1998).

### Effects of the Great Depression

The Depression of the 1930s had a major impact on the developing health care system. The federal, state, and local governments, which primarily had been concerned with quarantines, made relatively ineffective attempts to improve sanitation (Raffel, 1993). The government increasingly assumed responsibility for providing and funding services. Disease prevention and health promotion (primary care) became major goals in health delivery (Jonas, 1998). In 1935, the Social Security Act included provisions for the indigent and for the infirm elderly.

Accident and life insurance companies, which originally had covered the loss of earned income caused by diseases such as typhus, typhoid, scarlet fever, and smallpox, increased their hospital services. In 1939, the first Blue Shield plan for medical and surgical expenses was sponsored by the California Medical Society. However, because there was no coordination of growth, expansion was indiscriminate and often led to duplicative services.

## Health Care in the Mid- to Late 20th Century

After World War II, the rise of medical specialization led to fragmentation in the delivery of health care (Jonas, 1998). Governmental influence also increased in care delivery, and the belief that health care as an individual right of citizens arose. For example, the Hill-Burton Act (1946) stimulated hospital construction; creation of the Department of Health, Education, and Welfare in 1953 provided a mechanism to coordinate research and service programs; and Congress amended the Social Security Act (1965–1966) to include **Medicare** (basic federal government-sponsored health insurance plan for persons over age 65 years, who have retired or are disabled and receiving social security benefits) and **Medicaid** (a health insurance program for persons in poverty, administered by the states that receive federal funds for implementation). The federal government assumed major responsibility for providing health care for all elderly and most poor people by the end of the 1960s. Whereas the 1960s had emphasized equity and cohesion of services, the 1970s concentrated on access, with tremendous growth in the number of hospitals, hospital employees, ancillary services, and sophisticated technology. But the emphasis on research and technology led to specialization and depersonalization, as well as rapidly escalating expenses (Jonas, 1998; Kovner, 1999).

Rising health care costs also plagued Canadians, resulting in federal efforts to provide coverage for health expenditures for everyone. In 1947, the province of Saskatchewan legislated the Hospital Insurance Act that provided hospital insurance for all its residents. At the same time, the Canadian government offered grants to the provinces and public health agencies to meet health care of citizens as well as grants for hospital construction. In the 1960s, Saskatchewan expanded insurance coverage to include outpatient health care and by 1968, the Medical Care Act was enacted, thereby providing national health insurance for all Canadians (McIntyre & Thomlinson, 2003).

## The Rise of the Health Insurance Companies

The increasing cost of health care also was fueled by the developing health insurance industry. The first health insurance plan that covered hospitalization costs was Blue Cross of Dallas in 1929. By 1949, health insurance became part of collective bargaining contracts (Scofera, 1994). "The percentage of Americans covered by some form of health insurance rose from less than 20% prior to World War II to more than 70% by the early 1960s" (Torrens, 1978, p. 13). One hundred million persons were covered by major medical plans in 1951 and, by the end of 1960, 320 million persons had coverage (Scofea, 1994). In 1960, health care expenditures consumed 5.5% of the gross domestic product. Health insurance funded the increased costs caused by inflation and by additional optional services. A greater number of beneficiaries increased use of services, and all costs were essentially unmonitored.

The entire system became increasingly complex with the:

- Haphazard growth of nursing homes to provide care covered by Medicare and Medicaid.
- Expansion of military and veterans' hospitals to care for returning veterans and their families.
- Expansion of city and state hospitals.
- New construction of research facilities.

Although infectious illnesses were nearly eradicated because of the introduction of antibiotics in the 1940s, the fragmented and discontinuous health care delivery system continued to focus on curing all illnesses (Jonas, 1998; Kovner & Jonas, 1999). Thus, although chronic illnesses dominated health care needs, long-term illness, an area in which nursing has a great deal of expertise and potential power, was treated as a series of separate acute episodes.

## Focus on Cost, Not Care

By the late 1970s, spiraling and unacceptable health care costs became impossible to ignore. Emphasis shifted from access and quality to cost. The federal government established new regulations and began to reduce funding of social programs. The changes emphasized efficiency, rather than equity or quality, and competition, rather than access. Prospective payment reimbursement for hospital expenses for Medicare patients was instituted to significantly reduce hospital costs. **Prospective payment** set a pre-arranged reimbursement amount (by diagnostic category) that the federal government paid hospitals for the care given to patients covered by Medicare. The hospital received the prearranged amount, regardless of the actual cost of care for an individual patient. This initial change resulted in multiple ripple effects that are even now dramatically affecting the entire system, including the closure of some small hospitals.

Managed care plans started in the 1970s and flourished as health care costs continued to increase. Enrollment in managed care plans rose from 2 million persons in 1970 to more than 39 million persons in 1992. Managed care plans believed that they could reduce health care costs by promoting health (Scofea, 1994).

Canada also experienced problems with skyrocketing health care costs and limited public funding for care. The Canada Health Care Act of 1984 outlined the principles and conditions for health care delivery. Provincial governments rather than the federal government administer health care programs and specify the annual amount of funding for health care. The act provides for health maintenance and disease management. All Canadians have equal access to health care services and additional costs cannot be incurred by citizens for services covered by the provincial insurance plans. All Canadians are covered by the provincial policy plans. Finally, the Canadian plan is portable and covers citizens if they move from province to province or travel abroad. However, nonemergent and out-of-province services require preauthorization (McIntyre & Thomlinson, 2003).

### Costs Increase Despite Reform Efforts

The 1990s brought many changes in the health care delivery system. During the 1990s, health care expenditures outpaced inflation by more than 10% in some years. In 1994, health care expenses increased 13.7%, while the year's inflation rate was 3.5% (Jonas, 1998). In efforts to contain health care costs, acute care hospitals began the process of consolidation to avoid duplication of services within a geographical locale. Health care providers began looking at new methods for health care delivery to provide consistent cost-effective client care. These changes resulted in a highly complex, multifaceted health care delivery system.

Table 9-1 outlines the various settings where health care is delivered along with a definition of each setting. Table 9-2 specifies the various members of the **interdisciplinary health care team** and the contribution of each member. Table 9-3 presents the various methods that persons and society use to pay for rendered health care services. The three tables present a highly complex American health care system. When professional nurses understand how health care delivery occurs, they can assist persons in using the system.

## ● DIFFERENT HEALTH CARE DELIVERY SYSTEMS

Health care delivery systems vary from nation to nation. Some nations, such as the United States, rely heavily on private market forces for health care. In other nations, such as Canada, Australia, and the United Kingdom, government programs assure equal

TABLE 9-1

## Settings for Health Care Delivery

| Setting | Definition |
| --- | --- |
| Public hospital<br>  1. Federal hospital<br>  2. Nonfederal hospital | Nonprofit, government-owned institution that provides inpatient care<br>  1. Owned and operated by the United States government<br>  2. Owned and operated by a state or local government |
| Community hospital | A locally owned institution that offers short-term services that are accessible to the public |
| Specialized hospital | An institution that offers services in one specialty area of health care (e.g., oncology, mental health orthopedics, maternal–child health, children services) |
| General hospital | Offers a full scope of short-term services, including obstetric care |
| Teaching hospital | Provides medical education to undergraduate or graduate medical students, residents, or postgraduate medical fellows |
| Extended care facility | Institution that offers long-term care, also known as nursing homes (75% owned by for-profit companies) |
| Rehabilitation center | Institution that offers services to persons with a disability to become independent |
| Chemical dependence center | Institution that offers detoxification and rehabilitation for persons with drug or alcohol addiction |
| Neighborhood health center | Outpatient facility offering comprehensive primary care health services |
| Private physician office | Comprehensive ambulatory patient medical care provided by a single physician |
| Physician partnership office | Comprehensive ambulatory medical care provided by a pair of physicians |
| Group physician office practice | Comprehensive ambulatory medical care services provided by a group of three or more physicians |
| Managed care clinic | Comprehensive ambulatory medical care provided within the confines of an office or clinic operated by managed care |
| Public health clinics | State-, county-, or city-funded health services that focus primarily on prevention of or controlling communicable diseases |
| Ambulatory surgery center | Outpatient center where minor surgical procedures are performed |
| Specialty care centers | Outpatient offices or centers that offer full scope of ambulatory care services to persons with specific health problems (renal failure, cancer, diabetes, pain); may have for-profit status |
| Emergency department | Outpatient facility linked to a hospital where life-threatening health problems can be managed. Some emergency facilities have designated trauma center certification. Frequently used by persons to receive health care after office or clinic hours |
| Urgent care center | Outpatient facility (may be linked to a hospital) for health care consumers to receive medical care services for health-related problems when clinics or offices are closed or when they do not have an established health care provider. Usually have for-profit status |
| Hospital-based clinics | Outpatient comprehensive medical care services that are linked with a specific hospital. Many teaching hospitals hold resident clinics to provide health care to the poor |

## Settings for Health Care Delivery (Continued)

| Setting | Definition |
| --- | --- |
| Hospital outpatient departments | Ambulatory diagnostic testing or rehabilitation services that have connections to a specific hospital |
| Diagnostic testing centers | Ambulatory diagnostic testing services. Some have connections to nonprofit hospitals and others are run by for-profit companies |
| Industrial health services units | Employment-based health services to address job-related illnesses and injuries. Some industrial health service units provide health-promotion activities and health screenings for employees |
| School health clinics | Health care services offered to students in academic settings (health rooms in primary or secondary schools or university health clinics) |
| Home health care | Medical care and nursing services offered for persons who are homebound |
| Hospice | Comprehensive service to assist persons in receiving a "good" death. Services may be given in the home, extended-care, or acute care facility |

*Sources:* Jonas, S. (1998). *An introduction to the U.S. health care system* (4th ed.). New York: Springer Publishing; and Kovner, A. R., & Jonas, S. (Eds.). (1999). *Jonas & Kovner's health care delivery in the United States* (6th ed.) New York: Springer Publishing.

access for health care services. Nationally based health care systems rely on basic guiding principles that determine basic service coverage. Depending on the country, citizens may purchase private insurance to pay for services to gain immediate access to care. A **mandated insurance model** is used by Germany, Italy, and Spain. Under the mandated insurance system, everyone receives compulsory universal healthcare insurance coverage from nonprofit companies. Policies are purchased by employers and employees pay a portion of the coverage fees (Fried & Gaydos, 2002).

Differing modes of financing health care services are used. Countries with comprehensive national health insurance rely highly on general tax revenues. Compulsory mandated insurance programs use social insurance or social security systems. Individuals (and employers) pay for health care coverage in the voluntary insurance market system. Charitable donations from individuals or organizations (e.g., World Health Organization, United Nations, World Bank, churches, Planned Parenthood, and other nonprofit organizations) finance health care especially in poor, undeveloped nations. Finally, out-of-pocket payment for service appears in all health care delivery systems (Fried & Gaydos, 2002).

## The Canadian Health Care Delivery System

Like the United States, Canada has much wealth. Canada ranked twelfth of all nations in the World Health Organization's ranking of health systems. The life expectancy of Canadians is 79 years with citizens living in southern urban areas having a longer lifespan than persons living in the cold, rural northern areas (Fried & Gaydos, 2002).

Health care in Canada is directed by five key principles. First, provincial health insurance plans are administered and operated by a nonprofit public authority who answers to the provincial government. Second, each insurance plan covers all eligible

TABLE 9-2

## Members of the Interdisciplinary Health Care Team

| Member | Role |
|---|---|
| Client (consumer or patient) | Seeks out various health care services and makes decisions related to plan of care |
| Board of Directors (or Trustees) | Responsible for organizational mission, service quality, strategic planning, medical staff credentialing, evaluation and selection of the chief executive officer, self-evaluation and education, and financial status. For-profit companies report to stockholders. Nonprofit organizations usually have a variety of persons from the community with specialized expertise (e.g. lawyers) and philanthropists as board members |
| Chief Executive Officer (or Administrator) | Responsible for overall daily operation of the organization including implementation of board policies, addressing of health care concerns within the local community, and preparation and delivery of board reports |
| Administrative staff (managers or directors) | In large organizations, each department usually has someone responsible for its overall daily operations. In nursing, the head of the nursing department has the title of Chief Nursing Executive or Director of Nursing |
| Medical staff | Physician who may be independent practitioner or organizational employee who diagnoses and treats clients using medical therapies. |
| Nursing staff 1. Registered nurses 2. Licensed practical/vocational nurses 3. Unlicensed assistive personnel (care assistants) 4. Clerical assistants (unit clerk, secretary) | Responsible for execution of direct and indirect client care services. Registered nurses assess clients, diagnose human responses to illness, outline a care plan, implement the plan (including the delegation of tasks to others) and evaluate the effectiveness of nursing care |
| Case manager (for managed care organizations) | Advanced practice nurse or social worker who follows clients across the spectrum of health care settings. Most start the discharge process as soon as clients are admitted to acute care facilities |
| Dietitians | Baccalaureate-prepared nutritionists who have had internships to learn clinical nutrition. They outline specific client therapeutic diets and verify that client nutritional needs are met. They also provide client and family education related to therapeutic diets. Inpatient facilities have food service departments that prepare client and cafeteria meals |
| Pharmacists | Prepare and dispense medications, educate other help team members about medications, monitor controlled substance use, monitor client allergies, work to prevent medication errors, and monitor potential drug interactions |
| Paramedical personnel or Technologists | Highly trained experts who have specialized education or training. Examples include medical technologist (lab tests), radiology technologist (x-ray, CT scan, PET scan, etc.), respiratory therapist (breathing therapies, ventilator management, and oxygen therapy) |
| Social workers | Assist clients with social concerns that arise from illness, injury, or surgery. Help clients with financial issues resulting from disruption of work and insurance benefit gaps. Also refer them to community support agencies |

## Members of the Interdisciplinary Health Care Team (Continued)

| Member | Role |
| --- | --- |
| Therapists | Physical therapists assess function and provide restorative therapy for body movement, ambulation, and safety. Occupational therapists assess and provide restorative therapy for problems with activities of daily living as well as skills for employment. Speech therapists assess for swallowing difficulties, speech problems, and provide restorative therapy related to these areas |
| Medical Records or Health Information Services | Keep detailed and accurate medical records on clients |
| Business manager or office staff | Coordinates client appointments (outpatient settings) and keeps financial records for services rendered |
| Central supply or central products services | Warehouse and distribute client care products (not pharmaceuticals) per ordered request |
| Linen services | Provide client linen and gowns |
| Environmental or housekeeping services | Maintain a clean, safe physical environment |
| Biomedical engineering services | Maintain proper functioning of electronic client care machines (IV pumps, bedside monitors, thermometers, etc.) and verify electrical safety of client care equipment |
| Information services | Develop integrated computer systems and provide user support services (some may offer computer and software staff education) |
| Quality management | Monitors the quality of rendered services. Includes the risk management department that monitors actual and potential client care errors and financial losses. Outlines a plan for continuous quality improvement |
| Third-party payer | Pays for all or part of health care services used by the consumer. Various levels of government are third-party payers for tax-supported health insurance plans. Private insurance companies provide funding for plan enrollees. Frequently audit client records to verify rendered services |
| Utilization review | Set up in the late 1970s by the federal government to verify effective utilization of health care resources and avoid fraud |
| Spiritual support service (chaplain) | Inpatient settings usually have chaplain support services to provide spiritual and other support to clients and their significant others |
| Human Resources (Personnel department) | Hires new employees, tracks employee incidents, and coordinates employee fringe benefits. Payroll departments that issue employee paychecks may fall under this category |
| Foundation | Nonprofit organizations usually have services to coordinate private donations to the organization |
| Alternative care providers | Persons that provide alternative or complimentary therapy to clients such as chiropractors, herbalists, acupuncturists, massage therapists, reflexologists, and folk healers |

Adapted from Jonas, S. (1998). *An introduction to the U.S. health care system* (4th ed.). New York: Springer Publishing; Kovner, A. R., & Jonas, S. (Eds.). (1998). *Jonas & Kovner's health care delivery in the United States* (6th ed.) New York: Springer Publishing; and American Hospital Association. (1999). *Welcome to the board: An orientation for the new health care trustee.* Chicago: AHA Press.

TABLE 9-3

## Methods of Financing Health Care Services

| Method of Financing | Definition |
| --- | --- |
| Medicare<br>  1. Part A covers care received by clients in a hospital, extended care setting or home setting.<br>  2. Part B covers certain physician costs and other medical expenses. Participation in Part B is voluntary. | Federal program that provides a range of health care services for persons over age 65<br>  1. Part A is financed by payroll taxes.<br>  2. Part B is financed by general tax revenue and contributions of elderly participants in the program. |
| Medicaid | Jointly operated insurance program run by the federal and state governments that covers inpatient and outpatient hospital care, lab and x-ray services, physician services, and nursing care facility coverage for persons under the age of 21 years.<br>Each state has different qualifying criteria for participation |
| Veterans Benefits | Federal program for hospital and medical services for former members of the armed forces |
| Department of Defense | Federal program to provide health care services for current members of the military and their dependents |
| Worker's Compensation | State program to provide persons with income and payment for health care services as a result of an illness or injury arising directly from a person's employment |
| Women/Infant/Children Program | Federal and state program that provides compensation for prenatal, infant, and child health care |
| Public Health Service | Federal program that provides health care services to the poor as well as providing disaster preparedness and relief health services |
| Indian Health Service | Federal program that provides health care services to Native Americans |
| Out-of-pocket | Individuals pay for part of all of health care services received. Most insurance plans have individual deductibles or co-payments that persons pay to receive services |
| Fee for service | Insurance company pays a set amount for each health service that plan participant receives |
| Capitation | Insurance company pays a set amount to the health care provider for each program enrollee. This covers health care services for 1 year |
| Private health insurance | Insurance company provides coverage for health care expenses. Most plans are employment based, which means many Americans are at the mercy of employers for health insurance coverage |
| Preferred Provider Organization | Beneficiaries receive more coverage if they receive health care services from a list of providers who have negotiated with the insurer for group discounts. Beneficiaries may see provider of choice, but assume total or increased personal expense if provider is not on the list |
| Health Maintenance Organization | Health care providers receive capitated payments to maintain the health of program enrollees. Each enrollee selects a primary care health provider from a list of approved HMO providers |

## Methods of Financing Health Care Services (Continued)

| Method of Financing | Definition |
| --- | --- |
| Managed care | Insurance coverage in which approval of health services must be obtained through a managed care administrator or a primary care physician |
| Point of service plan | Another form of preferred provider coverage, but pays less for services rendered by out-of-network providers |
| Blue Cross and Blue Shield | A nonprofit pre-payment insurance system in which Blue Cross provides hospitalization coverage and Blue Shield covers other health care services |
| Commercial insurance | For-profit insurance companies that sell health care coverage to individuals, employers, or groups |
| Self-insurance plans | Claim risk assumed by an employer, union, or other group when the group has an established bank or trust account to finance health care costs |

Adapted from Jonas, S. (1998). *An introduction to the U.S. health care system,* (4th ed.). New York: Springer Publishing; and Kovner, A. R., & Jonas, S. (Eds.). (1998). *Jonas & Kovner's health care delivery in the United States,* (6th ed.). New York: Springer Publishing.

residents using uniform terms and conditions. Insurance coverage covers persons living in a province for at least 3 months, but not those covered by the Canadian government plan. Third, Canadians are covered when they travel across provinces or when traveling abroad. However, the plans have limited out-of-country coverage and provincial plan approval is required for nonemergency services when receiving care out of the province in which a citizen resides. Fourth, each plan covers "all medically necessary services" citizens may need from physicians and hospitals (no private room coverage unless someone has a severely suppressed immune system). Medically necessary services have been defined by the federal and provincial governments. Finally, the plan provides reasonable access to health services without discrimination. Provincial plans may require premiums from citizens, but care cannot be denied based on inability to pay fees for insurance coverage (Fried & Gaydos, 2002).

Funds for the Canadian health care system come from taxes (primarily payroll), health insurance premiums, and consumer out-of-pocket expenses. Tax credits offer relief for high out-of-pocket health care expenditures. For services not covered by government plans, some Canadians may purchase private health care policies. In recent years, government spending cutbacks have slowed the growth of the public sector of Canadian health expenditures (Fried & Gaydos, 2002).

### Research Brief 9-1

Sanmartin, C., Nge, E., Blackwell, D., Gentleman, J., Martinez, M., & Simile, C. *Joint Canada/United States Survey of Health.* Center for Disease Control, 2004. Available at: http://www.cdc.gov/nchs/data/hsis/jcush_analyticalreport.pdf.

This multinational study sought to compare the quality of health and satisfaction of health care delivery in the United States and Canada. In 2002 to 2003, 5,000 Americans and 3,500 Canadians were randomly selected to be interviewed over the telephone. Results revealed that Canadians and Americans report having similar access to a variety of health care services even though the systems of care differ. Both Canadians and Americans rely on insurance for dental care. Eighty-five percent of Americans and 88% of Canadians described their health as being good or excellent. Persons with low incomes in both countries reported poorer health status. Ninety percent of Americans and 87% of Canadians reported being very or somewhat satisfied with their current health care. Similarities in health status were noted in mobility, depressive episodes within the previous 12 months, percentage of persons seeing a physician within the previous 12 months, number of dental visits, and dental insurance coverage. Differences occurred in the following areas: Canada had a slightly higher percentage of daily smokers (Canada had a higher percentage of daily smokers among women over the age of 65 years); more Americans were found to be obese; poor persons in the United States reported more difficulty in accessing health care services; more Canadians reported having regular medical appointments for health promotion and maintenance; American women aged 50 to 69 years were more likely to have had annual mammograms; and Americans between the ages of 45 and 64 reported using more prescription drugs.

The investigators reported the following study limitations: data collection exclusively at national level, participants had household telephones, potential inaccuracies from self-reported information, potential misinterpretation of survey questions by respondents, potential sampling error, and no available data of characteristics of nonparticipants.

Implications for professional nursing practice include the need for increased education and follow up for Americans in seeing health care providers for health promotion and maintenance, targeted smoking cessation classes for older Canadian women, emphasis on reducing obesity in the United States, and advocating for increased access to health care services for Americans with low incomes.

## The Mexican Health Care Delivery System

Unlike Canada and the United States, Mexico has less money to spend on health care. The average lifespan for a Mexican man is 72.4 years and for a Mexican woman, 77 years. Rapid industrialization with increasing environmental pollution along with increasing tobacco and alcohol use, poor diet, sedentary lifestyle, and infectious diseases (in crowded urban areas) pose challenges to the health status of Mexicans. Not all Mexicans have equal access to health care services. The affluent purchase private health insurance plans; workers are covered through a social security system or purchase employment-based health insurance plans, and the poor rely on a public services system. The Ministry of Health manages health promotion and disease prevention for Mexican citizens. In addition, the Ministry of Health monitors and tests medications made by and sold in Mexico for quality, safety, and efficacy (Fried & Gaydos, 2002).

Affluent Mexicans receive the same quality of care enjoyed by Canadians and Americans. Services offered include traditional (scientific-based) medicine, homeopathy, chiropractics, Chinese medicine, self-help groups, and indigenous/religious health practices. The Mexican health care system consists of hospitals, outpatient facilities, and long-term care facilities. Modern medical centers are located in urban areas. Health care in rural areas frequently have problems with understaffing and rely on medical students as providers. In recent years, health delivery to Mexicans covered by public services has become decentralized and emphasis has been placed on a healthy municipalities program. Shifting the emphasis to health rather than treating chronic disease for poorer citizens has increased population access to health care services.

## ✦ FORCES INFLUENCING CHANGES IN HEALTH CARE SYSTEMS

Numerous forces influence recent and future changes within health care systems. Humans have control over some and remain powerless against others. Developing a health care system that effectively provides access, cost, and quality seems to be the greatest challenge confronted by the health care system. Professional nurses may seem to be an expensive resource and health care organizations may try to replace them with unlicensed care providers. This may change as nurses demonstrate their positive impact on the quality of client care.

### Demographic Forces

One of the most significant influences affecting health care delivery is the increasing population of older Americans. As a result of improvements in life expectancy at birth, the population 65 years of age or older in the United States is expected to grow from 12.3% in 2000 to 17% in 2020 and 30% in 2050 (United States Census Bureau, 2002). The ratio of people younger than 65 years to those older than 65 years will shrink from the current ratio of 9:1 to 5:1 by 2030. The United States Census Bureau (2002) projects that the population of those 85 years and older, mainly "frail elderly," will double from approximately 4.2 million people in 2000 to approximately 7 million in 2020, and then double again to 14 million by 2040 (Waite, 1996). Worldwide, the population of those older than 65 years is expected to grow from 10% in 1975 to 18% to 20% by 2030 (Bezold, 1982). Because older persons often have chronic conditions that require treatment and care, their increasing numbers will exert a continuing upward pressure on health care costs.

Other demographic influences include changes in geographic distribution and composition. Areas of the northeastern United States are losing population, whereas urban midsize cities in the South and Southwest are experiencing rapid growth, along with the need for health care delivery services for the very young and the elderly. The Baby Boom generation, born between 1946 and 1964, is settling into middle age and creating a wave of older persons who have higher incidences of chronic health conditions and use more health care resources.

Because of the increased pregnancy rate in teenagers with poor health habits, the continuing needs of infants with low birth weights have assumed major importance. In addition, immigration and population growth among ethnic minorities such as Hispanics, African Americans, and Asians present significant challenges for the provision of culturally acceptable health care. By 2025, the Hispanic and African American populations will together represent 32% of the U.S. population (United States Census Bureau, 2002). These groups currently are underserved by the delivery system and underrepresented in all the health professions.

Infant mortality continues to be of major concern, although there is evidence that primary care directed at high-risk mothers can be effective. Good prenatal care can prevent prematurity and low birth weight in infants. Health promotion efforts aimed at influencing high-risk behaviors among adolescents are especially needed.

## Age-Related Factors

The increasing numbers of older adults will fuel the need for "acute care hospitalization for diseases of the heart, malignant neoplasms, and chronic incurable diseases with multisystem failures and functional decline" (USDHHS, 1990, p. IIIB-3). Chronic disorders such as diabetes and osteoarthritis, cognitive impairment, and the increased fragility of advancing age are of major concern. Mental health and dental needs also will increase. Nursing home and home health programs are an especially high priority. Health promotion, illness prevention, and rehabilitative services are needed to enhance the quality of life for the elderly. Older adult caregivers (primarily women) of their frail elderly parents will need support and assistance. The increasing need for coordination and continuity of care provides an opportunity for managed care by professional nurses.

## The Impact of AIDS

Acquired immune deficiency syndrome (AIDS) is now a world pandemic. It is estimated that in 2000, an estimated 40 million people worldwide had HIV, with 90% of them in developing countries (UNAIDS/WHO, 2001). AIDS is now the leading cause of death in the United States among people 25 to 44 years of age (U.S. Department of Health and Human Services, 2000). A number of therapies have been developed, but no cure is known. In addition, many persons with AIDS have developed multidrug resistant tuberculosis, which may spread to others. Floyd, Blanc, Raviglione, and Lee (2002) predict that costs for managing global tuberculosis control will strain the economies of underdeveloped countries and that tuberculosis may emerge as a major global public health problem. There will be an increasing need for acute and community care, education, and counseling regarding HIV prevention, and nurses may be called upon to spearhead programs for HIV and other infectious illness prevention while providing holistic care for persons suffering with infectious diseases.

## Drug and Alcohol Abuse

Abuse of alcohol and other drugs is a causative factor in various severe health and social problems, including:

- Traffic accidents (implicated in 50%).
- Transmission of HIV through contaminated needles.
- Lost wages and productivity (an estimated 5% of the US gross national product).
- Increased pregnancy rates and infant mortality among teenagers.
- Increased numbers of neonates born addicted to cocaine and heroin.
- Increased homelessness, disability, poverty, and crime.

The inner-city poor are at particularly high risk for drug and alcohol abuse. Community health nurses, in particular, provide essential services for prevention, detection, referral for treatment, and education.

## Environmental Factors

Our industrial age is associated with numerous environmental problems that have an impact on health, including:

- Air pollution.
- The greenhouse effect.
- Acid rain.
- Deforestation.
- Increased ultraviolet radiation (associated with depletion of the ozone layer).
- Toxic and nuclear wastes.
- Lead-based paints and asbestos.

The health care system assumes responsibility for health promotion and disease treatment for all those who experience the ill effects of living in a sick environment.

## Science and Technology

Within the past century, medical science has focused on expanding the length of the human life span. Scientists have assumed that society wants the human life span extended. Sophisticated therapies for once fatal illnesses and injuries have prolonged life. As scientific knowledge and technology expand, even longer life spans can be predicted for those with access to these new therapies. However, scientific advances and increased use of technology add to the cost of health care delivery. Chapter 15 explains the impact of technology on health care delivery and nursing practice.

Scientific advances in medical therapies are expensive. Pharmaceutical companies expect to profit from newly developed medications. Within the past few years, pharmaceutical firms have begun directly advertising new products to consumers using various media formats. Although the United States ranks first in funding for biomedical research, the country ranks 24th in the attainment of health outcomes, as determined by the World Health Organization. The benefits of health care research remain unequally accessible to Americans. Wealthy citizens or those with insurance receive expensive therapies for illness. However, the estimated 44 million Americans without health insurance do not have access to complex, expensive health care (LeBow, 2003).

## Changing Attitudes

During the past two decades, the American public has become increasingly aware of and interested in promoting health. People are more aware of the relationship between lifestyle and the incidence of stress-related diseases, chemical and drug dependencies, and the predisposition to other diseases. To prevent illness and to promote health, many people have focused attention on moderating stressful aspects of their lifestyles; developing habits of good nutrition, adequate exercise, rest, and relaxation; and controlling the use of abusive substances, such as tobacco, alcohol, and other drugs.

People are seeking increased responsibility for personal health and self-care, requiring increased health education. As consumers have requested and received information, they have begun to question the adage that "the doctor (or nurse) knows best." Evidence suggests a shift in attitudes toward personal involvement in choices affecting health status. As informed consumers become more involved in health-related decision making, they increase the emphasis on expressive values, research on noninvasive (and cost-effective) preventive and therapeutic interventions, and the demand for mutuality, rather than paternalism, by health care professionals. This movement has created a real opportunity for nursing to:

- Disseminate information and promote an educated public.
- Strengthen the profession's influence on health promotion.
- Foster alliances with consumers and collaborative relationships with physicians.
- Become accepted as primary care providers for long-term care.

## The Nursing Shortage

A **nursing shortage** or an insufficient number of nurses to meet the health care needs of clients exists currently and is expected to worsen. The Bureau of Health Professions (2002) predicts a 12% shortfall of professional nurses in 2010, 20% in 2015, and 29% in 2020 in the United States. The supply of professional nurses also looks bleak in Canada where there has been a 5% decline in number of registered nurses from 1990 to 2000 (Fried & Gaydos, 2002). Currently, there are 126,000 unfilled registered nurse positions in the United States (Inglis, 2004). The decreasing number of nurses results from a variety of factors, including:

- Reduced number of people 18 to 24 years of age.
- Decreased interest in a nursing career because of career choices available to women (who comprise 97% of the nursing work force).
- Compressed salary and fewer promotions throughout a nursing career.
- Image problems, including an emphasis on nursing being hard physically, highly technical, low paying, limited career financial potential, poor investment for increased education, and low status.
- Increased labor intensity from increased acuity with chronic understaffing in acute and extended care facilities.
- Widespread fear of contracting AIDS and other contagious diseases.
- Perceived lack of hospital positions along with a lack of awareness of community-based employment.
- Reduced job satisfaction for nurses and nurses discouraging others from entering the profession.
- An aging registered nurse workforce (in 2004, the average age of an RN was 45.2 years).
- A projected nursing faculty shortage.

## The Perceived Physician Surplus

Since 1960, the number of physicians in the United States has climbed from 142 to 260 physicians per 100,000 people (Fried & Gaydos, 2002). Urban areas enjoy a **surplus of physicians** (more doctors than the market for medical services). However, a shortage looms in rural and impoverished areas. Health care reform has resulted in physician practice reorganization from individual offices to large group practices that negotiate discounted fees for service with health insurance companies. Physicians are increasingly working on a salary or capitation (fixed payment per person) basis, rather than the traditional fee-for-service basis.

The surplus of available physicians impacts nursing practice and other aspects of the health care delivery system. As competition among physicians has increased, the organized medical community has increased its opposition to nurses functioning in expanded roles. Physicians have become more active in prevention, elderly ambulatory care, and community settings that previously were less appealing. Currently 40% of physicians practice primary care medicine that emphasizes health promotion and illness prevention (Sultz & Young, 2004). Some physicians have relocated to rural and underserved areas that traditionally have been served by nurse practitioners.

Recently, the new role of hospitalist has emerged for physicians. Hospitalists are physicians (some of whom have direct employment status or contracts with the hospital) who manage client care in acute care settings for primary care physicians. Hospitalists devote 25% to 100% of their time managing inpatient client care. When clients are admitted to the hospital, the hospitalist becomes the physician of record for the hospital stay. The hospitalist refers clients for follow-up care with a primary care physician on an outpatient basis after dismissal. Hospitalists enable primary care physicians to focus on the ever-increasing complexity of health maintenance and promotion of clients in outpatient settings. Some integrated health systems and acute care facilities have reported reduced inpatient length of stay and savings of millions of dollars since introducing the hospitalist role. However, the hospitalist movement brings some disadvantages for primary care physicians, such as the potential loss of hospital privileges, reduced status within the medical community, and possible reductions in income. The hospitalist movement has resulted in reduced client satisfaction with health care because of a lack of medical care continuity across various health care settings (McDonald, 2001).

Current structural changes within the health care system may erode the power physicians have in the practice of medicine. Business managers and facility administrators could have the most powerful voices in health care delivery decisions. As health care costs continue to spiral, alternative ways to deliver health care may surface.

## Advanced Practice Nursing

Some physicians view advanced practice nurses as a threat to medical practice. The American Nurses Association (ANA) defines advanced nursing practice as registered nurses who have "the knowledge base and practice experience to prepare them for specialization, expansion and advancement in practice" (1995, p. 9). In the past, nurses could earn credentials for advanced nursing practice by attending special certificate programs and passing an examination. Currently, most nurse practitioners, certified nurse midwives, clinical nurse specialists, and certified registered nurse anesthetists receive education in graduate nursing programs before writing certification and licensing examinations. In states where laws demand preparation of advanced practice nursing at the graduate level, nurses who held advanced practice certifications received status through grandfather clauses (Snyder et al., 1999). Unfortunately, some physicians view advanced practice nurses as competitive providers of health care, rather than professional colleagues.

## Nurse Entrepreneurs

Nurses also can assume more control and accountability when they become entrepreneurs. The term entrepreneur is defined as "one who organizes, manages, and assumes the risk of a business or enterprise" (*Merriam-Webster's Collegiate Dictionary,* 1994, p. 387). As entrepreneurs, professional nurses create businesses to use personal and professional skills and talents more fully. Nurses with special knowledge and skills work as consultants or form private companies that offer nursing services to individuals and corporations. Current societal trends support entrepreneurs. Even during the Great Depression of the 1930s and big business era of the 1950s, American entrepreneurs survived and flourished. Individual business development and ownership accelerated in the 1970s. When nurses become disillusioned with the traditional system of health care delivery or when they see serious gaps in health care services, some turn to entrepreneurship, instead of leaving the profession (Vogel & Doleysh, 1994).

Outsourcing for specialized services has emerged as a recent business trend. Nurses possess highly specialized knowledge and well-refined communication skills. Many viable business options come from frustrations encountered in daily practice. Nurse entrepreneurs offer interactive video health education, case management, facility planning, foot care, enterostomal therapy, legal consultation, quality assurance, aromatherapy, massage, organizational reinvention, and general health counseling service programs.

## ✦ CHANGES IN THE HEALTH CARE DELIVERY SYSTEM: NURSING IMPLICATIONS

### Structure and Organization

The health care delivery system provides primary care for health promotion and prevention of illness, secondary care for treatment toward the cure of illness, and tertiary care for technologically complex diagnostic, treatment, and rehabilitative services. Although hospitals have been the dominant provider of care, alternative structures have been developed recently. Various categories and classifications designate the purpose of a health care providing organization. Table 9-1 outlines various types of settings where persons receive health care service, and the information that follows provides explanations of how each differ. Organizations offering health care services differ according to mission and philosophy. Although they exist to offer health care services, organizations differ from being proprietary (privately funded and for profit), governmental (publicly funded and not for profit), or voluntary (privately funded and not for profit) (Jonas, 1998). For-profit organizations tend to emphasize providing services while achieving a high profit margin. In some cases, for-profit hospitals rely more heavily on unlicensed care providers for the basic nursing care of inpatients. Registered nurses in these settings find themselves spending more time supervising others than giving direct client care.

### Alternative Delivery Systems

Alternative delivery systems, particularly for ambulatory secondary care, have developed during the past few years, primarily to provide care at a lower cost than is possible through hospital admission. Some examples of alternative ambulatory care systems include diagnostic, minor emergency, surgery centers, birthing centers, substance abuse facilities, and rehabilitation centers. Health care consumers also can receive health care services in outpatient clinics and urgent care centers located in shopping malls. Some mall clinics belong to an integrated health care delivery system, and others have no links to hospitals or a system. Consumers also may get annual influenza vaccinations at grocery stores, pharmacies, and or places of business. In addition, home health agencies and hospices provide continuity of nursing care to the home setting. Recognizing the need to offer more outpatient services, some hospitals have built plush outpatient centers complete with food courts and small shops. To promote health within the community, hospitals hold classes on health-promoting topics, such as smoking cessation, various types of exercise, weight reduction, and basic life support. Sometimes persons who attend these classes become future consumers of inpatient services.

## Physician Group Practices

Alternative delivery systems are being supplemented by a dramatic movement toward group practice by physicians. In 1980, it was estimated that 30% of physicians were in group practice, and 50% of licensed active physicians were on full-time salaries (Roemer, 1982). By 1996, more than 50% of physicians had joined group practices (Frenkel, 1996). The greatest growth in physician group practice is expected to be in either individual practice associations (IPAs) or PPOs, associated with an HMO or primary case management model.

A PPO or IPA enables a group of providers to negotiate fee schedules with hospitals and third-party reimbursers to reduce out-of-pocket expenses and receive rapid payment for claims. However, increasingly the financial risk has been shifted from health plans to physicians who are sometimes rewarded for efficient practice. The advantage to the system is the incentive toward decreasing the use of resources and thereby decreasing costs.

The HMO was designed to focus efforts and resources on health promotion, preventive care and consumer education to reduce the cost of treatment (including hospital admittance) for illness. The traditional group- or staff-model HMO is a vertically integrated organization that operates its own physical facilities in different geographic locations and whose salaried physicians work solely for the HMO. However, by the end of 1994, only 31% of HMOs were of this type. "Increasingly, HMOs are 'virtual organizations' or 'organizations without walls,' built on contractual relationships with community providers. . . . Today, most HMOs do not view themselves as HMOs but as managed care organizations that offer an array of managed care plans" (Gabel, 1997, p. 136).

## The Hospital Industry

Hospital industry employs 59.1% of registered nurses (1,593,655). As large integrated health care networks expand, future hospital closures are expected. Although occupancy rates have been decreasing, the severity of illness of clients who are admitted to the hospital has been increasing (Brewer, 1997).

Given that "the primary factor driving down hospital utilization is managed care" (Shindul-Rothschild et al., 1996, p. 26), hospital downsizing and restructuring are expected to continue. As a result, the Bureau of Labor Statistics (as cited in Shindul-Rothschild et al., p. 29) has estimated that "by 2005, the percentages of nurses employed in hospitals will decrease to 57.4% from 63.8%." In addition, "it's unlikely that every RN job lost in the hospital will be replaced" (Shindul-Rothschild, Berry & Long-Middleton, 1996, p. 35).

However, nursing practice is not confined to hospitals. As clients spend less time in hospitals, the need for professional nurses for home health services increases. Increased need for professional nurses is anticipated as the population ages to meet the projected demand for nursing care in extended care facilities. More nurses are also needed to promote health in communities in order to keep persons out of hospitals.

## ✦ INTEGRATED HEALTH CARE DELIVERY SYSTEMS

Kleinke (1998) proposes that health care delivery within the next few years may differ greatly. He advocates for a highly **integrated health care delivery system** that provides consumers with a high continuity of care. The proposed Emerging Healthcare Organization (EHO) combines dimensions of consumer preference, marketing efforts of providers, and economic reimbursement into a single package. The EHO structure will center around a large urban health care center that offers comprehensive, sophisticated, technological medical therapies and may offer complementary therapies. The large health care center may be associated with a national proprietary chain or a national not-for-profit organization or may be part of the government.

Consumers will select health care insurance coverage based on their preferred large health care center, personal health care provider, or out-of-pocket expenditures. Hospitals will transform into specialized intensive care units and negotiate special contracts with providers of pharmaceuticals and other client care equipment. Consumers will receive less expensive follow-up care at home or in subacute extended care facilities. Consumers will see nurse practitioners, physician assistants, or primary care physicians for routine health care maintenance. Consumers will see specialists only when advanced diagnostic services or complicated disease management needs arise. Under this system, care will be managed and emphasis placed on health promotion.

Health care providers will also work to continuously improve the quality of health care services provided to consumers. Nurses may be called upon to become primary care providers who emphasize health promotion leaving physicians to manage persons with ill health. The integrated health system approach also provides opportunity for tracking nursing sensitive client outcomes using multiple sites.

## ✦ COSTS OF HEALTH CARE

A plethora of changes have increased the cost of health care delivery. Most of the time, health care consumers rely on health care professionals for sound advice to maximize their health potential. Within the past 20 years, health care delivery shifted from being an altruistic service to a business. This section outlines how some societal changes have contributed to the escalation of health care costs.

### Economic Forces

In this century, health care costs have constituted an increasing percentage of the US gross national product, from 3.5% in 1929 to 15% in 2003. The United States spends close to one trillion dollars on health care (Sultz & Young, 2004). Inflation in health care costs continues to increase at a rate higher than that of general inflation. In the past 10 years, the inflation rate in health care costs has been more than twice the overall inflation rate. According to the United States Federal Health Care Financing Administration, health care expenditures fall into the following two categories: health-related research and facilities construction or payment for personal health care services and supplies. Payment for individual health care services and supplies costs more than new construction or research. Of the personal health care services, hospital costs constitute the greatest single health care expense (Thorpe & Knickman, 1999; Sultz & Young, 2004).

## Hospital Costs

Hospital costs have been a major component of increasing health care costs. Several factors have influenced hospital costs. The development and intense use of advanced technology was encouraged by federal money for medical research and by almost automatic insurance reimbursement. In the past, insurers unquestioningly paid costs, and consumers had limited out-of-pocket costs for health care. As a result, no group claimed responsibility for increasing costs.

Specialization of knowledge promoted the growth of medical specialties supported by a complex network of nonphysician health care workers. In the past, physicians and third-party reimbursement companies urged consumers to use hospital resources for diagnosis and treatment. Unnecessary costs were incurred for inappropriate hospital admissions, prolonged hospital stays, multiple laboratory and diagnostic procedures performed to avoid the threat of lawsuits. Although these practices have been changing, the costs of hospital care have continued to increase.

New technologies, such as magnetic resonance imaging, genetic engineering, the artificial heart, monoclonal antibodies for the treatment of cancer, and organ transplantation, create pressures on health care costs, just as hip replacement, long-term dialysis, coronary bypass grafts, and computed tomography scans did in earlier years.

## Physician Fees

High physician fees have been encouraged by lack of competitive pressures and by insurance reimbursement practices that allowed physicians to determine both fees and the level of insurer reimbursement. However, the physician surplus, along with prospective payment, caps on Medicare reimbursement for physicians, and changes in the structure of medical practice, have begun to moderate the increases in physicians' fees.

Despite resistance by organized medicine, in 1996, all states allow advanced practice registered nurses access to third-party reimbursement (Sultz & Young, 2004). Care given by nurse practitioners cost substantially less and consumers report high satisfaction. Nurse practitioners are unfairly reimbursed by Medicaid in most states at 60% to 100% of the physician rate. In July 1997, direct Medicare reimbursement for nurse practitioners and clinical nurse specialists was approved by Congress at 85% of the physician payment rate (Sharp, 1997). Current legislative efforts of the American Academy of Nurse Practitioners focus on increasing the number of states providing Medicaid reimbursement to all nurse practitioners, regardless of practice specialty area.

## Insurance

In the 1950s and 1960s, criticism of the cost of health care to the individual (and government) and the resulting low level of access to care stimulated the rapid growth of employer-provided and privately purchased health insurance, the initiation of federal government Medicare insurance for the elderly and disabled, and state government Medicaid insurance for the poor. However, the current health insurance system, which developed largely as a passive risk-sharing system, has contributed to overwhelming inflationary pressure on the costs of health care. Persons who have insurance hold coverage from private policies (personal or employment-based, or the government). Health insurance premiums have been rising over 11% annually since 2001 and are expected to rise at a higher rate in the future (LeBow, 2003).

Approximately 14% or 44.3 million Americans lacked health insurance (USDHHS, 2000) and another 50 million were underinsured (LeBow, 2003). The moral concern about access to care has contributed to major proposals for mandated national health insurance or other health care reform measures.

Many major health reform bills have been introduced in Congress, and there is a growing consensus on the need to deal with the problem of Americans who lack medical insurance and to develop a strategy to fill the gaps left by current public programs such as Medicaid. However, the cost containment, a lack of congressional commitment to health care reform, and public disagreement over the best design of any national health care plan indicate the enactment of comprehensive reform remains unlikely. Most likely, the health care industry and government may proceed with incremental changes by which citizens continue to have choices related to providers and services.

Corporations represent the largest purchasers of private health insurance. In an effort to contain costs, companies have:

- Limited consumer choice of providers through HMOs or PPOs.
- Increased cost sharing by shifting more cost to the consumer through larger premiums, deductibles, and out-of-pocket charges.
- Required authorization for hospital admittance and second opinions for medical treatments.
- Substituted ambulatory and home care reimbursement for hospital admissions.
- Encouraged reduced use of services.

Pressures for change in insurance policies have potential opportunities for nursing. Nurses serve as a competitive alternative choice as gatekeepers and care providers, decreasing costs and improving quality of care. As providers of primary health care, they educate consumers in reducing the unnecessary use of services and educate about the practice of healthful living to improve the quality of life and prevent illness. As responsible client advocates, nurses have a key role to play in the creation of new health care delivery systems, and they need to become active participants in this process.

## Competition

Increased competition as a cost-containment mechanism provides an opportunity for nurse practitioners to expand primary and secondary health care services with direct reimbursement from the client and from third-party insurers. The free market approach dominated the health care industry in the 20th century, and no sign of a different focus has emerged (Jonas, 1998; LeBow, 1993; Feldstein, 2002). However, the recent Medicare prescription coverage for the elderly is an example of an incremental change in the American health care system with the federal government assuming more responsibility for the health care of American citizens. For effective health care in a market driven by competition, consumers must be actively involved in choosing alternatives, and qualified providers must be willing to participate in a competitive environment.

Clearly, some physicians view advanced practice nurses as competitors even though nurses promote health rather than treat illnesses. This attitude has promoted resistance among organized medicine to impede independent advanced nursing practice. Although substituting nursing care for primary care services reduces costs, the concern is that providing third-party reimbursement to nurses ultimately will increase health care costs as additional health care providers, such as pharmacists and social workers, also seek direct reimbursement.

## Ethical Concerns

Ethical concerns have been raised by an increasing life span, the development of health care technology, and the increasing cost of delivering care. Curtin (1996, p. 19) states that "the critical ethical problem in health care today is that ability to pay determines the availability and quality of care."

Because it is not possible to meet all goals of accessibility, equity, and quality given available resources, difficult choices must be made among competing values and multiple desirable alternatives. According to Smelzer (2000), 54 million persons with disabilities in the United States fail to receive effective primary care, and most of these persons are women and children. One basic issue is the relative valuing of predictability and containment of the costs of health care versus the access to health care for all persons.

Ethical questions raised by these choices include:

1. How willing are some people to assume the costs to make the system affordable, acceptable, and available to all?
2. How much is health care a basic right?
3. If there are limits on access to health care, who should have priority?
4. What is an acceptable level of health care?
5. Should technology be available to all, regardless of cost, or should it be rationed?
6. What should be the criteria for rationing?
7. Who should determine the criteria?
8. How much choice should be determined by ability to pay?
9. What (and when) is death?
10. How much is the prolongation of life worth?
11. Does reducing costs reduce the quality of care?
12. What rights do clients have?
13. Is cure of all disease possible?
14. Is cure of all disease desirable at any cost?
15. Who needs professional nursing services?

"Treating health care primarily as a business and a commodity to be sold like cars is an impoverished notion of health care in relation to the concept of health care as a human service created by society to meet the needs of vulnerable people who are ill or at risk of becoming ill" (Aroskar, 1995, p. 65). It is critical that the voice of the nursing profession be added to that of the public in discussions of the philosophic considerations and values that will shape the decisions concerning the size, shape, and direction of the American health care system. Nursing focuses on health promotion and maximizing the quality of life for all.

## ● SUMMARY AND SIGNIFICANCE TO PRACTICE

As a result of significant demographic, economic, attitudinal, and available manpower forces, the health care delivery system is in the process of structural change and reorganization, raising multiple ethical considerations. Health care providers can use historical events to prevent repeating past mistakes. The nursing profession has the opportunity to influence the direction of change to ensure the improvement of health and health care.

### FROM THEORY TO PRACTICE

1. What are the current strengths of the American and Canadian health care delivery systems? Why are these strengths?
2. What are the current weaknesses of the American and Canadian health care delivery systems? Why are these weaknesses?
3. How can nurses work to improve health care delivery? What are the consequences if nurses do not get involved with changes in the health care delivery system?
4. Reflecting on the vignette, how should Jane explain to her father the benefits of a temporary stay in an extended care facility on his recovery? How would you explain the complex web of health care delivery to elderly clients? What type of help do they need to navigate their way through the health care system?

## WWW INTERNET EXERCISES

1. Visit the Health Insurance Association of America at http://www.ahip.org to learn about the complexity of the health insurance industry. The website contains the latest updates on legislative efforts to reform health insurance and provides consumers with information about the types of and how to enroll in health insurance plans.
2. To learn about issues confronting physicians in today's health care environment, visit the American Medical Association (AMA) at http://www.ama-assn.org. Look for the listing of a physician you know.
3. Visit the ANA at http://www.nursingworld.org to learn about issues confronting professional nurses in the health care system.
4. Compare and contrast the ANA and AMA websites. How could ANA improve its website? What are the consequences of having professional health care providers listed in a website directory?
5. To view how health care providers market services to the public on the Internet:
   a. Visit a for-profit integrated health care system site, such as Tenet Health at http://www.tenethealth.com.

      **b.** Visit a nonprofit health care system site, such as http://www.saint-lukes.org.

      **c.** Visit a large academic institution connected with a major research university, such as http://www.kumc.edu.

      **d.** Compare and contrast the various websites.

**6.** Using a search engine of your choice, type in the name of a local health department and see what services they offer.

## INTERNET RESOURCES

Agency for Healthcare Policy & Research: http://www.ahrg.gov.

American Nurses Association: http://www.nursingworld.org.

American Hospital Association: http://aha.org.

Health Care Financing Administration. (Medicare and Medicaid): http://www.cms.hhs.gov.

National Health Information Center: http://health.gov/nhic.

Health Insurance Association of America: http://www.ahip.org.

WebMD: http://webmd.com.

American Association of Retired Persons: http://www.aarp.org.

## REFERENCES

American Hospital Association. (1999). *Welcome to the board: An orientation for the new health care trustee*. Chicago: AHA Press.

American Nurses Association. (1995). *Nursing's social policy statement*. Kansas City: Author.

Aroskar, M. A. (1987). Fidelity and veracity: Questions of promise keeping, truth telling, and loyalty. In M. D. M. Fowler & J. Levine-Ariff (Eds.), *Ethics at the bedside: A sourcebook for the critical care nurse*,(pp. 72–83). Philadelphia: J. B. Lippincott.

Bezold, C. (1982). Health care in the U.S. Four alternative futures. *The Futurist, 16*, 14–18.

Brewer, C. S. (1997). Through the looking glass: The labor market for registered nurses in the 21st Century. *Nursing and Health Care Perspectives, 18*, 260–269.

Bureau of Health Professions (2002). National Center for Workforce Analysis. *Projected supply, demand and shortage of registered nurses 2000-2020*. U.S. Department of Health and Human Services, Health Resources and Services Administration, 2002. Available at: http://www.ahca.org/research/rnsupply_demand.pdf. Accessed June 30, 2005.

Curtin, L. L. (1996). The ethics of managed care-Part I: Proposing a new ethos. *Nursing Management, 27*, 18–19.

Feldstein, P. J. (2002). *Health policy issues: An economic perspective*, (3rd ed.). Chicago: Health Administration Press.

Floyd, K., Blanc, L., Raviglione, M., & Lee, J. (2002). Resources for global tuberculosis control. *Science, 295*, 2040–2041.

Fried, B. J., & Gaydos, L. M. (Eds.) (2002). *World health systems, challenges and perspectives*. Chicago: Health Administration Press.

Frenkel, M. (1996). Caveats for physicians in the financing of practice networks. *Journal of Health Care Financing, 22*, 49–51.

Gabel, J. (1997). Ten ways HMOs have changed in the 1990s. *Health Affairs*, 16, 134–135.

Inglis, T. (2004). Nursing the trends. *American Journal of Nursing. Career Guide 2004, 104*, 25–32.

Jamieson, E. M., & Sewall, M. F. (1954). *Trends in nursing history* (4th ed.). Philadelphia: WB Saunders.

Jonas, S. (1998). *An introduction to the U.S. health care system* (4th ed.). New York: Springer Publishing.

Kleinke, J. D. (1998). *Bleeding edge: The business of health care in the new century*. Gaithersburg MD: Aspen.

Kovner, A. R., & Jonas, S. (Eds.). (1998*). Jonas and Kovner's health care delivery in the United States* (6th ed.). New York: Springer Publishing.

LeBow, R. H. (2003). *Health care meltdown*. Chambersburg, PA: Alan C. Hood & Company, Inc.

Markowitz, G. E., & Rosner, D. (1979). Doctors in crisis. Medical education and medical reform during the progressive era, 1895–1915. In S. Reverby & D. Rosner (Eds.), *Health care in America: Essays in social history* (pp. 185–205). Philadelphia: Temple University Press.

McDonald, M. D. (2001). The hospitalist movement: Wise or wishful thinking? *Nursing Management, 32*, 30–31.

McIntyre, M. & Thomlinson, E. (2003). *Realities of Canadian nursing: Professional, practice and power issues*. Philadelphia: Lippincott Williams & Wilkins.

*Merriam-Webster's collegiate dictionary* (10th ed.). (1994). Springfield, MA: Merriam-Webster.

Raffel, M. W. (1993). *The U.S. health system: Origins and functions*. New York: Wiley.

Roemer, M. I. (1982). *An introduction to the U.S. health care system*. New York: Springer Publishing.

Sanmartin, C., Nge, E., Blackwell, D., Gentleman, J., Martinez, M., & Simile, C.(2004). *Joint Canada/United States Survey of Health*. Center for Disease Control. Available at: http://www.cdc.gov/nchs/data/hsis/jcush_analyticalreport.pdf.

Scofea, L. (1994). The development and growth of employer-provided health insurance. *Monthly Labor Review, 117*, 3–10.

Sharp, N. J. (1997). Personal Communication, November 10, 1997.

Shindul-Rothschild, J., Berry, D., & Long-Middleton, E. (1996). Where have all the nurses gone? *American Journal of Nursing, 96*, 25–39.

Smeltzer, S. C. (2000). Double jeopardy: The health care system slights women with disabilities. *American Journal of Nursing, 100*, 11.

Snyder, M., Mirr, M. P., Lindeke, L., Fagerlund, K., Avery, M., & Tseng, Y. (1999). Advanced practice nursing: An overview. In M. Snyder & M. P. Mirr (Eds.), *Advanced practice nursing: A guide to professional development* (2nd ed., pp. 1–24). New York: Springer Publishing.

Sultz, H. A. & Young, K. M. (2004). *Health care USA: Understanding its organization and delivery*. (4th ed.). Sudbury, MA: Jones and Bartlett.

Thorpe, K. E., & Knickman, J. R. (1999). Financing for health care. In S. Jonas & A. R. Kovner (Eds.), *Jonas & Kovner's health care delivery in the United States* (6th ed., pp. 32–63). New York: Springer Publishing.

Torrens, P. R. (1978). *The American health care system: Issues and problems*. St. Louis: Mosby.

United Nations Joint AIDS Program on HIV/(UNAIDS) and the World Health Organization (2001). *AIDS Epidemic Update*. Geneva: UNAIDS & WHO.

United States Census Bureau. (2002). *Statistical abstract of the US: 2002* (120th ed.). Washington, DC: Author.

United States Department of Health and Human Services (USDHHS). (1990). *Seventh report to the President and Congress on the status of health personnel in the United States*. Washington, DC: Author.

United States Department of Health and Human Services. (2000). *Healthy people 2010*. Washington, DC: Author.

Vogel, M. J. (1979). The transformation of the American hospital, 1859–1920. In S. Reverby & D. Rosner (Eds.), *Health care in America: Essays in social history* (pp. 105–116). Philadelphia: Temple University Press.

Vogel, G., & Doleysh, N. (1988). *Entrepreneuring: A nurses' guide to starting a business*. National League for Nursing Publication No. 41-2201. New York: National League for Nursing.

Vogel, G., & Doleysh, N. (1994). *Entrepreneuring: A nurses' guide to starting a business*. NLN Publication No. 41-2201. New York: National League for Nursing.

Waite, L. J. (1996). The demographic face of America's elderly. *Inquiry, 33*, 220–224.

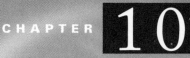

# CHAPTER 10

# Developing and Using Nursing Knowledge Through Research

## KEY TERMS AND CONCEPTS

Research

The Research Process

Quantitative Research

Qualitative Research

Research Critique

Variable

Independent Variable

Dependent Variable

Research Ethics

Informed Consent

Anonymity

Institution Review Board (IRB)

Research Utilization

Diffusion

Innovation

Diffusion of Innovations

Stetler Research Utilization Model

Research Utilization Facilitators

Research Utilization Barriers

Evidenced-Based Nursing

Scholar

National Institute for Nursing Research (NINR)

## LEARNING OUTCOMES

By the end of this chapter, the learner will be able to:

1 Describe how professional nurses contribute to research in nursing.

2 Outline the sequential steps of the research process.

3 Differentiate qualitative and quantitative research.

4 Debate the ethical considerations of nursing research.

5 Compare and contrast research utilization models.

6 Discuss the key elements of a research study critique.

7 Identify barriers to research utilization by the nurses in the clinical setting.

8 Identify strategies to facilitate clinical research utilization.

9 Differentiate research utilization from evidenced-based nursing practice.

10 Specify how using nursing research affects the public image of professional nursing.

**VIGNETTE**

Joan and Sandy work together on a surgical unit. Sandy has been practicing for 12 years, takes pride in her expertise, and practices nursing "the way that I was taught." Joan has read several research articles substantiating the effectiveness of noninvasive nursing interventions on reducing client need for postoperative narcotics for pain control. Joan is unsure if she should use these findings in practice and how Sandy will react if she suggests implementing these findings on a unit-wide scale. Joan also knows that current federal guidelines related to postoperative pain control specify that nurses should use other methods besides pain medication.

### Questions for Reflection 10-1

1. How do I feel about nursing research?
2. What research-based interventions have I used in my clinical practice?

In today's world, health care professionals and consumers rely on research-based interventions for health promotion and disease management. Discipline-specific research enables a profession to develop and validate its unique knowledge base. Research also validates principles and techniques of clinical practice. Because nursing primarily is a practice discipline, nurses need to understand research principles, critically analyze research study results, and use research findings to guide client care.

Florence Nightingale conducted research and published her findings in her book, *Notes on Nursing*. The information generated by her research transformed health care, changed nursing practice and provided a theoretical foundation for her nursing school in London. However, serious efforts to conduct nursing research and develop theory to guide practice began about 40 years ago when nursing scholars began the pursuit of establishing theoretical- and factual-based nursing practice, instead of perpetuating nursing practice based on personal opinions, longstanding traditions, and prescribed protocols from other disciplines. Martha Rogers, one of the nursing visionaries, said more than 30 years ago, "Only the most uninformed and those endeavoring to maintain a long obsolete hierarchal control would propose that in today's world society is better served by ignorance than by knowledge" (Rogers, 1967). However, a study of medical–surgical nurses found that many rely on information from individual patients, personal experience, and information gained during nursing school far more than on facts from journal articles (Baessler et al., 1994). Clinicians must appreciate that incorporation of research findings into practice is not an optional activity in which to engage when there is time, but is a critical element of professional practice.

Science seeks the truth and humans create science through research (Barrett, 2002). Therefore, nursing research should result in the creation of nursing science. **"Research is diligent, systematic inquiry or investigation to validate and refine existing knowledge and generate new knowledge"** (Burns & Grove, 2001, p. 3). Scholars debate over which of the following situations can be categorized as nursing research: a nurse or group of nurses conducting research, or studies based on nursing theories or to generate new nursing knowledge. Heitkemper and Bond (2003) identify two commandments, perhaps three, for nursing science: "contribute to science and contribute to patient care," and "contribute to theory development" (p. 152). When research-generated nursing knowledge results in improved client outcomes, enhances the professional practice environment, or contains health care costs, the research has practical applications for client care. When unresolved client care or professional nursing issues arise, nurses can conduct research to solve the problem. Therefore, research guides practice and practice generates new ideas for research.

The baccalaureate-prepared nurse can contribute to nursing research in several ways, including:

1. Reading and critiquing nursing research studies.
2. Using nursing research findings to guide nursing practice.
3. Valuing a sense of inquiry about the phenomena of nursing.
4. Participating in research projects as opportunity allows.
5. Refining the ability to collect, organize, categorize, and analyze data.
6. Suggesting nursing research questions that need to be addressed to improve practice.

To participate in these ways, the nurse must have an understanding of the research process and of strategies to overcome barriers and facilitate research utilization.

## ● RESEARCH PROCESSES IN NURSING

This section serves as an overview to facilitate understanding of the components of the research process. **The research process** consists of a series of logical steps of inquiry. Familiarity with the research process enhances the nurse's understanding of nursing research studies. Complete understanding of the research process and expertise in its execution improves as one develops as a nurse researcher, a process that requires much time and commitment.

Beginning with the nurse's query about some aspect of nursing, the research process structures the systematic investigation of that question and the reporting of the answers and new questions about that aspect of nursing. The research process follows the methods of science, which essentially means that the process:

• Has an identifiable order.
• Includes controls over factors not being investigated.
• Includes the gathering of evidence about the question.
• Is built on a theoretical framework.
• Operates for the purpose of applying results to improve nursing practice.

### Raising Questions

The most significant step in the nursing research process may be the first one—the nurse's identification and articulation of a question to be answered. When nurses seek to find the best way to practice, they become accountable for asking questions that reflect the sensitivity needed to better understand all that falls within the domain of nursing. Nurses identify potential research questions when they encounter clinical practice problems. Because nursing theory and practice are deeply intertwined, research questions also may arise when nurses identify a gap in theory and practice. Concrete examples for research studies include, but are not limited to, client health experiences, nursing professional characteristics and responsibilities, elements within the nurse–client relationship, environmental factors to promote health, health promotion, and client adjustment to illness and other life transitions. A clearly and concisely stated question provides direction for the entire study. The chance of executing clinically relevant nursing research studies increases when clinical nurses and nurse researchers collaborate.

## Quantitative and Qualitative Approaches

Two research approaches to developing nursing knowledge have emerged in recent years: the quantitative approach and the qualitative approach. In the earliest years of nursing research, valuing of the scientific method led to the use of quantitative approaches to develop objective information. However, nurse researchers currently accept qualitative approaches to develop subjective information while remaining open to quantitative approaches.

According to Haase and Myers (1988), quantitative and qualitative research approaches have a common purpose: to gain understanding. The difference between the approaches is one of emphasis. **Quantitative research** focuses on the "confirmation of theory by explaining," demonstrating an empirical analytical emphasis; **qualitative research** focuses on "discovery and meaning of theory by describing," demonstrating a human science emphasis (Haase & Myers, p. 131).

According to Guba and Lincoln (reported by Haase & Myers, 1988), the differences between the two approaches can be categorized in three ways according to the assumptions made by each approach: the nature of reality, the nature of relationships, and the nature of truth. The following comparison of quantitative and qualitative assumptions according to the three categories is presented from the work of Haase and Myers (1988, pp. 130–134).

1. View of reality

    Quantitative: Researcher focuses on objective reality seen as singular; the process for discovering reality is reductionistic; and it is believed that knowledge of the whole can be gained through knowledge of the parts.

    Qualitative: Researcher focuses on subjective realities seen as multiple and related; the process for understanding reality is ecologic; and it is believed that "the whole is greater than the sum of its parts" (p. 132).

2. View of relationships

    Quantitative: Researcher objectively distances self from subjects and believes that boundaries must exist to ensure objectivity.

    Qualitative: Researcher interacts with the subject and believes that a unity exists between them and that both are integral to the research process.

3. View of truth

    Quantitative: Researcher sees the world as stable and predictable and believes that the truth is discovered in common laws, principles, and norms. Thus, the researcher's goal is generalization.

    Qualitative: Researcher sees the world as dynamic and believes that truth is discovered in the changing patterns of the world. Thus, the researcher's goal is to discover uniqueness, valuing differences as well as similarities.

Appreciating the complexity of nursing phenomena and valuing subjective experiences as legitimate foci of nursing research, Artinian (1988) notes that nurses willingly use qualitative approaches, all of which use participant observation and in-depth interviewing. Cohen and Tripp-Reimer (1988, p. 226) support ethnography as a significant qualitative research approach to help nurses understand cultural differences, stating that "ethnography is a method designed to describe a culture. The ethnographer seeks to understand another way of life from the native's point of view."

Grounded theory methodology seeks to outline a basic social process or generate a new theory based on participant data. Using grounded theory methodology, Artinian (1988, pp. 138–149) describes four modes of inquiry the qualitative researcher can use.

1. Descriptive mode, which "presents rich detail that allows the reader to understand what it would be like to be in a setting or to be experiencing the life situation of a person or group" (p. 139).
2. Discovery mode, which "enables the researcher both to identify patterns in the life experiences of the subjects and to relate the patterns to each other" (p. 141).
3. Emergent fit mode, which is "used when a substantive theory has already been developed about the phenomenon under study" from which a research question "is formulated to extend or refine the previously developed theory" (p. 142).
4. Intervention mode, in which the researcher tries to answer the fundamental question of how to make something happen after the "phenomenon has been adequately conceptualized so that the conditions under which the basic social process takes place are understood" (p. 139).

The researcher decides which of the four modes of inquiry to use only after clarifying the purpose of the research and evaluating knowledge that is available on the topic.

Along with ethnography and grounded theory, nurse researchers use other qualitative research processes. Phenomenology looks at the "lived experience" of a particular life transition, clinical experience, or having a specific illness or surgery. Hermeneutic inquiry seeks to find the deep, personal meaning of an experience. Qualitative research enables nurses to discover individualized and human phenomena surrounding health and illness. Historical studies examine artifacts from a particular era to determine what persons did in the past that might have application for today.

## Steps in the Research Process

Whether the nurse researcher chooses the qualitative or the quantitative approach, the overall steps in the research process remain essentially the same. The research process is a sequence of eleven steps during which researchers make decisions to plan and execute a study. While engaged in the research process, the investigator may not necessarily complete a step, but rather may re-visit steps while planning and executing a study. The study question determines which approach would be best. Knowledge of the research process steps discussed in the subsequent sections will facilitate the nurse's use of findings in practice.

### Focus on the Clinical Problem Area

From where do the questions that need to be answered about nursing arise? Of these questions, which require research for adequate response? Which have sufficient data already available for effective problem solving? All nurses have the ability to identify problems in professional practice. While engaging in clinical practice, nurses frequently identify gaps between what is and what could be. The identified gaps become clinical problems that may be solved through nursing research.

Nurses also can focus on a problem area by reviewing the current research and other information in the literature on a topic of interest; by deriving questions from the theories or conceptual model used to guide practice in the nurses' practice setting or educational program; or by getting ideas from external sources such as faculty, peers, or priorities established for practice.

For example, some nursing organizations have determined areas of priority for research. The Oncology Nursing Society has ongoing research initiatives on pain control, prevention of nausea, optimal nutrition, and fatigue in persons with cancer. The American Nurses Association has ongoing studies related to workplace hazards for nurses. The American Association of Critical Care Nurses' priorities for clinical research focus on client pain, nosocomial infections, and ventilator weaning. Often, nursing organizations provide grants to researchers who conduct studies in the determined priority areas.

The development of the research problem, according to Polit and Beck (2003), incorporates the following sequential steps:

- Note a general area of interest about which you have some questions.
- Narrow the topic through critical evaluation of ideas with a mentor or expert. That evaluation must address feasibility and worth.
- Establish the benefit of the investigation of the selected problem to nursing by addressing who will benefit, what are the applications, what is the potential for the results to be relevant to theoretical bases of practice, and how important are the findings (in other words, so what?).
- Make certain that the selected problem is amenable to scientific methodology.
- Verify that the problem is not primarily a moral issue.
- Critique the feasibility of studying the problem in terms of time factors, availability of subjects, cooperation required, facilities and equipment needed, and costs.

The initial review of the literature helps researchers accomplish these steps in the early development of the problem.

## Initial Review of the Literature

Nurse researchers obtain a broad understanding and general background on the problem to be studied from an initial review of the literature. Once the researcher has raised a question, an initial review of the literature is helpful in:

- Identifying the major variables in the area of interest.
- Finding out what is already known.
- Gathering feasibility data on the needs for investigation of the question.
- Refining the focus of the problem to be investigated.

A review of the literature should make the researcher aware of all the possible relevant material available regarding a problem of interest. Along with reading the literature available on the research topic, researchers must appraise each research study by assessing its strengths and weaknesses. A **research critique** points out the strengths and weaknesses of a study and helps researchers discover gaps in the current literature. Helpful sources for locating resource materials include indexes from nursing, related disciplines, and popular literature; abstracting services from nursing and related disciplines; computer searches of appropriate databases; dictionaries; encyclopedias; guides; and directories. Reference librarians in most libraries provide tremendous help to the beginning nurse researcher in locating and using these materials.

In summary, the initial review of the literature should answer some questions about the topic of interest, describe other people's interests in the topic, and help the researcher develop a strong knowledge base of what has been written and reported on the topic. Frequently, qualitative research studies avoid reviewing the literature before collecting data to avoid developing preconceived ideas about the topic area. In quantitative research, such a knowledge base makes it possible for the researcher to proceed to the next stage of research: specifying the problem and defining the variables.

## Specification of the Problem and the Defining Variables

When the researcher has completed the initial review of the literature, gained a general understanding of the research topic and a sense of what is known about the topic, the researcher proceeds to more clearly delineate the problem to be investigated.

Decisions are made about exactly what is to be investigated or what part of the nursing domain is to be studied. The nurse researcher may be investigating some client aspect that is clearly important to understand in the nursing process; some client health phenomenon; some client outcomes associated with particular nursing interventions; some aspect of the nurse–client relationship; some aspect of the delivery of nursing care services; some aspect of the environment that affects the health status; or any combination of these factors in the nursing domain.

Clear articulation of the problem incorporates the identification of the phenomenon to be investigated. In quantitative research, a phenomenon of interest generally is called a "variable." A **variable** is a characteristic, a trait, a property, or a condition. If the variable is purposefully manipulated by the researcher to *have a direct effect on* another variable, it is an **independent variable.** The variable that *is observed, measured, and presumed to be influenced by or related in some special way to the independent variable* is the **dependent variable.** Variables do not exist in qualitative research because the purpose may be to identify key phenomena surrounding a client or nurse experience.

An example of an investigative problem with one variable that is manipulated and another that is observed and measured is: What is the relationship between specific parenting guidance by the professional nurse and the development of positive nutritional habits of the toddler? In this investigation, the independent variable is the specific parenting guidance, the dependent variable is the toddler's nutritional habits, and the approach to studying the variables is quantitative.

To make these variables measurable, the researcher must determine exactly what is meant by each variable: what constitutes parenting guidance and what constitutes positive nutritional habits in the toddler. The statement of the problem may be in the form of a question or a declaration. In both cases, this problem statement also must clearly identify who is to be studied and what is to be studied.

## Establishment of Tentative Propositions: Hypotheses and the Second Review of the Literature

After the nurse researcher has clarified the problem under investigation, studied the available data, and recalled observations from professional experience, he or she may formulate a hypothesis, a formal statement that predicts or explains the relationships between two or more variables (Polit & Beck, 2003). Not all studies require that the researcher generate a hypothesis; for example, descriptive, qualitative, and exploratory natured questions do not need hypotheses. However, for studies requiring manipulation of an independent variable and measurement of a dependent variable, hypotheses must be stated and tested.

Nurses have excellent opportunities to form some hunches about the relationships among variables they observe in practice. Thought of as bridges, hypotheses connect theory with observation and are derived from observations, reasoning, and theoretical bases.

Hypotheses in quantitative studies are tested statistically in relation to the laws of chance. Thus, they are based on statistical probability and incur an element of risk of reaching an incorrect conclusion. How much risk can be afforded is a judgment of the investigator, but when permanent or serious consequences are involved, the investigator cannot afford to take too many risks. Because hypotheses sometimes force the investigator to infer from the sample findings to an interpretation about the population, the researcher uses probability statistics (level of significance) to determine the likelihood that the relationship between the variables results from something other than chance.

When the researcher is determining hypotheses, additional review of the literature is used to evaluate testing procedures and to project a research design appropriate for investigating the variable(s). The review of the literature can be used to learn what investigative methods have been used, how data have been collected and analyzed, and what has and has not been successful in previous research.

In summary, in quantitative studies, hypotheses declare the researcher's proposition about the relationship between variables and then serve as the means for testing the proposed relationship. Hypotheses do not appear in descriptive, correlational, or qualitative research studies.

## Determination of a Suitable Research Design

The nurse researcher selects the type of research design suitable for the study based on the research question(s) or hypothesis(es). The descriptive design answers questions about the nature of presently occurring events. The experimental design tests the effects of manipulating one or more specific variables on other variables. The historical design is based on the desire to describe or evaluate past events. The researcher frequently acts as a member of or observes a group in ethnographic research. Detailed interviews followed by participant validation of data serve as the means to capture the essence of an experience in phenomenology.

## Development of Measurement Methods and Instruments

After the approach is selected for a particular study, the nurse researcher must decide on the appropriate method for gathering data about the variables. The investigator then selects instruments for data collection; the instrument chosen depends on the purpose of the research. Instruments generally are categorized under three methods: observation, questioning, and measurement.

Examples of data collection instruments from these categories include critical incidents, tests, interviews, questionnaires, checklists, records, scales, and physical measurement techniques. The researcher strives to select a measurement tool that is appropriate to answer the research question; that is not biased; and that has precision in measuring the variables being studied. For quantitative studies, the researcher carefully analyzes available measurement tools to determine instrument validity (the extent that it actually measured the variable of interest) and reliability (consistency of variable measurement). In qualitative studies, the researcher exercises caution to eliminate any personal biases that could interfere with objective data collection. The quality of data generated for a study relies on careful selection of data collection methods.

Knafl and Webster (1988, pp. 196–203) pointed out how the researcher's data collection, analysis of those data, and reporting are likely to vary, according to the purpose of the study. They describe four purposes of qualitative research.

1. Illustration, in which the researcher aims to identify qualitative examples of specific quantitative variables.
2. Instrumentation, in which the researcher aims to collect data that serve as the basis for developing an instrument to describe and measure perceptions of some phenomenon of interest to nursing.
3. Description, in which the researcher aims to "translate the data into a form that would facilitate an accurate, complete description" (p. 200) of a phenomenon of interest to nursing by identifying and delineating the major themes.
4. Theory building, in which the researcher aims to conceptually explain the phenomenon under study.

Knafl, Pettengill, Bevis, and Kirschoff (1988) reported that, although debate continues about the credibility of using either qualitative or quantitative approaches to study particular nursing phenomena, some nurse researchers are beginning to use both qualitative and quantitative methods in single studies. This process is known as method triangulation and it is believed that by integrating the two approaches, researchers can capitalize on the strengths of each approach while minimizing the weaknesses of each. For example, a nurse studying the effects of specific parenting guidance on positive toddler nutritional habits might want the mother's attitudes about specific guidance given to her, by the nurse.

In addition to selecting instruments for data collection during this stage of research, the nurse must determine the composition of the sample; establish a process for collecting data from the sample; and prepare a format for data collection (which may include designing specific forms), data classification, and data storage for later analysis. The sample subjects must be clearly described, and the method for choosing the subjects must be appropriate. The number of sample subjects must meet statistical requirements for the nurse to draw appropriate conclusions about the findings.

## Assurance of an Ethical Process

Research requires honesty and integrity. **Research ethics** are principles by which researchers abide to assure truth in scientific studies, protect the human rights of participants, balance risks and benefits of a study, and prevent exploitation of vulnerable persons. Research ethics became important after reports of inhumane and unethical treatment sustained by prisoners during Nazi Germany medical experiments. In 1949, the Nuremburg Code was established to protect human subjects in biomedical experiments. The researcher bears the responsibility for protecting human rights when persons participate in a research study. This protection is provided primarily through informed consent and protection from harm.

**Informed consent** means that the researcher provides subjects with a clear description about the study, how they meet study criteria, requirements for participation, and potential hazards. The subjects must understand and consent to their role in the study. Having given informed consent does not keep any subject from changing his or her mind anytime during the study and withdrawing from it.

Protection from harm means just that: the investigator will not knowingly do anything that will harm or abuse the subjects. Investigators also work to preserve subject **anonymity,** keeping the identification of all subjects confidential.

Most institutions where research is conducted have a formalized process for approving research proposals before implementation. An **Institution Review Board (IRB)** meets on a regular schedule to review research proposals to verify that investigators have considered research ethics and that the study meets scientific standards. In health care settings, nurses sometimes hold IRB membership. Because they are client advocates and have holistic views of health care, nurses sometimes identify potentially harmful research treatments that other IRB health team members may overlook.

To assure truth in research, the researcher assumes responsibility for honesty when collecting and analyzing data and when reporting research findings. For-profit and non-profit organizations frequently fund research studies. When corporations fund research projects, a conflict of interest may arise. Researchers have taken funds from sponsors for many years while remaining neutral when performing scientific studies. Corporations frequently fill in gaps in required funding so that research studies can be performed. When extramural funding has been received for the research study, the investigator has an obligation to report the source of funds within the written report (Blumenstyk, 2001).

## Collection of Data

After protection of human rights for all subjects has been ensured, data collection can begin. However, before any subject associated with an institution can be approached, the researcher must have approval from appropriate agency personnel.

The researcher or a specified data collector orients each subject clearly and concisely to the data collection method, then administers the data collection instrument to each subject in the same manner. Throughout this implementation stage, the researcher follows the written proposal (in the methodology) as closely as possible. While collecting data, the researcher records the data on the prepared forms. The data then are classified and organized for analysis.

## Analysis of Data and Report of Findings

Once data are collected, the researcher organizes data in a manner that makes them amenable to analysis. If the researcher's goal is simply to display the data collected, no analysis other than the narrative description of the displayed data is needed. However, if the researcher aims to infer some characteristics about a population or to evaluate some relationship among variables, the organized data must be subjected to statistical analysis. Computations are done. If hypotheses have been stated, statistical testing, by hand or by computer, of those hypotheses must be done.

Based on accurate data analysis, the researcher must report the findings exactly as they occurred. Summaries of the data must reflect the subjects' findings exactly. All data collected for purposes of testing the hypotheses must be reported. Tables, charts, and graphs used to present data should be pertinent, clear, and well labeled, and they should be discussed in the text of the research report. The reports of the findings are then used to draw conclusions.

## Conclusions and Implications

For quantitative research studies, the researcher must determine the meaning of the findings and their value to nursing with use of the theoretical foundation guiding the study. Findings are analyzed first by inspecting the statistical tests performed to test the hypotheses or evaluate the data. The researcher then interprets what the numerical analysis means. With hypothesis testing, the findings may support the predicted relationship with demonstrated statistical significance (the findings were not attributable to chance alone); the findings may not be in the predicted direction; the findings may be contradictory; or the findings may indicate an unpredicted relationship. Sometimes statistical significance has little practical significance. Practical significance indicates that the results add to the body of nursing knowledge or result in major changes in clinical outcomes. For example, the tobacco industry argued in the court system that cigarette smoking failed to cause lung cancer with statistical significance. However, research studies revealed a high degree if correlation (strong relationship) between smoking and the development of lung cancer.

For qualitative studies, the researcher determines the meaning of the study and its value to professional nursing by identifying the significance of the new knowledge generated by the study. The conceptual overview generated by a qualitative study may have profound importance when working with clients with similar conditions. Qualitative studies frequently provide a foundation for hypothesis generation and research instrument development for future quantitative research studies.

Based on the analysis and interpretation of data, the researcher might make generalizations about what the data mean and whether the data can be applied to groups different from the sample. Generalizations should emerge only from the findings, and the researcher should not go beyond the data as a result of the excitement generated by scientific discovery.

Study implications usually relate to one of the four aspects of professional nursing: clinical practice with clients, professional education, clinical practice environments, and ideas for additional nursing research. Researchers generally report implications in a section of a research study called "recommendations." The implications for practice (that is, how they affect the nursing process with clients) are discussed. Recommendations for the education of practitioners and future research are also usually given. If the recommendations are clearly and concisely stated and derived logically, clinical nurses can find the study valuable and consider using the findings in practice.

## The Written Report

Research completed but not compiled into a report is wasted. Some research experts argue that the research process is not complete until it is shared in writing or some other public medium. Characteristics of an effective research report are brevity, clarity, and complete objectivity.

Although there are variations on the form of the report that may be determined by faculty, a particular style manual, or other institutional requirements, the usual report follows the outline of the research process presented in this chapter. Most outlines include the problem statement, review of literature, methods of investigation, presentation of findings, discussion of the analyses and conclusions, bibliographic data, and appendixes. The reader is directed to a nursing research book or a writing style manual for specific guidance in developing each part of the written research report.

### Questions for Reflection 10-2

1. What questions do I have related to the research process and how to critique nursing research studies?
2. Who would be able and willing to help if I had questions when reading a nursing research report? How can I reach them?
3. Would I be interested in starting or participating in a nursing research journal club? Why or why not? If so, how could I make journal club participation a reality?

## ⊕ UTILIZATION OF NURSING RESEARCH

Nurses have used nursing research in practice for more than a century. Florence Nightingale used a systematic approach to collect data and presented detailed statistics using bar graphs, pie charts, and color-coded tables to highlight key points. She used these to present evidence of the benefits of sanitation, and trained nurses when she pleaded her case for increased funding for ill and infirm soldiers during the Crimean War. She published her findings in *Notes on Nursing* so that the knowledge she generated could be used in practice (McDonald, 2001). Nurses have been using research in practice for years, but frequently overlook its use. **Research utilization** is a systematic process used by nurses to incorporate research-based knowledge into professional nursing practice.

Every time nurses administer medications in the United States, the medication is subjected to randomized clinical trials. Because new knowledge is being generated rapidly, what nurses learn in an academic program may become obsolete within a few years. Professional nurses cannot plead ignorance of new knowledge and practices because part of professional accountability requires keeping up with new practice developments (Rambur, 1999). To stay abreast of new practices, professional nurses must read the research nursing literature and apply new knowledge appropriately in practice.

The use of a scientific base for clinical practice has a number of benefits, including:

- A sound foundation for practice.
- Enhanced self-confidence, autonomy, critical thinking skills, and professional self-concept.
- Cost-effective patient care.
- Increased patient and job satisfaction and quality of care.
- Improved patient outcomes.
- A stimulus for collaborative practice, retention, and recruitment.
- An improved image of nursing.
- An ever-increasing scientific nursing knowledge base (Goode et al., 1991, pp. 8–9).

---

**Case Study for Research Utilization**

Tony works on a rehabilitation unit with a variety of clients who have problems with activities of daily living, such as ambulation and feeding themselves. Because of staff shortages, he has noticed that there has been an increase in client impaired skin integrity. He would like to use the Braden scale, a research-based tool, to screen clients at risk for impaired skin integrity. When he suggests using research findings as the basis for nursing care protocols on the unit, his colleagues tease him and call him "professor". His work setting does not permit him time to prepare a proposal for using research-based findings on the job.

---

Research utilization may be as simple as one nurse changing the way in which care is given (Gennaro, 1994). However, despite the significant amount of available nursing research, there is a well-documented gap in the use of research findings to improve practice. This section describes two major theories of research utilization with Display 10-1 as an illustrative example, presents possible barriers, and describes strategies to facilitate the use of research findings in practice.

## Theories and Models of Research Utilization

The professional nurse can select from a variety of nursing research utilization models and theories to provide a conceptual basis for integrating research findings into practice. Since the 1970s, several nursing research models have appeared and have been useful for nurses who want to use nursing research findings in practice. Various research utilization models target different nurses. Research utilization theories that have been used with some success have been borrowed from the corporate world or developed by nurse researchers and collaborative nursing research projects. Some nursing research utilization models, such as the Iowa model, contain paths for nurses to follow when they cannot find adequate research upon which to base practice changes (Polit & Beck, 2003). The American Association of Critical Care Nurses has an ongoing collaborative research effort, the Thunder Project, to develop critical care nursing protocols based on research conducted at multiple clinical sites (Beyea & Nicoll, 1998). Because no single model fits each nurse's needs, nurses can find a variety of models for research utilization in nursing research texts, in professional journals, and on nursing specialty organization websites.

Tony, the nurse presented in the vignette, knows the key elements specified by many nursing research utilization models. To illustrate how to use them, the factors identified using the vignette appear in parentheses after each of the key areas to be addressed by nursing research utilization models. The following key elements appear in most of the nursing research utilization models:

1. Identifying a gap between desired outcome (skin integrity maintenance).
2. Articulating the clinical problem clearly and concisely (increased incidence of client impaired skin integrity).
3. Reviewing research literature (securing, reading, and critiquing research literature based on client risk factors for impaired skin integrity).
4. Preparing a comprehensive report outlining key research findings (preparing a table outlining the research findings from literature reviewed on risk factors

for impaired skin integrity, and drawing conclusions and forming clinical implications for a specific practice setting).

5. Selecting from one of the research-based innovations found in the literature review (selection of the Braden scale to monitor client risk for impaired skin integrity).

6. Developing specific practice outcomes for the proposed innovation (incidence of client impaired skin integrity will be reduced by 50% within 1 month of using the Braden scale to monitor clients at risk for impaired skin integrity).

7. Establishing an implementation plan for the innovation (staff education on the use and documentation of the Braden scale, securing staff acceptance of using the Braden scale, printing and distributing Braden scale assessment forms).

8. Creating an evaluation plan development to assess the effects or practice outcomes of the innovation (chart audits to verify staff use of Braden scale and identify episodes of skin development, summarize findings of audits, and note any changes from current incidence rate).

9. Implementing the innovation within a practice setting (using the Braden scale twice weekly to assess client risk for impaired skin integrity).

10. Evaluating the clinical effects of the innovation (seeing if Braden scale use reduced the incidence of client impaired skin integrity).

Once the effectiveness of the innovation has been demonstrated, agency policy and procedures may be revised to make using the innovation standard practice. To facilitate change and innovations to practice, many nurses desiring to make practice changes find using theories and models of research utilization helpful.

### Rogers' Theory of Diffusion of Innovations

According to Rogers (1983, p. 5), **"Diffusion** is the process by which an innovation is communicated through certain channels over time among the members of a social system."** Rogers (p. 11) defines an **innovation** as "an idea, practice, or object that is perceived as new." In Display 10-1 changing the method for screening clients for increased risk for skin integrity would be considered an innovation.

Rogers (1983) suggests **diffusion of innovations,** a five-stage process, is useful for deciding whether to adopt an innovation (something perceived as new by those who are considering adoption). The knowledge stage is the first awareness of the existence of the innovation (Tony's awareness of the Braden Scale as a research-validated instrument to assess impaired skin integrity risk that he shares with his colleagues). The persuasion stage occurs when the individual forms an attitude toward the innovation (Tony's willingness to ask his colleagues what they would think about trying the Braden Scale twice weekly for skin assessment). A decision occurs when the individual makes the choice for adoption or rejection of the innovation (Tony's staff decides to give the Braden scale a try to see if it makes a difference). In the implementation stage, the individual uses the innovation (staff use the Braden scale twice weekly for skin assessment and documentation), and in the confirmation stage, the individual seeks reinforcement of the decision (client incidence of skin breakdown decreases and staff like using the Braden scale). Reversal of the decision can occur at any time during the implementation and confirmation stages.

For an individual to consider adoption of an innovation, the person must be aware of the innovation. Rogers (1983) used the term diffusion to describe the dissemination of an innovation. The theory proposes that diffusion of an innovation is enhanced by face-to-face and mass media communication channels, time, and interaction within the social system. Adoption of an innovation is enhanced by persuasion by a peer colleague or by influence from opinion leaders within the social system. An outside change agent also may facilitate diffusion and adoption of an innovation.

The perceived characteristics of the innovation affect favorable or unfavorable attitudes toward the adoption. The probability and speed of adoption are enhanced if the staff perceives the innovation as being superior to current practice; the innovation is consistent with current values, experience, and priority of needs; the innovation is easy to learn, understand, or use, or can be tried out on a limited basis with the option of returning to previous practices; and the innovation causes visible results (Burns & Grove, 2001).

### The Stetler/Marram Decision-Making Model

Although Rogers' theory addresses the structure of diffusion of any innovation, including research findings, the revised Stetler/Marram model, now commonly called the **Stetler Research Utilization Model** (Stetler, 1994), refers to a six-phase, critical-thinking and decision-making process to assist the individual practitioner in using published research.

In Phase 1, preparation, the nurse determines the purpose for the research review (Tony identifies the problems of increased impaired skin integrity and decides to review research on risk factors for it). The purpose influences the development of measurable outcomes later in the process (desired outcome is to reduce the incidence of impaired skin integrity). In Phase 2, validation, the strengths and weaknesses of a research study are assessed to accept or reject findings based on their potential for applicability (Tony analyzes the research studies, and based on his findings he decides that the Braden scale may be a feasible way to screen clients on the rehabilitation unit for impaired skin integrity problems).

Phase 3, comparative evaluation, determines whether it is desirable or feasible to apply findings in practice. Criteria include similarity of the study sample and environment to the population and setting of the nurse; assessment of the effectiveness of current practice and whether or not theory would be an improvement; assessment of risk, need for resources, and readiness; and substantiating evidence. Multiple research articles with congruent findings or a meta-analysis are, of course, more desirable than one study. Table 10-1 presents considerations for examining the fit, flow, and feasibility of reported research that fits with Phases 2 and 3. (Tony looks at the research findings on the Braden scale use in long-term and rehabilitation settings and uses criteria found in the table to determine desirability and feasibility of using the Braden scale in his clinical practice setting.)

Phase 4, decision making, may result in the decision to use the new knowledge to change practice or modify a way of thinking without waiting for additional data. Another alternative is to consider use but continue to collect additional data. A third option might be to delay use until additional research has been conducted. A fourth alternative might be to reject or not use the information because of the risks or costs involved, lack of consistent, strong findings, or the strength of current practice (Stetler, 1994). (Tony decides that the research evidence provides a solid foundation to propose using the Braden scale on his unit.)

Phase 5, translation/application, involves generalization of the similarities or differences in the sources that were reviewed and identification of implications for practice (the "so what"). See Figure 10-1.

In Phase 6, evaluation, the expected outcomes are compared with the purpose that was defined in the preparation phase. Following this decision-making process, the nurse

TABLE 10-1

## Considerations for Preliminary Evaluation of Nursing Research for Use in a Particular Clinical Setting

| Fit to Clinical Setting | Flow of Research Study | Feasibility of Adoption |
|---|---|---|
| Purpose of study fits the clinical area where findings may be adopted | Research questions or hypothesis flows from the study's stated purpose | Innovation proposed legally permitted by State Nurse Practice Act |
| Study sample represents clientele of clinical setting | Researcher follows all steps outlined in the research process | Innovation is ethical practice |
| Sample size is appropriate | Variables are well defined | Acceptable costs to clients, third-party payers or institution |
| Enhances the fulfillment of the clinical area's mission | Measurements for the variables make sense | Enough staff and time to fully execute the proposed innovation |
|  | Validity and reliability of variable measurements presented | Innovation is congruent with nursing philosophy of the organization or unit |
|  | Efforts made to control factors that might affect the results | Any risks to clients, nurses or the organization? |
|  | Data presented accurately | Available resources needed are obtained |
|  | The correct statistics are used to answer the research question(s) or test the hypothesis(es): <br>• research purpose <br>• number and type of variables <br>• level of measurement for each variable | Staff ready to adopt the proposed innovation |
|  | Sample size is large enough to support the statistical test or researcher reports power level |  |
|  | Weaknesses of the study are reported |  |
|  | Logically and accurately generated study conclusions |  |
|  | Implications for practice logically flow from findings |  |

Source: Liehr, P., & Houston, S. (1993). Critiquing and using nursing research: Guidelines for the critical care nurse. *American Journal of Critical Care, 2,* 407–412; Burns, N., & Grove, S. (2001). *The practice of nursing research: Conduct, critique and utilization* (4th ed.). Philadelphia: Saunders.

**Important Note: Do not change practice on the basis of the findings of one study. Similar findings from multiple studies indicate that the findings were more likely not to be the result of chance.**

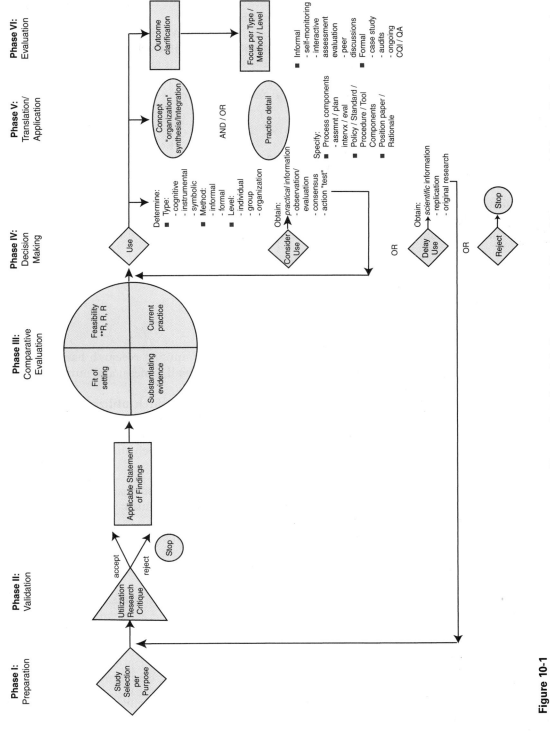

**Figure 10-1**

The Stetler/Marram research utilization model. (Stetler, C. B. [1994]. Refinement of the Stetler/Marram model for application of research findings to practice. *Nursing Outlook, 42,* 18-19. Used with permission.)

would implement a planned change model, such as Rogers Diffusion of Innovations or other planned change models presented in Chapter 19.

The process of research utilization is a continual one. Advances in the health science arena mean that nurses must stay abreast with changes in their clinical practice areas. New theoretical developments in nursing result in different approaches to client assessments, nursing interventions, and outcome evaluation. Nursing research utilization success relies on a variety of factors that facilitate use of research findings in practice.

## Facilitators to Research Utilization

Many factors influence the utilization of nursing research in clinical practice. **Research utilization facilitators** are any factors that promote the use of research-based knowledge into clinical practice. Individual nurse and employing organization factors can facilitate research utilization in clinical practice setting. Estrabrooks, Floyd, Scott-Findlay, O'Leary, and Gushta (2003) identified the following six categories of possible individual factors that promoted research utilization from a review of 22 studies:

1. Beliefs and attitudes toward nursing research.
2. Involvement in nursing research activities.
3. Information-seeking behavior.
4. Education level.
5. Professional characteristics.
6. Socioeconomic factors.

Table 10-2 summarizes facilitators of utilization of nursing research based on individual nurse factors. Cultivating these characteristics in all professional nurses remains a challenge for the profession.

Organizational factors also serve as facilitators to research utilization by nurses. Research utilization efforts require use of human and financial resources. Research utilization projects are time intensive. Nursing research utilization requires organizational commitment. The following strategies to facilitate research utilization have been used with some success in nursing departments:

1. Clear expectation of research utilization as part of a job description.
2. Staff educational programs on the process of research utilization.
3. Incentives, such as promotions or salary increases.
4. Formation of nursing research/research utilization committees.
5. Provision of time for nurses to read research reports while on duty.
6. Clinical career ladders requiring research utilization as criteria for promotion and maintenance of organizational position.
7. Organizational support to defray expenses for research utilization projects.
8. Formalized collaboration between nursing service and academia.
9. Library services for nurses to use to perform computerized literature searches and access needed materials.
10. Nursing unit based libraries and nursing journal subscriptions.
11. Sponsorship of nurses to attend professional nursing conferences.

Characteristics of published research studies also serve as facilitators of research utilization in nursing practice. Because many nurse researchers may not engage in clinical

TABLE 10-2

## Individual Nurse Facilitators for Utilization of Nursing Research

| Main Category | Facilitator |
| --- | --- |
| Beliefs and attitudes | Positive attitude toward nursing research<br>Self-expectation to use nursing research in practice<br>Interest in nursing research |
| Involvement with research activities | Perceived availability of research findings<br>Current collaboration or past participation on a research project<br>Collecting data for other researchers<br>Participation in a research study as a subject or participant<br>Previous use of nursing research<br>Experience with the research process |
| Information-seeking behaviors | Reading nursing journals as the top information source to stay current in practice<br>Regular reading of professional journals (*Nursing Research, American Journal of Nursing*)<br>Subscribing to professional journals<br>More time spent studying while off duty<br>Use of nursing school as a resource for nursing research materials and information |
| Education | Education preparation in the research utilization process<br>Attendance at professional nursing conferences<br>Attendance at more staff in-services<br>Bachelor of Science in nursing or higher degree<br>Perception of being well prepared in education process<br>Completion of a research and/or statistics course |
| Professional characteristics | Perceived organizational support for research utilization activities<br>Perception of an organizational policy for research use<br>Increased number of years experience in a nursing specialty areas or clinical unit<br>Nursing leadership or advanced practice nursing role<br>Membership in the American Nurses Association<br>Certification from the Oncology Nursing Society |
| Socioeconomic factors | Younger-aged nurses |

Adapted from Estabrooks, C., Floyd, J., Scott-Findlay, S., O'Leary, K., & Gushta, M. (2003). Individual determinants of research utilization: A systematic review. *Journal of Advanced Nursing, 43,* 506–520.

practice on a regular basis, performing clinically relevant studies may be challenging. However, nothing captures the interest of professional nurses better than a study that demonstrates substantial improvements in client outcomes or working environments. A well-written research study using clear, concise language enhances the ability of all nurses to read and understand published nursing research studies.

## Barriers to Research Utilization

**Research utilization barriers** are any factors that block or impede the use of research findings in clinical practice. "It has been found that although the majority of nurses are aware of research-based interventions, few use them even sometimes" (Miller, 1996, p. 175). Goode et al. (1991); Rutledge, Mooney, Grant, and Easton (2004), and Funk, Champagne, Wiese, and Tornquist (1991) identified a number of barriers to research utilization, including barriers from the researcher, the clinician, and the administration. Barriers to research utilization because of the nature of disseminated research studies include the following:

- Insufficient current research with solutions to address today's complex clinical problems.
- Failure of replicated research studies.
- Research reports that are difficult to read.
- Many unpublished or nondisseminated research reports (especially studies done to meet graduate and postgraduate program requirements).
- Lack of a central depository for nursing research studies.

Nursing practice should not be changed on the basis of a single study because of potential confounding factors that may have caused the study results. Unfortunately, few replication studies appear in the nursing literature. Either nurses are not performing replication studies or they are not being accepted for publication when they are submitted.

Barriers to research utilization based on characteristics of the clinician include the following:

- Lack of education in how to read, critique, conduct, and use research (most new nurses are being educated in associate degree programs that focus on technical skills).
- Negative attitudes among practicing nurses about using research findings in practice.
- Not enough time or commitment to implement research utilization projects.
- Failure of nurses to read nursing research articles or journals.
- Inability of nurses to understand statistical analyses contained within studies.
- Comfort with practice based on tradition, which is difficult to change, even if it is ineffective.
- Difficulty determining if studies are well designed and scientifically sound.
- Isolation from knowledgeable colleagues who could assist them in understanding research studies.

Nursing research utilization requires much time and commitment. In today's society, many nurses assume multiple roles that compete for their attention. Even though practice based on sound science is preferred, changing personal attitudes and the status quo remains difficult.

Barriers arising from nurse researcher characteristics include the following:

- Submission of studies for publication to journals not read widely by most nurses.
- Use of research jargon in publications that is not understood by clinicians.
- Failure to offer realistic implications for clinical practice because of either lack of patient care experience or current clinical experience.
- Presentation of findings in a format not conducive to clinical implementation.

Failure to understand statistics serves as another barrier for using research clinical practice. Researchers sometimes manipulate statistics to distort the truth (Best, 2001). Because the average nurse does not comprehend statistical tests presented in a research study, the nurse accepts the study's reported findings, even though the authors might make implausible claims. A common misconception related to statistics is that they "prove" something. A crucial approach to statistics avoids the extreme of naïve acceptance and cynical rejection. When reading statistics, the consumer of research must realize that researchers choose variable definitions, instruments for data collection, and samples for a variety of reasons (Best). Reported statistics represent a compromise among various choices that researchers make during a study. Critical analysis of a statistic found in a research report involves asking the following questions:

- Do they answer the question or issue outlined in the purpose of the study?
- What is the level of measurement of the research variables contained in the study?
- How many independent and dependent variables appear in the study?
- Is the sample size large enough to effectively use the statistical test?
- What instruments were used to collect data, and what is the level of measurement that these generate?
- How might the sampling techniques affect the study results?
- Are comparisons appropriate if comparisons are being made?
- How have the figures been generated, and have any techniques been used to alter the appearance of the data?
- What stakes does the researcher have if the statistical tests used are not significant?

Instead of being awestruck or overwhelmed by complex statistical tests found in research reports, nurses should read for logical, feasible, and appropriate findings. Many advanced practice nurses find great rewards in helping staff nurses understand research reports.

Barriers to research utilization from the health care agency administration include the following:

- Minimal value placed on research by many administrators and managers.
- No provision made for resources such as time, financial support, and education.
- Lack of nursing autonomy within a bureaucratic structure to implement data-based solutions to problems.
- Lack of incentives for nurses to participate in research utilization activities.
- Reliance on established policy and procedures, rather than openness to change.
- Lack of support for implementation of research findings by physicians and other staff.

Unfortunately, most clinicians are not familiar with research methods, language, and statistical methods because "almost half of the practitioners have never had a research course" (Cronenwett, 1995, p. 429). However, baccalaureate-educated clinicians should be able to raise questions during practice and recognize effective and ineffective interventions from experience. Strategies to address barriers and facilitate the utilization of research must build on basic professional education. The following section presents some strategies to facilitate research utilization in clinical practice settings.

## Strategies to Facilitate Research Utilization

"Prior research instruction, awareness of support for research, and positive attitudes toward research were predictive of nurses' participation in research activities" (Rizzuto, Bostrom, Suter, & Chenitz, 1994, p. 193). In the baccalaureate-degree program, students are exposed to the basics steps of the research process and how to effectively critique studies for use in clinical practice. Most baccalaureate graduates have a basic understanding of research terminology, and some (not all) can read and understand published research reports containing basic statistical analysis techniques (Hunt, 2001). Nursing students and professionals gain confidence and expertise in reading and understanding research with continuous practice. Upon graduation, beginning nurses focus on acquiring clinical competence, and they spend little or no time reading nursing research reports. Rutledge, Mooney, Grant, and Eaton (2004) found that when nurses received formal education in research utilization, oncology nurses could master the process well enough to design and implement nursing research utilization projects in clinical settings course.

## Research Brief 10-1

Rutledge, D., Mooney, K., Grant, M., & Easton, L. (2004). Implementation and refinement of a research utilization course for oncology nurses. *Oncology Nursing Forum, 31*, 121–126.

The investigators sought to determine the effectiveness of a short research utilization (RU) course presented at annual Oncology Nursing Society conferences from 1997 to 2001. The course covered information about systematic RU, research article critique techniques, RU models, strategies for computerized database literature searches, and preparation of a RU project. Participants presented proposals for RU projects during the course. The course was primarily held using director-led discussions. Twenty-two nurses attended the course, and course evaluations were collected at 6-month and 12-month intervals, and in summer 2002.

Findings from the interviews of 21 participants revealed that the nurses benefited more when they had precourse-mentored experiences in preparing a literature search and completing a set research critique tool for some of the articles. They identified the following facilitators for RU in clinical practice: institutional, peer, and interdisciplinary health team member support; nursing research departments within the work setting; role autonomy; and course knowledge and resources. Barriers to RU included lack of support in the clinical setting, staffing changes, increased client acuity or loads, competing time obligations, and difficulty of getting staff to learn and use new ideas from research in practice. Twelve participants reported that they had either completed or continued to work on their RU projects, six never completed them, two partially completed them, and seven began new projects. Of the nurses failing to complete their projects, two had taken medical leave, three had changed positions, and one nurse worked on a unit that had undergone restructuring.

Implications for practice identified by the investigators include the following: RU is hard to sell to nurses; most nurses fail to have a good grasp of the RU process, have no idea of RU models, find generating a literature review cumbersome, seem naïve about processes to facilitate practices changes, and become anxious when publicly presenting RU projects and proposals. However, attending a RU course seems to increase confidence and skill to promote RU in practice. Because of the small size of the study sample, more research is needed to determine the most effective ways to help nurses use research findings in clinical practice.

Researchers should make an effort to write for practicing nurses and to emphasize the meaning of the findings for practice in language that is understandable by most clinicians

(Hunt, 2001). Consultation with a master's degree–educated nurse serves as a useful method for understanding and interpreting complex statistical analyses. The clinical setting may employ a master's-prepared research facilitator who is available for consultation. Another source might be graduate students or faculty from a local school of nursing. Possibly, a group of nurses could work together with a consultant in locating and interpreting relevant literature.

To use research findings, practicing nurses must read professional journals, including research journals. A number of journals, including *Applied Nursing Research* and *Clinical Nursing Research*, now focus on use of research for practice. Many nursing specialty journals have adopted the practice of publishing research articles. Other means of finding research articles pertinent to one's areas of nursing practice is to use electronic databases such as Medline or Cumulative Index of Nursing and Allied Health Literature (CINAHL). Many hospitals have a basic medical (or health sciences) library that includes a core collection of nursing journals. Nurses also may visit a local college or university library. As state taxpayers, nurses may use public university and college libraries.

Nominal fees may be charged for book checkout privileges and for photocopying journal articles of interest. To save time, nurses should look for integrative reviews or meta-analyses that review a number of studies and provide information about the quality of the results.

Other ways of gaining access to research findings include a research bulletin board, newsletters, or research grand rounds, but these strategies need to be organized, maintained, and supported. Many institutions have a research committee that can take responsibility for coordinating the review of literature, exploring ideas, pilot-testing innovations, and developing and disseminating research-based protocols and policies.

Nurses also may find the inservice education or nursing staff development departments useful when seeking to establish nursing practice based on research. Master's-prepared clinical educators could evaluate and synthesize knowledge across studies and provide direction for clinicians. Practitioners need continuing inservice education to help with identifying and locating appropriate literature, evaluating the quality of research, understanding data analysis, and determining the relevance of research findings for practice modifications.

Even if resources are available to nurses, agency managers and administration must create an atmosphere where nurses are encouraged and supported to question and evaluate current practice protocols; to use research study findings as a basis for protocol revisions; and to be valued (and even rewarded) for using research in practice. Without a supportive environment, nurses who use research in practice may become discouraged and rely on agency traditions, or they may leave the work setting for an agency that supports research utilization. Managers and administrators who use research in their roles serve as role models for research utilization. They also should provide adequate funding for staff to have access to computerized databases, health sciences libraries, and research-based education programs (Hunt, 2001). When research is valued as a way of knowing, positive attitudes and tangible resources for research utilization become standard practice. Incentives and rewards for risk taking and creativity promote research utilization. Fostering peer collaboration and networking with other colleagues also provides impetus for research use in practice. Most of all, the atmosphere must be one of respect and encouragement for professional practice and delegation of authority so that nurses control nursing practice.

However, in the final analysis, the clinician has to value the use of research as the basis for practice enough to provide the effort and make the time for research utilization activities. When a significant number of nurses value scholarship enough to participate in creation, dissemination, and utilization, then and only then will nursing be viewed as a true profession.

## ⬥ EVIDENCE-BASED PRACTICE

Evidence-based practice recently has become a prevalent mode of care delivery among health care providers in all health care disciplines (Kirrane, 2000). Evidence-based practice may involve the entire health care team or be discipline specific, such as evidence-based medicine, evidence-based physical therapy, evidence-based nutrition, and **evidence-based nursing.** Nursing research provides nurses with the opportunity to supply evidence, and nursing research utilization facilitates the nursing research based on scientific findings. However, the evidence for evidence-based practice does not rely solely on research findings. Sources of evidence used for evidence-based practice include research findings, clinical experience, quality improvement data, logical reasoning, recognized authority, and client situation, experience, and values (Glanville, Schirm, & Wineman, 2000). Table 10-3 presents a comparison of research utilization with evidence-based practice.

### Questions for Reflection 10-3

1. What forms of evidence do I use to provide a basis for clinical decision making?
2. How are client care policies, protocols, and pathways developed where I engage in clinical practice?

**TABLE 10-3**

## Comparison of Nursing Research Utilization and Evidence-Based Practice

| | Nursing Research Utilization | Evidence-Based Practice |
|---|---|---|
| Purpose | Establish nursing practice based on scientific evidence | Establish best practice guidelines for various clinical problems |
| Participants | Professional nurses | Interdisciplinary health team |
| Sources of evidence | Quantitative or qualitative research study findings | Research study findings<br>Quality improvement data<br>Retrospective and concurrent chart audits<br>Risk management data Infection control data<br>Local, national and international standards<br>Pathophysiology of clinical problem<br>Cost-effective analysis data<br>Benchmarking data<br>Expert opinions<br>Logical reasoning |

## Comparison of Nursing Research Utilization and Evidence-Based Practice (Continued)

| | Nursing Research Utilization | Evidence-Based Practice |
|---|---|---|
| | | Clinical experience<br>Individual patient situations<br>Client preference data |
| Processes | Critiques of research reports of topic of interest<br>Integrative review of research reports<br>Innovation subjected to a planned changed process<br>Evaluation of results of care innovation | Group meetings of one component of the health care team for issues related to a specific discipline<br>Group meetings of interdisciplinary health team members to develop critical paths or other care pathways<br>Interdisciplinary review of current clinical needs, practices, established guidelines and care principles<br>Extensive systematic review of published research on issue to be addressed from all health care disciplines if the guideline will be interdisciplinary or from one health care discipline if guideline will be specific to a special group<br>Guideline review by experts, clinicians and clients<br>Guidelines are tested for effective clinical use<br>Guidelines are subjected to continuous review |
| Outcomes | Improve client outcomes<br>Improve professional practice<br>Research-based nursing care and clinical practice protocols | Improve client outcomes<br>Clinical guidelines for client care based on solid evidence that yield the most benefit for the least possible cost |
| Dissemination of information | Agency newsletter<br>Letters to staff<br>Staff electronic mail<br>Electronic or printed agency clinical policy manual<br>Staff inservices<br>Nursing publications<br>Nursing specialty organization websites | Agency newsletter<br>Staff electronic mail<br>Electronic or printed agency policy manuals<br>Professional publications<br>Web sites of professional organizations, large health care agencies, Agency for Healthcare Research & Quality, and the National Guideline Clearinghouse American Medical Association, American Association of Health Care Plans |

Sources: Burns, N., & Grove, S. K. (2001). The practice of nursing research: Conduct, critique & utilization, 4th Ed. Philadelphia: WB Saunders; Glanville, I., Schirm, V., & Wineman, N. M. (2000). Using evidence-based practice for managing clinical outcomes in advanced practice nursing. Journal of Nursing Care Quality, 15 (19), 1–11. Beyea, S. C., & Nicoll, L. H. (1998). Developing clinical practice guidelines as an approach to evidence-based practice. AORN Journal, 67, 1037–1038; Goode, C. J., & Piedalue, F. (1999). Evidence-based clinical practice. Journal of Nursing Administration, 29, 15–21; Jennings, B. M., & Loan, L. A. (2001). Misconceptions among nurses about evidence-based practice. Journal of Nursing Scholarship, 33, 121–127.

Proponents of evidence-based practice view it as a means to solve clinical practice problems by making the best possible decisions related to care based on client reports, clinician observations, and research data. Of the data used, valid and current research carries the most weight when developing guidelines (Goode & Piedalue, 1999; Soukup,

2000), with randomized clinical trials deemed to be the absolute best evidence (Slinger & Moher, 2001). Currently, many health care professionals use evidence-based clinical practice guidelines developed by the Agency for Health Care Policy and Research for treatment of urinary incontinence, low back problems, pain, depression, and prevention of and treatment for pressure ulcers (Beyea & Nicoll, 1998). When research data are not available on a specific clinical problem, professional experts who specialize in a specific area develop practice guidelines using consensus. Health care providers can access clinical practice guidelines from a variety of websites, such as the Agency for Healthcare Research and Quality, professional specialty organizations, and large health care organizations (Beyea, 2000a, 2000b; Glanville et al., 2000). Evidence-based practice enables health care providers to use objective and subjective ways of knowing when to make client care decisions.

Opponents of evidence-based practice in medicine and nursing suggest that the development of clinical practice guidelines, critical care pathways, and protocols entice practitioners of medicine and nursing to adopt a "cookbook recipe" approach to client care. The basic tenet to quality improvement initiatives specifies that elimination of variation in practice decreases the chance for error and improves quality (Glanville et al., 2000). Because quality improvement has it roots in industrial production, perhaps standardization may not be as desirable because clients have unique characteristics and needs that may be overlooked when practitioners adhere strictly to clinical practice guidelines. In addition, consumers and third-party payers may hold health care providers accountable for actions in addition to or for not strictly following established clinical practice guidelines (Glanville et al., 2000; Goode & Piedalue, 1999).

Health care organizations and individual health team members hold the key to the successful implementation of evidence-based practice. Organizations must display commitment to developing evidence-based care pathways and provide health care team members with the time and required resources. Time periods as long as 6 months may be required for development of a single evidence-based pathway (Kirrane, 2000).

## ✦ CREATING A PUBLIC IMAGE OF THE NURSE AS SCHOLAR

A **scholar** is someone who is an intellectual who has advanced study in a given field. Public perceptions of nurses tend toward the nurse as a person with technical expertise, a subordinate to physicians, and someone who cares for others. However, a visit to a college or university today reveals the strides that the nursing profession has made in developing a unique research base and expert researchers. In recent years, many nursing journals have become devoted to dissemination of research findings and nursing theory dissemination. Some journals devote space for research findings and methodological issues (*Nursing Research*, *Western Journal of Nursing Research*, *International Journal of Nursing Research*), and others have space for publication of research and nursing theory (*Journal of Nursing Scholarship*, *Journal of Advanced Nursing*, *Nursing Science Quarterly*). Some journals have print and online versions (*Evidence-Based Nursing*, *Nursing Research*). The journal published by the American Nurses Association, *The American Journal of Nursing*, recently has included original research studies as a regular feature. These journals reflect the advancing body of knowledge unique to nursing, an important element for an emerging profession.

Advanced technology offers great support for the nurse researcher today. The storage, retrieval, and analysis of data afforded by computer support make conducting research much faster and achievable by nurses. In most educational and practice settings, a researcher should not have to manually manage data. Another great help to research is the computer's ability to manipulate numbers, which allows almost unlimited analysis of data and the ability to use research findings to a fuller capacity.

In addition, it is anticipated that the word processing support and electronic transmission of information offered by computers will be helpful in sharing more research findings with clinicians in practice. Thus, nursing is moving into a period of valuing and conducting research at a time when technology greatly supports many aspects of the research process.

Traditionally, nurses have not been viewed as scholars. Nurses themselves sometimes fail to acknowledge advanced education of colleagues. Sometimes, health care-providing agencies refuse to place academic credentials on nurses' employment name badges. The public perception of nursing is highly affected by individual experience with nurses. With approximately 70% of nurses having less-than-baccalaureate preparation, nurses remain among the least educated members of the interdisciplinary health care team. Nurses and clients tend to value clinical practice over nursing scholarship. However, when (and if) nurses communicate to others the contributions of nursing research to health outcomes, the nursing profession will attain recognition as a scholarly, rather than an exclusively practice, discipline.

As nursing has developed its own theory base during the past 35 years, nurses have begun to value the scholarship role of the nurse. Most nurses today probably would agree that a practice based on research is desirable. Capitalizing on that consensus, the profession can begin to present a different image to the public. To help actualize the motivation to base nursing practice on research, educational programs need to prepare students in scientific inquiry while preparing them to apply theory in the conduct of professional roles.

Research in nursing also has been hampered by inadequate financial support. Between 1971 and 1981, the government awarded the National Center for Nursing Research $40 million. During the same period, the National Institutes of Health (NIH) received $1.7 billion for general biomedical research. Originally, the National Center for Nursing Research was established within the NIH. In 1993, the **National Institute for Nursing Research (NINR)** was established. The NINR identifies nursing research priorities, distributes grants to nurse researchers, and disseminates nursing research findings to health professionals and the public. Funding for the NINR has risen steadily since its inception. The NINR is funded through section 301, title IV of the National Public Service Act. In 2000, the NINR received more than $90 million in federal funding. The national budget for the fiscal year 2004 awarded over $134 million to the NINR. The NINR requests increases in federal funding annually and projected funding for the NINR is expected to increase steadily as nursing research provides crucial information that affects the health of Americans (NINR, 2004).

As nurses begin to feel and act like scholars, the public will begin to see a scholarly side of nursing. If the profession nourishes this scholarship in nurses, it undoubtedly will help change the image of the nurse. Because scholars accept that research is a vital component of nursing, the development of scholars will increase the supply of researchers to better serve the profession and the public.

## Questions for Reflection 10-4

1. How can I promote the image of nurses as scholars?
2. What are the potential consequences of changing the image of the nurse from caregiver to scholar?

## ⬥ SUMMARY AND SIGNIFICANCE TO PRACTICE

In the 1960s through the 1990s, many researchers and scholars provided a beginning theoretical base for nursing. Current trends toward providing the best possible health care to the most persons at the least possible expense provide nurses with an opportunity to demonstrate their contributions through nursing research. Through quantitative and qualitative research, nurses can capture a holistic picture of client responses to health, illness, and life transitions. The utilization of nursing research in clinical practice provides solid evidence for nursing actions in clinical practice. Recent public funding of nursing research initiatives show that the public values nursing research. In a postmodern society, researchers and scholars serve a vital role in establishing the basis for the emergence of nursing as an autonomous profession and to the provision of better nursing services to all global citizens.

### FROM THEORY TO PRACTICE

1. Reread the vignette at the beginning of the chapter. What strategies would you suggest to Joan to use in her attempts to integrate the research-based knowledge about alternative forms of pain control on her unit?
2. Outline a research utilization project for Joan to follow.
3. What forms of evidence are used as a foundation for currently used clinical policies and procedures in your area of clinical practice?
4. Who do you have available to help you if you encountered difficulty making sense of a published research study?

### WWW INTERNET EXERCISES

1. Visit The Royal Windsor Society for Nursing Research at www.geocities.com/researchnurses. Click on the icon, "Research Fun" and play Research Jeopardy. Learn about some interesting health care research findings.
2. Visit the National Institute for Nursing Research (NINR) at http://ninr-nih.gov/ninr/. Read about the mission and strategic plan of the NINR. Identify the research priorities of the Institute and bring them to class for discussion.
3. Peruse the online version of the journal, *Evidence-Based Nursing*, at http://www.evidencebasednursing.com. Read one or two selections from the journal. Answer the following questions:
   a. Do you believe the content contained in the summary of each research article and the commentary that follows it?

    **b.** What are the advantages of reading an entire research report?

    **c.** What are the disadvantages of reading an entire research report?

    **d.** Would you use information found in this journal in your clinical practice? Why or why not?

## INTERNET RESOURCES

National Institute for Nursing Research: http://ninr-nih.gov/ninr/.

The Canadian Health Services Research Foundation: www.chsrf.ca/.

The Royal Windsor Society for Nursing Research: www.geocities.com/researchnurses.

Nursing Effectiveness, Utilization and Outcomes Research Unit (NRU), a joint project of the University of Toronto & McMaster University School of Nursing in Ontario, Canada: nhsru.com/www.fhs.mcmaster.ca/nru.

American Nurses Foundation (ANF): www.nursingworld.org/anf.

Midwestern Nursing Research Society: www.mnrs.org.

Southern Nursing Research Society: http://www.snrs.org.

Agency for Healthcare Research and Quality: http://www.ahrq.gov.

National Institute for Clinical Evidence: http://nice.org.uk.

Centers for Disease Control and Prevention: http://www.cdc.gov.

Integrity in Science: http://www.cspinet/org.integrity. (Find the list of what corporations are currently funding or have funded research.)

## REFERENCES

Artinian, B. A. (1988). Qualitative modes of inquiry. *Western Journal of Nursing Research, 10,* 138–149.

Baessler, C. A., Blumberg, M., Cunningham, J. S., Curran, J. A., Fennessay, A. G., Jacobs, J. M., McGrath, P., Perrong, M. T., & Wolf, Z. R. (1994). Medical-surgical nurses' utilization of research methods and products. *MEDSURG Nursing, 3,* 113–117,120–121,141.

Barrett, E. A. M. (2002). What is nursing science? *Nursing Science Quarterly, 15,* 51–60.

Best, J. (2001). Telling the truth about damned lies and statistics. *The Chronicle of Higher Education, 47,* B7–B9.

Beyea, S. C. (2000a). Finding Internet resources to support evidence-based practice. *AORN Journal, 72,* 514–515.

Beyea, S. C. (2000b). More Internet resources for learning about evidence-based practice. *AORN Journal, 72,* 708, 711.

Beyea, S. C., & Nicoll, L. H. (1998). Developing clinical practice guidelines as an approach to evidence-based practice. *AORN Journal, 67,* 1037–1038.

Blumenstyk, G. (2001). A new web site details the corporate ties of some researchers. *The Chronicle of Higher Education, 47,* A25.

Burns, N., & Grove, S. K. (2001). *The practice of nursing research: Conduct, critique, and utilization* (4th ed.). Philadelphia: WB Saunders.

Cohen, M. Z., & Tripp-Reimer, T. (1988). Research in cultural diversity: Qualitative methods in cultural research. *Western Journal of Nursing Research, 10,* 226–228.

Cronenwett, L. R. (1995). Effective methods for disseminating research findings to nurses in practice. *Nursing Clinics of North America, 30,* 429–438.

Estabooks, C., Floyd, J., Scott-Findlay, S., O'Leary, K., & Gushta, M. (2003). Individual determinants of research utilization: A systematic review. *Journal of Advanced Nursing, 43,* 506–520.

Funk, S. G., Champagne, M. T., & Wiese, R. A., & Tornquist, E. M. (1991). Barriers to using research findings in practice: The clinician's perspective. *Applied Nursing Research, 4,* 90–95.

Gennaro, S. (1994). Research utilization: An overview. *JOGNN, 23,* 313–319.

Glanville, I., Schirm, V., & Wineman, N. M. (2000). Using evidence-based practice for managing clinical outcomes in advanced practice nursing. *Journal of Nursing Care Quality, 15,* 1–11.

Goode, C. J., Butcher, L. A., Cipperley, J. A., Ekstrom, J., Gosch, B. A., Hayes, J. E., Lovett, M. K., & Wellendorf, S. A. (1991). Video entitled, *Research utilization: A study guide.* Ida Grove, IA: Horn Video Productions.

Goode, C. J., & Piedalue, F. (1999). Evidence-based clinical practice. *Journal of Nursing Administration, 29,* 15–21.

Haase, J. E., & Myers, S. T. (1988). Reconciling paradigm assumptions of qualitative and quantitative research. *Western Journal of Nursing Research, 10,* 128–137.

Heitkemper, M., & Bond, E. (2003). State of nursing science: On the edge. *Biological Research for Nursing, 4,* 151–164, 170.

Hunt, J. (2001). Research into practice: The foundation for evidence-based care. *Cancer Nursing, 24,* 78–87.

Jennings, B. M., & Loan, L. A. (2001). Misconceptions among nurses about evidence-based practice. *Journal of Nursing Scholarship, 33,* 121–127.

Kirrane, C. (2000). Evidence-based practice in neurology: A team approach to development. *Nursing Standard, 14,* 43–45.

Knafl, K. A., Pettengill, M. M., Bevis, M. E., & Kirchhoff, K. T. (1988). Blending qualitative and quantitative approaches to instrument development and data collection. *Journal of Professional Nursing, 4,* 30–37.

Knafl, K. A., & Webster, D. C. (1988). Managing and analyzing qualitative data: A description of tasks, techniques, and materials. *Western Journal of Nursing Research, 10,* 195–218.

Liehr, P., & Houston, S. (1993). Critiquing and using nursing research: Guidelines for the critical care nurse. *American Journal of Critical Care, 2,* 407–412.

McDonald, L. (2001). Florence Nightingale and the early origins of evidence-based nursing. *Evidence-Based Nursing Online, 3,* 68–69. Available at http://ebn.bmjjournals.com/content/vol4/issue3/. Accessed June 15, 2004.

Miller, S. P. (1996). Dissemination and utilization of research: Outcome behaviours at the baccalaureate level. *Journal of Nursing Education, 35,* 175–177.

National Institute for Nursing Research (NINR). (2004). *Fiscal Year 2004 Budget, Congressional Justification.* Available at http://ninr.nih.gov/ninr/about/legislation/CJ2004.pdf. Accessed June 30, 2005.

Polit, D. F., & Beck, C. (2004). *Nursing research: Principles and methods* (7th ed.). Philadelphia: Lippincott Williams & Wilkins.

Rambur, B. (1999). Fostering evidence-based practice in nursing education. *Journal of Professional Nursing, 15,* 270–274.

Rizzuto, C., Bostrom, J., Suter, W. N., & Chenitz, W. C. (1994). Predictors of nurses' involvement in research activities. *Western Journal of Nursing Research, 16,* 193–204.

Rogers, E. (1983). *Diffusion of innovations* (3rd ed.). New York: The Free Press.

Rogers, M. E. (1967, February 3). Nursing science: Research and researcher. Presented at the Annual Conference on Research and Nursing, Teachers College, Columbia University, New York.

Rutledge, D., Mooney, K., Grant, M., & Easton, L. (2004). Implementation and refinement of a research utilization course for oncology nurses. *Oncology Nursing Forum, 31,* 121–126.

Slinger, R., & Moher, D. (2001). Evidence-based case review: How to assess new treatment. *Western Journal of Medicine, 174,* 182–186.

Soukup, S. M. (2000). The Center for Advanced Nursing Practice evidence-based practice model: Promoting the scholarship of practice. *Nursing Clinics of North America, 35,* 301–309.

Stetler, C. B. (1994). Refinement of the Stetler/Marram model for application of research findings to practice. *Nursing Outlook, 42,* 15–25.

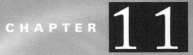

# CHAPTER 11

# Multicultural Issues in Professional Practice

## KEY TERMS AND CONCEPTS

Culture

Transcultural Nursing

Multicultural Nursing

Culture-Universal Care

Culture-Specific Care

Cultural Competence

Ethnocentrism

Cultural Relativism

Cultural Assessment

Culturally Congruent Care

International Nursing Practice

Folk Illnesses

Variations in Physical Appearance

Metabolism Variations

Multicultural Profession of Nursing

Culture Shock

## LEARNING OUTCOMES

By the end of this chapter, the learner will be able to:

1 Discuss diversity and assimilation issues for a shrinking world.

2 Compare and contrast theoretical frameworks addressing cultural competence in nursing practice.

3 Differentiate transculturalism and multiculturalism.

4 Specify strategies to address special cultural needs of nursing care consumers.

5 Outline strategies to create a multicultural nursing profession.

## VIGNETTE

Judy, a nurse administrator, cannot get American nurses to work in the small rural hospital where she works. The hospital has decided to send her and a group of nurses to the Philippine Islands to recruit Filipino nurses. Although she has reservations about hiring Filipino nurses and paying them for relocation and educational and licensure expenditures, Judy knows that she must have enough staff to provide effective client care. Judy wonders how her current nursing personnel will respond to having to work with foreign nurses. Judy has never been to the Philippine Islands and is very excited about the trip. She has a friend who works in a rural Filipino mission who would like to have Judy spend a few days working in the clinic. Judy wonders how she will be able to practice nursing in a foreign land, even if it is just for a few days.

Technology and transportation systems create opportunities for persons to experience the world. Technology, such as the Internet and fiberoptic cables, enables people to communicate instantly with each other despite vast differences in geographic locale. Within less than 24 hours, people can travel halfway around the world. This creates situations in which persons from different nations can meet each other. Sometimes persons from different nations meet and develop meaningful relationships that result in one person moving to another's country temporarily or permanently.

When visiting or residing in a foreign land, persons must abide by the laws of the country. For nurses, the shrinking world results in opportunities to care for persons in and from other lands. American nurses who plan to practice professional nursing in another country must learn the laws applicable to nursing practice along with the laws of the land. The United States Department of Health and Human Services (USDHHS) provides cultural education to persons from foreign countries living here and recently released recommendations for National Standards for Cultural Competence in Health Care (Abood & Gonzalez, 2001). Effective nursing care includes meeting special cultural care needs of clients.

## ⬥ DIVERSITY AND ASSIMILATION IN A SHRINKING WORLD

American culture values unity and equality. The United States consists of many immigrants who became assimilated into one culture. American national diversity has been represented on coins with the phrase *E Pluribus Unum* (out of many: one). In the United States, people tend to identify themselves in terms of economic status and geographical locale. However, sometimes as persons lose their ethnic identity, they yearn for it more. Some persons from immigrant backgrounds prefer to speak their native language at home.

Before 1930, immigrants frequently anglicized their surnames to hide their ethnic roots because Eastern Europeans were considered inferior to Western Europeans (Cose, 2000). With time, people from other areas of the world sought refuge in the United States. After World War II, many persons from Eastern Europe and the Soviet Union came to the United States to escape Communism. The American withdrawal from Vietnam resulted in increased immigration from Southeast Asian nations.

In recent years, persons from Mexico and South America have sought economic refuge in the United States. The populations of some towns in rural Kansas are 40% Latino (Campo-Flores, 2000). The population of the Silicon Valley is 49% white, 25% Hispanic, 23% Asian, and 3% African American (Breslau, 2000). Johnson (2004) reports that from 2000 to 2050, the nonwhite population of the United States will increase 30%. Within this increase, the Asian/Pacific Islander American population will increase 213.9%, the Hispanic population will increase 187.8%, the nonwhite Latino population will increase 217.1%, the African American population will increase 71.7%, and the white population will increase 7%. To provide effective nursing care to diverse cultural groups, nurses need to consider cultural and ethnic differences of the clients they serve. Because persons feel more comfortable with people like themselves, the profession of nursing needs to recruit persons of different cultures to join the profession.

### Basic Terminology to Understand Culture

Recently, confusion has arisen about the meaning of various terms to denote inclusion of culture in nursing care. In 1871, Sir Edward Taylor, a British anthropologist first used the term **"culture"** to refer to the complex whole, including knowledge, belief, art, morals, law, custom, and any other abilities and habits people acquired as societal members. In 1935, Margaret Mead expanded the definition of culture to include technological systems, political practices, and habits of daily life. Culture serves as a guide for determining the values, beliefs, and practices of individuals or groups of people.

**Transcultural nursing** uses the Latin prefix "trans," which means across, thereby referring to nursing across cultures. **Multicultural nursing** uses the Latin prefix "multi," which means many, denoting nursing of many different cultures. Finally, intercultural nursing uses the Latin prefix "inter," which means between, thereby meaning nursing between cultures (Andrews & Boyle, 1999).

Specific terminology must be understood to comprehend transcultural nursing principles. These terms come from the fields of sociology and anthropology and are summarized in Table 11-1. Most persons use culturally-based health practices before entering the formal health care system (Andrews & Boyle, 1999; Giger & Davidhizar, 1999; Leininger, 1995; Leininger & McFarland, 2002). Culture may include large numbers of

**TABLE 11-1**

### Basic Terminology to Understand Culture

| Cultural Term | Definition |
|---|---|
| Acculturation | Blending of two cultures by taking the best of each and combining them into one |
| Cultural accommodation | Allowing specific cultural practices within another culture |
| Cultural assimilation | Adoption of group culture by a member or members of a different culture |
| Cultural blindness | Ignoring cultural differences and acting as though they fail to exist |
| Cultural diffusion | Spreading out of cultural traits, patterns, and beliefs |
| Cultural competence | Integration of knowledge, attitudes, and skills that enable effective and appropriate communications and behaviors when working with persons from one or more cultures different from one's own |
| Cultural diversity | Differences in groups |
| Cultural empathy | Expressive concern and the ability to see the experiences as the client sees them |
| Cultural group | Two or more persons sharing the same ancestry, nationality, values, beliefs, or behavior |
| Cultural identity | Professed membership within a group |
| Cultural imposition | Forcing cultural beliefs, values, and patterns onto another from a different background |
| Cultural lifeways | Group beliefs about activities of daily living, inherited traits, and behaviors |
| Cultural maintenance | Continued practice of a specific culture |
| Cultural negotiation | Working with a person from another culture to determine what cultural practices can be used without jeopardizing effects |
| Cultural norms | Acceptable behaviors and practices |
| Cultural pluralism | Maintaining cultural differences after being assimilated into another culture |
| Cultural preservation | Continued practice of a specific culture |
| Cultural relativism | Acknowledging that other ways of doing things are different, but they are valid and may be superior |

*(continued)*

## Basic Terminology to Understand Culture (Continued)

| Cultural Term | Definition |
| --- | --- |
| Cultural repatterning (or restructuring) | Changing unhealthy cultural behavior patterns to promote better health |
| Culture shock | State in which one feels totally disconnected from the group because of extreme differences |
| Cultural values | Prevalent, powerful forces that provide meaning and direction to group actions, decisions, and lifeways |
| Culture | An integrated pattern of socially transmitted behaviors that includes all products of human work and thoughts specific to a group of persons that guide formulation of worldviews and decision-making processes |
| Emic perspective | An insider's view |
| Enculturation | Attempting to get one group to accept the ways of another group |
| Ethnicity | Sharing the same ancestral, physical, racial, and national origins along with the same language, lifestyle, religion, or other characteristics misunderstood by others |
| Ethnocentrism | Believing that one's way is best |
| Etic perspective | An outsider's view |
| Generalization | Oversimplified assumption about a group of persons |
| Rituals | Routine practices |
| Stereotype | Oversimplified idea, opinion, or belief about all members of a particular group of persons |
| Taboo | What is absolutely forbidden by a group |
| Transcultural nursing | Providing physical, psychological, and spiritual nursing care while considering specific cultural beliefs and practices when providing nursing services to clients from a different cultural background |
| International nursing | Providing nursing care services outside one's country of legal residence |
| World view | Personal perception of the universe that provides a foundation for values and beliefs about the world and life |

Adapted from Andrews & Boyle, (1999); American Association of Colleges of Nursing, (1998); Giger & Davidhizar, (1999); Leininger, (1995); Pedersen, Draguns, Lonner, & Trimble, (1996); and Purnell & Paulanka, (1998).

persons, as in the example of global or national culture, or it may incorporate small numbers of persons, such as a single-family unit or gang. Culture also can be differentiated by age, such as the youth culture and the old-age culture. Analysis of culture enables health care providers to understand the impact of lifeways (a way of life distinctly different in anthropology from lifestyle), rituals, and taboos when providing care.

As a nurse with advanced education in anthropology, Madeline Leininger founded the transcultural nursing movement. Leininger (1995, p. 4) defines transcultural nursing as "a formal area of study and practice in nursing focused upon comparative holistic cultural care, health, and illness patterns of individuals and groups with respect to differences and similarities in cultural values beliefs, and practices with the goal to provide culturally congruent, sensitive, and competent nursing care to people of diverse cultures." Leininger's writing justifies transcultural nursing by saying persons have rights and expectations to have their cultural values and beliefs respected and nurses have the obligation to meet the cultural needs of clients. Leininger suggests that efforts at being kind, relying on common sense, and ignoring prejudices fail to assure professional competence when nurses deliver care to clients with a cultural background different from that of the nurse. She proposes that nurses should receive formal education in transcultural nursing that begins with an analysis of one's own cultural values and beliefs.

Transcultural nursing blends nursing and anthropology in theory and practice. A provision of cultural-specific and cultural-universal care serves as the aim of transcultural nursing. "Care" refers to providing nursing services with consideration to particular values, beliefs, and behavior patterns unique to a specific group. These tend not to be shared with persons from other cultures. **Culture-universal care** denotes the commonly shared values, behaviors, and life patterns that appear among most cultures (Andrews & Boyle, 1999; Leininger & McFarland, 2002). Examples of culture-universal care include the formation of family, socialization of children into society, and basic physical survival needs.

**Culture-specific care** includes idiosyncratic practices of a particular cultural group. Cultural specific care practices may be similar across groups, but each group has slight differences in either the manner in which practices are implemented or the meaning behind them. Individuals from many cultural groups use folk (or generic) remedies and healers before seeking care from the medical health care system; sometimes they use folk care in conjunction with medical care. Table 11-2 lists some culturally-based healers and folk remedies and compares them to the culture of the American health care

**TABLE 11-2**

## Cultural Healers and Folk Remedies

| Cultural Group | Healer Title | Healer and Folk Remedies |
|---|---|---|
| Traditional Chinese | Physician<br>Acupuncturist<br>Herbalist | Physician diagnoses health problems by listening, questioning, and palpating, including feeling quality of pulse and sensitivity of body parts<br>Acupuncture<br>Herbal preparation (have used 5,767 documented herbs) |
| Eastern Indian | Ayurvedic medicine | Drugs used come from vegetable and mineral raw materials<br>Yoga<br>Meditation<br>Herbal preparations |
| Native American | Shaman<br>Singer or chanter (highest position in the Navajo tribe)<br>Crystal gazer, hand trembler, or diagnostician (one step below singer in the Navajo tribe)<br>Singer for healing ceremonies<br>Medicine man (Hopi tribe)<br>Herbalist | Sweating and purging usually done in a lodge<br>Herbal remedies from local environment<br>Healing ceremonies using the medicine wheel, sacred hoop, and singing (Lakota, Dineh, and Navajo tribes)<br>Stargazing and hand trembling for diagnosis (Navajo)<br>Herbalist prescribes herbs for symptomatic relief while members await healing ceremony (Navajo) |

*(continued)*

## Cultural Healers and Folk Remedies (Continued)

| Cultural Group | Healer Title | Healer and Folk Remedies |
| --- | --- | --- |
| Latin American | Curanderismo | Foods with qualitative (not literal) properties of "hot" and "cold"<br>Persons with "hot" diseases should receive "cold" foods and vice versa to restore a balance of hot and cold |
| Muckleshoots (Northwest Native Americans) | Nuclear and extended family | Mothers, grandmothers, and aunts are source of information related to pregnancy, birth, and childhood illnesses<br>Health care decisions are made by consensus of the family |
| American Jewish | Mohel | Performs the bris ceremony (infant male circumcision) |
| | Mother | Traditional folk remedies are passed down from many generations, such as cupping or charms to symbolize the "hands of God"<br>No consumption of meat and milk at the same meal |
| Mexican American | Family member<br>Curandera<br>Sobadora (massage and bone and joint manipulation specialist)<br>Espiritualista (spiritualist)<br>Yebero (herbalist) | *Curanderismo* is an eclectic, holistic, and syncretic compilation of beliefs from the Mesoamerican Spanish, spiritualistic, homeopathic, and modern medical beliefs<br>System is based on herbal preparations, Spanish prayers, altered states of consciousness, and healing rituals that blend Indian traditions and Catholic rituals<br>Herbal teas, ingestion or application of powdered substances, massage with warm oils, and skin popping on the small of the back |
| African American | Extended family members, friends and neighbors<br>Old Lady (experienced woman who successfully raised a family)<br>Folk practitioners<br>Faith healers (spiritualist)<br>Hougan (Voodoo priestess or priest) | Health clinic and physician visits occur when all folk remedies have been exhausted<br>Herbal remedies, potions, applications of heat and cold, crystals, massage, meditation, oils, powders, tokens, rites, and ceremonies<br>Oils, candles, soaps, and aerosolized sprays are used to repel evil forces |
| Philippine American | Family traditions<br>Folk healers | Based on hot/cold theory that requires persons to consume hot foods for a cold illness and cold foods for a hot illness<br>Widely use herbal remedies<br>Very quiet and passive when seeking health care |
| Japanese American | Kampo practitioners | *Kampo* is a holistic approach to illness and uses acupuncture, herbal medicines, moxibustion, and spiritual exercises |
| | Family members | For colds, use of ginger, sake, and egg; herbal teas for "cure-all"; headaches are treated by rubbing head with sesame or ginger oil; finger massage and exercise are used to stay well<br>Hot/cold (yin and yang) theory apply to health-related situations |

## Cultural Healers and Folk Remedies (Continued)

| Cultural Group | Healer Title | Healer and Folk Remedies |
| --- | --- | --- |
| Korean and Vietnamese American | Shamans | Serve as the mediator between people and the spiritual world to prevent, diagnose, and treat health problems<br>Principles of yin and yan (hot and cold)<br>Infections are hot and should be treated with a cold food such as fruit; cancers are cold and should be treated with hot food such as chicken soup<br>Strong herbal teas that may be dangerous if concurrently used with Western medicine<br>Dermabrasion, massage, acupressure, acupuncture, and moxibustion<br>Spiritual healing rituals (more commonly used by Vietnamese) |
| South African | Medicine men<br>Isangoma (diagnostician)<br>Inyanga (healer)<br>Midwives<br>Herbalists | *Ukincinda* (licking), *ukubhema* (inhalation of snuffing substances), *ukuhlanza* (emetics), *ukuchatha* (enemas), *ukugguma* (steaming), and *ukugcaba* (incisions made and medicine rubbed into them) are forms of traditional healing methods<br>Herbal preparations<br>Spiritual ceremonies and sacrifices to spirits<br>Goal of health is to achieve a balance with nature |
| Professional | Physician | Scientifically validated medication and therapies |
| American health care system | Nurse Practitioner<br>Nurses<br>Physical, occupational, and respiratory therapists<br>Social worker<br><br>Chaplain | Complex technological equipment for diagnosis and treatment<br>Some reliance on intuition<br>Effectiveness based on cost–benefit ratio<br>High degree of concern for timeliness of treatments and appointments<br>Spiritual needs of clients usually referred to chaplain |
| Puerto Rican American | Santiguadora<br>Spiritual healers | Herbal teas<br>Massage with warm oils<br>Spiritual rituals |
| Amish | Brauch or brauch-doktor<br>Lay midwife | Combination of many modalities, including manipulation of body parts, massage, herbs, herbal teas, reflexology, and other folk healing remedies<br>Midwife provides prenatal, birthing, and postpartum care |
| Greek American | Magissa<br>Bonesetters<br>Greek Orthodox priest | Magician, usually a woman, who cures "evil eye" and other disorders caused by spells<br>Bonesetters specialize in setting uncomplicated fractures<br>Ordained priest consulted for advice, direct healing, or exorcism |

system. The table only briefly summarizes cultural practices. Great differences may occur across various ethnic groups. Health care practitioners frequently impose their own cultural values, beliefs, and practices on clients receiving care. However, competent transcultural care blends the culturally-based practices with empirically-based medical practices. When these practices conflict with each other, the nurse (or other health care providers) works with the client from another culture to accommodate cultural practices with the medical plan of care so that the combination of remedies does not cause harm (Leininger & McFarland, 2002).

### Questions for Reflection 11-1

1. Have I used any folk healers or healing practices to enhance my health or recover from an illness or injury? How did I learn about these practices?
2. Have I ever encountered a folk healer in my professional practice? How did I react? How would I react if a family member or client insists that a folk healer practice folk medicine on a client to whom I am delivering nursing care?
3. What are the policies related to the use of folk healers in my clinical practice setting?

## ● ESTABLISHING CULTURAL COMPETENCE

Attainment of **cultural competence** is a lifelong journey that requires the elimination of **ethnocentrism** and an unconditional acceptance of **cultural relativism.** Establishment of cultural competence requires contact and interaction with persons from other cultures. Kavanagh and Kennedy (1992) propose that minority status is given to those who do not have power, status, and wealth within a given society (or situation), rather than being established by sheer numbers. Those with power, status, or wealth frequently may be viewed as being worthy of receiving health care services. In American culture, the ability to pay for the services rendered defines who is given access to health care services. In addition, the working poor may be seen as being more worthy of health care because they contribute valuable services and pay taxes to society. Health care professionals often expect minorities to adapt to the established norms and policies of the institution, rather than the institution adapting to the needs of the minority. To become minority friendly, health care institutions must have their professionals learn about the social organization and processes of each minority group served (Kavanagh & Kennedy, 1992). However, some persons who do not have societal power may find the term "minority" offensive.

### Steps to Acquiring Cultural Competence

Being culturally competent does not happen overnight, but rather takes time and commitment. Burchum (2002) defines cultural competence as a developmental process that builds continuous increases in knowledge and skill development in the areas of cultural awareness, knowledge, understanding, sensitivity, interaction, and skills. The following steps outline a process for nurses to follow to acquire cultural competence.

## Step 1: Examination of Personal Values, Beliefs, Biases, and Prejudices

The journey to cultural competence begins with an examination of personal values, beliefs, biases, and prejudices. Attitudes are most difficult to change because they have developed over time. Some attitudes become embedded in persons when they are children and others result from experience. Each person carries a set of values, beliefs, and biases. Those obtained in childhood may be transformed by experiences later in life (Andrews & Boyle, 1999; Purnell & Paulanka, 1998).

## Step 2: Specific Communication Strategies

Learning culturally-specific communication strategies serves as the second step toward attainment of cultural competence. Specific communication strategies affirm diversity. Verbal and nonverbal communication patterns indicate how well differences are respected. Learning about different cultures with the intent to understand them serves as the second step toward attaining cultural competence (Kavanagh & Kennedy, 1992; Leininger, 1995).

## Step 3: Interactions With Different Cultures

Engaging in interactions with persons from different cultures becomes the third step toward cultural competence. This requires risk taking. Respectful engagement during interactions with members of another culture or group provides opportunity for personal and professional expertise. Asking questions before acting serves as a useful tool. Sometimes, persons avoid others who differ from themselves. This practice creates minimization or denial that differences exist across various groups, such as race, class, nationality, or gender (to name a few broad differences in groups). Avoidance enforces the invisibility of sensitive issues (Kavanagh & Kennedy, 1992). However, most persons from different cultures send cues to each other during interactions. If heeded, the cues can guide the transcultural interaction, and errors can be avoided (Grossman, 1996; Yoder, 1996, 1997). Purnell and Paulanka (1998) strongly urge the use of an interpreter, rather than a translator, when clients and health care providers speak different languages.

### Questions for Reflection 11-2

1. How have I handled nursing care issues when taking care of clients who did not speak English?
2. What resources, policies, and procedures are available to me in my clinical setting to provide culturally competent care?

## Step 4: Mistake Identification and Acknowledgment

Mistake identification and acknowledgment serve as the fourth step toward cultural competence. Most persons from different cultural backgrounds accept sincere apologies when errors occur. Valuable lessons can be learned from communication and behavioral mistakes. Because literature on culturally diverse practices places persons into various groups, resulting in large clumps of cultural categories, errors of similarities may occur. These errors may have devastating effects (Leininger, 1995; Leininger & McFarland, 2002). For example, demographics related to Pacific Islanders represent 40 different cultural groups that speak 23 languages (Farella, 2001). Within this cultural group, health practices and taboos differ greatly.

Along with errors of similarity, errors of assumption frequently occur. Persons assume things about others based on outward appearances. Racial profiling results when persons assume that others who look alike share specific traits and behaviors. The population of the United States is a melting pot, and citizens often refer to themselves as African American, Japanese American, Italian American, Native American, Mexican American, or some other designation. Second- or third-generation immigrants may or may not abide by cultural practices of their ancestral homelands (Leininger, 1995). Likewise, as persons learn about health practices from other cultural groups, culturally-based folk practice may become intertwined with traditional Western medicine, resulting in an inability to know what individuals do to achieve and maintain health. For example, an American of German descent may or may not abide by the hot and cold food theory for illness treatment, although this is common practice in Germany. The best way to avoid the error of similarity is to perform a detailed, individually focused client health assessment.

Along with errors of assumption, nurses and other health care providers must understand that they hold membership in the American (or other national) health care provider culture. In the United States, health care delivery organizations value efficiency, quality, and empirical evidence. This culture often expects consumers to hold the same (or similar values) (Andrews & Boyle, 1999; Giger & Davidhizar, 1999; Leininger, 1995; Leininger & McFarland, 2002). Some clinics that serve diverse client populations hold clients to standards determined by the values of health care providers. For example, a teaching medicine clinic in an urban neighborhood sends clients a certified letter informing them of severing them from clinic services after they have missed three scheduled appointments without informing the clinic staff.

## Questions for Reflection 11-3

1. What policies in my clinical setting use American values or cultural values of the health care system as their foundations?
2. How have these policies obstructed culturally sensitive care?

## Step 5: Remediation for Cultural Mistakes

Remediation for cultural mistakes serves as the fifth step toward cultural competence. Correcting mistakes requires communication between both persons (and groups). Genuine dialogues result in the development of ideas for cultural accommodation and preservation. Because nursing focuses on client comfort, cultural-specific nursing interventions enhance client comfort by fostering maintenance of client cultural identity. In addition to enhancing client comfort, culturally competent nurses serve as a means for recruitment of health care consumers for a particular health care institution.

Once transcultural communication has been established, nurses and other health care providers can expand their knowledge related to cultural specific care practices. Andrews and Boyle (1999) identify examples of skills that are useful in transcultural nursing practice. These are assessment, communication, hygiene, activities of daily living, and religion. In relationship to assessments, nurses must consider biologic variations in signs of illness and health and ways to avoid cultural taboos when measuring the heads of infants, use separate charts for growth and development for children of Asian descent, modify childhood developmental screening tools, and use appropriate ways to conduct gynecologic examinations of women from various cultures.

Transcultural communication skills include speaking in the client's native language, providing health care information in the client's native language, and providing a language interpreter for clients. For hygiene, the nurse must become cognizant of specific hair and skin care needs for clients of various ethnic backgrounds. Nurses must be aware and capable of coaching clients who require special needs for activities of daily living (such as eating with chopsticks or using special assistive devices such as the West African "chewing stick" for oral hygiene).

Nutritional preferences also play a key role in health care. Providing hot and cold foods to clients whose cultures abide by this practice instills trust between nurses and clients. Finally, permitting clients to engage in their religious practices enhances spiritual well-being. Some religious ceremonies include the anointing of the sick (among Roman Catholics), circumcision and special rituals for the dead (among those of the Jewish faith), and cleansing before daily prayer (among practicing Moslems).

Several theories related to transcultural nursing have been published. Cultural phenomena that address the culturally unique individual vary slightly across these theories. Table 11-3 summarizes the key cultural phenomena addressed by major transcultural nursing theories. Because Leininger began cultural studies in the 1960s, the nursing profession sometimes refers to her as the founder of transcultural nursing. As members

**TABLE 11-3**

## Comparison of Transcultural Nursing Theories

### Leininger's Sunrise Model and Theory of Culture Care Diversity and Universality (1991)

Describes, explains, and predicts nursing similarities and differences focused on human care and caring in cultures

**Two Key Elements**

1. World view is the umbrella that encompasses the values and beliefs of the culture and person
2. Cultural and social structure is the dimension that includes the environmental context, language, and ethnohistory that influence care, expressions, patterns, and practices

Factors that influence care and holistic well-being (health) include technology, religion, philosophy, kinship, society, values and ways of life, politics, legal systems, economics, and education

The nurse serves as mediator to professional and generic (or folk) health care systems. The nurse preserves or maintains the client's culture by accommodating practices deemed safe and negotiating with the client not to abide by folk practices that interfere with or could be harmful with the professional health care system treatment(s)

At times, the nurse assists the client (or community) to establish different patterns and structures to more fully enhance health

First nurse to publish concepts related to cultural differences between nurses and patients when caring for emotionally disturbed children

Earned a doctorate in anthropology in 1965

Highly flexible theory and easily used with individuals, families, groups, communities, and institutions across diverse health care systems

*(continued)*

## Comparison of Transcultural Nursing Theories (Continued)

### Leininger (Continued)

Examines the culture of individuals, groups, families, institutions, regional communities, societies, nations, and global humankind

Outlines three phases for obtaining and using transcultural nursing knowledge:
1. Cultural awareness
2. Use of theory to guide cultural research and explain cultural behaviors
3. Use of cultural knowledge in nursing practice to provide culturally congruent care

### Purnell's Model for Cultural Competence (1998)

Cultural competence requires that the health care provider master the following tasks:
1. Development of a deep self-awareness of personal existence, feelings, ideas, and emotions and hold these from influencing actions and attitudes when working with persons from a different culture
2. Learning and understanding the culture of the health care client
3. Accepting and respecting cultural differences (p. 2)
4. Adapting usual care practices to become congruent with the culture of the client

Cultural competence is seen as a nonlinear conscious process

The individual is seen as the core of an ever-expanding network that includes the family, community, and global society

### Twelve Key Elements

1. Cultural overview and heritage includes the country of origin (climate and topography), heritage, residence, reasons for migration, economic factors, educational level, and occupation.
2. Communication encompasses the dominant group language, cultural communication patterns (eye contact, space, touch, facial expressions, separate ways to greet outsiders), temporal relationships (time orientation, social and clock time differences, importance of punctuality), and format for names (formal and informal use, sequencing of family, and individual names).
3. Family roles and organization include gender roles, accepted head of household, behaviors that are accepted or restricted, taboos, familial roles, familial priorities, alternative lifestyles, and nontraditional families.
4. Work force issues address immigration, temporary immigration for education, workplace, multicultural considerations, acculturation into the work group, native health care practices, issues related to professional autonomy, cultural gender roles, religious issues, perception of authority figures, and language barriers.
5. Biocultural ecology includes skin color, biological variations, culturally prevalent diseases, ethnic health conditions, and variances in medication metabolism.
6. High-risk behaviors include use of tobacco, alcohol, illegal drugs; sedentary lifestyle; and failure to use protective devices.
7. Nutrition considers the meaning of food, commonly consumed food, rituals, health-promoting dietary practices, nutritional deficiencies, and alterations in food metabolism.
8. Pregnancy and childbearing practices include cultural views and practices related to fertility control and pregnancy and any prescriptive practices, restrictions, or taboos related to pregnancy and childbearing.
9. Death rituals encompass cultural expectations of death, purposes behind death and mourning rituals, burial practices (including cremation), cultural expectations of grief, and cultural meanings about death and afterlife.
10. Spirituality considers the influence of the dominant religion on persons and families, the meaning of prayer, other religious rites and rituals, faith-based symbols (such as icons, statues, medallions), meaning of life, personal sources of strength, and the linkage of spiritual beliefs with health practices.

# Comparison of Transcultural Nursing Theories (Continued)

## Purnell (Continued)

11. Health care practices encompass predominant cultural beliefs that influence practices, especially those of health promotion and disease prevention, a curative or fatalistic focus for acute care, responsibility for health care, role of health insurance, over-the-counter medication use, folk practices, health care barriers, cultural responses to health, illness, and rehabilitation; cultural perceptions of the "sick role," and acceptance of blood transfusion and organ donations.
12. Health care practitioners includes an exploration of the roles of traditional, folk, and religious health care providers; acceptance of Western medicine health care providers, significance of health provider age, perception of various members of the health care team, status of various health team members, and perceptions of health team members of each other.

Theory acknowledges that health care providers' cultural competence falls into the following four categories: unconsciously incompetent, consciously incompetent, consciously competent, and unconsciously competent.

Emphasizes the use of interpreters over translators when health care clients do not speak the same language as the health care provider.

The 12 key elements of culture provide a comprehensive assessment of cultural care considerations.

Acknowledges workplace issues and the potential value conflicts between clients and providers and conflicts among health team members.

## Spector's Model of Heritage Consistency (1996, 2000)

Heritage consistency refers to the degree that a person's lifestyle reflects his/her traditional culture.

### Four Key Elements

1. Culture is a complex phenomenon that includes a connected web of symbols, a means for making and limiting human decisions, an extension of biologic capabilities, a medium for social relationship, and personhood. Only part of culture is conscious and exists in a person's mind as well as in the environment.
2. Ethnicity is the condition of belonging to a particular group that shares common characteristics, such as geographic origin, race, migratory status, religion, kinship, geographic locale, traditions, symbols, institutions, literature and other fine arts, values, food preferences, race, language, and dialect. Ethnicity provides an internal sense of distinctness as well as an external perception of distinctiveness. In the United States, a person may belong to different ethnic groups simultaneously.
3. Religion is the belief in a higher power to be obeyed and to worship that also provides a foundation for beliefs, practices, and ethics.
4. Socialization is the process by which persons are raised within a group and acquire group characteristics. Socialization results from the interactive effects of culture, ethnicity, and religion.

Socialization is the focal point of the model.

Factors indicating heritage consistency:
1. Childhood development within the country of origin or neighborhood of persons sharing same country of origin.
2. Extended family participation in cultural or religious activities.
3. Return visits to country or neighborhood of birth.
4. Regular contacts with extended family.
5. Extended family homes within the same community.
6. Individual participation in cultural and religious events.
7. Engagement in social activities with others from the same ethnic background.

*(continued)*

## Comparison of Transcultural Nursing Theories (Continued)

### Spector (Continued)

8. Personal knowledge of culture and language of origin.
9. Deep personal pride about heritage.
10. Surname not Americanized.
11. Extended family engaged in childrearing.

### Spector's Model of Heritage Consistency (1996, 2000) (Continued)

Heritage consistency occurs as a continuum.

Uses Giger and Davidhizar's six cultural phenomena that affect health: environmental control, biologic variations, social organization, communication, space perception, and time orientation

Views health providers as a special cultural group with values that frequently conflict with those of health care consumers

### Giger and Davidhizar's Transcultural Assessment Model (1995, 1999)

Provides a systematic approach for assessing culturally diverse clients

#### Six Key Cultural Elements

1. Communication is language spoken, voice quality, pronunciation, use of silence, and nonverbal behavior.
2. Space is action with personal space invasion, conversation distance, body movement, role of objects, and perception of space.
3. Social organization is the culture, ethnicity, race, role and function of family, work, leisure, religious practices, and friends.
4. Time includes how time is spent, measurement, definition, social, work, and orientation (future, past, or present).
5. Environmental control is cultural health practices (efficacious, neutral, harmful or uncertain effects), values and cultural definitions of health and illness.
6. Biologic variations include body structure, skin color, hair color, genetic makeup, enzymatic deficiencies, increased susceptibility to disease and chronic illness, nutritional preferences (and if these result in deficiencies) and psychological characteristics, including coping strategies and social support.

of the culture of health care providers, value conflicts frequently occur between nurses and health care consumers (Giger & Davidhizar, 1999; Leininger, 1995; Spector, 2000). Books written by these theorists provide more detailed descriptions of cultural traditions and taboos related to health protection, maintenance, and restoration.

## Hallmarks of Culturally Congruent Care

At times, nurses may be oblivious of cultural issues surrounding a client care situation. Failure to acknowledge and incorporate culture into client care increases the likelihood of distrust of the health care consumer and antagonism on the part of the health care provider. Trust and comfort, on the part of the client, increases when nurses consider cultural preferences during client care. Transcultural care considerations should not supersede the need for safe, effective client care (Andrews & Boyle, 1999).

Identification of cultural nursing considerations begins with the nursing assessment. **Cultural assessment** provides the nurse with the opportunity to learn about client lifeways. An individualized cultural assessment prevents the nurse from making cultural errors based on client appearance. Elements of the cultural assessment include family and kinship systems, social life, political systems, language, traditions, perception of the world, value orientation, cultural norms, religion and health beliefs, and practices. Table 11-4 presents information on each of these elements and suggests ways for nurses to collect data that may be relevant for nursing care. While performing a cultural nursing assessment, nurses must observe clients for cues that indicate discomfort with any questions asked. Sometimes, the nurse must rely on family members to supply information, especially in cultures in which a particular family member serves as the patriarch.

Along with verbal communication, the nurse can scan the environment for clues related to culture. In the home and inpatient settings, many persons have symbolic

**TABLE 11-4**

## Elements of Cultural Assessment

| Cultural Element | Description | Suggestion to Collect Data |
|---|---|---|
| Family and kinship system | Family structure, roles, and relationships | Describe your family to me. Who lives in your home? Describe the roles of each family member. Who provides support to you in the home? Observe the client as he/she interacts with family members. |
| Social life | Daily routine, group memberships, and recreation | Describe your typical day/week for me. To what groups do you belong? How do you spend your free time? |
| Political systems | Government, organizational, and economic affiliations | What support systems do you use outside of the home? Describe your work environment. What are your feelings about the government? Please share with me any economic concerns you may have related to this illness/injury or seeking health care. Please tell me what type of support you need at home. |
| Language | Language spoken inside and outside the home | What is your native language? Do you speak more than one language? |
| Traditions | Nonverbal communications, personal space, and other rituals that may have passed down from previous generations | Is there anything that I should share with other health team members with regard to your personal space or other aspects of communication? Do you have any rituals or habits that we need to consider in providing health care to you? |
| Perceptions of the world | Viewpoints on the meaning of existence and how the world operates | How do you view the world and your place in it? |
| Values orientation | What the person sees as being the most important things in life | What things in life matter the most to you? How can we see that these things are preserved for you? |
| Cultural norms | Cultural attitudes about food, time, work, and leisure | What are your attitudes about food, time, work, and leisure? (It may be useful to separate this into four separate questions.) |

*(continued)*

## Elements of Cultural Assessment (Continued)

| Cultural Element | Description | Suggestion to Collect Data |
|---|---|---|
| Religion | Spiritual beliefs including special beliefs and rituals surrounding life, health, illness, and death | Please tell me if there are any special spiritual needs that you have related to your life, health, illness, if you would have a terminal illness. Do you have a living will or advanced directive? |
| Health beliefs | Group attitudes about health and illness | What are your beliefs about health and illness? |
| Health practices | Behaviors and rituals surrounding health and illness including the use of folk healers and remedies | Tell me about the things that you do at home to maintain your health. What type of measures did you take to cope with this health problem before you sought health care? |

Adapted from Andrews & Boyle (1999).

objects to signify specific beliefs. Clients place these symbols in a prominent area so that they can be easily spotted. Sometimes, items such as charms or religious medals are worn and should not be removed without first asking the client. Displayed objects, such as statues, prayer beads, shrines, or special candles, may provide clues to nurses that special cultural health needs may surface. Polite inquiries related to unfamiliar objects may begin a dialogue about culture (Grossman, 1996).

Once the assessment is complete, the nurse proceeds with planning **culturally congruent care.** This may require referring to resources related to specific cultures and detailed information about the medical plan of care. Sometimes traditional folk remedies may interfere with ordered medications. When this occurs, the nurse must find ways to work with clients so that they understand the hazards of using folk remedies along with prescription medications. Some special rituals, such as providing clients with water for cleansing themselves before daily prayer, present no harm. However, the use of marijuana tea as a treatment for asthma poses great harm (Pachter, 1994). By engaging in respectful conversations, nurses and clients work together to make decisions related to accommodating lifeway practices with health care treatments.

When possible, interpreters should be used for health teaching unless the provider is fluent in the client's language. Conversational foreign language provides the nurse with an ability to meet the client's basic needs. Most persons who speak English as a second language find comfort with providers who speak to them in their primary language. However, mistakes can be made by the provider, and for critical information, interpreters are essential.

### Research Brief 11-1

Gil, K. M., Mishel, M. H., Belyea, M., Germino, B., Porter, L. S., La Ney, I. C., & Stewart, J. (2004). Triggers of uncertainty about recurrence and long-term treatment side effects in older African American and Caucasian breast cancer survivors. *Oncology Nursing Forum 31*, 633–639.

The investigators sought to discover triggers of uncertainty about breast cancer recurrence and long-term adverse effects of treatment in long-term survivors and see if there were any differences in the triggers between African American and white women. One hundred seventy-one white and 73 African American women from North Carolina participated in the study and were part of a larger National Cancer Institute study that was testing the effectiveness of uncertainty management using various cognitive behavioral skills. The women received four telephone calls during which they practiced one of the following four skills: relaxation, pleasant imagery, calming self-talk, or distraction. Techniques for these interventions along with an educational manual were given to the women using audiotapes or written materials. During the third and fourth telephone calls, the women were instructed on how to use the self-help printed manual. Then, the participants were called by an investigator to document information on triggers and symptoms associated with recurrence or adverse effects of breast cancer therapy. During these calls, the investigators were asked about a list of 10 potential triggers and six symptoms associated with previous breast cancer treatment that had been identified by three focus groups of women who had survived 5 to 20 years after initial diagnosis of breast cancer.

Results of demographic variables between the sample revealed that white women had higher educational levels, were more likely to be married, and had higher incomes than the African American women. The African American women were more likely to live alone, and had increased incidence of diabetes, hypertension, and glaucoma. Fifty-three percent of the white women had their breast cancer diagnosed at stage 1 compared to 41% of the African American women. Also, 42% of the African American women had diagnoses at stage II compared to 32% of the white women. Both women experienced the same number of symptoms per month (1.4), which were fatigue, joint stiffness, pain, and lymphedema. The researchers identified a weak, but statistically significant, correlation between other health problems and symptoms ($r = .34$, $P < .01$). There were no differences reported about the number of triggers for each group. Difference in the triggers reported are the following:

a.  Older women in the study reported fewer triggers related to uncertainty about recurrence.
b.  Women with higher education levels reported more triggers.
c.  New symptoms served as triggers for uncertainty more frequently in African American participants.
d.  Hearing about someone else having cancer or that their disease had worsened was the most reported trigger of uncertainty for white women.
e.  Other triggers for white women that differed from their African American women counterparts included environmental triggers (smells, sights, or sounds associated with the previous breast cancer experience), media coverage of controversy about breast cancer, and information about breast cancer from the Internet, magazines, radio, or television.

Clinical implications for this study reveal that many breast cancer survivors experience fatigue, pain, and joint stiffness and health care professionals need to address these symptoms when they are reported. In addition, health care providers should be made aware that environmental triggers can result in feelings of uncertainty about disease recurrence and should talk with survivors when they undergo diagnostic tests (especially mammography) about possible coping methods. Results of this study must be interpreted with caution because the data were retrospectively collected, there was no comparison group of women without a history of breast cancer to validate that symptoms occur only in breast cancer survivors or to determine if the triggers of uncertainty about recurrence could be applicable to fear of developing breast cancer, and perhaps, being asked about symptoms and triggers could have increased the incidence of reporting them. Results of this study reveal that fear of recurrence of cancer is always with cancer survivors. Additional research needs to be done with survivors of other forms of cancer and with more culturally diverse samples to see if different symptoms and triggers result in uncertainty about recurrence.

## International Nursing Opportunities

Disparities in access to health care occur across the globe. Many persons rely on the ability to pay to receive health care services (Alaniz, 2001; United States Department of Health and Human Services [USDHHS], 2000). Some developing countries have infant mortality rates exceeding 70% and life expectancies of less than 50 years, whereas other countries enjoy single-digit infant mortality rates and life expectancies that exceed 75 years. Most countries have a disparity in health care access for persons living in poverty. The World Health Organization and many state governments have documented evidence of positive contributions made by nurses in the areas of health maintenance, disease prevention, health promotion, and control of specific health-related problems. With formal recognition of the contributions that professional nurses can make toward improving the health of all citizens, nurses gain increased social status for nurses and reap increased governmental and nonprofit funding for nursing-based health care programs and nursing education.

Governmental, private, and religious organizations offer opportunities for **international nursing practice.** The United Nations has nursing opportunities for nurses in various areas, such as refugee support, immunization programs, AIDS prevention and treatment, and health promotion in developing countries. The Peace Corps provides nurses with the opportunity to improve health in developing countries under the sponsorship of the United States government. The United States Public Health Service offers assignments abroad. Private organizations, such as Doctors without Borders, seek the services of professional nurses for long- and short-term programs. The International Red Cross offers worldwide disaster relief, for which nursing services are needed. Various organized religions offer opportunities for missionary nursing.

The United States shares the current nursing shortage with other countries. Schiff (2001) reports that one in 27 nursing positions is vacant in the United Kingdom. Saudi Arabia frequently recruits professional nurses in nursing journals across the globe. When nurses accept employment for a foreign assignment, they become bound by the country's laws, cultural values, and norms. Lack of knowledge serves as no excuse for breaking laws, and in some cases, nurses have been subjected to corporal punishment for failure to abide by laws related to dress and being in public without escorts.

# ● STRATEGIES FOR MULTICULTURAL NURSING PRACTICE

When taking care of clients from multiple cultural backgrounds, the nurse must treat persons as individuals with unique personal needs. Some persons become assimilated to the culture of the nation in which they reside. Not only are there international differences, but there also may be geographical differences within a country. Differences also may occur within a state (or province), county, or city. Taking time to listen to clients as care is delivered and having a broad knowledge base of cultural preferences enables the nurse to increase client comfort.

## Challenges for Multicultural Nursing Practice

In relation to health promotion, knowledge of specific disease risks across various cultural groups provides useful information to the professional nurse. Table 11-5 summarizes some health risks and diseases that occur with higher incidence in various cultural groups in the United States. The governmental publication *Healthy People 2010* emphasizes disparities in the quality of health across various cultural groups in the United States, most of which arise from poverty and lack of access to health care (USDHHS, 2000). Burggraf (2000) noted that elderly persons of nonwhite backgrounds hold different attitudes and behaviors about health care. These include the following:

1. General distrust of health care systems, societal disadvantages, language problems, reliance on traditional or spiritual healing practices, discrimination based on race, ethnicity, gender or age.

**TABLE 11-5**

| Common Health Risks and Diseases Encountered by Various Cultural Groups in the United States | | |
| --- | --- | --- |
| **Cultural Group** | **Health Risks** | **Diseases** |
| African American | Higher incidence of homicide<br>Lower physical activity levels<br>Obesity<br>Cigarette smoking<br>Alcohol abuse<br>Incarceration<br>Unintended pregnancy<br>Untreated dental caries | Heart disease<br>Stroke<br>High blood pressure<br>Chronic renal disease<br>Cancer<br>Premature deaths associated with<br>  breast and prostate cancer<br>Sexually transmitted disease<br>HIV/AIDS<br>Cirrhosis of the liver<br>Arthritis<br>Asthma<br>Black out[a]<br>Low blood[a]<br>High blood[a]<br>Thin blood[a]<br>Disorders caused by spells or hexes (Voodoo)[a] |

*(continued)*

## Common Health Risks and Diseases Encountered by Various Cultural Groups in the United States (Continued)

| Cultural Group | Health Risks | Diseases |
|---|---|---|
| Native American or Alaskan | Highest infant death rate among cultural groups in the US<br>Unintentional injuries<br>Suicide<br>Cigarette smoking<br>Alcohol abuse<br>38% lack health insurance coverage<br>Home fire deaths<br>Gingivitis | Heart disease<br>Cancer<br>Diabetes<br>Chronic liver disease<br>Cirrhosis of the liver<br>Pneumonia/influenza<br>Chronic renal disease<br>Ghost affliction[a] |
| Pacific Island/Asian American | Cigarette smoking<br>Air pollution | Heart disease<br>High blood pressure<br>Diabetes<br>Cancer<br>Cervical cancer (Vietnamese)<br>Hepatitis<br>Arthritis[b]<br>Koro[a] (Southeastern Asian)<br>Wagamama[a] (Japanese)<br>Hwa-byung[a] (Korean) |
| Hispanic American | Low birth weight<br>Lower physical activity levels<br>Obesity<br>Cigarette smoking<br>Air pollution<br>33% lack health insurance coverage<br>Unintended pregnancy<br>Home fire death<br>Untreated dental caries<br>Gingivitis | High blood pressure<br>Diabetes<br>Tuberculosis (20% higher rate than European Americans)<br>Increased rate of cancer deaths<br>Cervical, esophageal, gall bladder, and stomach cancer<br>Increasing rates of breast and lung cancer<br>Sexually transmitted disease<br>HIV/AIDS<br>Asthma<br>Empacho[a]<br>Fatigue[a]<br>Mal ojo (evil eye)[a]<br>Pasmo[a]<br>Susto[b] |
| European American | Lower physical activity levels with increasing age<br>Obesity<br>Cigarette smoking | Heart disease<br>Alcohol abuse<br>Arthritis<br>Osteoporosis[b]<br>Asthma<br>Anorexia nervosa<br>Bulimia[a]<br>Hysteria[a] (Greek)<br>Evil eye[a] (Greek) |

[a]Culturally based syndromes.
[b]Health problem identified in elderly women of specified cultural group.
Adapted from U.S. Department of Health and Human Services (2000); Andrews & Herberg (1999); and Burggraf (2000).

2. Reduced satisfaction with health care plans and providers.
3. Abuse from family members who became acculturated to the American way of life.
4. Exposure to hazards in lower economic living areas and low paying jobs.

Burggraf (2000) notes that language barriers may be a deterrent to seeking health care in populations of older Hispanics and elderly Asian women. These groups of elderly women also tend to rely on folk and spiritual healing practices before entering the health care system (Burggraf, 2000).

Because all humans have similar biologic structure and basic physiology, nurses work to achieve cultural-universal care.

## Folk Illnesses

In addition to different risks for specific illnesses based on ethnicity, some cultures have **"folk illnesses"** that may require the use of culturally-based healers. Empacho is an infant gastrointestinal condition that occurs in Mexican culture. Empacho results in an obstruction in which food and other matter adheres to the walls of the stomach or intestines. Empacho occurs if the child swallows too much saliva during teething or when parents change formulas that do not mix well with each other. Symptoms include abdominal distention, pain, poor appetite, perceived stomach lump, and diarrhea. Infants are placed on a regimen of clear liquids and herbal teas to "refresh the stomach" (Pachter, 1994, p. 692). If the infant begins to lose too much weight, Latino parents may consult physicians so that they are not perceived as being neglectful by others. Successful blending of conventional medical therapy with folk remedies provides the family with culturally competent care. In addition, persons with medical illnesses go to "physicians" but may seek the advice of a folk healer to discover why the illness occurred. Some persons view medical illnesses as the result of an evil spell and need to seek treatment from a spiritual healer to be fully well (Pachter, 1994).

## Physical Appearance Variations

Along with increased specific health risks, persons from different ethnic backgrounds have **variations in physical appearance** (Andrews & Herberg, 1999; Pachter, 1994). The transculturally competent nurse considers physical appearance variations when performing health assessments. A general appearance scan reveals information related to gender, age, skin color, body structure, consciousness level, facial features, clothing, and behavior. Initial interaction with the client permits the nurse to collect information regarding orientation, speech patterns, facial expression, mood, and cognition. Choice of clothing determines the ability of the person to select appropriate clothing for the weather and social situation. Although a matter of personal preference, grooming also provides the nurse with cues related to client culture.

Clothing styles vary widely across cultures. Amish women usually wear solid color dresses, held together by pins or snaps and a bonnet. Mennonite women wear similarly styled clothing, but the dresses may be of printed material and have buttons. Islamic women wear clothing to cover all extremities and a veil. Arab-Muslim men sometimes wear a cloth headdress and long robe. Some Indian women wear saris. In certain instances, cultural and religious clothing may be concealed, as in the case of special white undergarments known as "temple garments" that are worn by members of the Church of

Jesus Christ of Latter Day Saints (Mormon) (Andrews & Herberg, 1999). Roman Catholics often wear religious medals or pictures of Jesus and the Blessed Virgin encased in plastic (scapulars) around their necks. When providing physical care to clients, the nurse should ask permission before removing specific items of clothing or jewelry.

Skin color varies among all persons and depends on melanin concentrations. Melanin protects the skin from ultraviolet radiation. Increased quantities of melanin protect persons from skin cancer (Andrews & Herberg, 1999). Because all persons have some level of melanin in the skin, all persons are people of color. When assessing for skin changes, the nurse must determine what the usual healthy shade is for the individual, rather than for the ethnic group. Specific skin variations for various ethnic groups may be found in physical assessment and transcultural nursing textbooks. Table 11-6 provides a brief summary of some key aspects for nursing assessments related to variations in

**TABLE 11-6**

## Nursing Assessment Considerations Based on Ethnicity

| Ethnic Group | Assessment Considerations |
|---|---|
| African | Mongolian spots and vitiligo more common |
| | Higher carotene levels in sclera may give them a yellow appearance |
| | Pallor appears as ashen or gray. |
| | Erythema difficult to see, but inflammation is more detectable by palpation for warmth, edema, and hardness |
| | Hard and soft palates may be the best place to see a macular rash |
| | Petechiae cannot be seen in some cases, and if seen, can be found on the buccal mucosa, conjunctiva, abdomen, buttocks, and volar forearm surface |
| | Tend to have stronger body odor |
| | Hair and scalp tend to be dry |
| | Copper color hair in children is an indication of severe malnutrition |
| | Less susceptible to noise-induced hearing loss |
| | Increased incidence of oral hyperpigmentation in older age |
| | Increased periodontal disease |
| | Highest bone density |
| Native Americans | Mongolian spots and vitiligo more common |
| | Pallor appears yellow brown |
| | Mild or absent body odor |
| | 18% have cleft uvula |
| | Eskimos have the largest teeth |
| | 30% of Navajo women have longitudinal vascular pattern on chest |
| | Eskimos have lower bone density than do whites |
| Asian | Mongolian spots and vitiligo more common |
| | Areola and genitalia are darker |
| | Pallor appears as pasty or nearly white |
| | Mild to absent body odor |
| | Hair usually silky, black, and straight |
| | Delayed hair graying |
| | Highest incidence of myopia (Japanese and Chinese) |
| | 10% have cleft uvula |
| | Lower bone density than whites |

## Nursing Assessment Considerations Based on Ethnicity (Continued)

| Ethnic Group | Assessment Considerations |
|---|---|
| European | Persons of Mediterranean descent frequently have blue lips, thereby negating reliance on circumoral cyanosis as a reliable indicator of poor oxygenation<br>Pallor appears as pasty or nearly white<br>Skin wrinkles appear at a younger age<br>Tend to have more moles than other groups<br>Tend to have stronger body odor<br>Hair turns gray at an earlier age<br>Smallest teeth, resulting in more tooth loss |
| Pacific Island | Higher carotene levels in sclera may give them a yellow appearance<br>Pallor appears yellow brown |
| Middle Eastern | Vitiligo more common<br>Persons of Mediterranean descent frequently have blue lips, thereby negating reliance on circumoral cyanosis as a reliable indicator of poor oxygenation<br>Pallor appears yellow brown |
| Hispanic | Pallor appears yellow brown |

Adapted from Andrews & Herberg (1999).

ethnic descent. If the nurse relies on assessment data information based on the skin color of whites, critical errors could occur. Along with skin color, specific hair care considerations surface. The hair of persons of African descent requires combing, gentle brushing, and oil application, rather than the frequent shampooing to eliminate hair oil that is practiced by persons of European descent (Andrews & Herberg, 1999).

## Variations in Physiology

In addition to skin color, physiology varies across various ethnic groups. Some of these result in the adjustment in "normal" reference laboratory values for blood tests. For example, the hemoglobin levels of African Americans tend to be lower than those of their African counterparts; Native, Japanese, and Hispanic Americans have higher blood glucose levels than do European Americans. African Americans have higher levels of high-density lipoproteins (HDLs) than do whites, and Hispanic Americans have lower levels of HDLs. The source of these variations may be genetic or environmental. The federal government has identified medical research across gender and ethnic groups as a research priority (USDHHS, 2000). Current trends indicate that a vast amount of data will be generated by genetic research.

**Metabolism variations** result in different responses to pharmacologic agents. Some of the known responses are summarized in Table 11-7. Some variations result from an inherited enzyme deficiency, whereas the source of other variations remains unknown. When providing care for a culturally diverse client population, professional nurses should be aware of differing responses to medications to anticipate potential adverse effects and different therapeutic responses that may require dosage alterations (Andrews & Herberg, 1999).

TABLE 11-7

## Cultural Variation to Pharmacologic Agents

| Cultural Group | Pharmacological Agent | Variations |
|---|---|---|
| African Americans | Analgesics | Reduced sensitivity to therapeutic effects<br>Increased gastrointestinal adverse effects, especially with acetaminophen |
| | Antihypertensives | Blood pressure responds better to single-agent therapy<br>Less responsive to beta blockers and angiotensin-converting, enzyme-blocking agents<br>Increase mood responses to thiazide diuretics |
| | Mydriatics | Less pupil dilation |
| | Psychotropics | Increased chance of extrapyramidal side effects |
| | Steroids | Increased chance of steroid-induced diabetes (especially with methylprednisolone in renal transplantation) |
| | Tranquilizers | 15%–20% poorly metabolize diazepam |
| Arab Americans | Antiarrhythmics | Some dose reduction may be needed |
| | Antihypertensives | Some dose reduction may be needed |
| | Neuroleptics | Some dose reduction may be needed |
| | Opioids | Higher doses may be required because this group may have diminished ability to metabolize codeine to morphine |
| | Psychotropics | Some dose reduction may be needed |
| Native Americans | Muscle relaxants | Alaskan Eskimos may have prolonged muscle paralysis with succinylcholine administration during surgery and may need mechanical ventilation for respiratory support |
| Chinese Americans | Narcotic analgesics | Less sensitive to respiratory depressant and hypotensive effects<br>Have a higher clearance of morphine |
| Asian Americans | Antihypertensives | Best response with calcium antagonists |
| | Neuroleptics | May need reduced dosage |
| | Psychotropics | May need reduced dosage and up to one-half the normal dose for tricyclic antidepressants and lithium |
| | Fat-soluble drugs | Increased dosages of fat-soluble drugs needed because of reduced percentages of body fat (especially vitamin K for Warfa reversal) |
| Hispanic Americans | Psychotropics | May need to reduce dosage as frequently have a higher incidence of adverse effects to tricyclic antidepressants |
| Americans of Mediterranean descent with glucose-6-phosphate dehydrogenase deficiency | Oxidating medications | Precipitation of a hemolytic crisis with primaquine, quinidine, thiazolsulfone, nitrofurazone, furazolidine, naphthalene, toluidine blue, phenylhydrazine, chloramphenicol, and aspirin |
| Jewish Americans (Ashkenazi) | Psychotropics | 20% experience agranulocytosis with clozapine treatment for schizophrenia |

Adapted from Andrews & Herberg (1999).

# ● CREATING A MULTICULTURAL PROFESSION OF NURSING

In an ideal health care system, health care providers should mirror the population that they serve. Surveys indicate less than 15% of nurses come from a minority background. According to the USDHHS (2000), only 6.9% of professional nurses are African American; 3.4% are Hispanic or Latino; 3.2% come from Asian or Pacific Island backgrounds; and 0.7% are Native American or Alaskan Natives. The Asian Pacific Island Nurses Association represents 40 nursing subgroups who speak 23 different languages (Farella, 2001). The proportion of minority members in the nursing profession varies across states.

To offer health care services to a diverse population, the creation of a **multicultural profession of nursing** must occur. Attracting persons from different cultural backgrounds to the nursing profession remains a challenge. The best and the brightest students often prefer to enter other professions (such as law, medicine, engineering, or teaching) because nursing sometimes is perceived by outsiders as an oppressed profession that holds a status that is subservient to physicians. Adding membership to one more oppressed group may be more than a person can bear. Nursing competes with other professions for the same students.

In addition to the perception of nurses being a less powerful member of the health care team, white women traditionally have dominated nursing. This dominance brings with it values, beliefs, and practices that reflect the socialization of white women. Current efforts to increase cultural diversity in the nursing profession include minority nursing scholarships, grant programs, and targeted recruitment efforts. The National Coalition of Ethnic Minority Nurses serves as a clearinghouse for information related to nursing education, leadership, practice, research, and health care policy initiatives (Farella, 2001).

However, once accepted into a nursing program, some minority nursing students experience **culture shock.** Most nurse educators come from a dominant group of nurses and expect students to abide by traditional cultural values of nursing. Faculty may make errors when working with students from various cultural groups. For example, punctuality is a highly valued work practice in nursing and in education. Students sometimes receive a grade penalty for arriving to class late or submitting assignments late, especially when faculty fails to explore reasons for a late assignment or fails to explain the reasons why punctuality is valued. Nursing students from differing cultures occasionally use different nonverbal behaviors when conversing with persons of authority. Students from Far Eastern countries tend to not make eye contact when conversing with teachers, supervising staff nurses, physicians, and older persons; for the students, this practice is a way of conveying respect, but some faculty and staff may label the student as being cold and distant. They question the student's ability to practice the profession of nursing with genuine compassion.

Upon graduation from a nursing program, the minority nurse may fall victim to incidences of racism and stereotyping, especially when nurses encounter stressful working relationships (Farella, 2001). Countries such as the Philippines produce a surplus of nurses. Many of these nurses seek employment in countries with nursing shortages, such as Canada, Great Britain, Australia, Saudi Arabia, and the United States (Alaniz, 2001). American nurses have a history of being less than hospitable to foreign nurses. Leininger (1995) and Farella (20010 report incidences in the 1980s in which Filipino nurses fell victim to racial slurs and stereotyping. Sometimes, European American clients and relatives accuse health team members from a different ethnic background of theft.

Professional nurses have an obligation to be hospitable to nurses and other health team members who are from different ethnic backgrounds. With increased client loads, nurses sometimes forget manners when distressed. Platz and Wales (1999) outline the various methods to make others feel welcome. First, good nurses make all clients and colleagues feel cared for and appreciated. Second, standards for business etiquette include greeting colleagues and all persons with each encounter, respecting the time of others, being prompt for meetings and appointments, calling to inform others if delayed for more than 5 minutes, sending thank-you notes, listening actively to others when speaking, respecting other's religion and culture, and considering other's privacy and the right to a neat, clean, and safe working environment.

## ✦ SUMMARY AND SIGNIFICANCE TO PRACTICE

Professional nurses face many challenges when working with persons from cultural groups different from their own. Errors frequently occur when a nurse provides care to and works with persons from a cultural background that differs from that of the nurse. Sometimes nurses make errors based on the outward appearance of the person. Nurses should take the time to ask questions related to cultural preferences, listen to individuals, consider cues given to them by persons from a different culture, and analyze the benefits (or hazards) of generic (or folk) health practices before outlining care plan strategies. Interacting with persons from cultural backgrounds different from their own means nurses must take risks, but nurses can learn from their mistakes. Nurses serve as client advocates when they see that specific client cultural needs are met. Authentic caring and effective communication skills enhance the development of therapeutic relationships with clients and collegial relationships with colleagues from different cultural backgrounds. Attainment of cultural competence takes a lifetime.

### FROM THEORY TO PRACTICE

1. Referring to the vignette at the beginning of the chapter, what do you think Judy could do to facilitate the teamwork for a multicultural nursing care team? Why is it important that team members of diverse cultural groups understand each other?
2. If you were Judy, what steps would you take to prepare yourself for nursing practice in a foreign country? Would you help your friend in the health clinic? Why or why not?

### WWW INTERNET EXERCISES

1. Using a search engine, type in the country or countries of your heritage. Visit a tourist site for the country or countries you identified and read a description of the people and any legal or cultural issues for which you may be held accountable. Bring these to share with your classmates.
2. Visit the Smithsonian Center for Folklife and Cultural Heritage (www.folklife.si.edu/index.html) and experience one of the posted Virtual Festivals

(Border festival, Hawaiian luau, or African naming ceremony). Write down your reactions as you proceed through each ceremony and listen to music. Click on the words "Folklife Festival." On the next screen, click on "Virtual Festival."

## INTERNET RESOURCES

To learn more about transcultural nursing, visit The Transcultural Nursing Society at: www.tcns.org.

To learn more about transcultural health care issues, visit the Center for Cross-Cultural Health (CCCH) careers at: www.crosshealth.com.

Visit the International Council of Nurses to find information and opportunities about international nursing and networking at: http://www.icn.ch.

To learn more about minority nursing information, visit: www.MinorityNurse.com and the following websites:

The National Black Nurses Association, Inc.: http://www.nbna.org

National Association of Hispanic Nurses: www.thehispanicnurses.org

For folkway and folklife information, visit one of the following websites:

The American Folklife Center at the Library of Congress: http://www.loc.gov/folklife, or the Smithsonian Center for Folklife and Cultural Heritage: http://www.folklife.si.edu/index.html/.

For a different look at health and healing, visit the Institute of Noetic Sciences at: http://www.noetic.org.

## REFERENCES

Abood, S., & Gonzalez, R. (Eds.) (2001). Cultural competence. *Capitol Update, 19*(1), 2.

Alaniz, J. (2001). Give-and-take. *Nurse Week Midwest, 2*(3), 14–15.

American Association of Colleges of Nursing (1998). *The essentials of baccalaureate education for professional nursing practice*. Washington DC: Author.

Andrews, M. M. & Boyle (1999). (Eds.). *Transcultural concepts in nursing care* (3rd ed.). Philadelphia: Lippincott Williams & Wilkins.

Andrews, M., & Herberg, P. (1999). Transcultural nursing care. In M. M. Andrews & J. S. Boyle (Eds.), *Transcultural concepts in nursing care* (3rd ed., pp. 23–77). Philadelphia: Lippincott Williams & Wilkins.

Breslau, K. (2000, September 18). Tomorrow land, today. *Newsweek, 68*, 52–53.

Burchum, J. (2002). Cultural competence: An evolutionary perspective. *Nursing Forum, 37*, 5–15.

Burggraf, V. (2000). The older woman: Ethnicity and health. *Geriatric Nursing, 21*, 183–187.

Campo-Flores, A. (2000, September 18). Brown against brown. *Newsweek, 68*, 49–51.

Cose, E. (2000, September 18). What's white anyway? *Newsweek, 68*, 64–65.

Farella, C. (2001). How we hurt our own. *Nursing Spectrum, 2*(2), 12–13.

Giger, J. N., & Davidhizar, R. E. (1999). *Transcultural nursing assessment and intervention* (3rd ed.). St. Louis: Mosby.

Gil, K.M., Mishel, M. H., Belyea, M., Germino, B., Porter, L. S., La Ney, I. C., & Stewart, J. (2004). Triggers of uncertainty about recurrence and long-term treatment side effects in older African American and Caucasian breast cancer survivors. *Oncology Nursing Forum 31*, 633–639.

Grossman, D. (1996). Cultural dimensions in home health nursing. *American Journal of Nursing, 96*, 33–36.

Johnson, A. D. (2004). In 2050, half of the U.S. will be people of color. *Diversity Newsletter*. Available at http://www.diversity.com/members/6550.cfm. Accessed March 18, 2004.

Kavanagh, K. H., & Kennedy, P. H. (1992). *Promoting cultural diversity: Strategies for health care professionals*. Newbury Park, CA: Sage.

Leininger, M. (1995). *Transcultural nursing* (2nd ed.). New York: McGraw-Hill.

Leininger, M., & McFarland, M. (2002). *Transcultural nursing: Concepts, theories, research & practice* (3rd ed.). New York: McGraw-Hill.

Pachter, L. M. (1994). Culture and clinical care: Folk illness beliefs and behaviors and their implications for health care delivery. *Journal of the American Medical Association, 271,* 690–694.

Pedersen, P. B., Dragunus, J. C., Lenner, W. J., & Trimble, J. E. (Eds.) (1996). *Counseling across cultures* (4th ed.). Thousand Oaks: Sage.

Platz, A., & Wales, S. (1999). *Social graces: Manners, conversation and charm for today.* Eugene, OR: Harvest House Publishers.

Purnell, L. D., & Paulanka, B. J. (1998). *Transcultural health care: A culturally competent approach.* Philadelphia: F. A. Davis.

Schiff, L. (2001). U. S. is not the only one facing a nursing shortage. *RN, 64*(19), 24.

Spector, R. E. (2000). *Cultural diversity in health and illness* (5th ed.). Upper Saddle River, NJ: Prentice Hall Health.

U. S. Department of Health and Human Services. (2000). *Healthy people 2010*: Volume II (Conference Edition in Two Volumes). Washington, DC: U. S. Government Printing Office.

Yoder, M. K. (1996). Instructional responses to ethnically diverse nursing students. *Journal of Nursing Education, 35,* 315–321.

Yoder, M. K. (1997). The consequences of a generic approach to teaching nursing in a multicultural world. *Journal of Cultural Diversity, 4,* 77–82.

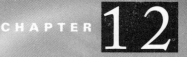

# Professional Nurse Accountability

## KEY TERMS AND CONCEPTS

Accountability

Responsibility

Answerability

Autonomy

Authority

Competence

Delegation

Professional Standards

Ethical Accountability

Nurses as Client Advocates

Shared Governance

Accountability Checklist

## LEARNING OUTCOMES

By the end of this chapter, the learner will be able to:

**1** Differentiate accountability from autonomy and authority.

**2** Identify the essential questions the professional nurse must answer to be accountable to the client and public.

**3** Relate current standards of professional nursing practice to accountability.

**4** List some current developments in nursing and health care that demonstrate an increased emphasis on accountability now and for the future.

**5** Identify some of the positive outcomes of the nurse becoming accountable to clients, profession, self, employing institution, managed care networks, and third-party payers.

**6** Evaluate oneself on professional accountability, using this chapter's checklist.

## VIGNETTE

Carol is a charge nurse of a neuroscience unit. This afternoon, Mr. Jones, who is 90 years old, has been admitted for dysphagia and left-sided weakness. Mrs. Jones wants absolutely everything done to make her husband well. She insists that the nursing assistant, Gloria, give him food and fluid to drink. When Gloria refuses, Mrs. Jones insists on seeing the nurse in charge. Carol is busy and cannot talk to Mrs. Jones. Mrs. Jones grows impatient and fixes coffee for her husband, then holds the cup to his mouth for him to take sips. Mr. Jones chokes violently. Martha, Carol's nursing colleague, runs into the room and finds that there are no suction catheters for the wall unit suction apparatus. As she delivers the Heimlich maneuver to Mr. Jones, she sends Gloria to the supply cart to get catheters; none are found there. Mr. Jones quits breathing, and Marie "calls a code." Unfortunately, Mr. Jones dies.

**Questions For Reflection 12-1**

1. List the mistakes and the persons who made them in the vignette.
2. What are the potential consequences of Mr. Jones' death?
3. How would I feel if a situation similar to this happened while I practiced nursing?

**Accountability** means being held responsible for having done something. In the early writings about the nursing profession, the term **responsibility** meant duty. Florence Nightingale's *Notes on Nursing* frequently emphasizes the responsibilities of professional nurses. She delineates the nurse's responsibility for the state of the sick room (Nightingale, 1946, p. 45), the need for careful observation on the part of the nurse to avoid patient accidents (Nightingale, p. 66), and mentions the fact that "I have often seen really good nurses distressed, because they could not impress the doctor with the real danger of their patients" (Nightingale, p. 68).

Perhaps private-duty nursing represents the epitome of nursing accountability to clients. In private-duty nursing of the past, a nurse took a "case," lived with the client, and remained until the patient no longer needed nursing services. The nurse assumed responsibility and was held accountable for the patient's life, space, and nursing care.

After the Depression of the 1930s, fewer nurses chose to practice private-duty nursing and nurses sought employment as staff nurses in hospitals or public health agencies (Dachelet & Sullivan, 1979). Nurses focused on care tasks and duties were assigned according to function at that time. Thus, the notion of accountability became tied to negative situations and earned a punitive connotation. Although they were unaware, nurses were legally liable for their actions or the omission of necessary actions. Many nurses believed that the ultimate liability remained with the institution, which would "cover" them in the event of a lawsuit. Accountability in the professional sense did not exist and the entire concept certainly had no positive attributes as far as the individual nurse was concerned. True professional accountability in nursing surfaced in the late 1970s (Clifford, 1981). In 1980, accountability first appeared as a free-standing topic heading in the Cumulative Index of Nursing and Allied Health Literature.

## ⊕ DEFINITION OF ACCOUNTABILITY AND RELATED CONCEPTS

To assume accountability, nurses must understand its definition. Accountability "is increasingly confused with and used in place of autonomy and authority, although it is synonymous with neither, but related to both" (Batey & Lewis, 1982, p. 13). The following section attempts to clarify and differentiate this trio of terms.

### Responsibility and Answerability

Accountability continues to retain its original meaning of responsibility but has an added dimension, that of **answerability,** the necessity of offering answers, reasons, and explanations to certain others. As the American Nurses Association (ANA) Code for Nurses states, this accountability

refers to being answerable to someone for something one has done. It means providing an explanation to self, to the client, to the employing agency, and to the nursing profession (ANA, 2001).

An additional dimension of accountability is its reporting aspect, embodied in the following definition:

(accountability is) . . . the fulfillment of a formal obligation to disclose to referent others the purposes, principles, procedures, relationships, results, income and expenditures for which one has authority. This disclosure is systematic, periodic, and carried out in consistent form. . . . Initiating the disclosure is the responsibility of the one accountable and not of others (Batey & Lewis, 1982, p. 10).

Currently, discussions of accountability for professional nursing revolve around interventions (nursing care), outcomes (results), and costs (expenditures). Because of legal, accrediting agency, third-party payer, and managed care requirements, documentation frequently serves as evidence that nurses either performed or did not perform specific nursing assessments and interventions. Currently, the health care delivery industry has higher error rates than other industries. Recent efforts by businesses, consumers, and the government to expect higher quality health care based on scientific evidence may result in increased areas of accountability for professional nurses.

Thus, accountability is the state of being responsible and answerable for the behaviors and their outcomes that fall into the realm of one's professional role. Professional nurses practice accountability each time they answer questions for reasons behind actions, document interventions and outcomes of delivered care, and participate in clinical competency programs.

## Autonomy and Authority

In distinction to accountability, **autonomy** refers to the independence of functioning. Autonomy means that one can perform one's total professional function on the basis of one's own knowledge and judgment and that one is recognized by others as having the right to do so. Obviously, this concept is related to accountability because one who functions autonomously must be accountable for his or her behavior (Holden, 1991; Hylka & Shugrue, 1991).

The final closely related term is authority. **Authority** can be defined as being in a position to make decisions and to influence others to act in a manner determined by those decisions. Again, this term is certainly related to accountability because those who are in authority are accountable for the decisions they make and for the actions of themselves and others who act on the basis of their decisions. In addition, authority relates to autonomy because those in authority often act autonomously in performing all or part of their respective roles.

One can see these relationships further developed in the nursing literature. According to Batey and Lewis (1982, p. 13):

Responsibility, authority, autonomy, and accountability are inextricably related. Responsibility and authority are necessary conditions for both autonomy and accountability. It is illogical and inappropriate for an organization to hold a department or an individual accountable for those activities over which the department or individual has no authority. . . . Autonomy within the areas in which nursing service has responsibility is also a necessary condition for accountability. . . . Accountability is an exercise in futility and an experience in failure unless it is linked to nursing service's autonomy. The process of fulfilling nursing's formal obligation to disclose requires that nursing services have the formal and legitimate power to carry out relevant actions. Without the opportunity to make binding decisions, accountability is a hollow concept.

Bergman sees this relationship somewhat differently by considering responsibility and authority (along with ability) as preconditions leading to accountability. As she states:

The basic precondition is to have the ability . . . to decide and act on a specific issue. One must be given or taken, the responsibility to carry out that action. Next, one needs the authority, i.e. formal backing, legal right to carry the responsibility. Then, with the preconditions, one can be accountable for the action one takes (Bergman, 1981, pp. 54–55).

Webb, Price, and Van Ess Coeling (1996, p. 29) discuss the relationship of accountability and several other concepts in a more contemporary form:

The professional elements of practice are authority, accountability, responsibility and decision-making; therefore, the professional nurse is described as one who is autonomous and who desires responsibility and accountability.

Krueger-Wilson and Porter-O'Grady (1999) propose replacing "responsibility" with "accountability" because responsibility historically has been tied to tasks and work processes, rather than outcomes. Job task and quality of work performance are the driving forces behind responsibility. Persons having responsibility tend to report to someone else, and such persons often can dodge the responsibility for poor work. In contrast, accountability focuses on outcomes of professional role performance. All persons in a living system such as a workplace assume ownership of various roles to attain desired outcomes. In this case, persons designated to fulfill a particular role also have the authority to design their work, clear expectations of their contributions, and an attitude to strive to do their absolute best to attain organizational outcomes. New relationships blossom among coworkers, and workers create meaningful partnerships with each other to fulfill specified outcomes. Workers become accountable for individual performance and outcomes, rather than being responsible to a superior (Krueger-Wilson & Porter-O'Grady).

Because professional nurses frequently delegate nursing responsibilities to practical/vocational nurses and unlicensed personnel, they become accountable for the outcomes of the actions of others. Before delegating a task to anyone, the nurse must ascertain that the person has the **competence** (or ability to) perform the delegated tasks. **Delegation** of tasks requires that nurses use professional judgment to decide what tasks can be safely done by another member of the nursing team. Most state nursing practice acts address the delegation process. Many of the directives regarding delegation leave room for the professional nurse to decide what tasks can be safely delegated to others. The following questions help professional nurses to decide what tasks can be safely done by another member of the nursing care team (Iowa Nurses Association, 1997):

1. What is the task/activity that needs to be done?
2. Can the task be performed by someone other than a registered nurse?

3. How stable is the client's condition?
4. What is the level of competence of the licensed practical/vocational nurse or unlicensed assistive care provider who will perform the task?
5. How experienced is the registered nurse with the procedure?
6. Which member of the nursing care team is best qualified to perform the tasks?
7. What is the potential for harm with the delegated task?
8. Does the task require any independent decision making?
9. What is the client ability for self-care?

The nurse may opt to perform a task usually delegated to an unlicensed care provider when client situations reveal a high potential for harm and quick independent decision making is required to avert a serious complication. For example, a registered nurse may decide to feed a newly admitted client who has difficulty speaking and a medical diagnosis of probable cerebrovascular accident because whether the client can safely swallow has to be established.

The agency that uses unlicensed personnel has the responsibility to verify that these persons receive adequate education and training before they assume work duties. Nurses who fail to respond to client problems reported by subordinates set up a potential violation to most state nurse practice acts. In addition, professional nurses, especially those serving as charge nurses and team leaders, have a duty to report any conditions that keep them from effectively performing their designated role.

Thus, accountability, responsibility, and autonomy are related, but not synonymous. However, each of these concepts projects an image of a responsible, independent individual, capable of making decisions and influencing others to act on them and who also is answerable for his or her behavior and the behavior of associates to attain specific outcomes. In the professional nursing context, the nurse becomes an autonomous practitioner who brings a different perspective and fulfills a particular role in the interdisciplinary health team. The nurse assumes responsibility for professional activities (including using research-based nursing actions, maintaining clinical competence, and staying abreast of new developments) and is held accountable for the outcomes of client care. This evolving image of a professional nurse demonstrates individual nurse consent to be held accountable for the outcome of actions thereby moving the profession toward distinction and status given to other health care professions.

## ● PROFESSIONAL ACCOUNTABILITY

As nursing evolves to fit all criteria for professional status, increased interest in and concern with accountability has arisen. Accountability has always been acknowledged as one of the hallmarks of a profession. Flexner (1915) supported this view when outlining characteristics of a profession. In that work, Flexner indicated that a profession is likely to be more responsive to public interest than are unorganized and isolated individuals.

In terms of nursing's involvement with its professionalization in the 1950s and 1960s, Bixler and Bixler (1959) stated that a profession functions autonomously to form professional policy and control professional activity. McGlothlin (1961) explains that a profession undertakes tasks that require exercise of judgment in applying knowledge to the solutions of problems and accepts responsibility for the results. Today, other emerging professions, such as social work and medical records professionals, have begun to address the issue of accountability. However, to be accountable, a profession must know that for which it is accountable. To do this, the profession must establish **professional standards** and attempt to enforce them. Professional standards outline the guidelines and principles of a specific line of work or career. The American Nurses Association (ANA), nursing's major professional organization, has done this with its standards of nursing practice, service, and education. In doing so, the ANA has complied with one of the functions of a professional organization, according to Merton (1958); that is, of providing the means by which members of the profession can judge the competence of its members. Through its standards, the ANA has contributed greatly to the ability of the nursing profession to be accountable.

By using the standards of practice (ANA, 1997) as a guide, the nurse can identify the scope and limits of professional nursing practice. Nurses can internalize that for which they are accountable. The National Council of State Boards of Nursing sets standards for "safe nursing practice." Individual State Boards of Nursing develop standards for professional practice and monitor professional nurse performance. In addition, a nursing service department monitors its collective accountability through the process of peer review.

Such monitoring has increased dramatically in recent years through the introduction of systematic nursing quality assurance and improvement activities with active participation by staff nurses in many institutions and agencies. In 1991, Joint Commission on Accreditation of Healthcare Organizations mandated (JCAHO, 1991) that quality assurance programs are requisite for accreditation. This action hastened the process of operationalizing the concept of accountability as quality assurance at the nursing service department level.

Nurses have another document to guide them for practice accountability—the *Code for Nurses*, which also was developed by the ANA. The code for nursing outlines terms for **ethical accountability** for professional nurses. **Nurses as client advocates** base professional decisions on what is best for clients. More in the nature of an ethical code, the *ANA Code for Nurses* provides a clear framework within which the nurse can seek to uphold the standards of care and protect the clients they serve. Should there be any doubt about accountability of the nursing profession, the Code lays this to rest by directly confronting the issue. As stated in item 4 of the code, "The nurse assumes responsibility and accountability for individual nursing judgments and actions" (ANA, 2001, p. 1).

Other items in the Code do not address the area of accountability directly, but by discussing various factors that are necessary underpinnings for accountability, indirectly support the concept. These factors include the presumed competence of the nurse, use of informed judgment, and use of nursing research.

Because society holds individual nurses accountable for professional actions, the profession is accountable for the nurse to establish and monitor standards for safe practice. Only nurses can determine the definition of "safe practice" and care standards. In some states, physicians routinely testify in court proceeding that a nurse displayed unsafe practice or deviated from the standard of care. Obviously, nursing is accountable as a profession and its individual practitioners also are accountable. It has been implied throughout this discussion that nurses are accountable to the public and to the profession itself. In addition, with most nurses remaining employed by health care agencies, rather than being independently employed, one must consider the area of accountability to the institution (Copp, 1988; Vaughn, 1989). In the current climate of cost control, the notion of accountability to managed care networks and third-party payers of health care has emerged. Finally, in light of the current emphasis on self-actualization and growth, it is important to add that the professional nurse must be accountable to oneself.

## Accountability to the Public and Client

A profession exists to provide service to the public. Although it may be intellectually stimulating, gratifying, and exciting to a professional to perform a role, ultimately the reason for that role lies in its service relationship with the public. Thus, almost by definition, a profession must be accountable to the public. The consumer has the right to receive the best possible quality of care—care grounded in a firm knowledge base and performed by those who can make use of that knowledge base through the application of sound judgment while using a clear and appropriate value system.

As consumers become more knowledgeable through formal education and access to information from many media formats, they know more about what the professions are supposed to be doing. The increased knowledge empowers consumers to demand more and to make those demands openly. Instead of assuming authority positions, nurses work collaboratively with clients to determine and attain health-related goals.

Nurses must be aware of increased consumer knowledge and sophistication and be prepared to respond to it in an equally knowledgeable and sophisticated manner. Nurses must demonstrate clearly the principles and concepts on which practice is based. They also need to access current information, use problem solving to effectively evaluate outcomes of care, and revise care strategies if desired outcomes are not achieved.

Society holds nurses legally accountable for professional practice. Each state has a Board of Nursing that monitors practice according the Nursing Practice Act (NPA). The NPA defines professional nursing practice, specifies the scope of practice, and distinguishes professional nursing from other health professions. Nurses must practice within these guidelines when working in a state. Thus, securing a copy of the NPA for states in which one practices is essential because ignorance of the law serves as no excuse for a professional nurse. Nurses can secure a copy of an NPA via the Internet, with a telephone request, or through a written request. When undesired client outcomes occur in health care, the law holds professional nurses to a standard of safe and prudent practice. Safe and prudent practice means that the nurse exercises reasonable judgment and delivers reasonable care (Kopp, 2001). Examples of reasonable actions and judgments include being competent in the area of current practice, securing help for situations in which one is unqualified to manage, and fulfilling professional duties as a nurse. Negligence occurs when a nurse commits a breach of duty; an example of this would be falling short of an acceptable standard of care through an action or omission (Kopp). When a nurse deviates from approved policies, procedures, or standards, the risk for being accused of malpractice or negligence increases. However, before legal action is taken, the plaintiff must demonstrate that the event caused some form of injury.

Documentation of care delivered serves as legal evidence when legal action is taken against nurses. Nurses must know the importance of documenting all work and the processes used when providing nursing care. Meticulous documentation of events enables the nurse to present a highly professional image and serves as one of the best defense resources during legal actions. When on the witness stand, the nurse must be able to formulate and present to others the theoretical and scientific bases for the judgment exercised in the performance of the role by indicating the depth and breadth of nursing science and of educational preparation.

In addition to legal accountability, nurses must be able to formulate and present to others the ethical code or value system to which they refer when making judgments and using knowledge. They must answer the questions from consumers and others of "Why did you do that?" and "How did you come to that decision?" and "What makes you believe that is the most effective course of action?" In addition, nurses must give responses to these questions without becoming defensive. Consumers have the right to know about all aspects of their nursing care and nurses who are truly professionals have the responsibility to know and provide the answers.

As knowledgeable professionals, nurses share accountability for the nation's health care delivery system with other health team members (Lane, 1985). When nurses blame others, such as physicians, administrators, or politicians, for the state of the health care delivery system or constantly look to others to improve the system, nurses weaken their position and power base. By accepting an appropriate degree of responsibility for the current situation and actively pursuing methods of improving it, nurses act on a more professional level and make their claim for a piece of the health care pie.

Nursing also is accountable to the public in guarding against ill-prepared coworkers being certified to give nursing care under the guise of a new category of health care worker (Wilkerson, 1988). Unlicensed assistive personnel, such as nursing technicians, currently provide complex nursing care. During times of nurse shortages and cost containment, some hospitals provide brief (4- to 6-week) training programs for unlicensed workers to prepare them to assume complex nursing care tasks. In some cases, the quality of care has been seriously compromised.

Considering pain as a fifth vital sign and delegating pain assessment to unlicensed personnel serves as an example of how nursing assessment may be compromised, resulting in potential client harm. Nurses must raise their collective voice to educate and inform the public about the dangers of designating nursing responsibilities to unlicensed personnel. Nurses also need to question and protest against policies that delegate "nursing" to unlicensed personnel. Professional nurse accountability to the public means that nurses must work cohesively to assure safe client care.

## Accountability to the Profession

The profession of nursing exercises its accountability toward itself in the performance of its duty to formulate its own policy and control its activities. Professional nurses determine standards for nursing licensure (National Council of the State Boards of Nursing and individual State Boards of Nursing) and those that exist for entry into a variety of professional groups and associations (such as the Association of Operating Room Nursing & the American Association of Critical Care Nurses). In addition, membership on the National Council of State Boards of Nursing and individual State Boards of Nursing consist primarily of nurses who set nursing standards for nursing practice, professional conduct, and discipline.

In connection with this aspect of accountability, the individual nurse must understand the necessity of being aware of and accountable for not only the nurse's own actions, but also those of colleagues. Chemical abuse in nursing is a complex problem (Lillibridge, Cox, & Cross, 2002). Often the professional nurse may be the only one who is present to observe the behaviors of another nurse or the only one competent to evaluate a professional colleague's care. Although sharing apparent evidences of poor practice or substance abuse with the appropriate authorities (within the agency or outside) may not be an attractive course of action, nurses must do so because it sometimes is the only possible act that can ensure quality care for all clients. Nurses move toward functioning in a truly professional manner when members of a profession monitor their peers. Approaching the culpable individual first with the evidence of practice shortcomings or professional misconduct serves to emphasize the observing nurse's empathy for and concern about the person and eliminates the secrecy or spying aspect that is so detestable in current society.

## Research Brief 12-1

Lillibridge, J., Cox, M., & Cross, W. (2002). Uncovering the secret: Giving voice to the experiences of nurses who misuse substances. *Journal of Advanced Nursing, 39,* 219–229.

The investigators wanted insight into the experiences of nurses who had substance misuse problems. They conducted personal and telephone interviews with 12 Australian nurses known to have substance misuse problems.

The study identified the following five key themes: justification for substance misuse, fear of discovery of the problem, personal meanings of the significance of misuse, impact on professional colleagues, impact on the nursing career, and turning point for recovery. The nurses reported being masters at masking their problems from others. They also reported amazement that their colleagues failed to identify or confront the problem. During the recovery phase, the nurses reported lack of collegial caring and support as they were treated with suspicion of relapse upon initial re-entry into the practice setting.

Because the study results are based on findings from 12 Australian nurses, results must be cautiously interpreted. However, efforts must be made to educate nurses on the signs of substance abuse and how to best confront the situation when it arises. This should also include promotion of work environments that prevent stress leading to abuse and collegial support for nurses who re-enter the workforce after receiving treatment for substance abuse. More research is needed to determine factors that prevent nurses from confronting colleagues with substance misuse problems.

Along with reporting deficiencies in clinical practice, some nurses participate in regular peer review programs. Benefits of peer review include increased self-awareness of practice, quality of client care, professionalism, and accountability. The JCAHO recommends that nurses engage in peer review as part of professional practice (Roper & Russell, 1997).

Nurses also bear accountability for determining the desired educational level for entry into professional practice. Since 1965, the profession has debated the issue related to requiring the baccalaureate degree for entry into professional nursing. With increased emphasis on evidence-based practice, nurses must become cognizant of how to assess research quality before deciding whether to use results from a research study in practice. Because nurses educated in associate degree programs receive no education in the art of research critique, they lack this essential skill. However, associate degree–prepared nurses can learn research critique skills by attending university classes or continuing education programs devoted to this topic.

## Accountability to the Interdisciplinary Health Care Team

As a professional in the interdisciplinary health care team, nurses have accountability for the unique contributions they make to client care. The nurse often spends more time with the client than any other health team member. Nurses who engage in holistic nursing care consider more than just client physiologic needs; they also identify psychological, sociocultural, and spiritual needs. Many times nurses identify obstacles for client self-care by spending time assessing, teaching, and evaluating client and family responses to what they need to know before discharge.

For example, when working on a rehabilitation unit, one nurse was caring for an elderly woman who was going to perform glucose self-monitoring at home. The diabetes nurse educator who provided the basic instructions on the procedure documented that the woman could effectively perform required tasks. However, 2 days before the client was to be discharged, the nurse observed that the woman failed to have the manual dexterity to manipulate the glucose monitoring equipment, the vision to read the results, and the fine hand control to record the results. The nurse inquired about the woman's discharge living arrangements and discovered she would be living alone and no family members would be available to assist with glucose monitoring. When noting the problem, the professional nurse had an obligation to document this information and share it with the woman's case manager, who then arranged home health care.

This example shows how professional nurses are accountable for sharing client information with other health team members and how in doing so, they fulfill obligations to the client system. In addition, the proactive steps taken by the nurse in this situation may have prevented poor blood glucose control for the client or an admission to an acute care hospital, thereby reducing health care costs for the consumer, third-party payer, or government.

## Accountability to Self

Although professional people perhaps display more commitment to their careers, they sometimes can be exploited by systems in which they work. In the early days of the profession, hospitals and clients expected nurses to live on the premises in which they work. Unlike the days of old, agencies no longer assume ownership of nurses and do not expect them to work long hours without breaks. Employers and clients see nurses as free and independent persons with multiple facets to life other than their professional role.

However, sometimes the job situation may cause nurses and others to overlook these basic facts. Staff shortages may keep nurses from fulfilling their basic needs for nutrition and elimination. In addition, nurses' other life roles may often affect professional performance. Therefore, nurses must be accountable to themselves for their actions both on and off the job because of the potential effects of their actions on themselves and others.

The nurse who appears for work still experiencing the effects of too much celebrating on days off may not be prepared to function as a safe professional. Fatigue, jet lag, minor illness, exhaustion, or the effects of alcohol or drugs make the nurse a liability, rather than an asset, in the work situation. Professional practice also may be hampered by nurses who put in too much overtime; allow themselves to be placed in a position far beyond their abilities and knowledge; and function in a constantly and highly stressed state. These nurses may find themselves too exhausted or unprepared to function ineffectively in professional and personal roles.

Significant others cannot always be expected to have lower priority than one's work, whereas work cannot always be expected to take second place to social and personal relationships. Nurses need to attain a certain balance. Overdoing the amount of time and energy expected on the job often leads to burnout, with the nurse becoming incapable of or unwilling to do adequate work. Burnout also may take a toll on personal and social lives (Chaska, 1983).

The nurse's accountability to self comes across clearly. Nurses must assume responsibility for their own physical, mental, and spiritual health by maintaining a balanced lifestyle. They must decide when to give more energy to work and when to devote more energy to other life areas. When nurses sacrifice wholeness of life, they lose capacity for optimal functioning as professionals and people. They must function at fullest capacity when on the job and yet set a pace to avoid despair and fatigue that come when the throttle is constantly at full speed ahead.

The nurse's accountability to self includes refusing to work in situations deemed unsafe. Each nurse defines unsafe situations individually. Some examples of unsafe practice situations include lack of knowledge or experience to work in an unfamiliar specialty area and insufficient staffing. Nurses must learn to see refusal to work in unsafe situations as the ultimate professional service to the consumer despite potential sanctions that may be applied as consequences for this action.

Accountability to self also involves acknowledging one's own limitations and knowing when additional education or assistance from other is needed for effective client care. Decisions by others must not guide a nurse's action. Questioning physician orders may sometimes require courage, but it protects both client and nurse. Deciding when to assume a new nursing position (such as promotion to a nurse manager) should be based on each nurse's appraisal of personal qualifications for the job rather than the opinion of other persons. Completing an academic degree (such as a bachelor's degree in nursing) does not automatically prepare all nurses to assume a managerial role. Other factors such as personality, job description, and career goals also play a role before an administrative position is assumed.

Because nursing and agency administration make decisions related to daily operations, professional nurses sometimes do not have full control over practice situations. Many agencies carry insurance policies to protect themselves when client care errors and other accidents occur. If professional nurses become involved in incidents in which client harm has occurred, the agency may support them or may use them as scapegoats. Accountability to self involves protecting oneself against financial loss should an unforeseen incident occur. Table 12-1 presents reasons for lawsuits filed against professional nurses. Client suits against nurses fall into two main categories: failing to do what is expected, and doing what is not expected (Aiken, 2003). Sometimes, a slight omission in documentation can precipitate legal action when harm comes to clients in a nurse's care. Table 12-2 presents arguments for and against purchasing individual professional liability insurance. Professional liability insurance pays for individual nurse legal defense costs should he/she be named in a malpractice suit. Liability coverage also pays damages to an injured party if the nurse is found negligent. As supervisors and coordinators of client care, the nurse may be held accountable for actions of unlicensed personnel, nursing assistants, other nurses, and clerical staff (Helm & Kihm, 2001; Croke, 2003.)

The average cost for $1,000,000 of professional liability insurance coverage is less than $90 a year (Helm & Kihm, 2001). Coverage terms vary according to type of policy

TABLE 12-1

## Reasons for Nurse Malpractice Suits

| Reason | Example |
| --- | --- |
| Failure to document | Procedures, medications, and physician interactions not documented are considered not done in a court of law |
| Therapy error | Incorrect medication or treatment |
| Failure to follow standards of care | Using alternative treatments or procedures and/or failing to follow guidelines outlined by institutional policy and procedure manuals |
| Communication failure | Not listening intently to client concerns, inaccurate discharge instructions, not notifying a physician in a timely manner |
| Omitted assessment | Not performing routine assessments for various medical conditions or procedures, or forgetting to document a required assessment |
| Forgetting to be a client advocate | Not questioning physician orders when needed or not providing a safe environment |
| Breach of confidentiality | Sharing of private information with others |
| Invasion of privacy | Failure to provide drapes for procedures requiring physical exposure |
| Release of medical information without permission | Failure to get written permission from clients when sharing medical information with others |
| Assault and battery | Performing invasive procedures without client-informed consent |
| False imprisonment | Inappropriate use of physical or chemical restraint |
| Discrimination | Unequal treatment based on particular group membership or specific disease |
| Defamation | Harming the reputation of another person |
| Slander | Saying false statements or misrepresentations that harm the reputation of another |
| Libel | Any written or oral statement or other representation published without just cause for the purpose of exposing another to public contempt |

Adapted from Helm & Kihm (2001); and Croke (2003).

purchased. Claims-made policies cover the nurse for the time when the plaintiff files a court claim. In contrast, occurrence policies cover the nurse for the time in which the situation happened that resulted in litigation. The nurse should know which type of policy he or she carries. When a nurse has claims-made coverage, the policy needs to be active until all chance of litigation has expired. Each state determines the time when persons can file legal claims for health care providers for undesirable care outcomes.

The nurse's accountability to self was tested dramatically in the late 1980s and 1990s with the advent of the human immunodeficiency virus (HIV) epidemic. Some nurses expressed great fear, and some even refused to provide care for persons with HIV. To protect health care workers, health care agencies and the Center for Disease Control, established universal precaution guidelines. Despite these efforts, some nurses contracted

TABLE 12-2

## Reasons for and Against Nurses Carrying Individual Liability Insurance

| Reasons For | Reasons Against |
| --- | --- |
| Employer language may cover the facility but not individual employees. | Attitude of being not at risk for malpractice |
| Employer policies may be insufficient to cover all claims, leaving the nurse responsible for the amount that exceeds the facility policy limits. | Perceived adequate coverage from employer |
| Hospital insurer might seek indemnity from nurse after lawsuit is settled. | Clients may file malpractice claims several years after an incident, and the nurse may change jobs, or the facility could close or change its malpractice policy. |
| Personal policies provide legal defense for the nurse, and some include costs for time off work and transportation during legal proceedings. | Nurse could be caught in a facility's decision to side with a physician during legal proceedings, holding the nurse responsible for malpractice. |
| Facility policy may have coverage gaps. | Perception that carrying own insurance policy increases the likelihood of being sued. |
| Most jurors assume nurses carry individual liability insurance. | |

Adapted from Helm & Kihm (2001).

HIV. With meticulous use of appropriate precautions, nurses are able to effectively prevent transmission of the disease to their patients; however, nurses with HIV also must be aware of the danger to themselves of secondary infections and adjust work time, setting, and duties accordingly. Sometimes the nurse encounters situations when accountability to the public and self overlap. When this happens, nurses must recognize when they are too ill (or incapable) to continue to practice safely and remove themselves from client care.

Finally, nurses are accountable to themselves to do their own personal best (Styles, 1985). Factors outside nursing can influence this aspect of accountability. Government can aid or hinder nurses' abilities to do their best through legislation, funding (or lack of it) of health care, education and research, reimbursement policies, and health care priorities. Managed care networks and third-party payers strive to provide health care services to subscribers at the least possible cost. The nurse must consider political activism a means to the end of accountability to self, as a method of bringing public policy and the most expert care into congruence.

## Accountability to the Employing Agency

Yet another domain of the nurse's accountability is the agency in which that nurse is employed. Employees, even those with professional status, have responsibilities and must answer for actions taken on the job. Although not unimportant, accountability to the agency rightfully takes a back seat to the client, public, profession, and nurses themselves.

A health care agency is accountable to the public for the care provided under its auspices. Agency administration must verify that they have competent persons providing health care to consumers. Thus, the agency has the right to expect the nurse to be accountable to that agency. The following section discusses how the nurse is accountable to the employing agency.

## Quality of Work

The agency holds nurses accountable for the quality of work (nursing care). This includes their preparation for the job and their fitness each time they report for work. The agency has contracted with nurses for a specific job to be done at a specific time and place for a specific wage. Nurses must uphold their end of the bargain in all of these areas. They also have accountability for the nature of the performance of their peers. In addition, professional nurses are accountable for those whom they supervise in the work setting and must be aware of what they are doing and how they are doing it, to exercise that accountability.

## Unsafe Practice Situations

Recent legislation has resulted in legal protection for nurses who report unsafe practice situations. Sometimes the agency may refuse to correct what the nurses perceive as an unsafe practice situation. Nurses must refuse to work in areas and situations that they consider unsafe. This further fulfills accountability to the agency (as well as self) because such nurses are saying, in effect, "I will not put the agency in the position of giving unsafe care." However, sometimes refusal to provide client care as designated by terms of employment may result in dismissal from the agency.

## Attitude Conveyed About Agency

An additional aspect of the nurse's accountability to the agency involves the attitude toward that agency that the nurse projects to clients. The attitude should be one of objectivity and honesty. Nurses who find joy in working for a particular agency may appropriately and honestly promote the agency's strengths. However, if confronted with an agency shortcoming, nurses must be honest in their responses. Sometimes, in the heat of the moment, when particularly taxed or following a disagreement, a nurse may denigrate an agency. In this case, the nurse has not acted maturely and has no awareness of the impact of such statements on the client, visitors, or the agency.

## Use of Outside Agency Personnel

Concerns have arisen recently regarding accountability to the employer because of a large and growing number of nurses employed by nursing agencies and then essentially "rented" to hospitals on a per-diem basis. In most cases, agency nurses possess high levels of clinical competence. However, they may be unfamiliar with an employing institution's policies and procedures. Some agency nurses rely on nurses who are employed by the institution to help them access information and guide them through institutionally set care standards. Agency nurses may have more accountability to the nursing agency, thus diminishing some of the support they might be offering the hospital, or they feel primarily accountable to the hospital and wish to provide effective client care. When the allegiance to the employing institution supersedes that to the agency, the nurses may run the risk of being dropped by the agency.

Nurses have, for too long, maintained their accountability to their employing agency above their accountability to all others. This has detracted from a desirable image of nurses as working primarily in the public interest and instead has fostered the impression of the nurse as being subservient to and totally under the control of the employing institution. Now is the time to fully recognize and implement nursing's accountability toward its primary foci (the client and public, the profession, and the self) without losing sight of the nurse's accountability toward the employing agency.

## The Groundwork for Accountability

From this description of accountability, it should be evident that this professional attribute requires intense preparation and does not magically appear. It is necessary to provide a substantive service about which to be accountable and to possess a variety of skills and attributes that enable one to exercise that accountability. A definite foundation or groundwork must be in place.

## Research and the Establishment of a Theoretical Base for Nurse Accountability

One of the major factors in the accelerating pace of nursing's movement toward professional status is the growth of its theoretical and conceptual base for practice. It is this growth that allows the nurse to be truly accountable in this technological and scientific era (Copp, 1988). Theory-based knowledge is now available in some practice areas and will be available increasingly in others as the result of nursing research.

However, nurses in practice must use knowledge generated through research to substantiate nursing actions. Research demonstrates that professional nursing care makes a difference in the lives of clients. Doran (2003) identifies the following nursing-sensitive client outcomes: functional status, self-care ability, symptom control, safety, adverse occurrences, and client satisfaction. Nurses have access to online and printed research findings. However, finding time to read and analyze nursing research results poses a dilemma for many nurses. Some nurses (especially those educated in associate degree programs) have received no formal education on how to evaluate research findings for use in practice.

The dissemination of nursing research results to practicing nurses occurs very slowly. Some nurses use research findings to develop clinical practice policies and procedures. With the advent of evidenced-based practice and quality improvement initiatives, the use of research findings has become more desirable and acceptable in many practice settings.

Among the reasons for limited use of nursing research in practice is the inability of many nurses to comprehend and evaluate the research studies they may read. These professional nurses desperately need help to understand available research reports and apply the findings to work situations. Some health care agencies have nursing research committees and offer resources to help nurses use research findings in practice. These can be provided under the auspices of staff development departments, nursing associations, continuing education departments, or degree programs. However, until nurses and health care organizations value nursing research use, nurses will continue to practice on the basis of tradition.

## Clinical and Professional Competence

The public, consumers, health care agencies and physicians expect nurses to have clinical competence. Different specialty areas of practice have different knowledge and skills for competent practice. However, all areas of practice require that nurses understand and apply principles and techniques of asepsis, physical assessment, nursing process, pathophysiology, pharmacology, human growth and development, psychology, sociology, spirituality, and safety. Because all nurses hold their clients' lives in their hands, whatever a nurse does, it must be done well.

Currently, with many levels of nursing being reflected in the composition of the health care team, nurses at each level should have a clear idea of the scope of practice at their level, and responsibly perform to the maximum limit of that level. The nurse's accountability may be called into question if he or she is functioning beyond the scope of practice at a particular level. It is no more appropriate for nurses who have been educated at the baccalaureate level to restrict professional activities to those they may have exercised at the associate degree level than it is for them to assume the role of the master's-prepared practitioner.

The key to expertise in practice lies in both knowledge and skill, a somewhat artificial distinction that nevertheless allows for more clarity in this discussion. Nursing has always had a strong manual skills component. To the extent that the nurse is in a role that calls for these skills, activity, gentleness, quickness, and accuracy remain hallmarks of excellence. Where the skills required are in the areas of communication, teaching, leadership, management, and research (the so-called hands-off skills), the matter of expertise is no less pressing.

Underlying all skills is excellence in terms of command of "nursing knowledge." Nurses can never expect to contribute significantly to health care in its assessment, planning, implementation, and evaluation aspects if they do whatever they do in a mediocre manner. Competence is an absolute prerequisite for accountability.

## Leadership Skills

Leadership development frequently brings questions and puzzlement when first introduced to nursing students. A frequent response is, "Not everyone can be a head nurse or a supervisor, or wants to be an instructor. I don't want to be a leader; I just want to be a nurse." The fact is that the elements of leadership are inherent in the nurse role.

Leadership ability is one of the most important areas in laying the groundwork for accountability. The nurse's accountability extends into the areas of health maintenance and promotion, as well as the area of promoting self-care by the ill as long as possible. The nurse is a constant catalyst in the process of change, at this highly individual level at the very least, especially if she or he is "just" a nurse.

To satisfactorily fulfill the leadership portion of the role, a nurse must be well versed in the theory and practice of change, which is practically synonymous with saying a nurse must be able to exercise leadership. Nurses are leaders in working with patients, their families, and significant others. They are leaders with regard to health care in contacts with friends and acquaintances in the community. They are leaders in performing and making certain that they are permitted to perform their roles as professionals involved in health promotion, maintenance, and restoration. Accountable nurses cannot function without leadership skills.

## Ethical Framework

Nurses are accountable within an ethical framework. They cannot be accountable in a moral vacuum. They must have as their guide standards and values in which they believe and to which they refer. To some extent, these are determined by the collective values of the profession, and these, in turn, are partly determined by what the public expects of that profession and partly by what the profession demands of itself.

In nursing, these professional values are formalized by the *Code of Ethics for Nurses* (ANA, 2001). However, in large measure, this ethical code is a personal one, developed in the course and context of the individual's total life experience. It includes values learned in the home, in schools, from social groups, during religious training, in the work setting, and from the activities and contacts of daily life. It is influenced by the nurse's ethnic and religious background, the area of the country in which he or she lives, and the nurse's personality. It is highly individual.

A person's ethical code often is something of which he or she is relatively unaware. It is unconsciously used in making decisions and running one's life, but is rarely, if ever, pulled out and scrutinized or even acknowledged as existing. It is this code that is so essential in the professional nurse. A nurse must be aware of his or her code, how it affects decisions and actions, and where it is congruent with or departs from standard codes of the profession. Thus, these conflicts must be worked through and compromise sought so that the nurse can feel comfortable with and confident in the ethical basis in which the practice is rooted.

## Baccalaureate Nursing Education and Beyond

It is obvious from the discussion thus far on laying the groundwork for accountability that this is neither a simple nor a short-term task. Accountability cannot be accomplished in a weekend or, for most individuals, on one's own. Rather, it is a task that continues over a long time, during which various ideas are explored, analyzed, tested, and absorbed into the individual's make-up. It is a task that is partially contributed to, at times guided by, and discussed and shared with others. It is a task most ideally accomplished within the context of a higher education (Hegyvary, 1991).

Although most educational programs in nursing are based on a conceptual framework, baccalaureate programs devote significant time to understanding some of the outstanding conceptual and theoretical frameworks for nursing practice, and examining the relationship between these frameworks and the research process. The research course often included in a baccalaureate program provides an opportunity for learning how to read research, adequately evaluate it, and judge its potential applicability within a work setting. When nurses can knowledgeably read and interpret research findings, then they can use them to improve practice. Referral to and use of research findings increases professional nurse accountability.

Leadership truly comes into its own in the baccalaureate and higher degree programs. In nursing programs located in institutions of higher learning, students learn about styles of leadership behavior, health care delivery systems, the economics of health care, characteristics of bureaucracies, and change theory. They also receive a liberal education that helps them not only to communicate more effectively with other, more highly educated health team members, but also to have the resources for living out a balanced life. Here nurses, who in practice may already be in leadership positions, learn how to function more effectively and with more accountability in their professional nursing roles, and how to inculcate greater levels of accountability in staff. They also learn about the basics of institutional accountability (or lack of it) regarding the care they and others provide. Finally, in collegiate nursing programs, they work with and analyze the professional behavior of leaders in nursing, role models from whom they can learn accountability—for it is a learned behavior (Clifford, 1981).

Finally, in the area of ethics and values, nurses attending university level programs can and are encouraged to contemplate their value systems, to uncover such systems, and to see their relationship to practice and to the other aspects of life. Through the liberalizing influence of baccalaureate and higher degree programs, nurses learn about different value systems and how other nurses have sought to make their ethical codes complementary to those of the profession.

In summary, it takes all of what the nurse is and does as a person to prepare for functioning in an accountable manner (Lanara, 1982). It is a lifelong process engaged in with others in both structured and unstructured ways and is interwoven with the nurse's preparation as a professional person.

## ✦ ACCOUNTABILITY IN AN ERA OF COST CONTAINMENT

Health care costs continue to outpace the inflationary rate of other goods and services. Prospective payment systems serve as the major reimbursement method for many health care services. Public support for imposing controls on costs for health care continues to increase. Managed care has rapidly expanded and may soon become the primary mode of delivering cost-effective health care. Health care practices deemed to be effective will be increased and retained while those determined to be ineffective will be decreased or discarded. Professional nurses must substantiate the benefits they provide to health care consumers.

All too often in health care, "effective" seems to mean "cost-effective." The idea of a universal right to top quality care for all is being diluted to a standard of adequate care to those who meet specific criteria set by third-party payers. Nurses are now asked to be accountable for the care they give and for giving that care in the least expensive manner possible, often in a setting or time frame severely limiting the comprehensiveness of that care.

### The Unlicensed Health Care Worker

Professional nurses (registered nurses [RNs]) have always been held accountable for the work performed by those with lower level credentials whom they supervise, such as the licensed practical/vocational nurse and the nurse's aide. In the past, these workers performed functions that, for the most part, the RN felt were within the workers' range of capability, had little potential for client harm, and for which their relatively short training programs had adequately prepared them. However, in the current climate of cost containment and the looming nursing shortage, more unlicensed workers are assuming functions once reserved for professional and licensed nurses. The nursing technician, nursing assistant, or unlicensed assistive personnel currently receives training to perform functions and skills that have the potential to harm clients. Some RNs express great concern at having these workers perform "under" the RN's license, carrying out the implementation phase of many complex nursing functions without having the concomitant assessment or evaluation skills to maintain client safety.

However, when more closely examined, this situation is not very different from the past. The unlicensed worker has always worked under the supervision of a professional nurse who has always performed the assessment and evaluation aspects of care. The RN has always instructed the unlicensed worker as to who needed care and when. The RN has always been accountable for the care given.

In addition, the unlicensed worker has always been accountable for proper performance of assigned duties and for knowing when other workers must be consulted for situations determined to be beyond the limits of the worker's knowledge and training. Unlicensed workers must earn the trust of the professional nurse. Although the legal doctrine of respondeat superior (let the superior answer) still applies, unlicensed workers do bear some accountability for their actions.

Thus, principles that have guided nursing care for years still apply. The RN is still accountable for the client's overall care. However, the current situation requires that the RN broaden the scope of supervision and be more vigilant. The RN must be more aware of the unlicensed worker's abilities and activities while increasing availability for consultation. The concept of accountability for self and others must be made clear to every prospective nurse and reinforced for the new graduate nurse. After all, accountability is a hallmark of professional activity.

## Managed Care and Third-Party Payers

Managed care has been seen by some as the mode of health care delivery that will monitor access to services, eliminate redundancy, reduce overuse of services, and control health care costs. Managed care companies rather than nurses and other health care professionals make decisions related to health care delivery. Those without the appropriate knowledge base or with cost containment focus actually determine the type and amount of health care consumers receive.

With managed care, the nurse's role as a client advocate becomes vital. The nurse advocate pays attention to and acts in instances in which clients are being denied access to essential care or seem to be short-changed by policies and actions directed primarily at cost containment (Aroskar, 1992; Stevens, 1992). The issue of access to care has been a legitimate one for nurses to address for years, as succinctly stated in the *Code of Ethics for Nurses*:

The nurse assumes the responsibility and accountability for individual nursing judgments and actions. . . . The nurse collaborates with members of the health professions and other citizens in promoting community and national efforts to meet the health needs of the public (ANA, 2001, p. 1).

This notion has been reiterated and emphasized by its inclusion in the ANA's *Nursing Policy Statement* (1995) and *Nursing's Agenda for Health Care Reform* (1991b). There can be no doubt that the nurse's accountability extends into exerting efforts to respond to the health care needs of the public in a collective sense.

Along with doing what is right for clients, nurses play a key role in reimbursement to the employing agency from managed care and other third-party payers. Meticulous documentation of all supplies and interventions provides evidence that consumers received care. Third-party payers frequently audit charts in efforts to disallow charges appearing on consumer bills.

## ⬤ ACCOUNTABILITY IN THE FUTURE

The future relies on current actions. The nursing profession has renewed its interest in accountability and practice changes have occurred to increase nurse accountability.

Nurses have assumed control of practice by adopting **shared governance** models that increase nurse participation in shaping professional practice. Nurses assume responsibility and accountability for developing unit-based and institutional-wide procedures for clinical practice and quality improvement.

The JCAHO has added quality improvement and reporting of sentinel events as criteria for accreditation. Because quality improvement efforts require that the persons engaged in the work develop work processes and monitor effectiveness, nurses become more active in devising and evaluating activities that fall within the realm of professional nursing. Instead of being used as punishment, incident reports provide clues to needed changes in work processes. Health care delivery (especially in hospitals) relies on many team members to execute physician orders. Each member of the health team makes a contribution and all assume accountability for actions.

Advanced technology has provided the means for nursing to become more accountable. Using technology, nursing can clearly show what it does: the care it delivers, its cost and outcomes. Nursing must be rescued from burial in the category of "room and board" in budgets and on client bills. Once nursing services departments control their budgets, they will be empowered to make decisions and be accountable for them.

Nurses must ultimately decide that for which they want to be accountable. How much will nurses shoulder individually and as a group (Hegyvary, 1991)? The concept of ownership has entered the scene. Jackson (1989) suggests that nurses do not take on problems that do not belong to them. Jackson also proposes that nurses must improve the quality of nursing care by assuming ownership of all aspects of care (including menial tasks). However, the recent thrust toward more multidisciplinary cooperation, planning, documentation, action, and evaluation may cloud attempts to define that area for which nurses, and nurses alone, are truly accountable. Nursing may have to learn to be accountable within a more ambiguous, multidisciplinary framework.

## ⬤ CHECKLIST FOR ACCOUNTABILITY

Preparation for accountability for action requires that nurses evaluate personal actions periodically. The following questions serve as an **accountability checklist** for nurse self-assessment of professional accountability. The list is not all-inclusive; but offers a beginning tool for working the concept of accountability into one's life and work.

### Accountability to the Client

- Am I providing the best care of which I am capable?
- Is that care sufficient to meet the needs of the client in this situation?

- Is this client entitled to more than I can offer, and am I turning elsewhere to obtain the needed, additional dimension?
- Am I incorporating what I know of nursing theory and research into my practice in this situation?
- Am I using my leadership skills to encourage others to function at their optimal ability levels in the care of this patient?
- Am I acting in accordance with my own ethical code and that of the profession?
- If, by meeting the needs of this client, am I in conflict with my personal ethical code, and am I seeking some alternative method or person to satisfy those needs?
- Have I given clients information that they want or need to know about their health status, while considering the effect on them of that knowledge?

## Accountability to the Public

- Am I seeking to improve health and nursing care?
- Am I speaking out against abuses I see in health and nursing care?
- Am I acting as a community resource in the areas of health and nursing?
- Am I remaining an active and contributing member of the profession after using public funds to finance my education?
- Am I attempting to increase the knowledge of the public to enable it to make more knowledgeable choices about health and nursing care?
- Am I recruiting others to enter the profession to have future health care needs of the clients met?

## Accountability to the Profession

- Am I fulfilling my professional role in accordance with the requirements of the profession?
- Are other nurses in my setting doing the same?
- If I am not performing satisfactorily, or if others are not, am I taking steps to remedy that situation?
- Am I willing to help other nurses in my work setting?
- Am I a participant in professional meetings, organizations, seminars, conferences, and so forth, so that I may express my views on nursing to those in nursing?
- Am I working within the profession to improve practice, education, or research?
- Am I complying with the ethical code of the profession?

## Accountability to Self

- Am I satisfied with my chosen profession?
- Am I performing my professional role in the best way I can?
- Should I seek additional preparation for that role?
- Should I withdraw from that role until I receive additional preparation?
- In areas where I am dissatisfied, am I seeking alternative modes of action or thought?
- Am I comfortable, ethically, with the way in which I am performing my professional role?
- Am I shortchanging my patients, my significant others, or myself in the way I am performing my professional role?

- Do I have adequate financial protection for myself and family if I were to be involved in a professional litigation case?
- Am I satisfied with the position this role assumes within my total lifestyle?

## Accountability to the Agency

- Am I performing in accordance with the job description for the position for which I was employed?
- If I am not satisfied with that job description, am I seeking appropriate ways to change it?
- Am I seeking to ensure that I am practicing under safe, if not optimal, conditions?
- Am I giving the institution its money's worth in terms of my work?
- Am I working in accordance with the policies and procedures of the institution?
- If I am not satisfied with those policies and procedures, am I seeking to change them using principles of leadership and change and with the total mission of the institution in mind?

Because of the magnitude of this checklist, only a super person could look through this checklist and confidently say he or she fulfills all criteria. Some activities are more appropriate than others for nurses in different settings and at different times. However, nurses who are to act in an accountable manner or increase the accountability of their decisions and actions must consider these and other questions. Those who wish to call themselves professional nurses must consider these questions to live a life of accountability.

## ⊛ SUMMARY AND SIGNIFICANCE TO PRACTICE

As changes in health care delivery occur, nursing accountability issues fluctuate. Because of its breadth and depth, professional accountability takes time to develop. As nurses achieve accountability in one aspect of practice, they can continuously extend their scope of accountability throughout an entire career.

### FROM THEORY TO PRACTICE

1. Review the vignette at the beginning of the chapter. List the persons who made mistakes in the care of Mr. Jones and the mistakes that they made. Who has accountability for their actions? How could this unfortunate incident been avoided? What steps should be taken by everyone involved in the incident to avoid repeating the same errors with a future patient?
2. Do I currently carry professional malpractice insurance? Why or why not?
3. Answer the questions contained in the chapter accountability checklist. Note areas for future growth in areas of accountability to the client, public, profession, self, and agency for which you work.
4. How are student accountabilities addressed in your professional nursing program? How are they communicated to students? What are the consequences for a student breach of accountability?

## WWW INTERNET EXERCISES

1. Visit the National Council of State Boards of Nursing website at http://www.ncsbn.org. Click on "About NCSBN" and read the NCSBN mission, vision, and purpose. Go back one screen. Click on "Boards of Nursing" to access your State Board of Nursing. Find your state in the list and click on the website address to discover specific information related to professional nursing in your state.

2. View a sample nurse's malpractice insurance policy by visiting the website of the Nurses Service Organization at www.nso.com. Click on the words "Professional Liability Insurance." Under Individuals, select either "Nurses" or "Student Nurses." Select your state. Then Click on NSO's Professional Liability Insurance Program to get a sample of terms of liability coverage from this professional liability insurance provider.

## WWW INTERNET RESOURCES

The American Nurses Association: www.nursingworld.org.
Code for Nurses with Interpretive Statements:
   http://www.nursingworld.org/ethics/code/protected_nwcoe303.htm.
International Council of Nurses: http://www.icn.ch/.
ICN Code of Ethics: http://www.icn.ch/icncode.pdf.
ICN Scope of Nursing Practice: http://www.icn.ch/psscope.htm.
Nurses Protection Group: http://nursesprotectiongroup.com.
American Association of Colleges of Nursing: http://www.aacn.nche.edu/.
National League for Nursing: http://www.nln.org.
National Council of State Boards of Nursing: http://www.ncsbn.org.
American Association of Legal Nurse Consultants: http://www.aalnc.org.
Medical-Legal Consulting: http://www.legalnurse.com.
Nurses Service Organization: http://www.nso.com.

## REFERENCES

Aiken, T. M. (2003). Nursing malpractice: Understanding the risks. *Travel Nursing 2003, 7*–12.

American Nurses Association (1991). *Nursing's agenda for health care reform*. Washington DC: Author.

American Nurses Association (1995). *Social policy statement*. Washington DC: Author.

American Nurses Association (ANA). (1997). *Scope and standards of college health nursing practice*. Washington, DC: American Nurses Publishing.

American Nurses Association. (2001). *Code of ethics for nurses with interpretive statements*. Washington, DC: American Nurses Publishing.

Aroskar, M. A. (1992). Ethical foundations in nursing for broad health care access. *Scholarly Inquiry for Nursing Practice, 6*, 201–205.

Batey, M. V., & Lewis, F. M. (1982). Clarifying autonomy and accountability in nursing service: Part 2. *Journal of Nursing Administration, 12*, 10–15.

Bergman, R. (1981). Accountability—definition and dimensions. *International Nursing Review, 28*, 53–59.

Bixler, G. K., & Bixler, R. W. (1959). The professional status of nursing. *American Journal of Nursing, 59*, 1142–1147.

Chaska, N. L. (1983). *The nursing profession: A time to speak*. New York: McGraw-Hill.

Clifford, J. C. (1981). Managerial control versus professional autonomy: A paradox. *Journal of Nursing Administration, 11*, 19–21.

Copp, G. (1988). Professional accountability: The conflict. *Nursing Times, 84*(3), 42–44.

Croke, E. M. (2003). Nurses, negligence and malpractice. *American Journal of Nursing, 103,* 54–64.

Dachelet, C. Z., & Sullivan, J. A. (1979). Autonomy in practice. *Nursing Practice, 4,* 15–16, 18–19.

Doran, D. (Ed.) (2003). *Nursing-sensitive outcomes: state of the science.* Sudbury, MA: Jones & Bartlett.

Flexner, A. (1915). Is social work a profession? In *Proceedings of the National Conference of Charities and Correction* (pp. 576–590). Chicago: Heldman.

Hegyvary, S. T. (1991). Education: Freedom and responsibility. *Journal of Professional Nursing, 7*(1), 8.

Helm, A., and Kihm, N. C. (2001). Is professional liability insurance for you? *Nursing, 31,* 48–49.

Holden, R. J. (1991). Responsibility and autonomous nursing practice. *Journal of Advanced Nursing, 16,* 398–403.

Hylka, S. C., & Beschle, J. C. (1995). Nurse practitioners, cost savings, and improved care in the department of surgery. *Nursing Economics, 13,* 349–354.

Hylka, S. C., & Shugrue, D. (1991). Increasing staff nurse autonomy. *Nursing Management, 22,* 54–55.

Iowa Nurses Association (1997). *Delegation decision-making grid.* Available at: http://www.ioanurses.org/grid.htm. Accessed June 30, 2005.

Jackson, B. S. (1989). Ownership imbalance. *Journal of Nursing Administration, 19,* 4–5.

Joint Commission on Accreditation of Healthcare Organizations (JCAHO). (1991). *Nursing cared accreditation manual for hospitals, 1991,* (p. 94). Chicago: Author.

Kopp, P. (2001). Fit for practice. Legal issues in accountability. *Nursing Times, 97*(5), 45–47.

Krueger-Wilson, C., & Porter-O'Grady, T. (1999). *Leading the revolution in health care: Advancing systems, igniting performance* (2nd ed.). Gaithersburg, MD: Aspen.

Lanara, V. A. (1982). Responsibility in nursing. *International Nursing Review, 29,* 7–10.

Lane, C. A. (1985). Exercising professional accountability. *Oncology Nursing, 12,* 12–14.

Lillibridge, J., Cox, M., & Cross, W. (2002). Uncovering the secret: Giving voice to the experiences of nurses who misuse substances. *Journal of Advanced Nursing, 39,* 219–229.

McGlothlin, W. J. (1961). The place of nursing among the professions. *Nursing Outlook, 9,* 214–216.

Merton, R. K. (1958). The functions of the professional association. *American Journal of Nursing, 58,* 50–54.

Nightingale, F. (1946). *Notes on nursing: What it is and what it is not.* Philadelphia: J. B. Lippincott (facsimile of 1st ed., London: Harrison & Sons, 1859).

Roper, K. A., & Russell, G. (1997). The effect of peer review on professionalism, autonomy and accountability. *Journal of Nursing Staff Development, 13,* 198–206.

Stevens, P. E. (1992). Who gets care? Access to health care as an arena for nursing action. *Scholarly Inquiry for Nursing Practice, 6,* 185–200.

Styles, M. (1985). Accountable to whom? *Nursing Mirror, 160,* 36–37.

Vaughn, B. (1989). Autonomy and accountability. *Nursing Times, 85*(3), 54–55.

Webb, S. S., Price, S. A., & Van Ess Coeling, H. (1996). Valuing authority/responsibility relationships. *Journal of Nursing Administration, 26,* 28–33.

Wilkerson, I. (1988, June 30). AMA backs new category of hospital workers. *New York Times,* p. B8.

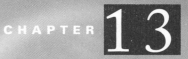
# Environmental and Global Health

## KEY TERMS AND CONCEPTS

Environment
Global Environment
Environmental Health
Ecocentric
Pollution
Environmental Surprises
Discontinuity
Extinct
Synergism
Unnoticed Trend
Positive Feedback
Cascading Effects
Multiple Chemical Sensitivity
Community Environment
Work Environment
Home Environment

## LEARNING OUTCOMES

By the end of this chapter, the learner will be able to:

1 Explain the role that the global, community, work, and home environments play in human health.

2 Identify elements within one's personal environment that are noxious to the global environment.

3 Identify factors within the environment that are health-promoting.

4 Integrate personal behaviors that foster a health-promoting environment.

5 Outline noxious environmental factors that may impair human health.

6 Relate environmental quality to the quality of human health.

## VIGNETTE

Emily has come to the emergency department of a teaching hospital reporting an intense headache and an inability to concentrate. As the triage and charge nurse, Barbara asks Emily questions related to her medical history. Emily states that she is allergic to a long list of medications, cleaning products, and foods. Emily begins to hyperventilate and whispers when responding to questions. Barbara becomes suspicious of all of Emily's allergies and seeming overdramatization of her symptoms and decides that Emily must be mentally ill. As Barbara searches for the pager number of the psychiatric resident, Emily's allergist arrives, orders epinephrine, and mentions that Emily has multiple chemical sensitivity syndrome, a rare disorder that the allergist says is becoming more prevalent in her practice.

Objects, conditions, and circumstances create the environment. Living organisms depend on the environment for formation and survival. Not all environments possess the capability of sustaining life. Multiple environmental systems must remain in balance to sustain life. For the purpose of this chapter, **"environment"** refers to the conditions by which one is surrounded (*Merriam-Webster's Collegiate Dictionary,* 1994). The environment consists of physical domains (air, water, soil) and social domains (land use, industry, housing, transportation, agriculture). Depending on the context, environments may be miniscule or enormous. The **global environment** refers to the conditions on the planet earth.

Humans rely on an external environment for air, water, and food. Within a systems framework, interacting groups create a unitary whole. When the balance is altered, the unitary whole experiences changes, some of which may lead to destruction of life. How persons use the physical environment results in exposure to health hazards, such as accidents, chemical exposures, violence, and psychological distress (United States Department of Health and Human Services, 2000). **Environmental health** refers to conditions in the environment that preserve the balance of nature. This chapter examines the effects of the global, local community, working, and home environments on human health and offers strategies for professional nurses to create a sustainable future.

## ✦ THE GLOBAL ENVIRONMENT

Florence Nightingale linked environmental quality to the health of soldiers during the Crimean War. As a diligent supporter of germ theory, her writings emphasized the importance of cleanliness and adequate ventilation with fresh air to prevent mortality and promote healing and disproved conventional nursing practices of her time (Dock, 1912). In Victorian times, persons tended to look at local, rather than global, environmental conditions. Nurses lost Nightingale's passion for the environment as they developed the profession and as women fought for equal social status (Kleffel, 1994). In the 1970s and 1980s, nurses again included the environment as part of nursing theories. Fawcett (1984) delineated environment as an essential element when developing a metaparadigm for nursing (man, health, environment nursing). Definitions of the environment depend on the philosophical stance of each theorist. Rogers, Leddy, and Newman define the environment as an energy field. However, Watson, Neuman, and Roy define the environment as an open system. Neuman further separates the environment into internal and external domains that interact with each other. Humans have come to know much more about the environment through the advancement of scientific technology. When the world saw pictures of the earth from outer space, people acknowledged the interconnectedness of nations and how regulations (or lack of them) could potentially affect everyone. The future of human civilization relies on a safe and clean environment. As people realize the importance of the environment on human health, an **ecocentric** (the perspective of the environment as being whole, interconnected, and alive) approach to health care delivery becomes a societal priority (Kleffel, 1996). The professional nurse needs to understand principles related to exposure sources, dosage, and toxicity to appreciate the complexity of the environmental impact on human health (Green, 2000).

The earth is a delicate planet that has the conditions to support many varieties of life. Balanced ecosystems provide the resources to sustain life. Most of the time, humans cause environmental **pollution** from waste products from manufacturing products, energy production, or burning wood or petroleum products; chemicals used to control pests (animals, insects, or plants); and widespread use of plastic products. Pollution disrupts the usual natural balance. When the balance becomes disturbed, **environmental surprises** emerge. Bright (2000) identifies the following three forms of environmental surprises: discontinuity, synergism, and unnoticed trends. An abrupt shift in a trend or steady state constitutes a **discontinuity.** Forest habitat loss causes some animals to seek refuge elsewhere or travel to human populated areas for food. The species (e.g., bears) becomes a menace to persons by scouring human garbage cans for food; local governments spend money to control them; some people get harmed, and in extreme cases, the species becomes endangered or **extinct** (ceases to exist). Simultaneous changes in several natural phenomena with greater-than-expected environmental effects define **synergism.** The combined effects of a heavy rainstorm, cutting trees on a hillside, and people moving to an identified flood plane resulting in a catastrophe with a high human death toll is an example of a synergism. An **unnoticed trend** develops when an event occurs undetected but does considerable damage to an ecosystem. Nonnative weed invasion of fertile farm acreage in the United States displaced native plants that facilitated the balance of natural fire cycles that destroyed 9,884 acres of farmland during a 30-year period before it was detected. To further complicate the earth's balance, synergisms can produce discontinuities (ozone depletion combined with acid rain and other atmospheric aerosols results in increased depth penetration of ultraviolet radiation in water, which results in the destruction of microorganisms essential for the survival of coral reefs and fish). Alternatively, discontinuities can produce synergisms, such as pesticide-resistant insects carrying plant viruses that destroy crops (Bright, 2000).

Along with the three types of environmental surprises, positive feedback loops can create discontinuities. In a **positive feedback** loop, the cycle of change continues to amplify itself. Global warming provides a prime example of the positive feedback loop. The Arctic ice cap is melting as the result of global warming. Even a thick ice cap absorbs only 10% of the sunlight, and the ocean absorbs the rest. As the ice mass dwindles, the ocean becomes warmer, which results in even faster warming (Bright, 2000).

In addition to positive feedback loops, cascading effects occur, leading to more environmental changes. **Cascading effects** happen when a change in one component of a system results in a change in another component, which sets up a change in yet another component, with multiple changes occurring throughout various components. Cascading effects can produce discontinuities and synergisms. The Alaskan coastline provides an example of a cascading effect. When the Alaskan perch and herring population declined, sea lions and seals starved. As the population of sea lions and seals declined, killer whales had to resort to finding new prey to survive. The sea otter was the ideal candidate. However, the sea otter feasted on sea urchin. As the sea urchin population exploded, they demolished kelp forests. Now, many species of fish, marine invertebrates, marine mammals, and birds are at risk because they rely on kelp for food (Bright, 2000).

Brown (2000) identifies seven key environmental trends that shape the future of humankind. These are a growing human population, rising global temperatures, falling water tables, declining croplands, diminishing fisheries, shrinking forest, and the loss of plant and animal species. The population is expected to increase from 6.1 billion to 8.9 billion by 2050. With increased carbon dioxide emissions from the Industrial Age, the global temperature has risen 44° Celsius (0.8° Fahrenheit) since 1969 and continues to rise, especially as people across the globe burn fossil fuels. China, India, North Africa, Saudi Arabia, and the United States continue to pump more water than what is returned from rain and melting snow.

The rising population creates more demand for food. Farmers overpump water for crops, and many industries (such as the paper industry) use enormous amounts of water for production. Crop and livestock production result in increased release of nitrogen and phosphorus into the atmosphere and trigger acid rain (Tilman et al., 2001). Trees become more susceptible to disease and damage from extreme temperatures associated with the effects of acid rain (Krajick, 2001). In addition, urban sprawl impinges on available cropland and results in deforestation.

Urbanization increases the consumption of fossil fuels that have been determined to contribute to global warming. Higher global temperatures result in increased ocean temperatures that destroy plankton and coral that fish rely on for survival (Barnett, Pierce, & Schnur, 2001). From 1957 to 1997, the annual oceanic fish catch increased by 71 million tons, from 19 to 90 million tons. Many marine biologists theorize that the ocean cannot sustain an annual fish catch of more than 95 million tons (O'Meara, 2000). In addition, rising atmospheric carbon dioxide levels may be leading to increased ocean acidity, which may further deplete fish supplies (Feely et al., 2004).

As a global society, international efforts for global preservation have been formed by governmental, international, and private organizations. Governmental agencies and nongovernmental organizations frequently exert pressure on companies to clean up their acts. Ann Florini, an Environmental Protection Agency (EPA) official, dubs this approach "regulation by revelation." The EPA releases an annual Toxic Release Inventory, and the United States government offers incentives for companies to reduce pollution. Between 1970 and 1997, total emissions of air pollutants decreased 31% (United States Department of Health and Human Services, 2000). However, the planet requires a global effort to preserve conditions suitable for life (Bright, 2000; O'Meara, 2000). Tough national standards can be undermined by less vigorous standards abroad. Deforestation in South America and Asia results in local and global environmental changes. Wood burning in China results in acid rain in Japan (French, 2000).

American hospitals produce approximately 6,000 tons of medical waste per day. According to the Environmental Protection Agency, the health care industry is one of the major sources of mercury (found in medical equipment such as thermometers, sphygmomanometers, and endoscopes) and dioxin (from polyvinyl plastic materials) pollution.

Other pollutants attributed to health care organizations include dead batteries, old computers, hazardous chemicals (cleaning products), and pharmaceuticals (chemotherapy, radioactive isotopes) (Shaner & Botter, 2003).

In addition to formal governmental and international global efforts, nongovernmental organizations serve as environmental caretakers. Table 13-1 outlines several global environmental networks. Global networking among environmentalists provides the opportunity for global solutions to global problems. When environmental watchdog groups post information on the Internet, the information has the potential to reach a vast number of people (O'Meara, 2000). In addition to special interest groups, research universities such as the University of Michigan devote resources to ecosystem toxicology. By exploring microscopic changes in the environment, such as measuring the content of specific pesticides in marine life and avian eggshells, damage to the environment can be discovered before deformed animals are found and freshwater sources become hazardous to drink (Scully, 2001). Nurses can use information from these organizations to increase their awareness of global pollution, take steps to minimize pollution-promoting behaviors, and educate others about behaviors that may contribute to global pollution and destruction.

Environmental degradation indicates that the earth has undergone and is currently undergoing many changes as the result of human habitation. Ancient Greeks, Romans,

**TABLE 13-1**

## Global Environmental Organizations and Networks

| Organization/Network | Purpose | Website |
|---|---|---|
| Environmental Defense Fund | Monitors and communicates the status of the environment. Creates an online data scorecard that ranks facilities, revealing the most offending polluters | www.scorecard.org |
| Association for Progressive Communications | Links nongovernmental organizations that promote human rights and environmental concerns with each other | www.apc.org |
| OneWorld Online | Links many websites to provide information on economic development | www.oneworld.net |
| UNEPnet | United Nations Environmental Programme (UNEP) offices are linked with other partner institutions by satellite to improve the flow of environmental data | www.centre.nep.net |
| Global Urban Observatory | Links researchers to a global network of data, statistics, and examples of best practices in urban management | http://www.unhabitat.org/programmes/guo/ |
| HORIZON Solutions | Case studies on solutions related to water, waste, energy, transportation, toxic pollutants, public health, industrial, biodiversity, air pollution, and agricultural issues | www.solutions-site.org |

Adapted from O'Meara, M. (2000). Harnessing information technologies for the environment. In L. R. Brown, C. Flavin, H. French, S. Postel, & L. Starke (Eds.), *State of the world 2000* (pp. 138-139). New York: W.W. Norton & Company.

Asians, and Native Americans viewed the world as a living organism. Traditional Native American and Eastern philosophies still espouse this belief. The Gaea hypothesis proposes that the difference between living and nonliving things is one of graded intensity and that the Earth remains the sole provider of resources for humans. Many environmentalists profess a worldview of wholeness, in which each cell has equal value and is reflective of the entire cosmos. All cells within the environment interact and achieve a balance. Because everything is interconnected, all parts of the universe are equally important, and no organism should receive special status (Kleffel, 1994). Unfortunately, human beings have appropriated a special status for themselves, and the environment has been the casualty of our self-interests.

## Global Environmental Factors Threatening Health

Many global environmental factors threaten the health of people, plants, and animals. Professional nursing practice focuses on health promotion, as well as caring for the infirm. Nurses must become aware of environmental health risks. Many people drink chemical soups when they partake of water from local water supplies. Persons living in urban locales inhale chemical vapors, which results in an increased incidence of asthma, lung cancer, and other chronic pulmonary diseases. Agricultural workers have an increased incidence of lymphoma and other cancers that are linked to herbicide and pesticide exposure (McGinn, 2000).

Infectious diseases also pose health risks to persons. Many diseases have a higher prevalence in various geographical locations. For example, 23 million persons in sub-Saharan Africa have the human immunodeficiency virus (HIV). Cohen (2003, 2004a, 2004b) reports that more than 5 million persons in Asia (India, 3.8 to 4.6 million; China, 840,000; Myanmar, 687,000; Cambodia, 259,000; Thailand, 163,827; and Vietnam, 130,000) have HIV, and Asia has the potential to surpass the sub-Saharan African epidemic. Unprotected sex and contaminated needles serve as the primary means of HIV infections for Asians and Africans (Brown, 2000; Cohen, 2003).

Besides HIV, other infectious illnesses threaten humans. Human Ebola virus outbreaks over the past 4 years have been confined to the Republic of Congo, Sudan, and Gabon where hunters were infected by handling dead primates and subsequently spread it to other humans (LeRoy, et al., 2004). West Nile virus originated in Africa, but appeared in the United States when infected birds migrated to the United States. The birds transmitted the virus to mosquitoes that then transmitted the virus to humans. However, documented cases of infection with West Nile virus have been linked to blood transfusions, organ donation, and breast milk (Bender & Thompson, 2004). Severe acute respiratory syndrome (SARS) is a human form of an avian flu that originated in the Chinese province of Guangdong. SARS spread rapidly across the globe because it is transmitted from human-to-human by inhaling respiratory droplets from infected persons. The close contact of humans during air flights facilitated its spread in 2003. Antibiotic-resistant bacteria (methicillin-resistant *Staphylococcus aureus* and vancomycin-resistant enterococcus) have arisen because of indiscriminate use of and client noncompliance with antibiotic therapy. Professional nurses and all health care workers bear the responsibility to contain the spread of infectious disease.

Along with infectious disease detection and containment, nurses and other health care providers must be aware of potential environmental health hazards. Table 13-2 outlines

TABLE 13-2

## Environmental Health Hazards and Potential Remedies

| Health Hazard | Geographical Locale(s) | Potential Remedy |
|---|---|---|
| Overpopulation | Ethiopia, Pakistan, Nigeria, India, South and Central America | Education about birth control<br>Limitations on number of children<br>Sterilization<br>Abortion<br>Drugs to prevent conception or induce abortion |
| Human immunodeficiency virus (HIV-AIDS) | Sub-Saharan Africa | HIV prevention education |
| Shrinking crop lands from soil erosion, persistent plant disease, and soil pollution | Worldwide | Environmentally sound agricultural practices |
| Deforestation | Brazil, Indonesia, Malaysia | Reduce demand for paper, lumber, and fuel wood |
| Increasing carbon dioxide atmospheric concentrations | Worldwide | Human population control<br>Reduce demand for fossil fuel<br>Reforestation |
| Global warming | Worldwide | Reduce demand for fossil fuel<br>Reforestation<br>Reduce demand for paper, lumber, and fuel wood |
| Reduced fish population | Worldwide with profound implications in the East | Curb release of industrial waste chemicals into oceans, lakes and waterways<br>Judicious use of pesticides<br>Reduce global warming<br>Enforce fishing catch limits |
| Falling water tables | China, India, North Africa, Saudi Arabia, United States | Find ways to reduce use of water in industrial production; water conservation efforts; paper recycling; and reduce agricultural crop irrigation |
| Ozone depletion | Worldwide | Limit demand for fossil fuel<br>Avoid use of aerosol products containing fluorocarbons<br>Eliminate freon from air conditioning and refrigeration systems |
| Air pollution | Worldwide | Reduce use of coal, wood, and petroleum products for fuel sources<br>Use hydrogen as an alternative fuel source<br>Use solar and wind power plants.<br>Consider taxation for usage of polluting fuels |

*(continued)*

## Environmental Health Hazards and Potential Remedies (Continued)

| Health Hazard | Geographical Locale(s) | Potential Remedy |
|---|---|---|
| **Malnutrition** | | |
| Undernourished | Africa, Asia, Latin America, the Caribbean, and especially Bangladesh, India, Ethiopia, Vietnam, Nigeria, Indonesia | Promote breastfeeding efforts, improve prenatal care, find a way to alleviate poverty, examine and correct food distribution problems |
| Overnourished | United States, Russian Federation, United Kingdom, Germany, Columbia, Brazil (adults) | Educate about health hazards of fast and highly processed foods, reduce food portion sizes, limit advertisements of food aimed at children, adopt a "junk food" tax |
| Persistent organic pollutants (dioxins, polychlorinated biphenyls, and furans) | Russia, Japan, Holland, Belgium | Intensive recycling of batteries, electrical wiring, transformers, computers; limit use of incinerators; institute laws for business and agricultural use of these products; paper recycling; autoclaves for sterilization; barriers such as nets or steel meshes for insect control; larvae-eating fish, selected natural pests for agriculture; use of environment-friendly pesticides |
| Chlorine (plastics, polyvinyl chloride) | Worldwide | Recycle products containing plastic and reduce demand for products made from plastic |
| Latex | Health care institutions, day care centers, schools | Latex-free health care products; ban latex balloons |
| DDT | Central Asia, India, China, Columbia, Ecuador | Crop rotation and use of environmentally-friendly pesticides and herbicides |

Adapted from Brown, L. R., Flavin, C., French, H., Postel, S., & Starke, L. (Eds.). (2000). *State of the world 2000*. New York: W.W. Norton & Company.

some environmental health hazards and potential remedies. Awareness of exposure to environmental toxins provides nurses with the ability to teach clients about ways to avoid long-term exposure to pollutants that sometimes result in devastating health consequences.

Global industrialization and urbanization affect the quality of the air and water. People become exposed to a variety of chemicals no matter where they live. The quality of air and water relies on international efforts. Irrigation and the use of herbicides and pesticides along the Colorado River in the Rocky Mountains affects the quality of water in Mexico. Industrial pollutants, medical waste, and other garbage dumped into the ocean near the United States may wash onto Canadian coastlines.

Some persons experience severe reactions to chemical exposures. Ordinary persons experience chemical injuries, environmental illnesses, and chemical hypersensitivities and allergies. Some persons experience sensitivities to many chemicals found in the environment; this condition is known as **multiple chemical sensitivity** (MCS) and is a recognized form of physical disability (Gibson, 2000). For unknown reasons, persons with MCS have sustained "systemic damage that causes them to react negatively to common chemicals in ambient air" (Gibson, p. 8). Reactions range from slight drowsiness to potentially fatal asthmatic attacks. Table 13-3 outlines the criteria for MCS as determined by group consensus of 34 researchers and clinicians who treat MCS. Sensitivities frequently result from exposure to solvents, pesticides, formaldehyde, fresh paint, new carpets, gas exhaust (diesel, car, propane, and natural gas appliances), perfumes, scented cleaners, air fresheners, and food additives. Even processed lumber products used in new construction and electromagnetic fields from appliances can trigger reactions (Gibson). Gibson estimates that 11 million Americans have MCS and that 2% of these persons have lost jobs because of it. Persons with MCS frequently receive psychiatric diagnoses from health care providers. Reports of chemical sensitivity have been published in Denmark, Sweden, Norway, Finland, Germany, Holland, Belgium, Greece, and Great Britain (Gibson).

The cause of MCS appears to have a physiologic basis. For unknown reasons, the human body becomes damaged in response to repeated chemical exposures. The following physiologic theories related to the etiology of MCS have been proposed:

1. Nervous system damage as a result of repeated exposures.
2. Limbic kindling through the olfactory-limbic system, resulting in triggered responses to repeated chemical exposure.
3. Depletion of or damage to enzymatic production within the body.
4. Repeated immunologic insults.
5. Airway and neurogenic inflammation.
6. Chronic candidiasis.
7. Carbon monoxide poisoning.
8. Electrical changes in the brain.

Along with the physiologic theories, the following psychological theories have surfaced:

1. Psychological and behavioral conditioning.
2. Odor conditioning.

**TABLE 13-3**

## Criteria for Multiple Chemical Sensitivity Diagnosis

Identical symptoms are reproduced with repeated exposure to the same chemical.

Reactions are chronic.

Low levels of exposure to the offending chemical produces manifestations of the reactive symptoms.

When the offending chemicals are removed, the symptoms lessen or resolve.

Reactions occur to multiple, unrelated chemical substances.

Reaction symptoms affect multiple organ systems.

Adapted from Gibson, P. R. (2000). *Multiple chemical sensitivity: A survival guide* (p. 9). Oakland, CA: New Harbinger Publications, Inc.

3. Increased vulnerability related to preexisting anxiety and depression.
4. Amplification of symptoms.
5. Negative affectivity.
6. Personality disorders.
7. Somatization disorder.
8. Childhood trauma.
9. Excessively focused thought patterns and cognitions on chemicals.

Practitioners who espouse a physiologic theory think that avoidance of chemicals is the only way to avoid continued health deterioration. Some health care professionals believe that MCS is a psychiatric disorder. They think that chemical avoidance enables persons with MCS to obsess about their disorder and become socially isolated. However, personality disturbances and panic attacks have been documented in workers exposed to organic solvents, and these problems may be the result of nervous system injury (Gibson, 2000).

Foods consumed by humans (especially those in developed countries) contain an array of additives and contaminants. To increase crop yields, many farmers use a variety of herbicides and pesticides; farmers also genetically manipulate crops. To improve meat production, some farmers use bovine growth hormone feed to maximize livestock growth and development. Many preservatives protect the consumer from foodborne infections. Persons who try to lose weight consume artificial sweeteners, such as aspartame and saccharin. To increase the visual appeal of food, some manufacturers use artificial dyes. Some foods contain flavor enhancers such as monosodium glutamate. Although some food chemicals reduce the risk of foodborne disease, others merely create another human chemical exposure (Gibson, 2000).

## The Professional Nurse's Role in Promoting a Healthy Global Environment

Musker (1994) proposes a life of voluntary simplicity—a holistic, ecologically-based lifestyle—to create a healing environment. In the voluntary simplicity outlook, "less is more," and persons focus on the quality of life, rather than quantity of consumer products (contrary to Western culture in which some think "more is better"). Voluntary simplicity consists of inner and outer processes. The inner process consists of the process of "mindfulness" and requires deep self-reflection to attend to personal needs and to separate them from personal desires. In this inner process, persons discover their genuine, authentic self and discard the illusion of their preconceived self. Some persons keep journals to discover patterns of behavior. The external process consists of the process of "doing," which results in responsible life behaviors that serve the world, rather than pure self-interest. Eventually, the inner and outer processes fuse. Being becomes doing, and doing becomes being. Voluntary action involves the elimination of automatic responses and choices. Simplification of life involves reducing overall consumption, purchasing durable and easily repaired products, consuming a more natural diet, pursuing work that contributes to the world while using more individual creativity and capacities, and changing transportation habits. Simplification also means releasing mental clutter, emotional baggage, useless worries, and other concerns that distract from seizing the enjoyment of the present.

As individual global citizens, professional nurses can model environmentally-friendly behaviors. Table 13-4 offers some suggestions for preventing pollution and conserving environmental resources. When possible, nurses should look for ways to reduce energy consumption, recycle discarded products, and limit purchases to reusable items.

TABLE 13-4

## Suggestions to Curb Pollution and Conserve Resources

| Environmental Goal | Suggestions |
| --- | --- |
| Clean air | Reduce gasoline vapors by replacing cracked gas caps and do not top off fuel tanks |
| | Refuel vehicles in the evening, decreasing exposure of gas vapors to sun |
| | Repair any systems in vehicles or appliances that leak |
| | Carpool |
| | Avoid purchasing products with chlorofluorocarbons, polystyrene, methyl chloroform, and freon |
| | Use a push or electric powered lawn mower |
| | Mow lawn in the evening |
| | Use water-based rather than latex paints |
| Oil conservation | Use fuel with octane rating recommended for vehicle and not a higher one |
| | Limit vehicle warm-ups to 30 seconds |
| | Recycle oil and purchase recycled oil |
| | Keep tires inflated to manufacturer's specifications |
| | Carpool |
| | Purchase vehicles with best available mileage ratings |
| | Keep vehicles tuned up |
| | Fit vehicles with radial tires |
| Land | Purchase products containing at least 25% recycled materials |
| | Buy canned soup instead of instant soups |
| | Buy products made of wood, cotton, or wool instead of plastics |
| | Use a durable shopping bag |
| | Reuse shopping bags |
| | Choose cloth, instead of paper napkins and cleaning rags |
| | Wrap sandwiches in wax paper instead of plastic wrap |
| | Use reusable food containers, plates, and utensils |
| | Purchase a reusable coffee filter rather than paper ones |
| | Compost vegetable scraps with yard waste |
| | Use unbleached paper items when paper products are used |
| | Buy pet food in bulk |
| General resources | Consume less meat and eat foods lower on the food chain |
| | Use durable coffee mugs and drink containers |
| Energy | Seal any appliance seals that contain cracks |
| | Bake in glass or ceramic dishes |
| | Thaw frozen foods in the refrigerator |
| | Cool leftovers before refrigeration |
| | Use self-cleaning oven cycle immediately after baking |
| | Clean clothes dryer filter and hoses regularly |
| | Dry several loads of clothes in succession or hang clothes outside to dry |
| | Use natural sunlight for lighting |
| | Close blinds, shades, and curtains during the summer |
| | Place air conditioners in a shady location |
| | Keep air conditioner vents free of debris |
| | Service furnaces and air conditioners regularly |
| | Change furnace and air conditioner filters every 4 months |
| | Keep freezers full of food |
| | Cap stored liquids in the refrigerator |
| | Install a hot water tank timer |

*(continued)*

## Suggestions to Curb Pollution and Conserve Resources (Continued)

| Environmental Goal | Suggestions |
|---|---|
| Energy (continued) | Wrap an insulation blanket around hot water heater<br>Attach a timer to home thermostat<br>Install solar panels<br>Turn off unused lights and appliances<br>Install compact fluorescent bulbs in light fixtures<br>Tighten and insulate cooling and heating ducts<br>Keep attic well ventilated by using turbine or screen vents<br>Repair foundation cracks<br>Use air drying setting on dishwasher<br>Use short cycles for laundry and dishwasher loads whenever possible |
| Forests | Recycle paper<br>Buy recycled paper products<br>Use durable cups and drinking containers<br>Use both sides of paper<br>Institute a sharing program for books, magazines, and other periodicals<br>Store information on computers rather than on hard copies<br>Check out books and periodicals from the library |
| Water | Water lawn only when absolutely necessary and use a deep soak watering technique<br>Drip irrigate gardens<br>Mulch around trees and plants<br>Use natural pesticides and herbicides<br>Leave grass clippings on lawn<br>Turn off water when brushing your teeth<br>Install low-flow shower heads and aerators on faucets<br>Rinse razor in a filled sink rather than a running tap<br>Inspect toilets and faucets for leaks and fix them promptly<br>Clean driveways and garages with a broom instead of a hose |

Adapted from *Simple Steps for Individuals*, a publication from Choose Environmental Excellence, which is part of Bridging the Gap Inc. Kansas City, MO.

### Questions for Reflection 13-2

1. Do I have any personal habits that may be potentially toxic to the global environment?
2. What could I do differently to change my environmentally unsafe behaviors?

## ● THE COMMUNITY ENVIRONMENT

Multiple environmental factors affect the health of the community. Community services that enhance health include public health departments, disease prevention services, and social support services. The individual health status of community residents relies on the quality of the physical and social community environments. For the purposes of this discussion, the **community environment** refers to the geographical location where people live and work.

## Community Environmental Factors Threatening Health

Although the local community provides health services to promote community health, most communities also have environmental factors that threaten the health of citizens. Heavy traffic and industrial fumes pollute the air. Some municipalities and counties use pesticides to prevent the spread of insect-borne illnesses. High-tension power lines and power stations emit electromagnetic fields (Gibson, 2000).

Along with business and industry, the level of affluence within the community affects the health of individuals and families. The income of citizens enables communities to maintain infrastructure and provide services to enhance health. However, affluence can negatively affect health. Since 1980, Americans have increased the annual mileage on their cars by 80%. Many persons have long commutes from their suburban homes to their workplaces. Traffic jams contribute to road rage and increased pollution.

Automobiles make it convenient to drive short distances, resulting in individuals getting less exercise from walking or cycling. For many Americans, the ease of obtaining high-calorie foods quickly contributes to an unhealthy diet. The combination of physical inactivity and excessive food intake has resulted in 23% of adults and 16% of children in the United States having a body mass index 30% or higher than the criteria for obesity. Reasons for obesity include heredity, metabolism, behavior, environment, culture, and socioeconomics (United States Department of Health and Human Services, 2000).

The United States Department of Health and Human Services (2000) reported that 120 million Americans lived in areas where exposure to air pollutants including ozone exceeded governmental health standards. The same report indicated that a disproportionate number of Hispanic and Pacific Islanders lived in these areas.

Although pesticides may result in environmental pollution, they play a key role in preventing infectious disease epidemics. Surveillance and control of insect-borne illnesses requires expenditures of public revenue. Revenue for epidemic prevention comes from federal, state, and local sources. In recent years, the West Nile virus has been linked to insects that infect birds, and Lyme disease has been linked to insects that infect deer (Enserink, 2001). Professional nurses frequently participate in the development of community educational programs or community service announcements to help citizens avoid contracting these infectious diseases. The proper application of pesticides limits environmental damage. Responsibility for the proper use of pesticides lies with companies who secure community contracts and homeowners.

To eliminate the risk of foodborne illness, local health departments license businesses and organizations that serve food. Poor hand washing by persons handling food has led to outbreaks of hepatitis A, salmonella, and *Escherichia coli* infections. Foodborne illnesses also occur when persons fail to abide by guidelines for food storage and safe preparation.

The potential for the spread of infectious illnesses, such as tuberculosis, influenza, and viral or bacterial meningitis, is increased in persons subjected to overcrowded conditions. College dormitories, schools, and child day care centers also provide residence for a variety of disease-causing organisms.

In addition to the threats to the physical integrity of communities, social problems also threaten human health. Poverty, substance abuse, incivility, and moral decay have led to a decline in communities. Violence occurs in urban, rural, and suburban settings. In urban areas, violence is the leading cause of death in young African American men. Among industrialized nations, the United States has the highest rate of childhood homicides (United States Department of Health and Human Services, 2000). In most instances, victims of homicide know their killers. Domestic, child, and elder abuse occur in all socioeconomic groups but occur more frequently when families struggle to have basic human needs met (food, water, shelter). In addition to economic factors, the media exposes persons to acts of violence in movies, fictional television programs, cartoons, and newscasts, and some computer and video games use violence as entertainment. As individuals are repeatedly exposed to images of violence, victims of violent crime become depersonalized, and violence becomes a part of life.

School shootings have occurred across the United States (Colorado, Oregon, Arkansas, Tennessee, Georgia, Kentucky, and Mississippi). Most of the shooters came from middle-class homes with two parents, and most used guns found in their homes. Preventive measures against teen violence focus on parents and include limiting teen exposure to violent movies, television programs, and video games. Experts place emphasis on parents spending quality time with their children, serving as role models for them, and teaching them ethical and moral behavior (Steger, 2000).

Social interactions vary according to the type of communities in which persons reside. Persons tend to socialize more with persons who share similar life situations. In working-class neighborhoods (especially when adults of households are both employed), relationships tend to be more casual. Time constraints present challenges for maintaining relationships with neighbors. Schools and churches provide opportunities for persons with similar values to develop relationships.

## The Professional Nurse's Role in Promoting a Healthy Community Environment

Professional nurses play key roles in promoting a healthy community environment. Nurses assess communities for actual and potential factors that are noxious to human health and well-being. When noxious factors are identified, nurses can inform community members about them, provide community education to eliminate them, and take action to eliminate them. Nurses can also inspire other community members to incorporate health promotion activities into their lives. Reporting local health hazards, such as deteriorating road conditions, the need for reduced speed limits, or dangerous intersections that need traffic signs or signals, helps to prevent motor vehicle and pedestrian accidents. Nurses, like all citizens, have the freedom and obligation to attend local governmental meetings to express concerns related to community development projects. By participating in community cleanup programs, nurses reduce the community's risk of injury from exposure to broken glass, used needles, sharp metal objects, and of infectious illnesses from exposure to rotting food.

Nurses also can become active participants in local school, civic, and church activities to foster mental health and offer safe recreation for persons of all ages. As an act against societal violence, nurses can refuse to purchase products that use violence as entertainment, buy products from companies that advertise their products during violent television programs, or attend movies or plays that glorify violence. When working with teens, nurses should be alert to any precursors of imminent violent acts, including inappropriate angry outbursts; cruelty to animals; essays with violent themes; fascination with weapons (especially firearms); obsession with playing violent computer games; threats to harm self or others; vandalism (even of their own property); assumption of the victim role; involvement in fringe groups or gangs; behavior with the goal of getting suspended or expelled; and incidents of bringing weapons to show to other students. Teaching violence awareness, stress management, self-esteem, gun safety, substance abuse, and cultural diversity classes in the community serves as a means to eliminate violence in society (Steger, 2000). Nurses also can serve as resources to local schools for violence prevention, violence recovery, and other health promotion programs. Finally, nurses can lobby local, state, and federal legislative bodies to protect environmental health.

### Questions for Reflection 13-3

1. How would I rate the health of my local community based on the information presented previously?
2. What community resources are available to me as a citizen and professional nurse to improve the environment of my local community?
3. What strategies could I use to promote a healthy community environment?

## ● THE WORK ENVIRONMENT

Many persons spend more time in the workplace than they do at home. The quality of the **work environment** relies on physical and cultural factors. National, state, and local laws protect worker safety. Individual organizations have policies that guide worker behaviors and inform them of potential health hazards.

### Work Environmental Factors Threatening Health

Many offices and work settings contain factors that threaten the physiologic, psychological, and spiritual health of employees and consumers. Some industries and manufacturers rely on chemicals and solvents to produce products. Some jobs require workers to perform repetitive movements. According to the United States Occupational Safety and Health Administration (OSHA), each year 1.8 million workers in the United States experience work-related disabling musculoskeletal disorders. Nelson, Fragala, and Menzel (2003) report that nursing-related back pain occurs in 47% of all American nurses. They also project that nurses will have more back pain as they care for more obese clients. Other common injuries sustained by nurses in clinical practice include overexertion (including lifting too much), falls or slips, twisting injuries, bruises or lacerations from being struck by or against objects, injuries from violent acts, harmful substance exposure, transportation accidents, repetitive motion insults, and compression injuries. Nurses also have a six times higher suicide rate than that of the general population (Belanger, 2000).

Tasks required for patient care performed by professional nurses in hospitals create an "ergonomic nightmare" (Trossman, 2000, p. 1). Many nurses work 12-hour shifts and experience repetitive movement stress from lifting and turning patients, pumping up sphygmomanometers, resetting monitor alarms, and moving heavy equipment (Trossman, 2000).

In addition to the potential for disabling musculoskeletal disorders, nurses are exposed to dangerous chemicals in the work setting. In recent years, an increase in latex allergies in health care providers, ancillary personnel, and clients has been reported. Currently, there are more than 40,000 consumer products containing latex including gloves, clothing, intravenous supplies, medication vials, urinary catheters, feeding tubes, endotracheal tubes, carpeting, furniture, blood pressure cuffs, tape, balloons, condoms, and chewing gum (Dyck, 2000; Kellet, 1997; Kim, Graves, Safadi, Alhadeff, & Metcalfe, 1998; Lee & Kim, 1998). Since 1998, most medical devices containing latex must be appropriately labeled to protect persons sensitive to latex (Kim et al., 1998). Just using a latex-containing product exposes the professional nurse at risk for latex sensitization and future latex allergy (Lee & Kim, 1998). Kim, Wellmeyer, and Miller (1999) report that as many as 17% of health care workers may have a latex allergy. Most have cutaneous allergic responses, but 1.3% of health care workers with latex allergy have allergic asthmatic responses with exposure. However, vinyl gloves tend to tear more readily than do latex ones. In addition, vinyl gloves release toxic environmental substances such as dioxin. Nitrile, neoprene, and thermoplastic gloves offer protection equal to that offered by latex gloves. However, like latex, these products may trigger allergic reactions, because their chemical composition is similar (Worthington, 2000). Because of recent increases in the incidence of latex allergies in health care providers and consumers, some health care organizations are striving toward creating a latex-free environment.

Depending on their practice area, nurses are exposed to dangerous chemicals other than latex. These are summarized in Table 13-5. OSHA has published standards for safe handling of all dangerous chemicals used in the workplace. In addition, nurse specialty organizations publish guidelines for safe practice use, which usually are covered in nurse specialty certification examinations. Antineoplastic agents may cause birth defects, allergic reactions, and skin, eye, and mucous membrane irritation. Chemicals used for sterilization and anesthesia have been associated with cancer development, birth defects, spontaneous abortion, respiratory tract irritation, central nervous system symptoms, dermatitis, eye irritation, liver dysfunction, and renal disorders (Pope et al., 1995).

In addition to chemical and radiation exposure, infectious diseases pose a hazard to nurses and other health care workers. Nurses have the potential to contract hepatitis B and HIV from a percutaneous stick with a contaminated needle or other sharp implement. Strategies for preventing such an event include strict adherence to OSHA Bloodborne Pathogen Standards and hepatitis B vaccination. Nurses may encounter hepatitis A if they work in places where personal hygiene may be poor. Effective hand washing serves as the best method for preventing contraction of this virus. In recent years, nurse exposures to pulmonary illnesses such as SARS and tuberculosis (TB) have increased. Contributing factors for resurgence in cases of TB include the acquired immunodeficiency syndrome epidemic, immigration, homelessness, and the development of drug-resistant strains. Diligent attention to isolation procedures and wearing special ventilation masks decreases the chance of contracting TB. SARS is contracted

**TABLE 13-5**

## Strategies to Prevent Health Hazards in Nursing Environments

| Health Hazard | Prevention Strategies |
|---|---|
| Needle stick injuries | Use needleless systems for IV therapy when possible<br>Use syringes with recapping devices for intramuscular, subcutaneous, and intradermal injections<br>Replace containers for used needles before they become more than two-three full |
| Back and shoulder injuries | Evaluate all clients for weight-bearing status and mobility before moving or lifting them<br>Use assistive devices (such as mechanical lifts, slide boards, and sheets) and engineering controls properly<br>Verify that enough help is present before lifting, transferring, or ambulating clients<br>Take time to raise beds and equipment to a comfortable working level<br>Provide training on proper body mechanics from physical therapy departments for employees<br>Redesign work stations to provide ergonomically sound charting stations for standing and sitting<br>Provide supportive chair for seated activities<br>Negotiate for ergonomically sound workplace practices<br>Lobby state legislators to enact ergonomic legislation |
| Repetitive stress injuries | Increase worker and administrator awareness on how repetitive movements may result in musculoskeletal injury |
| Carpal tunnel syndrome | Avoid long time periods for computer data entry<br>Provide wrist support devices for computer mouse and keyboards<br>Teach employees wrist-stretching exercises |
| Blood-borne infections | Use needleless and recapping syringe devices |
| Air-borne infections | Use and change masks<br>Provide respirator masks for specific infections<br>Separate ventilation units for isolation rooms |
| Other infections | Make soap and water accessible for handwashing<br>Make alcohol-based hand cleansers accessible |
| Latex | Persuade employer to remove as many latex-containing supplies from the organization as possible<br>Use latex-free gloves exclusively<br>Follow extensive rinse procedures for any equipment rinsed with gluteraldehyde solutions and wear gloves not containing vinyl or latex<br>Encourage co-workers to refrain from touching telephone, intercom, and other equipment buttons and light switches while wearing latex gloves |
| Hazardous chemicals<br>  Antineoplastics | Follow OSHA and Oncology Nurses Society guidelines for safe handling of chemotherapeutic agents |
|   Ethylene oxide, formaldehyde and glutaraldehyde (sterilization chemicals) | Follow OSHA guidelines |
|   Anesthetic gases (especially nitrous oxide) | Follow National Institute of Occupational Safety and Health recommendations for exposure limits |

*(continued)*

## Strategies to Prevent Health Hazards in Nursing Environments (Continued)

| Health Hazard | Prevention Strategies |
| --- | --- |
| Mercury | Do not touch mercury with hands. Request published standards for mercury disposal from environmental services or housekeeping departments |
| Bleach and other disinfectant cleaners | Wear gloves when cleaning surfaces containing bleach and be certain that the work location is well ventilated |
| Radiation | Limit exposure by using lead shields, keeping distance between self and radiation source, and limiting time spent in areas where radiation exposure may occur. The Nuclear Regulatory Commission (NRC) has set maximum exposure at 3 rem every 3 months for safe exposure. If radiation dose exceeds exposure limit, workers are to be reassigned to work without radiation exposure risk. OSHA has guidelines for workers not covered by the NRC |
| Suicide | Monitor self and others for addictive behaviors (including cigarettes) Talk to colleagues when intensively critical situations arise or when they are resolved Be alert for colleagues who appear preoccupied with death or say they wish they were dead Practice stress management and relaxation techniques Do not be afraid to confront colleagues when suicidal warning signs occur and refer them to mental health professionals |

Adapted from Shaner, H. (1994). Environmentally responsible clinical practice. In E. A. Schuster & C. L. Brown (Eds.), *Exploring our environmental connections practice* (pp. 233–251). NLN Publication No. 14-2634. New York: National League for Nursing. Belanger, D. (2000). Nurses and suicide: The risk is real. *RN, 63,* 61–64. Kim, K. T., Graves, P. B., Safadi. G. S., Alhadeff, G., & Metcalfe, J. (1998). Implementation recommendations for making health care facilities latex safe. *AORN Journal, 67,* 615–632. Trossman, S. (2000). Moving violations: Working to prevent on-the-job injuries. *The American Nurse, 32,* 1, 12–14.

from infected persons via inhaled respiratory droplets. Measles, rubella, mumps, and influenza also threaten the health of nurses as they engage in professional practice. To protect nurses, determination of immune status and offering appropriate immunizations eliminate the risk of contracting most of these diseases (Pope et al., 1995). However, nurses bear the responsibility for protecting their health by following specific isolation techniques when caring for clients with potentially contagious diseases.

Along with contracting illnesses from clients, nurses come into contact with many organisms that cause nosocomial infections. Vancomycin-resistant enterococcus and methicillin-resistant *S. aureus* thrive in hospital environments. Frequently, nurses may

### Questions for Reflection 13-4

1. How would I rate the health of my work environment based on the information presented previously?
2. In what ways have I promoted a healthy work environment within the past month?
3. What are factors in my work environment that negatively affect the health of me and my coworkers?
4. What strategies could I take in the future to promote a healthy work environment?

be colonized with these organisms but because of immunocompetence, infection does not develop. Other infections that threaten the health of nurses include herpes zoster, *Clostridia difficile*, and *S. aureus*. Diligent isolation practices, meticulous handwashing, and habits to promote immunocompetence protect nurses from catching infectious diseases from clients or the work environment.

Many nurses accept professional positions on the day shift with the knowledge that they will be required to work later shifts as needs arise. Circadian rhythms can be disrupted by some work schedules, such as those that include rotating shifts. Lack of sleep and rest takes a toll on the immune system.

Nurses also experience stress in the workplace. The following workplace factors contribute to the work-related stress encountered by nurses:

1. Making decisions that may result in life or death.
2. Working with clients in pain.
3. Working with demanding clients.
4. Understaffing.
5. Rotating shifts.
6. Working long shifts (12 hours or more).
7. Completing client documentation in a timely fashion.
8. Keeping current in the areas of pharmacology, technology, and procedural changes.
9. Dealing with authoritative managers.
10. Working with unlicensed personnel.
11. Being eliminated from participating in decisions that affect nursing care delivery.
12. Coping with client deaths.
13. Feeling unappreciated by other health team members.
14. Practicing nursing without the time to establish meaningful and therapeutic client relationships.
15. Delegating tasks that serve as a source of accomplishment.
16. Dealing with reduced client length of stay (inpatient settings).
17. Working in uncivil work settings.

In any setting, people cannot avoid stress. However, individuals perceive stress differently (Lazarus & Folkman, 1984), and those perceptions may affect physical and mental health (McLean, 1974).

## Violence in the Workplace

Recent initiatives by health care administrators, nurses, and collective bargaining units have resulted in zero tolerance for workplace violence. In previous years, nurses considered working with violent patients to be part of the job. However, when a nurse sustained a severe head injury after being assaulted by a mental health patient, the Illinois Nurses Association informed the media and legislators. The Illinois Department of Human Services began exploring incidents that threaten the safety of mental health care providers and patients in state facilities. The mental health facility where the nurse was injured has implemented the following reforms: giving nurses more freedom to use professional judgment to place violent patients in restraints; forming a patient-monitoring team to identify potentially violent patients; providing staff with personal alarm devices that can be used when a staff member feels he or she is in danger; providing two-way radios for contacting security; and assuring security personnel are available at all times. Along with reforms, the mental health facility provided mandatory staff education on violence theory and prevention and psychological support from an 11-member "debriefing" team (Trossman, 2001).

In addition to being injured by patients, nurses can be assaulted by patients' family members or friends. Gang members frequently accompany victims of violent crime to the emergency department. On rare occasions, nurses and other health team members have been assaulted by a member of the patient's gang or a member of a rival gang. Isolated incidents of nurses being assaulted or shot by patient visitors have also been reported (Carroll, 2004).

## The Professional Nurse's Role in Promoting a Healthy Work Environment

Before a nurse can promote a healthy work environment, he or she must become cognizant of actual and potential hazards in the workplace. The nurse should assess the work setting systematically to identify the quality of the work environment, paying close attention to its impact on worker physical, mental, and spiritual health. When nurses identify actual or potential health hazards, they should educate staff about them and make referrals to persons who can eliminate them. The nurse has an ethical obligation to protect the health of all health team members. The nurse should validate that governmental guidelines to protect workers and clients are followed and take risks to advocate for change when needed.

Along with protecting the physical health of co-workers, nurses play a key role in promoting the mental and spiritual health of colleagues and client care team members. Health team members sometimes encounter ethical dilemmas especially when they work in health care organizations that emphasize profits over client care quality, find themselves being unable to provide services to all persons in need of health care, and have to make decisions on how best to use new technology in clinical practice. These conditions create an unhealthy work environment characterized by little or no commitment, worker rebellion, deflated morale, workplace anger, worker disengagement, inferior problem solving, and sloppy client care (Wilson & Porter-O'Grady, 1999). Hierarchical relationships among health team members (physicians, nurses, administrators, unlicensed personnel) compound the problem of unhealthy work environments (Watkins & Mohr, 2001; Wesorick, Shiparski, Troseth, & Wyngarden, 1997; Wilson & Porter-O'Grady, 1999). When persons deeply connect with each other to do important work, a healthy work environment emerges (Watkins & Mohr, 2001; Wesorick et al.,1997). Client care in any setting is important work. When nurses and other team members focus all efforts on what is best for clients, they become united in purpose. Finding meaning in one's existence nourishes the human spirit (Frankl, 1970). When coworkers share the same meaning in work, they connect on a spiritual level (Wesorick et al., 1997).

Efforts to create this healthy work environment require personal commitment, cooperative efforts with others, and a courageous attitude to express genuine authenticity. Unfortunately, current clinical environments exert much pressure to do more with less. Threats of mergers and downsizing create fear in nursing staff members (Wilson & Porter-O'Grady, 1999). Instead of keeping the client's best interest at the center of care, nurses find themselves having to please administrators, physicians, or unlicensed assistive personnel. Wesorick and colleagues (1997, p. 9) have identified the following three characteristics to connect souls and create healthy work cultures: (1) shared meaning and purpose in work, (2) healthy relationships, and (3) meaningful conversations. Identification of shared meaning and purpose in work requires that everyone working together is aware of and agrees to what matters most in their work. Wesorick and colleagues (1997, pp. 14–15) define healthy relationships as partnerships and outline the following six basic partnership principles:

1. Intention: a personal decision to connect with another at the deepest level of humanness.
2. Mission: a calling to live out something that deeply matters or is meaningful.
3. Equal accountability: mutual ownership of the mission without one person having power over or instilling fear in another.
4. Potential: the human capacity of all (including oneself) persons to continuously learn, grow, and create.
5. Balance: harmonious relationships with self and others required to attain the mission.
6. Trust: synchronous sense on important things or issues that matter.

Wesorick and colleagues (1997) outline meaningful conversation as the vehicle for developing healthy and meaningful relationships in work settings. Participants engaging in dialogue feel welcomed and honored while they share ideas, thoughts, and feelings. In dialogue, messages are deeply listened to and not judged. The partnership approach to clinical practice has the potential to transform a toxic work setting for all health team members to one that promotes health in body, mind, and spirit.

The American Academy of Nursing has embarked on identifying "magnet" hospitals that deliver excellent client care, recruit and retain professional nurses, and provide a nice working environment for nurses. Using descriptive research methods, the American Academy of Nursing derived eight essential elements that distinguished magnets from other hospitals. According to Kramer and Schmalenberg (2004, p. 50), the eight essentials are (1) support for education, (2) working with other nurses who are clinically competent, (3) positive nurse/physician relationships, (4) autonomous nursing practice, (5) a culture that values concern for the patient, (6) control of and over nursing practice, (7) perceived adequacy of staffing, and (8) nurse-manager support (enumeration added).

When nurses look for employment, they might want to consider working for a magnet hospital because the hospital values these eight essential elements.

## Research Brief 13-1

Kramer, M., & Schmalenberg, C. (2002). *Essentials of magnetism.* In M. McClure, & A. Hinshaw (Eds.). *Magnet hospitals revisited: Attraction and retention of professional nurses.* Kansas City, MO: American Nurses Publishing.

The investigators sought to distinguish the differences in work environments for nurses in hospitals with magnet status (16), hospitals aspiring to attain magnet status (8), and other hospitals (6). A total of 4,607 nurses responded to a survey that was mailed or posted on the Internet. Survey data included 3,602 staff nurses.

Statistically significant differences occurred in the number of nurses working in magnet hospitals reporting more positive responses toward the following factors:

perceived hospital valuing of nurse continuing education, increased availability of programs, more rewards for attending continuing education programs, more financial assistance to attend continuing education, increased collaborative and collegial relationships with physicians, better rating of collegial competency, hospital rewards for competency, recognition of specialty certification as evidence of competency, perception of autonomy in clinical practice, perception of patients being the top priority, shared governance structures that provided evidence for nurse control of and over professional practice, perceived adequate staffing levels, and perceived support from nurse managers and nursing administration. These identified differences reveal that there is a difference in the working environments among magnet, magnet-seeking, and other hospitals according to the nurses survey.

Implications for practice for this study reveal that nurses from many hospitals value similar conditions in an acute, inpatient work setting. Hospitals creating this work environment are able to recruit and retain professional nurses. When a hospitals achieves and maintains its magnet status, prospective nurses can be assured the "it is a good place to work." Nurses can use magnet status to determine where they want to engage in clinical practice.

## ✦ THE HOME ENVIRONMENT

The **home environment** plays a key role in human health. A family's home creates a haven for individual autonomy and control. Some consider the home as an extension of their personal identity. The quality of the physical structure, general cleanliness, storage of chemicals, and interpersonal relationships affect the health of individual family members.

### Home Environmental Factors Threatening Health

Persons seek safe living quarters. Even the homeless find some way to stay warm and dry. Persons with established residences live in single or multiple family dwellings. Homes may be purchased or rented. The home's arranged floor plan provides family members with space for privacy, sleeping, and interaction. In American culture, social status and self-esteem are linked to the home. Homeowners (or landlords) bear the responsibility for repairs to maintain environmental safety.

Accidents occur frequently in the home. The types of accidents vary according to the age and developmental level of family members. The structural integrity of stairs, railings, ceilings, walls, and furniture must be assessed periodically to prevent injury. Safe storage and proper labeling of cleaning products and medications is critical in homes with young children. Homes with throw rugs create hazards for falls, especially for the elderly. Fire safety relies on periodic inspection and maintenance of household appliances, working smoke detectors, storage of paper and flammable materials away from furnaces or other appliances that could generate sparks, and clear home entrances and exits.

The home can be a source of illness, as well as the scene of accidents. Problems with cleanliness and personal hygiene result in outbreaks of infectious disease. An estimated 30 million cases of foodborne illnesses, resulting in 9,000 deaths, occur each year in the

United States. Salmonella, *E. coli* (especially *E. coli* 0157:H7 found in raw ground beef), and *P. aeruginosa* thrive on many kitchen counters (Rutala, Barbee, & Aguiar, 2000). Adequate water supply, plumbing, refrigeration, garbage disposal, and general household cleaning practices assure reduced infections in the home. Handwashing after using the toilet and before food preparation and eating remains the most effective measure for the prevention of infectious illness in the home. Proper kitchen counter cleaning using commercially prepared disinfectants (such as Lysol, Lysol antibacterial spray, Mr. Clean) or a 10% bleach solution effectively destroy bacteria when left on surfaces for at least 30 seconds. However, vinegar and baking soda fail to provide effective disinfection (Rutala et al., 2000).

Indoor air pollution and allergens set the stage for the development of allergic disorders, especially asthma. Smoking has been named the main source of indoor air pollution. Sources of indoor allergens include house dust mites, cockroach particles, pet dander, rodent dander, and mold. Limiting smoking to the outdoors and regular house cleaning eliminate these factors that could potentially impair respiratory health.

Pets and insect infestation also may serve as vectors for infectious diseases. To control lawn and household infestations, people use pesticides. Organophosphate insecticides kill insects by inducing muscle paralysis. Organophosphates can be absorbed through inhalation, ingestion, and dermal and optical contact. Symptoms of insecticide poisoning may occur when humans are exposed (Melum & Kearney, 2001). In addition to direct contact, organophosphates contaminate freshwater supplies, especially if applied too heavily.

Many potentially noxious substances can be found in the home. Household chemicals, fixtures, and even construction materials contain organic compounds that contaminate the indoor environment (Gibson, 2000). Benzene, a known human carcinogen, is present in synthetic materials, plastic, cleaning solutions, and tobacco smoke (Friedman & Morgan, 1992; Gibson, 2000). Construction materials such as particleboard and plywood emit formaldehyde, especially during the first year after construction. Most new carpeting contains a latex back, and latex carpet pads also are common. Newly poured concrete, fresh mortar, and paint emit gases (Gibson, 2000). Most commercial cleaners contain petrochemicals, fragrances, dyes, organophosphates, or bleach, which also contribute to environmental pollution. Tap water contains pollutants such as bacterial colonies, nitrates, pesticides, particulates, and metals. Radon gas may seep into basements from rock foundations (Gibson, 2000).

In addition to indoor pollution, people are exposed to chemicals and vapors used by neighbors. Propane cookers, gas-powered lawn tools, gas appliances, and fresh paint emit fumes (Gibson, 2000). Many people apply dangerous herbicides and pesticides on lawns to make lawns look thicker and greener.

Along with pollutants, the home contains many sources for accidents. Home power sources such as natural gas and electricity can pose health hazards if basic rules for each are not followed. Appliances provide another source for accidents, especially in households where children reside. Hot water may cause burns, especially if the hot water tank is set above 140° F. Along with sources of power and appliances, stairs and throw rugs provide opportunities for falling. Fireplaces and improper storage of paper, rags, and combustible materials may create fire hazards.

Psychological health requires privacy. Persons need to have a place for emotional release, to feel independent, and to express affection toward those they love. When persons have time to recharge emotionally, the threat of domestic violence is reduced.

Factors contributing to domestic violence include household weapons, pregnancy, and drug or alcohol abuse. Many batterers have a history of violent behavior outside the home, depression, chemical dependency, and posttraumatic stress disorders. Children from homes where domestic violence occurs are at risk for being victims or perpetrators of violence. In addition, a history of head trauma has been associated with intense jealousy and violence (Gerard, 2000).

## The Professional Nurse's Role in Promoting a Healthy Home Environment

The professional nurse detects home health hazards by performing a comprehensive environmental assessment. When hazards are identified, the professional nurse provides education and support to help clients eliminate them. Sometimes, especially when nurses work with the disabled, community resources can be obtained to assist persons with housekeeping and home maintenance.

Because 35% of emergency department clients are victims of domestic violence, nurses should routinely screen all persons for its signs. Nurses should ask direct questions about abusive behaviors in a private, safe place. Both written and photographic documentation of injuries provides victims of abuse with substantial evidence if they decide to press charges. Once violence has been confirmed, the professional nurse's priority is to ensure the safety of the victim and any dependents. Sometimes immediate referrals to social workers, police departments, or domestic shelters may be needed to protect the victim(s). If danger to immediate safety poses no threat, the nurse should outline a plan for safety if the violence escalates (Gerard, 2000). In some states, professional nurses have a legal duty to report incidences of child and elder abuse but not domestic violence between intimate partners.

### Questions for Reflection 13-5

1. How would I rate the environment of my home based on the information presented previously?
2. What things could I change in my home to promote a healthy home environment?

## ⬤ COMPREHENSIVE ENVIRONMENTAL HEALTH ASSESSMENT

Before professional nurses can take action to promote a healthy community environment, they must identify environmental factors that affect health. Shaner (1994), and Pope, Snyder, and Mood (1995) have outlined various elements of an environmental health history; these elements are summarized in Table 13-6. The age of residences and their proximity to military installations and industries provide clues to potential exposure to substances and chemicals that impair health. Because persons might be exposed to health hazards within work settings, information about occupations also provides information about environmental health hazards. Workers in many businesses that prepare foods for consumption (restaurants and grocery stores) use latex gloves to prevent

TABLE 13-6

## Elements of a Comprehensive Environmental Assessment

| Location or Activity | Key Questions |
| --- | --- |
| Home | Where do you live? |
| | What is the distance from a major thoroughfare, industrial complex, or military base? |
| | If close to an industry, what type of industrial plant is it? |
| | What is the drinking water source for your residence? |
| | What types of cleaning agents do you use for housework and laundry? |
| | What types of chemicals do you use for yard care? |
| | What insecticides do you use inside the home? |
| | How old is your home structure (house, condo, or apartment)? |
| | How is your home heated? |
| | How is your home cooled? |
| | What is your fuel source for cooking? |
| | Have you tested your home for radon gas? |
| | Do you have a carbon monoxide alarm and smoke alarms in your home? |
| | Do you purify your home air or water? |
| | Have you recently acquired new furniture or carpeting? |
| | What type of paint is used on the exterior and interior of your home? |
| | Have you ever or recently refinished furniture or wood items in your home? |
| | What are the occupations of other household occupants? |
| | Do household occupants come into contact with chemicals as part of employment or leisure activities? |
| | Does anyone living with you smoke? |
| Work | List your past jobs (including military experience) and if you were exposed to any chemicals. |
| | Describe any work-related health problems or accidents. |
| | Did any of your co-workers have similar health problems or accidents? |
| | Where do you currently work? |
| | Are you employed full-time or part-time? |
| | How does your employer inform you of potentially hazardous chemicals, equipment, or procedures used in the workplace? |
| | Describe your work safety education programs (if any available). |
| | What protective devices are available for your use? |
| | Do you use the protective devices? |
| | How old is the building in which you work? |
| | Do you have any symptoms associated with your work setting? If so, please describe them. |
| Hobbies | What hobbies do you have? |
| | Are there any chemical agents used while engaging in the hobby? |
| Symptom assessment | What symptoms do you currently have? |
| | When did they start? |
| | When do they occur? |
| | Where do they occur? |
| | Does anyone who works with you or lives with or near you have the same symptoms? |

Adapted from Shaner, H. (1994). Environmentally responsible clinical practice. In E. A. Schuster & C. L. Brown (Eds.), *Exploring our environmental connections practice* (pp. 233–251). NLN Publication No. 14-2634. New York: National League for Nursing; and Pope, A. M., Snyder, M. A., & Mood, L. H. (Eds.). (1995). *Nursing, health, and the environment*. Washington, DC: National Academy Press.

food-borne infections (Dyck, 2000; Kellet, 1997; Kim, Wellmeyer, & Miller, 1999; and Lee & Kim, 1998). Along with home and work settings, hobbies such as photography, furniture restoration, and gardening may result in exposure to hazardous chemicals. Household and lawn chemicals used on a regular basis also serve as a source of exposure to substances that may affect health. Finally, nurses should assess persons for being potential perpetrators or victims of violence.

## ● SUMMARY AND SIGNIFICANCE TO PRACTICE

Professional nurses have the responsibility to assess global, community, work, and home environments for factors that affect health. In addition to discovering actual and potential factors that affect health, nurses can take action to create a more health-promoting environment. Nurses serve as role models for global environmental preservation. They use education and political activism to promote changes within the communities in which they reside. Nurses assess factors that threaten worker health and provide worker education to prevent work-related injury and illness. In addition, professional nurses create clinical practice environments that enhance the mental and spiritual health of all health team members by discovering purpose in and meaning of client care, practicing principles of partnership, and engaging in meaningful conversation. Nurses also assess client home environments and educate clients on how to create a health-promoting home. Finally, nurses take action in their personal lives to promote the health of the global, community, work, and home environments.

### FROM THEORY TO PRACTICE

1. After reading this chapter, how would I handle a client like Emily presenting in the emergency department with breathing difficulty? What advice would I give to a nurse providing care to a client like Emily? Why is it important to look for environmental factors contributing to client symptoms?
2. What workplace environmental hazards can I identify in my clinical practice setting? What are the procedures for making changes in my health care organization? Why is it important to know the established policies and procedures for making changes in a workplace setting?
3. What individual behaviors could I change to promote a more healthy global, community, work and home environment? What would be the consequences for making these changes?

## WWW INTERNET EXERCISES

1. Visit the Scorecard Organization at http://www.scorecard.org. Type in your zip code to get answers to the most frequently asked questions about the major polluters and polluting agents found in your community. Click "Get Report" after entering your zip code. Make a list of the top polluters in your county and the top chemicals released in your county. Learn about local lead hazards in houses and if your area has a worst toxic site. Bring this information to share in class with your colleagues.

**2.** Visit the National Institute of Occupational Safety and Health at http://www.cdc.gov/niosh/homepage.html. Read down the page and click on "Health Care Workers." On the next screen, scroll down to see the various topics covered. Select a topic of interest and click it. Read the information. Compare your current clinical practice agency's policies and procedures on the topic. Also, note the compliance level of health team members with the policies and procedures in your agency. Outline areas of compliance and areas of noncompliance. Develop a report about noncompliant practices to submit to the appropriate administrator in your clinical practice agency.

## INTERNET RESOURCES

### Resources for Mapping the Environment: Global Digital Data Sets on the Internet
For population distribution, visit www.ciesin.org/data.html.
For oceans and sea surface temperatures, visit the University of Wisconsin Space Science and Engineering Center at www.ssec.wisc.edu/data/sst.html.

### Websites for Information Related to Environmental Health
Environmental Protection Agency: http://www.epa.gov.
Health Care Without Harm: http://www.noharm.org.
Center for Disease Control: http://www.cdc.gov.
National Center for Environmental Health: http://www.cdc.gov.nceh
National Institute of Occupational Safety and Health: http:www.cdc.gov/niosh/homepage.html/
National Library of Medicine: http://www.nlm.nih.gov.
Nightingale Institute for Health and Environment: http://www.nihe.org.
Toxnet: http://toxnet.nlm.nih.gov.
Toxic Release Inventory: http://www.epa.gov/tri.
U.S. Environmental Protection Agency, Persistent, Biocumulative & Toxic Chemical Program: www.epa.gov/pbt

### Resources for Workplace Safety
Visit www.osha-slc.gov/index/html. Type in "workplace violence," then click on the title "Guidelines for Preventing Violence for Health Care and Social Service Workers."
Visit OSHA's ergonomic web site at www.osha-slc.gov/SLTC/ergonomic/index.html.
Visit the Clinical Practice Model Resources Center to learn more about Partnership, Dialogue and Healthy Workplace Development at www.cpmrc.com.

## REFERENCES
Barnett, T. P., Pierce, D. W., & Schnur, R. (2001, April 13). Detection of anthropogenic climate change in the world's oceans. *Science, 292*, 270–274.
Belanger, D. (2000). Nurses and suicide: The risk is real. *RN, 63*, 61–64.
Bender, K., & Thompson, F. (2003). West Nile Virus: A growing challenge. *American Journal of Nursing, 103*, 32–40.
Bright, C. (2000). Anticipating environmental 'surprise.' In L. R. Brown, C. Flavin, H. French, S. Postel, & L. Starke (Eds.), *State of the world 2000* (pp. 22–38). New York: W. W. Norton.
Brown, L. R. (2000). Challenges of the new century. In L. R. Brown, C. Flavin, H. French, S. Postel, & L. Starke (Eds.), *State of the world 2000* (pp. 3–21). New York: W. W. Norton.

Carroll, V. (2004). Preventing violence in the healthcare workplace. *The Missouri Nurse, 2*, 12–13, 31.

Cohen, J. (2003). Asia: The next frontier for HIV/AIDS. *Science, 301*, 1658–1662.

Cohen, J. (2004a). Poised for takeoff? *Science, 304*, 1430–1432.

Cohen, J. (2004b). HIV/AIDS India's many epidemics. *Science, 304*, 504–509.

Dock, L. L. (1912). *A history of nursing* (Vol. 3). New York: G. P. Putnam's Sons.

Dyck, R. J. (2000). Historical development of latex allergy. *AORN Journal, 72*, 27–29, 32–33, 35–40.

Enserink, M. (2001). Infections diseases. West Nile researchers get ready for round three. *Science, 292*, 1289–1291.

Fawcett, J. (1984). *Analysis and evaluation of conceptual models of nursing.* Philadelphia: F. A. Davis.

Feely, R., Sabine, Cc. Lee, K., Berelson, W., Kleypas, J., Fabry, V., & Millero, F. (2004). Impact of anthropogenic CO2 on CaCO3 system in the oceans. *Science, 305*, 362–366.

Frankl, V. (1963). *Man's search for meaning.* New York: Washington Square Press.

French, H. (2000). Coping with ecological globalization. In L. R. Brown, C. Flavin, H. French, S. Postel, & L. Starke (Eds.), *State of the world 2000* (pp. 184–202). New York: W. W. Norton.

Friedman, M., & Morgan, I. (1992). The health care function. In M. Friedman (Ed.). *Family nursing: Theory and practice* (3rd ed.) 291–313. Norwalk CT: Appleton & Lange.

Gerard, M. (2000). Domestic violence: how to screen and intervene. *RN, 63*, 52–56, 58.

Gibson, P. R. (2000). *Multiple chemical sensitivity: A survival guide.* Oakland, CA: New Harbinger Publications Inc.

Green, P. M. (2000). Taking environmental health education seriously. *Nursing and Health Care Perspectives, 21*, 234–239.

Kellet, P. B. (1997). Latex allergy: A review. *Journal of Emergency Nursing, 23*, 27–36.

Kim, K. T., Graves, P. B., Safadi, G. S., Alhadeff, G., & Metcalfe, J. (1998). Implementation recommendations for making health care facilities latex safe. *AORN Journal, 67*, 615–618, 621–624, 626.

Kim, K.T., Wellmeyer, E.T., & Miller, K.V. (1999). Minimum prevalence of latex hypersensitivity in health care workers. *Heray and Asthma* Proceedings *20*, 387–391.

Kleffel, D. (1994). The environment: Alive, whole and interacting. In E. A. Schuster & C. L. Brown (Eds.), *Exploring our environmental connections* (pp. 3–15). NLN Publication No. 14-2634. New York: National League for Nursing.

Kleffel, D. (1996). Environmental paradigms: Moving toward an ecocentric perspective. *Advances in Nursing Science, 18*, 1–10.

Krajick, K. (2001). Long-term data show lingering effects from acid rain. *Science, 292,* 195–196.

Kramer, M. & Schmalenberg, C. (2002). Staff nurses identify *Essentials of magnetism,* in M. McClure & A. Hinshaw, (Eds.) *Magnet hospitals revisited: Attraction and retention of professional nurses.* Kansas City, MO: American Nurses Publishing, pp. 25–59.

Kramer, M. & Schmalenberg, C. (2004). Essentials of a magnetic work environment, part 1. *Nursing, 34*, 50–54.

Lazarus, R. S., & Folkman, S (1984). *Stress, appraisal and coping.* New York: Springer.

Lee, M. H., & Kim, K. T. (1998). Latex allergy: A relevant issue in the general pediatric population. *Journal of Pediatric Health Care, 12,* 242–246.

Leroy, E., Rouquet, P., Formenty, P., Souquiere, S., Kilbourne, A., Froment, J., Bermejo, M., Smit, S., Karesh, W., Swanepoel, R., Zaki, S., & Roullin, P. (2004). Multiple Ebola virus transmission events and rapid decline of central African wildlife. *Science, 303*, 387–390.

McGinn, A. P. (2000). Phasing out persistent organic pollutants. In L. R. Brown, C. Flavin, H. French, S. Postel, L. Starke (Eds.), *State of the world 2000* (pp. 79–100). New York: W. W. Norton.

McLean, A. (1974). Concepts of occupational stress: A review. In A. McLean (Ed.), *Occupational stress* (pp. 3–14). Springfield, IL: Charles C. Thomas.

Melum, M. F., & Kearney, K. (2001). Organophosphate toxicity. *American Journal of Nursing, 101*, 57–58.

*Merriam-Webster's collegiate dictionary* (10th ed.). (1994). Springfield, MA: Merriam-Webster.

Musker, K. (1994). Voluntary simplicity: Nurses creating a healing environment. In E. A. Schuster & C. L. Brown (Eds.), *Exploring our environmental connections* (pp. 195–212). NLN Publication No. 14-2634. New York: National League for Nursing.

Nelson, A., Fragala, G., & Menzel, N. (2003). Myths and facts about back injuries in nursing. *American Journal of Nursing, 103*, 32–41.

O'Meara, M. (2000). Harnessing information technologies for the environment. In L. R. Brown, C. Flavin, H. French, S. Postel, & L. Starke (Eds.), *State of the world 2000* (pp. 121–141). New York: W. W. Norton.

Pope, A. M., Snyder, M. A., & Mood, L. H. (Eds.). (1995). *Nursing, health and the environment.* Washington, DC: The National Academies Press.

Rutala, W. A., Barbee, S. L., Aguiar, N. C., Sobsey, M. D. & Weber, (2000). Antimicrobial activity of home disinfectants and natural products against potential human pathogens. *Infection Control and Hospital Epidemiology, 21*, 33–38.

Scully, M. G. (2001). Taking the pulse of the Kalamazoo. *The Chronicle of Higher Education, 47*, B16.

Shaner, H. (1994). Environmentally responsible clinical practice. In E. A. Schuster & C. L. Brown (Eds.), *Exploring our environmental connections practice* (pp. 233–251). NLN Publication No. 14-2634. New York: National League for Nursing.

Shaner, H. & Botter, M. (2003). Pollution: Health care's unintended legacy. *American Journal of Nursing, 103,* 79, 81, 83–84.

Steger, S. (2000). Killed in school! *RN, 63,* 36–38.

Tilman, D., Fargione, J., D'Antonio, C., Dobson, A., Howarth, R., Schindler, D., Schlesinger, W. H., Simberloff, D., & Swackhamer, D. (2001). Forecasting agriculturally driven environmental change. *Science, 292,* 281–284.

Trossman, S. (2000). Moving violations: Working to prevent on-the-job injuries. *The American Nurse, 32*, 1, 12–14.

Trossman, S. (2001). Illinois RNs win workplace safety measures. *The American Nurse, 33*(1), 1, 8.

United States Department of Health and Human Services. (2000). *Healthy people 2010.* Boston: Jones & Bartlett.

Von der Werf, G., Randerson, J., Callatz, G., Gigio, L., Kesibhatla, P., Arelloro, A., Olsen, S., & Kassichke, E. (2004). Continental-scale partitioning of fire emissions during the 1997–2001 El Nino/La Nina Period. *Science, 303,* (5654), 73–75.

Watkins, J. M., & Mohr, B. J. (2001). *Appreciative inquiry.* San Francisco: Jossey-Bass/Pfeiffer.

Wesorick, B., Shiparski, L., Troseth, M., & Wyngarden, K. (1997). *Partnership Council field book.* Grand Rapids, MI: Practice Field Publishing.

Wilson, C. K., & Porter-O'Grady, T. (1999). *Leading the revolution in health care* (2nd ed.). Gaithersburg, MD: Aspen.

Worthington, K. (2000). Seeking the perfect fit. *American Journal of Nursing, 100,* 88.

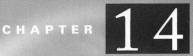
# Community Health

## KEY TERMS AND CONCEPTS

Community

Population

Community Health Problem

Demography

Epidemiology

Community Assessment

Community-Based Nursing

Community Health Nursing

Systems Model for Geopolitical and
Phenomenological Communities

General Systems Theory

Lundy-Barton's General Systems Model for
Community and Population Assessment
and Intervention

Community as Partner

Dimensions Model

## LEARNING OUTCOMES

By the end of this chapter, the learner will be able to:

1 Define the terms community, community health, and community health nursing.

2 Compare and contrast the following models for community health nursing: systems model for geopolitical and phenomenological communities; Lundy-Barton's general systems model for community and population assessment and intervention; community as partner model; and the dimensions model.

3 Outline the roles of the community health nurse.

4 Summarize key elements of professional nursing within various community settings presented in the chapter.

## VIGNETTE

Paula works as the nursing director of a county public health department that receives 3,000 free flu vaccines annually from a federal government program. Last year, she had to return 1,000 doses because they were not used. She noticed that there were four small towns in the county in which no residents took advantage of the free flu vaccine program. She noticed that these towns were more than 20 miles from the health department office. To make it easier for residents of the small towns, Paula decides to hold a free immunization clinic in each town. She schedules the clinics on a Wednesday from 8:00 AM to 4:00 PM. Even though each of the towns has a population of 1,500 persons, only a total of 150 vaccines were given. Paula asks herself "Why didn't more people come for free vaccines?" What assumptions did Paula make regarding the lack of participation in the free vaccination program? How could she have elicited better participation of these small town residents in the program?

Community health nursing originated in the Middle Ages when persons opened their homes to care for the infirm (Anderson & McFarlane, 2000; Jamieson & Sewall, 1954; Lundy & Janes, 2001; Stanhope & Lancaster, 2002). Before 1965, most clients received nursing care in the home. Nursing care delivery shifted primarily to acute care settings during the mid-1960s through 1980. During the 1980s, escalating health care costs resulted in changes in third-party reimbursement to hospitals. The federal government initiated a prospective payment system known as diagnosis-related groups, whereby predetermined reimbursement schedules were set for payment for services rendered by hospitals to persons covered by Medicare and Medicaid. To reduce health care costs, health care services— especially nursing care—have shifted back to community settings. Nurses who work in community settings need to display competence in client physical care, teaching, communication, and management (Hunt, 2001). They also must look beyond individual and family client systems and consider the global nature of community health issues.

## ● KEY CONCEPTS OF COMMUNITY HEALTH

Community health nursing differs from other forms of professional practice because the focus of care shifts from individuals to groups. To develop an understanding of community health nursing, the professional nurse must have a clear understanding of key definitions.

### Community

Sources of community health nursing information have varying definitions of the term "community." *Merriam-Webster's Collegiate Dictionary* (1994, p. 233) defines **community** as "1. a unified body of individuals . . . 2. society at large . . . 3. joint ownership or participation." Scholars of community health nursing define community in various ways. Leonard (2000, p. 93) defines community as a web of persons "shaped by relationships, interdependence, mutual interests and patterns of interactions." He proposes that a community encompasses "people at a particular time and place" (p. 93). Lundy, Janes, and Hartman (2001, p. 12) define a community as "a group of people who have something in common, and interact with one another, who may exhibit a commitment to one another and may share a geographic boundary." Hunt (2001, p. 9) defines community as "a people, location, and social system." Smith and Maurer (2000, p. 342) define community as "an open social system that is characterized by people in a place over time who have a common goal." All these definitions agree that a community consists of a group of persons who share a common interest and interact with each other.

A community need not have specific geographic borders (Hunt, 2001; Leonard, 2000; Lundy et al., 2001). Communities may encompass persons from a particular profession, such as the nursing community; a specific faith community; a specific cultural group, such as the Hispanic community; or persons living within a geographical area, such as a local community. Schools also may be considered a community. As a species, all persons have membership in the global community (Hunt, 2001; Lundy et al., 2001). In community health nursing, professional nurses target a specific group of persons or a geographical locale to serve; this group or location is known as "the **population**." For example, the population served by school nurses includes all persons who provide and receive school services, such as students, parents, teachers, counselors, administrators, clerical workers, and service workers (janitorial, food). The *Healthy People 2010* initiatives of the United States Department of Health and Human Services (USDHHS) target all American citizens.

The holographic community described by Davis (2000) expands the definition of community to one of multiple dimensions that include the following concepts: community consciousness (awareness), community heart (values), community soul (service), community voice (power), community body (structure and relationships), community mind (learning and development), community spirit (celebration and ritual), and community vision (health and survival) (Leddy, 2003).

The profession of nursing fits the definition of a holographic community because its members are connected to each other (belong to a profession); have shared values (caring, compassion, altruism); possess moral integrity (code of ethics); strive for unity (work toward providing the best care possible); create learning environments (client and professional educational programs); and work as individuals and collectively to achieve a better level of health for all.

Other approaches to community define community as place, social interaction, and political and social responsibility. As a place, the essential element includes a specific designated area where persons live and engage in various types of activity. Sharing a common purpose to communicate and work together to attain the goal denotes community as a social interaction. When considered as a political and social responsibility, community involves dynamic interactions and social relationships to form a sense of mutual obligation, solidarity, and responsibility to assure social survival (Leddy, 2003).

## Healthy Community

The healthy city/community movement began in the middle 1980s in Europe. Hancock and Duhl (1986) specify that the following must be present for a community to be classified as healthy.

1. A clean, safe, ecologically stable physical environment.
2. Resident access to resources that promote and maintain healthy, diverse, vital, and innovative economy.
3. A strong, supportive, nonexploitative community.
4. Basic human needs met for all members (food, water, shelter, income, safety).
5. Access to a wide variety of experiences and resources (communications, cultural events, diverse contacts, and communications).
6. A connection to community's heritage and past.
7. Equal access to public health and illness care services.
8. Good health status of citizens.
9. High levels of public participation in and control over decisions that affect individual citizens' lives, health, and well-being.

Morse (2004) denotes characteristics of successful communities that plan for and adapt to change. Healthy communities have members who understand their relationship and responsibility to others rather than focusing on individual pursuits. By strategically planning for change, communities assure their survival and brighter futures for members following in their footsteps. Morse identifies the following seven key points that result in successful community adaptation to change:

1. Making the right investments/decisions the first time.
2. Working together instead of as individuals or special interest groups with specific agendas.
3. Building on current community strengths.
4. Using a democratic process.
5. Preserving the community's history.
6. Growing their own leaders.
7. Inventing a better and brighter future.

In an ideal world, nurses working in community health help communities become better and use nursing skills to help them achieve health for all their members.

## Community Health Problem

Hunt (2001, p. 384) defines a **community health problem** as a "health need identified in a community assessment." Lundy and Barton (2001) and Anderson and McFarlane (2000) would equate community health problems to the concept of nursing diagnosis. When a gap exists between ideal community health and current community health, a community health problem exists.

## Demography

**Demography**, the science of human populations, traces population size, characteristics, and changes. Shifts in demographics may have profound implications for health care delivery and professional nursing, as in the case of the graying and increasing cultural diversity of American citizens (Anderson & McFarlane; Hunt, 2001; Lundy & Janes, 2001; *Merriam-Webster's Collegiate Dictionary*, 1994; USDHHS, 2000).

## Epidemiology

Along with demographic trends is **epidemiology,** the study of factors that promote wellness or cause illness and help delineate the health of a community. Because illness is easier to measure, the focus of epidemiology tends to be on factors such as morbidity (illness), mortality (death), incidence (number of persons in a population who have a condition develop during a specified time frame), and prevalence (number of persons in a population who have a condition within a given time). Epidemiology views health and disease as a composite state of the three following variables: agent, host, and environment. These three variables create the epidemiologic triangle. In the case of altered health, an agent (or combination of agents) may result in the development of a specific health problem. Before the health alteration occurs, there must be a host, or person who contracts the health problem. Finally, environmental factors contribute to the development of a health problem (Anderson & McFarlane, 2000; Lundy & Janes, 2001; *Merriam-Webster's Collegiate Dictionary*, 1994; Smith & Maurer, 2000; USDHHS, 2000).

For example, for tuberculosis (TB) to develop, a person must come into contact with the *Mycobacterium* tubercle. The environment must have conditions for the tubercular bacillus to thrive (crowded conditions), and an available person must be susceptible to contract the illness (host). Many community health nurses spend much time tracking down cases of infectious diseases, and in some cases, they monitor client compliance to prescribed therapies.

## Community Assessment

To determine the health of a specific community, community health care nurses assess the community in terms of status, structure, and process. Because of the breadth of **community assessment** in each of the terms, the following list provides brief examples of each.

- Status assessment includes reported statistics related to birth, death, poverty, crime, and incidence of mental and physical illness.
- Structure assessment includes inpatient and outpatient health care facilities, local government structures, schools, law enforcement agencies, retailers, roads, and population demographics (socioeconomic status, gender, age).
- Process assessment includes factors such as member commitment; communication patterns; relationships of the community with the larger society; how well the community voices need for, accesses, and uses resources (Anderson & McFarlane, 2000; Clark, 1999; Hunt, 2001; Lundy & Janes, 2001; Smith & Maurer, 2000).

## Community-based Nursing

Hunt (2001) defines **community-based nursing** as delivery of nursing care within the context of a family's home and community. Community-based nursing facilitates continuity of care across the spectrum of consumer health care services, thus enabling health care professionals to meet the needs of people as they move from acute care to the community and vice versa. Community-based nursing refers to where nursing care is delivered. Nurses who deliver nursing services away from acute or extended care institutions practice community-based nursing.

## Community Health Nursing

**Community health nursing** encompasses more than where nursing care is delivered, but represents a specialized area of professional practice. As a more comprehensive concept, Anderson and McFarland (2000) expand the concept of community health nursing to include the following dimensions of nursing practice: (1) assessment of populations; (2) development of partnerships with community members and stakeholders; (3) emphasis on health promotion (primary prevention); (4) creation of health environmental, social, and economic conditions in a community; (5) outreach services for community members in need; (6) focus on the group as a whole rather than individual members; and (7) judicious allocation of resources and wise stewardship.

## ✦ CONCEPTUAL MODELS FOR COMMUNITY HEALTH NURSING

A variety of nursing models may be used by community nurses to guide clinical practice. Community nurses select models to guide clinical practice based on their world views.

Models commonly used by nurses in community settings are the **systems model for geopolitical and phenomenological communities** (Smith & Maurer, 2000), the Lundy-Barton general systems model for community and population assessment and intervention (2001), and Anderson and McFarlane's (2000) community as partner model. These models base theoretical relationships on general systems theory.

## General Systems Theory

In **general systems theory,** the universe is composed of interacting elements of various sizes known as subsystems, with the individual's cells being the smallest element. Each system has boundaries that separate it from other systems. Subsystems increase in size and complexity, include persons, groups, towns, states, and nations, and expand to encompass the entire universe. All subsystems receive energy, resources, and information (input) that are transformed (throughput) for the maintenance of a steady state or for subsystem growth and development. Results of resource and energy use then return to the system (output). Resources used by subsystems (individuals, groups, or society) may result in waste products that may be beneficial or noxious to the environment and other subsystems. In the general systems theory, a change in one subsystem results in cascading changes for the entire system, thus necessitating adaptation. System disorganization (entropy) results from demands of continuous readjustment for effective adaptation to change. For systems to meet goals, increasing order (negentropy) occurs so the system can attain a steady state. Systems strive for balanced steady states but must experience disorder for growth and development. Subsystems continuously receive feedback from each other when the output of one becomes the input for another (Bertalanffy, 1968).

## Systems Model for Geopolitical and Phenomenological Communities

The systems model for geopolitical and phenomenological communities uses a systems analysis framework to guide nurses in data collection and organization. Smith and Maurer (2000, p. 348) designate the following seven key components.

1. Boundaries: factors that separate the community from the environment and maintain the integrity of the community.
2. Goals: The purpose or reason for which the community exists.
3. Set factors: The physical and psychosocial characteristics of the community that affect behavior.
4. Inputs: External influences from the suprasystem.
5. Throughputs: The internal functioning of the community divided into four functional subsystems (economy, polity, communication, and values).
6. Outputs: The health behavior and status of the community.
7. Feedback: The information that is returned to the system regarding its functioning.

Nurses using the systems model for geopolitical and phenomenological communities assess these seven components when collecting data about the community that receives professional nursing services. Smith and Maurer (2000) advocate for the following three different approaches to community assessment: the comprehensive needs assessment, in which community members are asked what they need; the problem-oriented approach, in which the nurse addresses a particular health concern; and the familiarization approach, in which the nurse studies existing data about a community to determine the presence of a special group that has specific health care needs.

Once the community assessment is completed, the nurse analyzes the collected data to determine the level of community health according to environmental safety, social structure, available energy and resources, and health status behaviors. When problems arise in any of these areas, the professional nurse works in partnership with community representatives to set priorities and design a plan of care with a goal of maximizing health for all community members. Professional nursing interventions include providing health education, screening persons for health problems, developing and implementing policies, fostering community self-help, and looking for ways to empower the disenfranchised community members. Once the nurse has implemented nursing interventions, the nurse evaluates the community care plan in terms of outcome attainment, appropriateness, adequacy, efficiency, and process. Evaluation of the effectiveness of each is performed.

## Lundy-Barton General Systems Model for Community and Population Assessment and Intervention

**Lundy-Barton's general systems model for community and population assessment and intervention** offers a global systematic approach for professional nurses to use when practicing community health nursing. The Lundy-Barton model incorporates the steps of the nursing process to identify community health issues and take action to remedy them. (Table 14-1 summarizes the model in detail.) The Lundy-Barton model provides a comprehensive approach to community health nursing and effectively addresses individual, family, health care delivery, political, social, educational, economic, and religious systems within a community. The model serves as one template that community nurses may use on which to base their professional practice. However, before using the model, professional nurses must define the target community or population that receives nursing services. Then, the nurse considers the subsystems within the community and how the target community interacts with larger systems (suprasystems) and compares with communities of similar size and structure (Lundy & Janes, 2001).

## Community as Partner Model

Another nursing model commonly used to direct community health nursing is the **community as partner** model. Anderson and McFarlane (2000) adapted the Neuman systems model (see Chapter 5) to communities. Anderson and McFarlane identify eight areas for community assessment and care: physical environment, health and social services, communication, economics, safety and transportation, politics and government, education, and recreation. Nurses assess community stressors and buffers (flexible lines of defense, normal lines of defense, and lines of resistance) that the community uses to reduce the impact of stressors. The model considers individual and group reactions to stressors. Based on assessment, nurses generate community-nursing diagnoses in collaboration with community members. Nurses and community members work together

**TABLE 14-1**

## Summary of the Lundy-Barton General Systems Model for Community and Population Assessment and Intervention

| Nursing Process Step/Model Phase | Elements for Nursing Consideration |
| --- | --- |
| Assessment/database | Compile a database that includes community demographics, psychological climate, nutritional status, physical fitness, geographical boundaries, location, environmental conditions, safety practices, health care delivery services, political systems, dominant social system, communication patterns, and educational systems |
| Diagnosis/problem list | Generate a community problem list based on assessment findings |
| Planning/problem assessment and plan formulation | Determine an action plan for identified community problems in partnership with members of the community. Community members and the nurse work together to set priorities for action, long- and short-term program objectives, and specific actions |
| Implementation | Execute the action plan with continued community participation while documenting progress notes |
| Evaluation/progress notes | Review documented progress notes to determine effectiveness of the action plan as the plan is executed so that changes in approaches may be made and again at completion of the action plan to determine its effectiveness |
| Restart process | Reassess the community and proceed with steps of nursing process |

Adapted from Lundy and Janes, 2001.

to determine primary interventions to promote community health (e.g., *Healthy People 2010*, routine vaccinations); secondary interventions to address stressor penetration (e.g., screening people for exposure to an infectious disease, vaccination, or prophylactic antibiotic administration to persons exposed to an infectious illness and treatment of ill community members); and tertiary interventions to promote community recovery from stressor penetration (education, counseling, and support services for members living in fear of the contagious illness for which interventions have occurred). Anderson and McFarlane emphasize that community feedback and changes in community processes provide the basis for evaluating community health nursing interventions.

## Epidemiology

Although humans acknowledged the contagious dimension of many illnesses during the time of Hippocrates, William Farr, a London physician, developed a system of tracking births, illnesses, and deaths that started the discipline of modern epidemiology (Harkness, 2001; Jamieson & Sewall, 1954; Anderson & McFarlane, 2000). Florence Nightingale used the epidemiologic principles of cleanliness, fresh air, and optimal nutrition to reduce the fatalities during the Crimean War (Harkness, 2001; Jamieson & Sewall, 1954).Work of pioneers in the field of epidemiology resulted in the development of the epidemiologic triad: host, agent, and environment. The epidemiologic triad evolved into the epidemiologic model that acknowledges that disease is multifaceted and that the three factors—a susceptible host (humans), an offending agent (something that causes a disease or illness), and an environment (physical, chemical, biologic, and social climate)—must all be present before a health-related problem can occur (Harkness, 2001; Parrish, 1969). In recent years, epidemiology has expanded from the study of infectious illnesses to include the critical influences that lead to chronic illnesses, crime, lifestyle, and other factors that result in less-than-optimal health.

Epidemiology, like professional nursing, has a process that is used to solve health-related problems. The following steps occur in the epidemiologic process:

1. Define the problem.
2. Gather information from a variety of reliable sources.
3. Describe the problem by identifying people, time, and places.
4. Formulate a hypothesis to speculate who, what, where, why, and how the problem occurred.
5. Compile descriptive data analysis to test the generated hypothesis.
6. Develop a plan to control the problem.
7. Implement a controlled plan.
8. Evaluate the controlled plan.
9. Prepare a report that includes the scope of the problem, control plan development, implementation, and evaluation, as well as prevention strategies for problem recurrence.
10. Conduct additional research on the identified problem (Harkness, 2001).

The science of epidemiology is divided into two branches: descriptive epidemiology and analytical epidemiology.

## Descriptive Epidemiology

Descriptive epidemiology focuses on statistics to describe the state of health for a given population. Persons with particular health problems are identified. Risk factors for a particular health problem result when persons with the problem share common characteristics (e.g, risky sexual practices and the development of sexually transmitted diseases). Epidemiologists frequently use rates, which are fractions, to describe the incidence of a health problem during a specified time (105 cases/100,000 persons). Incidence refers to the occurrence of new cases in a previously disease-free population for a specific time. Prevalence rates indicate the number of persons within a given population who have an existing health problem within a specified time.

Along with rates, epidemiologists become concerned with place and time when the health condition occurs. In the fall of 2001, several letters contaminated with anthrax entered the United States Postal Service system in the eastern part of the United States. The letters contaminated equipment, resulting in contamination of mail that was processed at the same time. In addition, the Postal Service unknowingly shipped contaminated equipment to other areas of the country. Persons who had contact with contaminated postal equipment or mail from postal centers where the letters had been processed were closely monitored for signs and symptoms of cutaneous and inhaled anthrax. Epidemiologists track trends or long-term changes to forecast future health care needs.

### Analytical Epidemiology

Analytical epidemiology focuses on the why, or determinants, of the health-related problem. Sometimes determinants surface when descriptive data are analyzed. However, analytical epidemiology sometimes reveals that more descriptive data need to be collected. Analytic epidemiologists conduct the following four types of studies.

1. Cross sectional surveys: Data collected at one point in time to describe current health status and to determine possible hypotheses for a particular health problem.
2. Retrospective studies: Study a group of persons to trace past experiences to determine reasons for a health problem.
3. Prospective, cohort, or longitudinal studies: Determine/compare the incidence of a health-related problem in persons who were exposed to that of persons who were not exposed to a specific factor.
4. Therapeutic, intervention, or prevention trials: Randomized studies to determine the persons who will benefit from specific interventions to prevent the health-related problem.

In the anthrax situation described above, the Centers for Disease Control (CDC) served as a resource for local health departments and health care professionals who monitored persons known to be in contact with contaminated mail and equipment. In addition, the CDC developed recommendations for prophylactic antibiotic therapy for persons who had contact with levels of anthrax known to result in the disease.

## The Dimensions Model

Using concepts derived from epidemiology, Clark (1999) developed the **dimensions model** to guide community health nursing practice. The dimensions model uses dimensions of nursing, health, and health care as interacting elements to determine a state of health or illness. The dimensions of nursing, health, and health care are outlined in Table 14-2. The nurse uses the dimensions of professional nursing outlined by Clark when working with individuals, families, or communities. The dimensions of health determine the quality of individual, family, and community health. Finally, the level of prevention determines specific strategies used by the nurse to prevent health problems, treat them when they arise, and support persons to attain the best possible health state after experiencing a health problem.

The dimensions model emphasizes the importance of the role of the professional nurse in helping persons to obtain and maintain optimal health by providing a holistic approach to care. Along with individual and family factors, the model also incorporates the health care system as a determinant of health status for individuals, families, and communities.

Other nursing models also provide a conceptual basis for community health nursing. Leininger's sunrise model (see Chapter 11) for transcultural nursing focuses on specific considerations when nurses provide professional service to clients from various cultural groups. Pender's health promotion model (see Chapter 8) also provides a solid foundation for promoting wellness when working with individuals and groups.

TABLE 14-2

## The Dimensions Model

| Nursing Dimensions | Health Dimensions | Health Care Dimensions |
|---|---|---|
| **Cognitive dimension** | **Biophysical dimension** | **Primary prevention** |
| Knowledge | Age<br>Genetic heredity<br>Physiological function | Health promotion<br>Disease prevention |
| **Interpersonal dimension** | **Psychological dimension** | **Secondary prevention** |
| Interaction skills<br>Affective elements | Internal psychological<br>　environment (ideas<br>　about self)<br>External psychological<br>　environment (ideas<br>　derived from others) | Early detection of health<br>　problems<br>Treatment of existing<br>　health problems |
| **Ethical dimension** | **Social dimension** | **Tertiary prevention** |
| Ethical decision-making<br>　skills and processes<br>Client advocacy | Social structure<br>Norms<br>Attitudes<br>Social action | Return to highest functioning level<br>　after health problem treatment<br>Prevent further health deterioration<br>Prevent health problem recurrence |
| **Skills dimension** | **Behavioral dimension** | |
| Manipulative skills (clinical skills)<br>Intellectual skills | Diet<br>Exercise<br>Recreation<br>Substance use (and abuse)<br>Sexual habits<br>Use of protective devices | |
| **Process dimension** | **Health system dimension** | |
| Nursing process<br>Epidemiology<br>Health education<br>Home visits<br>Case management<br>Change<br>Leadership<br>Group process<br>Political action | Availability<br>Access<br>Affordability<br>Appropriateness<br>Adequacy<br>Acceptability<br>Use | |
| **Reflective dimension** | | |
| Theory development<br>Research<br>Evaluation of care | | |

Adapted from Clark, 1999.

# ● COMMUNITY LEVEL NURSING INTERVENTIONS

Health promotion within a community encompasses collective efforts. Community nursing interventions work best when the community assumes ownership of the plan, responsibility for community health program maintenance, and control for planning future programs. Nurses use multiple strategies to help communities improve their health. Nurses empower, collaborate with, build capacity for, and advocate for individual members and the entire community (Leddy, 2003). Nurses empower communities by investing time and resources to enable communities to assume control over their destiny. Community members view the nurse as a health expert who has much knowledge and expertise in developing programs and supporting others to attain better health. Poverty-stricken communities perceive a lack of control over their destinies and feel powerless because they may not be valued by others, have few (or no) resources, lack economic and political power, have no experience in making decisions, and have learned helplessness. Sometimes, community members have a history of fighting with each other. Nurses can serve as mediators to settle long-standing disputes so that the community members can determine which programs are needed. Nurses also serve as consultants, coaches, and cheerleaders as community members plan, implement, and evaluate community health programs.

Collaboration with the community requires that the nurse and community members share information and resources with each other, but above all, trust each other. The nurse's ability to effectively listen to member concerns enables the nurse to identify key community health problems. The nurse may assume a coordination role for work in the beginning. However, once work processes are standardized, community members receive education or training, and common values and beliefs about a project are shared by all, then the nurse can serve primarily as a resource person. For an effective program, the nurse must collaborate with community workers, health groups, traditional folk healers, and community leaders (Leddy, 2003).

Capacity building occurs with individual members, small groups, and the entire community. Capacity building involves building upon the current strengths, resources and abilities already present in the community. Individual capacity building involves: changing personal values for health enhancing outcomes; having a positive attitude toward collaboration; deciding things using consensus; sharing power and information; showing respect; giving support; participating in egalitarian relationships; perceiving self-efficacy; setting future goals; feeling a sense of coherence; identifying with others with similar problems; feeling able to help others; and understanding community member roles and responsibilities. Small group capacity building includes interacting with others to help them assume control; fostering a sense of connectedness; establishing trust; and creating positive interactions. Capacity in building communities involves helping members and the community to articulate health problems and potential solutions, providing them access to information, supporting current community leadership, and assisting them to overcome obstacles to action. While building capacity within a community, the nurse may act as a strategist, coach, meeting facilitator, mediator, and developer of community leadership (Leddy, 2003).

Once the community has mobilized its internal human and physical resources, the community shares a group consciousness. With a united purpose, the community becomes capable of taking social and political action to obtain more resources for use in community building and improvement. Disenfranchised persons may not have the ability to independently develop as a community. The nurse helps these persons achieve community-building skills through role-modeling, providing support, and listening to them share their problems and concerns.

# ✦ CAREER OPPORTUNITIES IN COMMUNITY HEALTH NURSING

Many opportunities for nurses to engage in community nursing exist. Sometimes, as members of a community apart from an employment setting, community members who know the professional nurse ask for health advice and information. Professional nurses may be employed in community settings, such as public health departments, factories, businesses, camps, homes, homeless shelters, prisons, schools, parishes, and the armed forces. However, some nurses elect to use professional skills to serve communities and engage in volunteer nursing. Nurses who give health-related advice to friends and acquaintances are practicing nursing and assume accountability for actions. Thus, the professional nurse should keep a record of nursing actions (including consultations with neighbors) and evaluate outcomes of health education, advice, recommended consultations, and nursing procedures.

Because of the array of nursing opportunities, the subsequent section briefly describes selected practice areas for community health nursing. More detailed information regarding community nursing opportunities may be found by consulting chapter website resources or references.

## Public Health Nursing

Since 1893, public health nurses have been serving individuals, groups, communities, and populations. Public health nurses respond to societal health needs. Public health nurses focus on promoting and protecting the health of populations. Frequently, public health nurses collaborate with world organizations (the United Nations), national governments (the United States Public Health Services Department), and state and local (county or city) governments. Public health nurses also may be employed by capitated health systems to meet the needs of members of a population with the same health-related problem. Health promotion and protection are the top priorities for public health nurses (Quad Council of Public Health Nursing Organizations, 1999).

When public health is the goal of professional practice, the Quad Council of Public Health Nursing Organizations (1999) stipulates the baccalaureate degree as the practice entry level. They recommend the master's degree for disease prevention and health promotions for populations at risks. However, when practice focuses on health and illnesses of individuals, less highly educated nurses may appropriately practice public health nursing.

Public health nurses provide many essential services to protect and promote health for citizens. Public health nurses provide services to meet government-specified health objectives as outlined in *Healthy People 2010*. Essential services offered by public health service nurses include (1) monitoring the health states of a particular population; (2) diagnosing community health problems; (3) identifying community health hazards; (4) investigating community health problems when they arise; (5) developing partnerships with those whom they serve; (6) solving community health problems; (7) developing policies and action plans to support community health; (8) enforcing laws and regulations to assure public safety and health; (9) linking persons to appropriate health care services; (10) educating current and future public health personnel; (11) evaluating the effectiveness and quality of public health services; (12) identifying future health threats; and (13) researching to find innovative solutions to maximize the health and safety of the public (Bender & Salmon, 2001; Clark, 1999; Smith & Maurer, 2000; Quad Council of Public Health Nursing Organizations, 1999).

## Questions for Reflection 14-1

1. Do I know how to contact the closest local public health department?
2. What services does my local public health department offer?

## Community Mental Health Nursing

Promoting mental health of citizens is extremely important for the quality of life in a community. Many countries, including the United States, provide mental health services for citizens who need them. The civil rights movement of the 1960s transformed the delivery of mental health care in the United States. Many mentally ill persons were freed from institutions that provided chronic mental health services. They became part of local communities and were no longer required to conform to the restrictions required by shelters and group homes. Many homeless persons suffer from mental illness. When left to fend for themselves, some mentally ill persons have no access to mental health services to receive the psychotropic medications necessary to function effectively as a citizen. Some communities have civil ordinances against persons living on the streets; some provide homeless shelters; other communities rely on private agencies or churches to provide shelter for the homeless. Some homeless shelters provide mental health services for their clients. Community mental health nurses sometimes work in homeless shelters or provide outreach mental health services to persons living on the streets.

Violent crimes usually occur when someone (or group) is out of control. The American (and other country) legal system offers persons accused of crimes to use insanity as a defense for committing crimes. Many times persons who commit crimes cannot be held accountable for their actions. For every crime, there are victims (those directly affected by the crime and those indirectly affected by it.) Unfortunately, the homeless mentally ill often fall victim to acts of violence, especially when they live on the street. Crime also instills fear in persons living in the community, because all persons may become a crime victim. Some persons living in high crime areas become isolated because of their fear for their safety or the safety of their home and its contents. Not all public health departments provide mental health services for their communities. When they do, community health nurses provide mental health services to clients who seek care in public health clinics. If the public health department does not offer mental health services, then community members receive mental health services from free-standing government-supported, nonprofit, or for-profit mental health centers. Separation of mental health services from public health departments increases the complexity of delivery of mental health services to the community because community members must go to a different location for mental health services. In addition, community members must be informed of the location and nature of mental health services offered by each center to access care. If a major event occurs within a community that has the potential to affect the mental health of its members, coordinated efforts from all facilities offering mental health services is required. For example, community mental health nurses from various mental health facilities may be consulted to support students and teachers in schools after an act of violence or student loss of life has occurred.

Many mentally ill rely on substantial public assistance because they cannot hold a job. Most states bear the brunt of expenses to provide basic needs and services for the mentally ill. Community mental health nurses work in interdisciplinary teams to maximize use of available resources. Often community mental health nurses share clients with other interdisciplinary mental health team members. In these cases, nurses assess the client for therapeutic and potential adverse effects of medications, monitor mental status, and contact physicians for medication adjustments. The social worker provides clients with information and assists them in receiving required resources such as free medication, food stamps, and housing assistance (Haque, Nolan, Dyke, & Khan, 2002). Community mental health nurses may visit mentally ill persons in their homes (group home or private residence). Depending on the community, these nurses may be employed by a public health or a private visiting nursing agency.

The United States Government specified goals to improve and increase access to quality mental health services in *Healthy People 2010*. Mental health services targeted for improvement include preventative services for suicide, adolescent suicide attempts, and eating disorders. Increased efforts aimed at providing employment of persons with serious mental illnesses is another goal. The initiative also hopes to improve services for serious mental illnesses among homeless adults. Areas for treatment expansion for mental health and illness include the following: (a) primary care including screening and assessment for mental disorders, (b) pediatric mental health problem treatment, (c) screening for mental disorders in juvenile justice facilities, (d) treatment for adults with mental and co-occurring disorders, and (e) providing adult jail diversion programs (USDHHS, 2000). More community mental health nurses are and will be needed to attain these goals.

*Healthy People 2010* also challenges the states to track consumer satisfaction with offered mental health services, create means to address cultural competence, and develop plans to address the mental health needs of the future burgeoning elderly population (USDHHS, 2000).

## Research Brief 14-1

Minhard, H. A., & Blanchard, M. (2004). Older people with depression: Pilot study. *Journal of Advanced Nursing, 46,* 23–32.

Using a convenience sample of 24 elderly persons who regularly attended a community day center in Great Britain, the investigators wanted to identify the incidence of depression and its precipitating factors in elderly residents living in the community. Data were collected over 3 months from four men and 20 women, age range 65 to 90 years. Participants completed the Geriatric Mental State-Automated Geriatric Examination for Computer Assisted Taxonomy, Satisfaction with Life Scale, Social Support Questionnaire, and London Handicap Scale to provide study data.

The study yielded higher rates of depression in this group of elderly men and women. Results revealed statistically significant corrections among depression and increased loneliness scores and depression and reduced life satisfaction scores. However, the study found no significant relationships among depression, physical handicap, and social support.

This study reveals that there may be a role for community mental health nurses in community centers providing activities for the elderly living in the community. Depression may be more widespread than previously thought among elderly living in the community. However, the results of this study must be interpreted with caution because the daycare director hand-picked elderly persons who participated in the study. Perhaps, she targeted elderly clients who she thought could benefit from study participation. Also, the study was performed in Great Britain and may not be applicable to other countries because of cultural variations in attitudes toward and support services for the elderly. Community mental health nursing in adult day centers may become a useful way for early assessment and intervention for depression in the elderly.

## Electronic Community Health Nursing

Internet chat rooms create a gathering place for persons with similar interests or conditions. When a chat room is formed for a specific purpose, such as providing support, education, and resource information for persons with a similar condition or life situation, the purpose is consistent with the American Nurses Association *Scope and Standards of Public Health Nursing* (1999a). When nurses participate in chat rooms with the aim of promoting and protecting the health of its members, they could be providing community nursing services. In chat rooms, nurses may provide social support to other members, model therapeutic communication techniques, reinforce positive behaviors among group members, offer self-care or health-promoting advice, provide health-related information, and monitor group dynamics (Copeland, 2002).

Before electronic community health nursing can be recognized, current international, national, and state laws require changes. The following questions about professional nursing practice must also be addressed:

1. How (or will) professional nurses receive compensation for their services?
2. What accountability will the nurse have to the members of the electronic community?
3. What are the roles of the professional nurse providing *e-Community Health Nursing* services?
4. If the nurse shares a similar condition as other chat room participants, how are professional and personal boundaries delineated?

## Disaster Nursing

The education of professional nurses arms them with useful knowledge and skills to help others in times of disaster. In addition, the public perceives nurses as persons with knowledge and expertise with an obligation to provide care to them in times of distress.

Nurses have a detailed understanding of first aid principles, helping victims of trauma, and preventing the spread of contagious illnesses. Professional nurses also have well-refined teaching, organization, and leadership skills. Professional nurses have knowledge of what physicians and surgeons can realistically accomplish within a given time. Finally, professional nurses have expertise in therapeutic communication skills to help provide psychological and spiritual support to persons during times of uncertainty. Thus, professional nurses play a key role in helping persons prepare for, survive during, cope with, and adapt to life after a disaster.

Veenema (2003) defines a disaster as "any destructive event that disrupts the normal functioning of a community" (p. 4). Disasters come in many forms. They may arise suddenly without warning (terrorist attack, plane crash, subway accident, earthquake), occur with warning (hurricane, flood, tornado, blizzard), or evolve over a long period (drought, famine). Disasters can be caused by nature (natural) or by humans. Disasters caused by humans fall into three broad categories: complex (e.g., multiple causation, such as a drought leads to a famine that stimulates political unrest and relocation of large numbers of people); technologic (e.g., destruction of community infrastructure, industrial accidents, massive power failure), or human settlement (e.g., migration of an entire ethnic group to avoid persecution). The magnitude of a disaster depends on its location. Disasters in highly populated areas affect more people and strain more resources than those occurring in rural areas. A medical disaster occurs when a catastrophic event creates more casualties than the health care resources within a community can effectively accommodate (Veenema, 2003).

Veenema (2003) developed a disaster nursing timeline that starts with preparation and ends with recovery. The first phase occurs before the disaster and encompasses planning/preparedness, prevention, and warning. In the first phase, communities identify hazards and make attempts to remove them. If they cannot be removed (such as weather), then the community develops early warning systems, evacuates members at risk, institutes public awareness campaigns, performs disaster drills, develops nursing databases (mass casualty plans), and devises means to evaluate all components of the disaster response. The response phase (phase 2) occurs with disaster onset and lasts 72 hours immediately following its end. The second phase consists of response, emergency management and mitigation. In the second phase, the disaster response plan is activated; potential and ongoing hazards are identified and action is taken to relieve human suffering (mitigated); public health needs are anticipated; victims are triaged for effective use of available health care resources; emergency food and water distribution centers are established; and alternatives for sanitation and waste removal are established if the community infrastructure has been damaged. The third and final phase focuses on recovery, rehabilitation, reconstruction, and evaluation. This phase starts after 72 hours of the disaster. In this phase, victims receive medical and nursing care; disease surveillance continues; public health infrastructure is restored; family members are reunited; victims are monitored for long-term physical and psychological injuries; disaster responders attend debriefing and counseling sessions; and the disaster team evaluates the disaster plan and revises the original disaster preparedness plan as needed (Veenema, 2003). In developed countries, most communities have a disaster preparedness plan. However, these plans remain intact only in those with stable governments.

Professional nurses play key roles in each of the disaster states. Professional nurses who are uninjured at the disaster site offer basic first aid to victims. Some nurses, especially those working in emergency departments and as flight nurses, have special certification in trauma nursing and find themselves assisting in the rescue of victims in the field, triaging persons for appropriate treatment, or treating victims in first aid stations or emergency departments. Nurse administrators participate by assisting in communicating information about victims to families. Some nurses may assume the responsibility of reuniting family members and friends who became separated during the disaster. Mental health nurses offer counseling to victims and relatives of victims. Acute care nurses may find themselves mobilizing supplies, adjusting staff assignments, and determining which patients can be discharged early to make room for victims. If the prospect of spread of infectious disease surfaces, other nurses may participate in mass vaccination programs. Finally, nurses may become involved with shelter supervision.

The American Red Cross offers professional disaster nursing certification programs for nurses who wish to become professionally prepared to assist during a disaster. The program provides education for nurses to assist with damage assessment, case management, triage displaced persons for illness and injury, and administer first aid. The American Red Cross employs nurses and has more than 40,000 nurse volunteers available for immediate assignment in the event of a disaster (Schmidt, 2004). The United States Government also provides specialized training for multidisciplinary health care teams to act as first responders in the event of a major disaster.

The White House Homeland Security Council plans to have a functional model mobilizing 20,000 health care workers capable of responding to a mass casualty event affecting 100,000 to 200,000 persons. States have been assigned to create individualized data banks to establish the Emergency System for Advance Registration of Volunteer Healthcare Personnel. Each state will develop an individual data bank that will be linked to the Health Resources and Services Administration. Health care personnel, including nurses, would volunteer to serve in a capacity based on levels of expertise including nursing specialty certification. An incident commander could identify and mobilize health care personnel with the skills to handle specific types of incidents (Vogt, 2004). Lundy and Butts (2001) outline the following approaches for community health nurses to use to be prepared for a disaster.

1. Personal preparation: be aware of potential disasters; maintain personal emergency equipment and supplies; keep first aid supplies and skills up to date; remind family members of what to do in the event of a disaster; and evaluate the location of a house before making it a home.
2. Community involvement: familiarize yourself with local disaster and local evacuation plans; become involved in community activities related to disaster preparedness and recovery; support leaders who promote long-term solutions to reduce loss and promote emergency preparedness; assist in passing ordinances and modify the use of land that has the potential for flooding, mud slides, or collapse; assist in educating the public about disaster preparedness; visit schools to prepare children who will become accustomed to disasters throughout their lives.
3. Professional preparation: obtain disaster nursing certification by your local American Red Cross Chapter; become involved in the development of disaster plans; support efforts to increase disaster preparedness; and write articles for and letters to lay and professional publications to increase the awareness of disaster preparedness.

However, all professional nurses, not just community health nurses, should be educated for and capable of providing nursing services to anyone in need during a disaster. Other ways to promote personal disaster preparedness are to purchase handbooks that cover first aid techniques and wilderness survival (especially if power plants become inoperable), participate in wilderness survival programs, teach classes related to disaster preparedness, and learn specific techniques to provide support for persons with posttraumatic stress disorder. To increase the profession of nursing's disaster preparedness, nurses could work toward changing the standards of nursing education programs to include curriculum content related to disaster preparedness and response and by attending continuing education programs related to disaster preparedness.

## Camp Nursing

Camps are temporary, small communities. "Like all communities, camps provide basic services for their members, including food, shelter, socialization, protection from harm, meaningful activity, and the other necessities of life" (Lishner & Bruya, 1994, p. 7). Although seen primarily as a form of recreation, camps offer opportunities for nurses to practice first aid skills and care for the injured and infirm in more rustic settings, thereby providing practice in skills that might be required to respond to and care for disaster victims (Erceg & Pravda, 2001).

Camp nurses work toward attaining a healthy camp community. Camping allows individuals of all ages to experience nature; escape the stress of a fast-paced, highly technological society; and learn self-reliance while learning skills for survival and recreation, depending on the type of camp. Camp enables persons to live with others unlike themselves and shows them how to establish a community for a prescribed time. Skills learned at camp transfer to other settings.

Professional nurses have opportunities to participate in a variety of camping experiences. Day camps provide sessions of varying lengths, but the participants and staff return home at night. Resident camps require participants and staff to live on site for a few days or up to 2 months. Resident camps assume great responsibility to assure the safety and health of participants and staff. Travel camps involve some form of motorized transportation so that participants can move from site to site. Trip camps use individually guided vehicles or animals (such as a horse, bicycle, or canoe). Special needs camps serve persons with special physical, cognitive, or emotional needs and provide an opportunity to reap the benefits of camp life. Special needs camps include the various members of the interdisciplinary health care teams on staff to assure that special health needs are met (Erceg & Pravda, 2001).

Camp nurses confront a variety of health care needs in professional practice. Generally speaking, camp nurses provide the following:

1. Emergency care for accidents and acute care for minor illness and injuries (such as insect bites, sore throats, or cuts).
2. Plans to avoid spread of contagious illnesses (foodborne illness, athlete's foot, plantar warts).
3. Health education for campers and staff.
4. Screening and eliminating health hazards from the camp environment (insects; snakes; mice; and poison ivy, oak, and sumac).

5. Verification of healthy diet offerings and daily camp schedules.
6. Supervision that persons abide by health-related rules.

Nurses working or volunteering in special needs camps find themselves providing direct care to campers by administering medications, performing specialized procedures and therapies, and monitoring the effects of interventions and the camping experience on those with special needs. Camp nurses also must be aware of, develop relationships with, and secure camp contracts for emergency care with health care providers located in the camp's vicinity (Erceg & Pravda, 2001).

## Occupational Health Nursing

Because employers and employees in work settings share a common goal and spend time together, workplaces fit the definition of community. Occupational health nursing provides primary, secondary, and tertiary care to persons in the work setting. Occupational health nurses assure employee safety by collaborating with agencies that set standards for safe, healthy working environments. Federal guidelines for worker safety specify that employers bear responsibility for deleterious effects encountered by workers for occupational and environmental hazards (Clark, 1999; Rogers, 2001). Large businesses may have an occupational health department that employs many nurses; small businesses may employ only one nurse or contract with health care providers to provide occupational health services for employees.

In addition to providing direct care services, occupational health nurses may provide health education to employees. They also compile statistical reports summarizing the annual incidence of employee occupational illness and injuries. By law, these reports are submitted to federal, state, and local agencies and made available to employees. Commonly occurring occupational illnesses include repetitive stress injuries, allergic and contact dermatitis, respiratory disorders caused by inhalation of toxic agents, poisoning, hearing loss, low back disorders, hearing loss, traumatic injuries, fertility problems, and pregnancy abnormalities (Clark, 1999; Rogers, 2001).

In 1999, the American Association of Occupational Health Nurses developed 11 standards for occupational and environmental health nursing practice. These standards are summarized here. The entire document is available from the American Association of Occupational Health Nurses. According to these standards, occupational health does the following in clinical practice:

1. Assesses the health status of clients, workforce, and work environment using a systematic approach.
2. Analyzes the health data from the assessment to develop nursing diagnoses and plans for interventions.
3. Develops specific expected outcomes based on the attained nursing diagnoses.
4. Creates a goal-directed plan with comprehensive interventions and therapies to achieve goals.
5. Implements the plan of care to promote health, prevent illness and injury, and facilitate rehabilitation of injured or disabled workers.
6. Uses best practice standards to systematically and continuously evaluate responses to the developed plan of care.

7. Manages and uses corporate resources to meet the health care needs of the workforce.
8. Assumes responsibility for professional self-development and continuing education.
9. Collaborates with employees, managers, other health care providers, professionals, and community representatives to assess, plan, implement, and evaluate care and services.
10. Uses research findings in practice.
11. Acts as a client advocate by assuring equal access, equitable services, and high quality to all; establishes a safe and healthful work environment; and uses an ethical framework to guide ethical decision making in practice.

Occupational health nursing provides nurses with an opportunity to improve the health of employees and the work environment. By screening employees for various health problems related to their work before they occur, occupational health nurses not only improve the health of workers, they reduce long-term health care costs for employers (AAOHN, 1999).

### Questions for Reflection 14-2

1. What are some of the occupational health hazards that are present in my current work setting?
2. What are some of the health hazards that are present in my position as a student and in the building where I attend classes?
3. How can I reduce health hazards that I find in my work or school setting?

## Home Health Nursing

Nurses engaged in home health nursing provide nursing services to a client within the confines of the client's residence. Although home health nursing practice focuses primarily on individuals, the home health care nurse considers the needs of the family and designated caregivers. Home health nurses view the client, family, and designated caregivers as partners when planning and implementing nursing care. The nurse performs a detailed home assessment to determine the safety of the home for the client (Clark, 1999). In addition, the home health nurse performs a community assessment in which the client's home is located to determine access to services and availability of resources for client support. The home health nurse provides direct care; educates the client, family, and caregivers how to independently meet health care needs; counsels the client and family; and coordinates community resources and benefits. Home health nurses continuously evaluate the effectiveness of planned intervention and community resources as nursing care is delivered (American Nurses Association [ANA], 1999).

The nurse–client relationship differs in home health nursing because the client (and family) considers the nurse as a guest (ANA, 1999). This perception of the client sets up vastly different dynamics for the nurse–client relationship. The nurse must diligently work to assure that he or she is welcomed while helping the client and family assume responsibility for meeting individualized health needs. The nurse exercises special care not to offend the host or disaffirm client and family self-determination. Sometimes, the nurse must politely refuse client requests when they fall outside of the arena of professional nursing practice (Clark, 1999). When such requests are made, the nurse might consider referring the client to appropriate community resources or set up visits by a homemaker or unlicensed care provider.

Home health nurses frequently supervise visits by unlicensed care providers and coordinate the schedules of other members of the health care team and home services so that the client has someone making a visit each day of the week. Home health care nurses frequently take calls on weekends and holidays so that homebound clients have access to a nurse should health care problems arise.

Recent advances in technology enable home health nurses to have daily contact with clients. Telehealth and satellite home monitoring systems enable home health nurses to check client weight, blood pressure, pulse, peripheral blood glucose, and prothrombin times. Some home monitoring systems set alarms and verbally prompt clients when it is time to get connected and send physical assessment data to the home health care agency. Certain systems offer direct video monitoring of clients. Because of computer technology, the home health agency can create printed records of client data using tables or graphs to detect trends toward meeting expected outcomes or that indicate deteriorating parameters. Some systems even have the capability to ask a client specific questions to assess for potential disease complications. Home health nurses stress to clients that the home monitoring system does not replace calling 911 or an ambulance when an emergency arises. Home health nurses use these systems for planning the sequence of daily visits. They also can telephone clients when they fail to perform required, daily monitoring tasks. Medicare covers home monitoring systems as long as clients have been certified for home health nurse visits. Once clients no longer need home health care, the monitoring system may be removed from the home. Some clients with financial resources elect to keep the system in their home using private funds to pay for continued home monitoring.

For home health agencies to be reimbursed for services, the professional nurse maintains detailed records of home health visits. Complete, accurate documentation of the visit serves as data for third-party payer reimbursement, validation of services rendered, and data for nursing research. The professional nurse completes approval and recertification forms to validate the need for nursing services.

## Hospice Nursing

Hospice care nurses frequently make home visits. For terminally ill clients who reside in extended care or residential facilities, hospice nurses visit clients where they live and assist care providers with end-of-life care issues. Starting in 1983, Medicare began covering home health services for the terminally ill (Lundy & Janes, 2001; Smith & Maurer, 2000; Stanhope & Lancaster, 2002).

Nurses have a long history of caring for the dying. In 1950, Dr. Cicely Saunders founded the hospice movement at St. Christopher's in London. Hospice aims to add more life to each day when medical science cannot add additional time to a person's life. Hospice uses a team approach to maximize the quality of life for the terminally ill client and caregivers. Hospice provides the following services: (1) intermittent nursing services; (2) physician services aimed at alleviating human suffering; (3) medications for relieving pain, nausea, and other discomforts associated with the dying process; (4) home health aides; (5) medical equipment and supplies; (6) pastoral services for spiritual support; (7) continuous care when crises arise; and (8) follow-up bereavement services for the family for as long as a year after the client has died.

Hospice nurses receive special education on the dying process, grief, and bereavement management. To effectively care for the terminally ill client and caregivers, hospice nurses must have confidence in their clinical skills and spiritual beliefs. Much of the nursing care focuses on helping the terminally ill and their families find meaning in their past, present, and future lives. As a team member, the hospice nurse frequently spends more time with clients and families and shares comprehensive information with other members of the hospice care team (Lundy & Janes, 2001; Smith & Maurer, 2000; Stanhope & Lancaster, 2002).

## Nursing the Homeless

Homeless persons are humans who lack a fixed, regular nighttime residence or use a shelter, mission, welfare hotel, or other physical place not designed for human slumber. For some persons, homelessness may be temporary (has no home, but community membership remains), episodic (several bouts of having no home), or chronic (no home as a way of life). Homelessness is not confined to single adults; children appear among the ranks of the homeless. During times of economic recession, the number of homeless families increases. Reasons for homelessness include poverty, lack of affordable housing, unemployment, lack or inadequacy of government financial support, crime, violence, lack of kin support, mental illness, substance abuse, de-institutionalization of the mentally ill, and socially stigmatized infectious diseases (Butts, 2001; Clark 1999). In American life, securing a job, societal privileges, or government-sponsored social services require a permanent address.

Access to health care services creates problems for the homeless. Frequently, homeless persons use emergency rooms for treatment of illnesses or enter the health care system as a victim of crime. They receive emergency and acute care for sustained injuries in acute care facilities. Once they recover, placing them in a safe situation where they can meet the demands of follow-up care poses a great challenge to social workers and case managers.

Homeless persons rarely have a consistent primary care provider because of their inability to pay for rendered services. When health care is needed, some homeless persons rely on community free health clinics or homeless shelters. Unfortunately, some of these health care providing organizations depend solely on volunteer health care providers and the consistency of seeing the same client over time becomes problematic. Nurses also see homeless clients in soup kitchens and on urban streets. However, homelessness is not confined to urban settings. Migrant workers also fit the definition of homelessness. Rural county health departments frequently serve as the vehicle for health care for transient farm workers and homeless persons seeking refuge in rural areas.

For effective nursing practice with the homeless, the community health or volunteer professional nurse must develop and maintain a realistic understanding of the world of homelessness. Many times, homeless persons lack the knowledge of available local programs and services to which they are entitled. Sometimes, homeless persons become so overwhelmed in securing food and shelter they lose hope. To survive, some homeless individuals develop street-smart behaviors that include manipulation, lying, and panhandling. Sometimes homeless alcoholics and drug addicts use money received to purchase alcohol or elicit drugs. Some churches give homeless persons food when they ask for cash.

Professional nurses may play a variety of roles when working with and for the homeless. Nurses, when working with persons in clinical practice and in social activities, can work with clients to prevent the factors contributing to homelessness. Nurses also can lobby for legislation that increases services to homeless persons and provide government officials with information about the plight of the homeless. Professional nurses can provide direct care and health screening to persons who seek help at public health departments, free health clinics, homeless shelters, churches, or soup kitchens. Finally, professional nurses can refer the homeless to mobile treatment centers, mental health facilities, and drug and alcohol rehabilitation programs.

## Nursing the Incarcerated

As punishment for crimes, individuals become incarcerated in jails, prisons, and juvenile detention facilities. Professional nurses do not participate in procedures exclusively for correctional purposes. However, professional nurses working in such facilities engage in primary, secondary, and tertiary interventions for the those who are incarcerated. Professional nursing practice in correctional facilities emphasizes disease prevention, promotes health enhancement activities while recognizing and treating physical and mental illness and injuries from an accident or act of violence. Nurses also evaluate the effectiveness of care and look for ways to improve prison health services (ANA, 1995). In prisons, nurses make most health care decisions. They work with medically approved care protocols. Correctional registered nurses have the opportunity to work with diseases rarely seen in the general population (such as TB). Before becoming incarcerated, prisoners frequently pursued high-risk lifestyles that included drug and alcohol abuse, poor living conditions, lack of effective parenting, and poor access to preventive health services (Stringer, 2001).

Watson, Stimpson, and Hostick (2004) report that as many as 90% of incarcerated persons may have mental health problems, 80% smoke, 12% may be infected with HIV, and 8% may have hepatitis. As prison sentences lengthen, nurses in prison encounter older inmates and as many as 85% of them may have more than one chronic major illness. Although not common, some terminally ill prisoners may be seen by prison hospice workers or volunteers (Watson, Stimpson, & Hostick).

Security systems at correctional facilities apply to health care professionals and other staff members. Security systems protect staff, volunteers, and visitors from acts of violence. Prison officials have corrections officers stand outside examination rooms and accompany nurses to cells as they deliver health care to inmates who have a history of violence (Stringer, 2001). Some inmates receive outpatient care in prison clinics and if 24-hour nursing care is needed, most prisons have an infirmary. Prisons frequently develop partnerships with university health care centers and the private sector to obtain medical staff coverage for clinics. However, prisons staff infirmaries with nurses and other unlicensed care providers are employed by the prison system (Watson, Stimpson, & Hostick, 2004).

The nurse in the correctional institution must display self-confidence and strength. Correctional nurses also must avoid performing favors for inmates because inmates frequently try to take advantage of anyone who displays kindness toward them (Stringer, 2001).

## Forensic Nursing

The scientific study of death, or forensics, has been a vital arm of law enforcement. In recent years, the application of forensic science to investigate trauma in emergency departments has created the need to secure reliable evidence and support victims of violent crime. The practice of forensic nursing includes forensic nursing sexual assault examiners, forensic nursing educator/consultant, nurse coroners, nurse death investigators, legal nurse consultants, nurse attorneys, correctional nurses, clinical nurse specialists, forensic pediatric nurses, forensic gerontology nurses, and forensic psychiatric nurses. Forensic nurses use the nursing process to determine the occurrence of sexual assault, homicide, physical assault, spouse abuse, and child abuse (International Association of Forensic Nurses & American Nurses Association, 1997).

Forensic nurses identify injuries with forensic implication. Using strict protocols, they collect evidence when evidence of a crime has occurred. Nurses who collect evidence frequently provide expert witness testimony to the integrity of the evidence. They also meticulously document client interactions and evidence collection because the documentation will be used in court as trial evidence. Forensic nurses also interact with the victims of crime and their grieving families. Finally, forensic nurses may consult with other agencies and law enforcement personnel when forensic interests are shared (International Association of Forensic Nurses & American Nurses Association, 1997).

## Armed Forces Nursing

The United States Armed Forces work and live together to protect the country. Each branch has a specific area of expertise in defense. The armed forces share a common purpose. Each branch fits the definition of community. Armed forces nursing provides nurses with the opportunity to work with military personnel and families. The United States Army, Navy, and Air Force each have Nursing Corps. Nurses may serve the military by enlisting for active duty, reserve status, or in the National Guard. Military nurses have the opportunity to work with neonates, children, adolescents, adults, and the elderly. Armed forces nurses work in ambulatory clinics, community hospitals, large medical centers, hospital ships, field hospitals, and aircraft. Military nurses receive comparable compensation to nurses in civilian practice settings. Branches of the armed services offer generous signing bonuses, offer a full array of benefits and an option to retire with full benefits after 20 years of service. Nurses have lots of upward mobility potential in all branches of the armed forces (Marquand, 2004). Professional practice responsibilities vary according to assignment. However, no matter where nurses practice they look for ways to promote health and meet the health care needs of military personnel and their dependents during war and in times of peace.

Armed forces nursing provides professional nurses with opportunities for advanced education. Nurses can earn graduate degrees in nursing, receive specialty education, and pursue graduate degrees outside the discipline of nursing. Military nurses have opportunities for teaching patient care skills to corpsman and leadership classes to future officers (Marquand, 2004). A recent interest of the armed forces is conducting nursing research related to issues of deployment, needs of military personnel and their beneficiaries in times of war and peace, and cultural aspects of military nursing (Committee on Military Nursing Research, 1996; Marquand, 2004).

Military nursing provides the opportunity for nurses to work with other health team members as equal partners. The camaraderie among health team members is high because everyone focuses on what is best for the soldier, sailor, airman, or marine receiving care. Physicians and nurses have weapons training together. In some circumstances, nurses may outrank physicians. When armed forces deploy active duty and reserve nurses during times of war, they expend energy and resources to recruit civilian nurses to fill vacancies left in state-side hospitals and clinics (Marquand, 2004).

## School Nursing

Schools are organizations that focus on the education of persons of all ages. Within a school, many persons work together to attain the goal of imparting cognitive, affective, or psychomotor knowledge and skills to others. Thus, all levels of schools meet the definition of a community. Many persons tend to view school nursing as confined to the kindergarten through high school levels. However, many colleges and universities also provide health services to students, and some nurses work with college students. The role of the school nurse remains consistent across all levels of education. However, when nurses work with children and minors, they spend much time working with the parents of these younger clients (Lundy & Janes, 2001; Novak, 2002; Smith & Maurer, 2000).

School nurses have various roles in clinical practice. They provide student health care directly when using clinical knowledge and nursing process in meeting the health care needs of students when they have bouts of acute physical illness, chronic illness, or when special health care needs are the result of a disability. In addition, professional school nurses also administer first aid; administer medications; screen students for health problems, general fitness, and for signs of abuse; monitor vital signs; participate in case management activities; change dressings; and perform urinary catheterizations. School nurses develop individualized nursing care and health educational plans for students with chronic illness or those who need to learn complex self-care skills to cope with a disability. Along with providing services to students, school nurses engage in enhancing the wellness of teachers; administrators; counselors; and nutritional, janitorial, and clerical staff. School nurses perform periodic environmental assessments to assure a safe and health-promoting environment of the school. School nurses also may review the daily menu schedules for school cafeterias to verify that healthy meals are being served. When specific health cares needs arise, school nurses make referrals to local health care providers (Lundy & Janes, 2001; Novak, 2002; Smith & Maurer, 2000).

In some school systems, nurses frequently develop the health education program in collaboration with school administration, teachers, and parents. Health education programs may be tailored to meet an individual school's needs or be developed to meet health education needs and concerns for a school district. Many times, the school nurse teaches health education classes to students, parents, school staff, or community groups (Lundy & Janes, 2001; Novak, 2002; Smith & Maurer, 2000).

School nurses spend much time maintaining student health records. They verify that all students have received required immunizations and that students have received screening for visual, hearing, and skeletal deformities. When students make visits to the school nurse, the nurse documents the reason for the visit, interventions performed, parental contact (if needed), and referrals made (if required). Most school health programs have protocols indicating actions that can be taken by nurses without parental consent. Many schools have parents sign forms specifying particular over-the-counter medications (such as acetaminophen, antibiotic or steroid ointments, antihistamines, and decongestants) the nurse may administer to their children. School nurses also receive detailed information about routinely prescribed medications that students may require. Because of the prevalence of drug abuse, students taking prescription medications must visit the school nurse to receive their scheduled doses (Lundy & Janes, 2001; Novak, 2002; Smith & Maurer, 2000).

The school nurse serves as a resource of health information for students, faculty, and staff. Sometimes, faculty and staff consult the school nurse when they suspect a potential health-related problem among students. The nurse develops several approaches to the problem and consults with school administration before activating a plan. Sometimes nurses work collaboratively with teachers and administrators to develop plans for students with learning disabilities and mental health problems. In some cases, the school nurse assumes responsibility for monitoring school compliance to specific portions of student disability regulations.

School nursing is a specialized area of nursing practice, and additional education beyond the baccalaureate degree is recommended for optimal clinical effectiveness. School nurses may become certified through the National Association of School Nurses and the ANA. Many states also have certification requirements for school nursing.

In addition to providing nursing services and health education, the school nurse participates in research, investigates cases, and delegates health-related tasks to unlicensed persons. Unfortunately, not every school has a nurse on campus, and certain tasks must be delegated to school staff members. When this happens, the professional nurse must provide the staff members with education to safely accomplish health-related tasks.

College health nursing focuses primarily on the health care needs and concerns of persons between the ages of 17 and 24 years. Nurses working with college students emphasize self-care and wellness. College nursing services vary in size and scope. Some college health programs offer ambulatory care services with scheduled office hours exclusively, whereas others provide an infirmary for acute care staffed by a multidisciplinary health team. The American College Health Association Review Group in collaboration with the ANA has published guidelines for collegiate nursing practice. Many colleges and universities provide clinics for students that have an advanced practice nurse on staff to deliver required health services (ANA, 1997).

Regardless of student age group, school nurses use the nursing process to guide client care activities. They also systematically evaluate the effectiveness of nursing practice and health care services. School nurses also must abide by various state regulations where they practice. They bear responsibility for the following: (1) maintaining competence; (2) remaining current in regard to knowledge and issues affecting their student populations; (3) providing ethical care; (4) using research findings in practice; (5) conducting research studies when gaps in practice are identified; (6) using school resources judiciously; and (7) collaborating with others to develop relevant health care services (ANA, 1997; Lundy & Janes, 2001; Novak, 2002; Smith & Maurer, 2000).

**Questions for Reflection 14-3**

1. What are the health services offered at the college where I attend classes?
2. What health-promoting factors are present within the college where I attend classes?
3. What are my major health-related concerns as a nursing student? Why are these important to me?

## Parish Nursing

Parish nursing provides nurses with an opportunity to practice within faith communities. Faith communities are people who share a common faith tradition and meet in a house of worship (church, mosque, or synagogue) (Berry, 2002). In 1984, Granger Westberg started a parish-nursing program at Lutheran General Hospital in Chicago. The International Parish Nursing Resource Center offered the first continuing education program in parish nursing in 1987. Unlike other community-based health programs, parish nurses hold the spiritual dimension of persons as the main focus of nursing practice (McDermott, Solari-Twadell, & Matheus, 1999). In 1998, the ANA published *Scope and Standard of Parish Nursing Practice*, thereby acknowledging parish nursing as a distinct specialized area of professional practice (ANA, 1998).

Berry (2002) identifies two models for parish nursing. In the congregational model, the nurse acts autonomously and nursing and health programs arise from the community in which the nurse serves. The nurse is held accountable to the congregation and the governing body. In the institutional model, the nurse collaborates more closely with local hospitals, medical centers, extended care facilities, and educational institutions. Sometimes the parish nurse holds contracts with the collaborating agencies. The nurse works in partnership with the local health care and educational institutions to meet the needs of parishioners.

Nurses holding membership in a faith-based community frequently serve as the first responder when a congregational member has a health-related problem during a service or activity. However, a parish nurse expands the role and engages in health ministry. Health ministries may or may not need the expertise of a professional nurse and include activities such as visiting homebound congregational members, providing meals for families in times of crises, forming prayer circles or chains, serving healthy church meals and refreshment at congregational activities, and volunteering for local community care groups (Berry, 2002). In some parishes, nurses provide volunteer service. Other parishes have formalized programs staffed by paid directors, coordinators, and nurses. Some parish nursing programs allow the nurse to run clinics to serve poor, marginalized congregations. These clinics are staffed by nurse practitioners (Boss, 1999).

As a specialized area of professional practice, the following factors distinguish parish nursing from other practice areas:

1. The client spiritual dimension is the core and central dimension of parish nursing practice.

2. The parish nurse balances knowledge of nursing science, humanities, and theology as nursing services are delivered.
3. The faith community and its ministry become the focus of practice.
4. The parish nurse emphasizes individual, family, and faith community strengths.
5. Spiritual health, health, and healing are viewed as dynamic ongoing processes (Solari-Twadell & McDermott, 1999).

Nursing skills used when providing care to faith-based communities vary across parish nursing programs. Solari-Twadell (1999, p. 249) emphasizes that "parish nursing cannot be all things to all people." The eight key functions of the parish nurse have been identified: health education, personal health counseling, health care referral services, support group development, volunteer facilitation, volunteer training, faith and health integration, and health care advocate. In 1984, Westberg envisioned the parish nurse as a 20-hour nursing role assumed by a baccalaureate-prepared nurse (Solari-Twadell, 1999).

Education preparation for parish nurses has evolved from a 1- or 2-day continuing education seminar into more formalized programs. Nurses can attend a 1-day continuing education program or take a formal course of study lasting several years to earn a master's degree in nursing or a graduate degree in divinity. A standardized curriculum for parish nursing has been developed based on the needs assessment of 50 parish nurse coordinators in 1996. Curricular content addresses the church's role in health; health theology, history, and philosophy of parish nursing; models of parish nursing practice; the teaching, counseling, referring, and educating functions of the parish nurse; integration of faith and health; parish community assessment; health promotion and maintenance; families and faith communities as client; parish nurse self-care; working with churches and within a ministerial team; legal and ethical issues; accountability, documentation techniques; prayer, worship leadership; and how to start a parish nursing program. Additional content for parish nurse coordinators includes budgeting, writing grants, managing human and fiscal resources, developing spiritually, and planning continuing education for parish nurses (McDermott et al., 1999). Berry (2002) suggests that advanced practice and specialty practice education along with practical experience in community health nursing enriches parish nursing services.

Parish nursing offers an avenue for development of new spiritual (or religious), community, and interpersonal nursing diagnoses and interventions. Proposed new nursing diagnoses include the potential for enhanced acceptance, disabling image of God, spiritual concern, altered spiritual development, spiritual isolation, altered spiritual ritual patterns, risk for cultural incongruity, ineffective boundaries, ineffective meditation skills, and communication enhancement. Spiritual nursing interventions focus upon enhancing health through strengthening faith and hope while preventing religious addiction. Parish nurses empower parish communities to engage in unified political actions on health-related legislation; support and teach each other to provide volunteer assistance to ill and frail parishioners; and promote health by enhancing the spiritual dimensions of congregation members (Burkhart & Kellen, 1999).

## Volunteer Nursing

Many nurses volunteer to provide nursing services in community settings. Some nurses routinely schedule volunteer activities into life routines. Examples of scheduled volunteer activities may be serving on organizational or institutional boards, monthly or weekly duties at a free health clinic, and regularly scheduled community health screening activities. Other nurses may provide volunteer service for episodic events such as health fairs, camps, community service projects (e.g., nursing services for a Habitat for Humanity group), church activities, and community events. When volunteering, professional nurses have an obligation to have adequate knowledge about actual and potential situations that may arise.

When providing services, the professional nurse assumes responsibility for providing accurate health information and assuring that those served receive the care they require. In the case of blood pressure screening, the professional nurse must establish guidelines for persons who require emergency treatment, those with dangerously high or low blood pressure measurements, those who need medical referral for high or low measurements, and those with borderline measurements. Nurses who engage in blood pressure screening can use the client interaction to teach persons about blood pressure and ways to avoid hypertension. Sometimes, nurses provide clients with a form containing the client's blood pressure reading and recommended actions for various readings. The professional nurse cannot force anyone to seek immediate treatment for blood pressure problems or verify that clients participating in the screening follow through with referral recommendations.

Family members, friends, neighbors, and other acquaintances often consult the professional nurse for health-related concerns. When this occurs, the nurse assumes responsibility for health care advice. The nurse must acknowledge his or her limitations to knowledge and expertise. The professional nurse safeguards the person asking questions by giving advice that is more cautious and making referrals when uncertain. When giving out health advice, some nurses keep personal notes as to the advice they give family, friends, and acquaintances. Recordkeeping enables the nurse to make additional inquiries regarding the results of advice given.

## ● SUMMARY AND SIGNIFICANCE TO PRACTICE

Professional nurses have an array of opportunities to engage in community health nursing. Community health nursing requires that the nurse and community members collaborate and establish partnerships with each other to establish effective and relevant health programs. Professional nurses use nursing process, communication skills, and knowledge of the political process to plan, establish, and provide effective programs to promote community health in a variety of community settings.

### FROM THEORY TO PRACTICE

1. Reread the vignette at the beginning of the chapter. After reading the chapter, what ideas can you generate as possible reasons for lack of community participation in the annual flu vaccine program developed by Paula?
2. Generate a plan to improve turnout for next year's program. In this plan, include specific details, such as ways to entice each small town community member to participate in the plan.
3. What are some community health problems that you can identify in the community where you live? What community services are available to address the problems that you identify? If no services are available, how would you go about to develop a community health program to address them?

# WWW INTERNET EXERCISES

## Exercise 1

Visit the CDC Emergency Preparedness and Response home page at http://www.bt.cdc.gov/.

1. Click on "Recent Outbreaks & Incidents" to learn about recent public health hazards. Select a topic of interest and prepare a brief summary to share with your colleagues in class.
2. Return to the home page and click on "Bioterrorism Agents" to learn about potential agents that could be used in a bioterrorist attack. Do you think that you would recognize an act of bioterrorism? Why or why not?
3. Return to the home page and read about "Chemical Emergencies" and "Radiation Emergencies." Has your local community had a release of a toxic chemical or radiation?
4. Return to the home page, click on "Natural Disasters & Severe Weather. "List the disasters and severe weather incidents that are possible in your area. Check with your clinical agency to see if the Mass Casualty and Disaster Plan has procedures to follow for each disaster/severe weather incident that might occur in your area.

## Exercise 2

Visit the American Public Health Association: http://www.apha.org. Quickly skim the home page. When finished, click on the words Site Search. Enter the word "nursing" in the blank space provided to search American Public Health Association documents. Once the documents appear, select the latest edition of the Public Health Nursing Newsletter and read it. Make a list of the key topics and issues contained in the newsletter. Compare these issues to issues and concerns in your current area of professional nursing practice.

# WWW INTERNET RESOURCES

Healthy People 2010: http://health.gov/healthypeople.
Morbidity and Mortality Weekly Report: http://www.cdc.gov/mmwr.
American Public Health Association: http://apha.org.
The American Red Cross: http://www.redcross.org and http://www.redcross.org/services/disaster.
The International Parish Nurse Resource Center: http://ipnrc.parishnurses.org.
Johns Hopkins University Center for Civilian Biodefense Strategies: http://www.hopkins-biodefense.org.
American Psychiatric Association: http://www.psych.org.
Association of Camp Nurses: http://www.campnurse.org.
Occupational Safety and Health Administration: http://www.osha.gov.
American Association of Occupational Health Nurses: http://www.aaohn.org.
American Correctional Health Services Association: http://www.org/achsa.
The International Association of Forensic Nurses: http://www.forensicnurse.org.
National Association of School Nurses: http://www.nasn.org.
Armed Force Nursing:
  U.S. Army Nurse Corps http://www.goarmy.com.amedd/nurse/index.jsp/
  U.S. Navy Nurse Corps http://www.navy.com/healthcare/nursing.
  U.S. Air Force http://www.airforce.com.

# REFERENCES

American Association of Occupational Health Nurses (AAOHN). (1999). *Standards of occupational health nursing practice*. Atlanta: Author.

American Nurses Association. (1995). *Nursing social policy statement*. Washington, DC: Author.

American Nurses Association (ANA). (1997). *Scope and standards of college health nursing practice*. Washington, DC: American Nurses Publishing.

American Nurses Association (ANA) (1998). *Scope and standards of parish nursing practice*. Washington, DC: American Nurses Publishing.

American Nurses Association (ANA). (1999). *Scope and standards of home health nursing practice*. Washington, DC: American Nurses Publishing.

American Nurses Association (ANA). (1999a). *Scope and standards of public health nursing practice*. Washington, DC: American Nurses Publishing.

Anderson, E. T., & McFarlane, J. (2000). *Community as partner* (3rd ed.). Philadelphia: Lippincott Williams & Wilkins.

Bender, K. W., & Salmon, M. E. (2001). Public health nursing: Pioneers of health care reform. In B. S. Lundy, & S. Janes (Eds.), *Community health nursing: Caring for the public's health* (pp. 866–879). Sudbury, MA: Jones & Bartlett.

Berry, R. (2002). Community health nurse as parish nurse. Chapter 26 in M. Stanhope, & J. Lancaster (Eds.), *Foundations of community health nursing: Community-oriented practice* (pp. 449–461). St. Louis: Mosby.

Bertalanffy, L. von. (1968). *General systems theory*. New York: George Brazziller.

Boss, J. G. (1999). Parish nursing practice with underorganized, underserved, and marginalized clients. In P. A. Solari-Twadell, & M. A. McDermott (Eds.), *Parish nursing: promoting whole person health within faith communities* (pp. 55–65). Thousand Oaks, CA: Sage.

Burkhart, L., & Kellen, P. (1999). Proposed diagnoses and interventions. In P. A. Solari-Twadell, & M. A. McDermott (Eds.), *Parish nursing: Promoting whole person health within faith communities* (pp. 257–267). Thousand Oaks, CA: Sage.

Butts, J. B. (2001). Urban and homeless populations. In K. S. Lundy, & S. Janes (Eds.), *Community health nursing: Caring for the public's health* (pp. 594–617). Sudbury, MA: Jones & Bartlett.

Clark, M. J. (1999). *Nursing in the community* (3rd ed.). Norwalk, CT: Appleton & Lange.

Committee on Military Nursing Research, (1996). The program for research in military nursing: Progress and future direction. Available at: http://www.nap.edu/catalog/5257.html. Accessed July 5, 2005.

Copeland, M. (2002). E-Community health nursing. *Journal of Holistic Nursing, 20*, 152–165.

Davis, R. (2000). Holographic community: Reconceptualizing the meaning of community in an era of health care reform. *Nursing Outlook, 48*, 294–301.

Erceg, L., & Pravda, M. (2001). *The basics of camp nursing*. Martinsvlle, IN: American Camp Association.

Hancock, T., & Duhl, L. (1986). *Healthy cities: Promoting health in the urban context*. (Healthy Cities Paper No 1.) Copenhagen: World Health Organization Europe.

Haque, M., Nolan, P., Dyke, R., & Khan, I. (2002). The work and values of mental health nurses observed. *Journal of Psychiatric and Mental Health Nursing, 9*, 673–680.

Harkness, G. A. (2001). Epidemiology of health and illness. In K. M. Lishner, & M. A. Lishner (Eds.), *The camp community* (pp. 100–117). Martinsville, IN: American Camp Association.

Hunt, R. (2001). *Introduction to community-based nursing* (2nd ed.). Philadelphia: Lippincott Williams & Wilkins.

International Association of Forensic Nurses & American Nurses Association (1997). *Scope and standards of forensic nursing practice*. Washington, DC: American Nurses Publishing.

Jamieson, E. M., & Sewall, M. F. (1954). *Trends in nursing history* (4th ed.). Philadelphia: WB Saunders.

Leddy, S. (2003). *Integrative health promotion*. Thorofare, NJ: Slack.

Leonard, B. (2000). Community empowerment and healing. In E. T. Anderson, & J. McFarlane (Eds.), *Community as partner* (3rd ed., pp. 92–115). Philadelphia: Lippincott Williams & Wilkins.

Lishner, K. M., & Bruya, M. A. (Eds.). (1994). *Creating a healthy camp community: A nurse's role*. Martinsville, IN: American Camping Association.

Lundy, K. S., & Barton, J. (2001). Community and population health: Assessment and intervention. In K. S. Lundy, & S. Janes (Eds.), *Community health nursing: Caring for the public's health* (pp. 30–69). Sudbury, MA: Jones & Bartlett.

Lundy, K. S., & Butts, J. B. (2001). The role of the community health nurse in disasters. In K. S. Lundy, & S. Janes (Eds.), *Community health nursing: Caring for the public's health* (pp. 546–573). Sudbury, MA: Jones & Bartlett.

Lundy, S. & Janes, S. (2001) (Eds.). *Community health nursing: Caring for the public's health*. Sudbury, MA: Jones & Bartlett.

Lundy, K. S., Janes, S., & Hartman, S. (2001). Opening the door: Community and public health nursing. In K. S. Lundy, & S. Janes (Eds.), *Community health nursing: Caring for the public's health* (pp. 4–29). Sudbury, MA: Jones & Bartlett.

Marquand, B. (2004). An army (and navy and air force) of opportunities. *Minority Nurse,* (Spring, 2004), 26–30.

McDermott, M. A., Solari-Twadell, P. A., & Matheus, R. (1999). Educational preparation. In P. A. Solari-Twadell, & M. A. McDermott (Eds.), *Parish nursing: Promoting whole person health within faith communities* (pp. 269–276). Thousand Oaks, CA: Sage.

*Merriam-Webster's collegiate dictionary* (10th ed.). (1994). Springfield, MA: Merriam-Webster.

Minhard, H. A., & Blanchard, M. (2004). Older people with depression: pilot study. *Journal of Advanced Nursing, 46,* 23–32.

Morse, S. (2004). *Smart communities*. San Francisco: Jossey-Bass.

Novak, J. (2002). Community health nursing in the schools. Chapter 28 in M. Stanhope, & J. Lancaster. *Foundations of community health nursing: Community-oriented practice* (pp. 487–510.). St. Louis: Mosby.

Parrish, H. M. (1969). Epidemiologic and public health aspects of disaster. In S. Garb, & E. Eng (Eds.), *Disaster handbook* (pp. 20–25). New York: Springer.

Quad Council of Public Health Nursing Organizations. (1999). *Scope and standards of public health nursing practice*. Washington, DC: American Nurses Publishing.

Rogers, B. (2001). Occupational health nursing. In K. S. Lundy, & S. Janes (Eds.), *Community health nursing: Caring for the public's health* (pp. 942–967). Sudbury, MA: Jones & Bartlett.

Schmidt, C. (2004). American Red Cross nursing: Essential to disaster relief. *American Journal of Nursing, 104,* 35–38.

Smith, C. M., & Maurer, F. A. (2000). *Community health nursing theory and practice* (2nd ed.). Philadelphia: WB Saunders.

Solari-Twadell, P. A. (1999). Nurses in churches: Differentiation of the practice. In P. A. Solari-Twadell, & M. A. McDermott (Eds.), *Parish nursing: Promoting whole person health within faith communities* (pp. 249–256). Thousand Oaks, CA: Sage.

Solari-Twadell, P. A., & McDermott, M. A. (Eds.). (1999). *Parish nursing: Promoting whole person health within faith communities*. Thousand Oaks, CA: Sage.

Stanhope, M., & Lancaster, J. (2002). *Foundations of community health nursing: community-oriented practice*. St. Louis: Mosby.

Stringer, H. (2001). Prison break. *Nurse Week, 2,* 24–25.

U. S. Department of Health and Human Services. (2000). Healthy people 2010. (Conference Edition in Two Volumes). Washington, DC: U. S. Government Printing Office.

Veenema, T. (2003). *Disaster nursing and emergency preparedness for chemical, biological, radiological terrorism and other hazards*. New York: Springer.

Vogt, R (2004). Message from the president: Continuing the plan for national security. *Missouri State Board of Nursing Newsletter, 6,* 1.

Watson, R., Stimpson, A., Hostick, T. (2004). Prison health care: A review of the literature. *International Journal of Nursing Studies, 41,* 119–128.

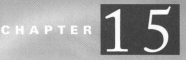
# Informatics and Technology in Nursing Practice

## KEY TERMS AND CONCEPTS

Informatics

Nursing Informatics

Personal Digital Assistants (PDA)

Electronic Health Records (EHR)

Informatics Nurse Specialist

Telehealth

Robotics

Genomic Medicine

Stem Cells

Optical Technology

Cyberstalking

## LEARNING OUTCOMES

By the end of this chapter, the learner will be able to:

1   Discuss the role of informatics in nursing practice.

2   Specify the educational preparation and roles of the informatics nurse specialist.

3   Outline current technology used in clinical practice.

4   Debate the advantages and disadvantages of complex technology used in clinical practice.

5   Specify how technology is used in nursing practice and education.

6   Discuss the implications for technological advances for professional nursing.

7   Identify key ethical considerations as technological advances become the standard practice in professional nursing.

## VIGNETTE

John, Susan, and Amy graduated from the same nursing program several years ago. They now are employed at three different health care facilities. John works at a large university medical center where he enters information related to client care into a computer. Susan, a director of nursing at a rural hospital, is exploring the feasibility of starting a computerized client care documentation system. Amy works in a home health care agency that provides nurses with personal computers to record home visits. When they meet at a college alumni event, they compare notes about the strengths and weaknesses of the current documentation systems they use in practice. Susan poses the following questions during the discussion: I know that computers are wonderful, but how can I get my older staff members to overcome their computer phobia? How can we assure confidentiality of client information with computerized medical records? What are the key elements that need to be included in an employee policy related to computer use and confidentiality of information? How will client care documentation occur when the computer system fails or during a power failure? How much time will be required of staff for computer documentation?

Like the nurses in the vignette, many professional nurses raise practical questions about the use of computer technology and complex information systems in practice. The complexity of managing information requires competent information specialists. Nursing information systems are just a small piece of a complex health care system (Ammenwerth & Haux, 2000).

This chapter provides an overview of the informatics, computers, Internet capability, and technological advances that affect professional nursing practice. Key computer competencies for professional nursing and advances in technology for clinical practice are presented. Finally, the chapter challenges professional nursing students to consider the advantages, disadvantages, and ethical issues of technology use for client care.

Changes in technology occur quickly. Faster, improved models of computer equipment seemingly come out just as the latest model has been bought. Some of the information contained in this chapter may be obsolete by the publication date. Since 1970, microprocessor power has increased by a factor of 7,000. Computing tasks that took a week in 1970 now can be performed in a minute (Rauch, 2001).

## ✦ INFORMATICS AND TECHNOLOGY IN NURSING PRACTICE

Nurses must know how to effectively use computer technology. Professionals have developed a working knowledge of technology because informatics has had an impact on the health care system. **Informatics**, the science of information (*Merriam-Webster's Collegiate Dictionary*, 1994), is an integral part of managing health care technology. Thede (2003) expands the definition of informatics that encompasses "the management of information, using cognitive skills and the computer" (p. 5). Because many fields of study and professionalism have embraced computers and complex information management systems, the term health care informatics focuses the broad field of informatics into a specialized field. **Nursing informatics** is a subspecialty of health care informatics that addresses issues surrounding nursing practice.

### Computer and Informatics Competencies for Professional Nurses

Computers and software programs play key roles in the delivery of client care. Consumers of health care expect nurses to know what they are doing. Nurses must display competence in using computers, software, and machinery that uses computer chips to deliver safe, effective care. Use of technology has become a critical component of basic and continuing education for nurses. The American Association of Colleges of Nursing (1998) recommends that nursing students be taught to:

- Use information and communication technology to document and evaluate patient care, advance patient education, and enhance the accessibility of care.
- Use appropriate technologies in the process of assessing and monitoring patients.
- Work in an interdisciplinary team to make ethical decisions regarding the application of technologies and the acquisition of data.
- Adapt the use of technologies to meet patient needs.
- Teach patients about health care technologies.

- Protect the safety and privacy of patients in relation to the use of health care and information technologies.
- Use information technologies to enhance one's own knowledge base.

In 1999, the International Medical Informatics Association (IMIA) drafted a list of 41 recommendations to integrate informatics into health care delivery. The IMIA suggests that two areas of specialization be developed in medical informatics: one that focuses on informatics, and one that focuses on health care delivery. Informatics specialists would design software programs and computer systems to manage information related to clients and health care. Examples include information related to specific clients (medical history, diagnostic test results, insurance information, and billing information), and reference materials regarding medications, governmental regulation guidelines, current changes in health problem management, and professional organization information. Specialists who focus on the health care delivery aspects would design software and create integrated systems that would facilitate health care delivery by nurses and other health care providers.

Components of the integrated delivery system would include hyperlinks to the latest information related to client care, nursing care planning programs, specific client teaching materials, and online clinical practice manuals containing evidence-based nursing care protocols, data collection for best health care practices, client billing systems, and health care insurance reimbursement programs. The IMIA also proposes standardized, global curricula for educating both specialists.

The American Medical Informatics Association (AMIA) assembled an expert panel of nurses to develop and refine necessary competencies for nurses. The panel identified 313 different competencies for beginning nurses, experienced nurses, informatics nurse specialists, and informatics innovators.

Sample competencies for the beginning nurse include use of administrative applications, telecommunication devices, e-mail, database management programs, and the Internet. The beginning nurse also should be able to operate the appropriate devices required to capture patient data (such as peripheral blood glucose monitor), and find available resources to assist with ethical decision making as it relates to computing.

The experienced nurse must be able to use applications for diagnostic coding, evaluate computerized assisted instruction as a teaching method, and integrate selected resources into a client file. The experienced professional also can define how computerized information affects the nurse's role, assess the accuracy of health information posted on the Internet, and serve as an advocate to client system users.

The informatics nurse specialist has a graduate education and can integrate established technologies into clinical practice. The informatics innovator holds a doctorate and designs new technological systems, techniques, and conceptual models for databases. The innovator evaluates the safety, effectiveness, cost, and social impacts of the technological systems and researches theoretical foundations of the specialty itself (Staggers & Gassert, 2000).

## Informatics and Technology Applications in Direct Client Care

Professional nurses use a variety of technological tools in clinical practice. Many pieces of client care equipment have computer chips and frequently nurses are unaware when sophisticated medical devices are used. Technology has revolutionized client care delivery. For client assessment, nurses use bedside and handheld monitors to collect a variety of information, including blood glucose level, clotting time, electrocardiograph rhythm, cardiac output, blood pressure, oxygen saturation of hemoglobin, and temperature. Some monitoring systems require that the client be connected in some way to the device, and others require a drop or two of blood. Point-of-care testing enables nurses to receive instantaneous results for peripheral blood glucose levels for diabetics and activated clotting time for clients receiving anticoagulation therapy (Nelson, 2001). Client monitoring systems that use wireless technology enable automatic nurse paging capability when client measurements fall outside normal parameters.

For example, a client connected to a centralized telemetry system experiences a run of multifocal premature ventricular contractions. The monitoring system immediately pages the nurse. If the nurse fails to respond in a specified time, the system sends pages to other nurses working on the unit (McConnell, 2001). These improved assessment techniques enable nurses to act more quickly to abnormal findings.

Nurses and other health care providers also have access to computerized clinical decision-making support systems. Decision-making support systems help nurses define clinical problems, generate potential solutions, and select the best solution based on the likelihood of success. Many decision-making models use spreadsheets with formulas to predict the results of specific actions in a given client care situation (Thede, 2003). Nurses also have access to decision-making algorithms when clinical practice guidelines and procedures have been entered into computer systems.

At the University of Virginia Medical Center, Suzanne Burns, RN, MSN, ACNP, CS, developed the Burns Weaning Assessment Program, which can be loaded onto handheld computer devices for clinical use. Her program contains key concepts and decision-making strategies for weaning clients from ventilators. Other computer software for personal digital assistants includes book-length medical dictionaries, drug reference guides, and clinical drug calculation programs. Patient helper software enables nurses to enter client laboratory test results and be cued to the best clinical decision to fit a given situation (Dickenson-Hazard, 2001).

Along with improved client assessment, many nurses use computers to plan client care. Some health care institutions have software that enables nurses to enter care plans by selecting a specific nursing diagnosis. The software provides the nurse with expected outcomes and nursing interventions related to the identified nursing diagnosis. Some software programs enable the nurse to input individualized nursing actions to communicate client care preferences. Computer software programs also organize client care and teaching protocol information. Various software programs offer different features, including the capability to translate client education materials into Spanish or other languages. Some institutions place clinical practice guidelines and employee policies onto a mainframe that can be accessed by using any computer connected to the local area network.

In addition to providing client care and educational information, wireless handheld computer devices or **personal digital assistants (PDAs)** may serve as a valuable clinical reference. Currently available software for handheld devices consists of pharmacology, medical terminology, and pathophysiology programs. Some of these devices have electronic-mail access, Internet capability, and signaling devices to track the location of health personnel. Some PDAs have the capability to send prescriptions to pharmacies, access recent online medical and nursing journals, send faxes, and access e-mail (Thede, 2003).

Nurses can also access an array of reference materials for client education, professional information, and institutional policies by using computers. Computer software programs support clinical decisions and facilitate development of client nursing care plans. Internet access permits nurses to stay abreast of current research findings. Some businesses and nurse specialty organizations offer online continuing education programs. Computerized documentation systems provide a wealth of information about client outcomes related to nursing care and provide a means for monitoring quality of nursing care.

Nurses also use technology for nursing interventions. Most intravenous pumps contain computer microprocessors for effective operation. Computerized intravenous pumps enable nurses to program administration rates for ordered medications. Patient-controlled analgesia pumps have been programmed so nurses can select the type of drug and its concentration before inputting an intermittent or continuous infusion rate. In critical care, pumps with the ability to run three or more medications sometimes are used. When using these complex pumps, nurses can program an infusion of medications at specified times.

In addition to IV pumps, other nursing care devices use computer technology. Even some air mattresses use computer components and software to regulate the amount of air inflation. Implantable subcutaneous pumps deliver local anesthetic along surgical incisions and have the computer technology to regulate the rate of subcutaneous drug administration. Computerized medication–dispensing stations prevent nurses from making medication errors while automatically notifying the pharmacy when the stocked medications need to be replenished.

### Questions for Reflection 15-1

1. How do I currently use technology in client care?
2. What does it mean to use complex technological equipment in professional nursing practice?
3. Why does the introduction of new equipment create distress for some professional nurses?
4. What is the impact of new technology on the cost and quality of health care?

## Applications in Recordkeeping and Documentation of Care

For care evaluation, some health information systems (HIS) can be used to track care delivery. HIS integrate various aspects of care delivery. For example, a physician enters an order for a diagnostic test into a computer. Almost instantaneously, the order request appears in the department that performs the test. The department schedules the test and sends computer-generated information to the nursing unit to notify staff and client of any required, special client preparation. Once the test is performed, the business office receives notification for billing. Test results are entered into a computer and health care providers can access test results almost instantaneously. Along with test results, nurses enter client assessments, interventions, and therapeutic effects into the client record using a computer and all health care providers can view specific client information on a computer screen. HIS also track client medical history and can double check the safety of ordered medications for clients based on information of drug allergies, currently ordered medications and IV therapy, and what over-the-counter medications the client was taking before entering the hospital. HIS may also be linked to outpatient facilities to provide seamless access to client information to streamline health care delivery.

HIS require that nurses become adept with computer technology. Documentation can be performed with a personal computer located in a central area, with laptop computers, or PDAs. However, nurses must also know what to do to document client care activities and provide care when computers are not functioning because of routine maintenance, software updating, or a power failure. **Electronic health records (EHRs)** are computerized client documents that contain complete and accurate data about a client's past and present health. EHRs also may possess practitioner's alerts, reminders, and clinical decision-making systems. In addition, EHRs have links to bodies of medical knowledge and health information databases (Thede, 2003). In 1992, the Institute of Medicine formed the Computer-Based Record Institute to promote the development of computerized patient records to capture a comprehensive record of an individual's health status over a lifetime. Persons could carry such information on a card no larger than a credit card and have it with them at all times.

As health care delivery complexity increases, universal access to a client's health record by all members of the health care team improves care quality, safety, and efficiency. EHRs can alert care providers to drug incompatibilities, allergies, and scheduled cancer and heart disease screenings. EHRs also can provide information related to regional differences in health care delivery, track health care costs, identify areas of best practices for certain procedures, and provide clients with one health record that could be used anywhere when health care needs arise. Staff members need time to master electronic documentation systems. Notable improvements in client care documentation may not be apparent for as long as one year after an electronic documentation system is introduced (Ammenwerth & Haux, 2000).

## Applications for Communication

The use of wireless telephones reduces the time spent by health care professionals in trying to reach each other ("playing telephone tag"). Wireless telephones also decrease the need for overhead paging, which sometimes disrupts client rest. Physicians can call nurses directly. Alphanumeric pocket pagers enable staff members to inform each other of specific events or assistance needs. Handheld computers can record nursing assessments, laboratory results, and nursing progress notes. Once downloaded into a cradling station, client information becomes available immediately to all health care providers. Nurses or clerical staff can print out hard (paper) copies of entered information as needed for the client's medical record (Platt & Reed, 2001). Electronic mail also can be used to send messages about patients to physician's offices (McConnell, 2001) or inform staff of continuing education opportunities, special institutional events, and personal messages.

Integrated health care service organizations look for ways to improve health care for all member institutions. Digital video cameras and client monitoring devices can be linked to complex networks, making off-site client monitoring and consultations possible. For example, rural critical care units linked to a central monitoring location have access to a critical care physician specialist and a critical care nurse to facilitate client monitoring and more rapid interventions for seriously ill clients. A neonatologist consults with a rural emergency department physician who has just delivered a preterm infant.

Along with enhanced communication among health team members, providers and clients can use electronic communication devices. Digital video cameras permit home monitoring of clients. For example, a home health agency provides a digital video camera and the client connects to the agency making a nurse's visit to his or her home unnecessary. The nurse assesses the client from the beamed video signal, receives client vital signs from client self-monitoring devices, provides client education, and evaluates client progress toward expected outcomes without leaving the agency office.

## ● THE INFORMATICS NURSE SPECIALIST

Because of technological advances, the human species generates vast volumes of information in a relatively short time. Management of this information requires special expertise. To use information effectively, it must be organized, accessible, and relevant. **Informatics nurse specialists** are nurses with special education and experience who develop nursing computer applications, and analyze technology and informatics to improve nursing practice and the quality of care.

### Responsibilities of the Informatics Nurse Specialist

The American Nurses Association (1994) defines nursing informatics as nursing-related information management. Nursing informatics enables nurses to access databases to improve client care. In 2001, the American Nurses Association (ANA) developed *Scope and Standards of Nursing Informatics Practice*. Informatics nurse specialists work as "project managers, systems specialists, consultants, system educators, researchers, policy developers and product developers" (Thede, 2003). Some informatics nurse specialists work for health care organizations; others are employed by product vendors, and others work as entrepreneurs. Some informatics nurse specialists manage large databases specific to a specialty area of practice. Because of the rapid advances in technology, all informatics nurse specialists must engage in lifelong learning. Knowledge of computers and information systems comes through formal education (collegiate and continuing education programs) as well as practical experience (Thede).

Informatics nurse specialists serve as integral parts in the development of health information systems. Their perspective gives the technological development team a working knowledge of the nursing profession so client care information can be better managed. Without input of nursing, created health information systems may miss critical aspects of client care and may create procedures that reduce nursing effectiveness.

### Education of the Informatics Nurse Specialist

The education of nursing informatics specialists varies. Table 15-1 outlines the educational preparation and role description for a nursing informatics expert. This area of nursing practice requires a thorough understanding of clinical practice and detailed computer expertise. Because nursing informatics is a new area of specialty practice, the preparation and roles vary.

As a nursing specialty, the ANA offers certification examinations to validate competence in nursing informatics. To stay abreast of changes in the practice of nursing informatics, the ANA requires certified informatics nurse specialists to engage in clinical practice and complete continuing education. Hours of clinical practice vary. An informatics

TABLE 15-1

## Education and Role Description of the Nursing Informatics Specialist

| Education | Role Description |
| --- | --- |
| Hold an active professional nursing license[a] | Understand the current use of nursing process in the clinical setting |
| Baccalaureate degree or higher in nursing[a] | |
| At least 2 years of clinical nursing practice[a] | Thorough understanding of clinical practice to develop, implement and maintain information systems that are relevant to clinical nursing practice |
| Successful completion of the ANA Certification Examination in Nursing Informatics [a] | Provides evidence for competence in the area of nursing informatics |
| Computer system design and analysis[b] | Develop novel system designs to meet nursing information needs<br>Analyze hardware and software available to design a comprehensive nursing information system<br>Recommend hardware and software to develop a system<br>Develop proposals for acquisition of resources needed for a system or system revisions<br>Program computers to meet the needs of the health care organization |
| Information and support of systems [b] | Develop, plan and implement education for nurses who use the information system<br>Develop and implement policies and procedures for system use<br>Develop documentation for staff education and support services<br>Maintain collegial relationships with system users<br>Outline strategies for implementation of system<br>Provide ongoing technical and clinical support for system users |
| Testing and evaluation of systems | Implement testing of system to verify functioning<br>Develop and implement system evaluation plan to detect strengths and weaknesses<br>Assess current system and new products for potential updates |
| Managing information and databases [b] | Collect and analyze aggregate data<br>Transform data into meaningful presentation format<br>Plan future updates to system |
| Professional practice, issues and trends [b] | Role components: nurse, information expert, computer expert, educator, and researcher<br>Financial issues related to system development, utilization, and updates<br>Future developments in technology<br>Ethical issues, such as confidentiality of client information<br>Federal regulations<br>Interdisciplinary organizations for health informatics<br>Professional standards for health and nursing informatics |

## Education and Role Description of the Nursing Informatics Specialist (Continued)

| Education | Role Description |
|---|---|
| Theoretical foundations for practice[b] | Concepts of nursing informatics<br>Nursing Taxonomy and Nomenclature (e.g., NANDA, Nursing Interventions Classification System/Nursing Outcomes Classification System, Nursing Management Minimum Data Set, Omaha System, Patient Care Data Set, Nightingale Tracker)<br>Mental models of data and information processing<br>Nursing decision making models and decision support systems |

[a] Certification requirements from the American Nurses Credentialing Center, 2000.

[b] Topics covered the American Nurses Credentialing Center Examination, 2000.

Information adapted from Thede (1999), *Computers in nursing: Bridges to the future* (pp. 289–293). Philadelphia: J. B. Lippincott; and Turley, J. P. (2000). Informatics and education: The start of a discussion. In B. Carty, (Ed.), *Nursing informatics education for practice* (pp. 271–293). New York: Springer Publishing.

nurse specialist may have 2,000 hours of clinical practice or 1,000 hours with 12 semester hours of academic credit within 5 years. In addition, the specialist must complete 20 contact hours in continuing education in nursing informatics within 2 years (American Nurses Credentialing Center, 2000; Thede, 2003).

### Role of the Informatics Nurse Specialist in Technological and Health Care Development

Software developers and computer programmers have expertise in computer systems, but lack familiarity with clinical nursing practice and health care delivery. Thus, to develop software and computer systems that are compatible with nursing care delivery and facilitate, rather than hinder, client care, health care systems and software companies seek nurse consultants or hire nurses with special education in nursing informatics. Nurses contribute critical information that affects client care. They also field test software programs to determine the ease of use and the feasibility for implementation in client care settings.

Nursing informatics is an exciting nursing specialty practice area. As computer technology and complex information systems permeate health care, more informatics nurse specialists will be needed to verify that systems address key nursing practice considerations and facilitate, rather than hinder, nursing care delivery. Table 15-2 outlines the complex nature of health information systems currently in use. Nearly every application has implications for professional nursing practice. As the need for automated systems to manage health care and document client health information increases, the need for computer analysts, computer support personnel is expected to rise. The United States Department of Labor Bureau of Labor Statistics (2000) projects a 102% increase in the need for computer support specialists, a 94% increase for systems analysts, and a 22% increase for registered nurses. Computer support personnel and computer analysts will communicate with nurses in health care systems. Nurses with advanced education in informatics will be able to design nurse-friendly systems and direct nurses effectively in the use of computer and information systems.

**TABLE 15-2**

**Components of a Health Information System Currently Employed by Health Care Providing Institutions**

| Health Information Component | Function Descriptions |
| --- | --- |
| Admission, discharge and transfer application | Tracks patient demographic data, insurance information, responsible parties, medical record number, care provider, and dates of admissions, transfer and dismissals |
| Financial application | Keeps records related to billing information for medical supplies and services rendered, tracking of accounts receivable, general ledger, and institutional costs for care delivery |
| Physician order entry application | Provides computer order entry and almost instant notification of orders to ancillary departments. Sometimes, information related to specific test preparation is immediately sent to the unit |
| Ancillary department application | Shares information among various departments to facilitate scheduling of entered orders. These applications also provide information related to quality control |
| Documentation application | Consist of pop-up screens that enable care providers to select assessment parameters, document care delivered and evaluate client response by using checklists. These also have the capability of free text entry should the need arise |
| Care planning application | Allows the nurse to select appropriate nursing diagnoses, expected care outcomes and nursing interventions for any client |
| Scheduling application | Enables patient scheduling of radiographic, nuclear medicine, and other specialized diagnostic tests and surgery. In addition, provides a means to schedule staff. Both systems are integrated into the financial information system |
| Acuity application | Provides a summary of the client care needs based upon the acuity of illness and in some cases, the project hours of nursing care in order to verify adequate staffing levels to fulfill client care needs |
| Specialty practice application | Provides health care providers within a specific specialty practice area to collect specific client data. Unfortunately, many of these systems fail to integrate data with other components of the health information system |
| Decision support application | Provides algorithmic decision making related to specific health problems, client demographics, and laboratory test results |
| Communication application | Provides e-mail and Internet access. Some institutions publish policies and procedures in this system component |

| Components of a Health Information System Currently Employed by Health Care Providing Institutions (Continued) | |
|---|---|
| **Health Information Component** | **Function Descriptions** |
| Critical pathways applications | Streamline the efforts of the interdisciplinary health team by focusing on specific care outcomes. Because all members document on the same form, a more coordinated approach to care results. When documentation is done by computer entry, comparisons of clinical data related to intervention, outcomes and multidisciplinary approaches become possible. |

From Hassert, M. (1999). Information systems. In Thede, L. Q. (1999). *Computers in nursing: Bridges to the future* (pages 237–247). Philadelphia: J. B. Lippincott.

## TECHNOLOGICAL CHANGES AFFECTING NURSING PRACTICE AND HEALTH CARE

In the late 1950s and early 1960s, businesses used computers for financial record management. Computer use accelerated in health care after the enactment of the Social Security Act that provided Medicare and Medicaid because data were required to document care delivered for governmental reimbursement.

### Lawrence Weed

In 1968, Lawrence Weed, gynecology department head at the University of Vermont, designed the first computer system for client care. The system was based on Weed's problem-oriented medical record and was named the Problem-Oriented Medical Record Information System (PROMIS). With PROMIS, all health care professionals gained access to information, such as costs of procedures, lists of patient problems, and client outcomes (Thede, 1999). Computers also made it possible to organize large volumes of data, giving professionals greater knowledge of disease management and prevention.

### Telehealth

**Telehealth** enables health care providers to "see" clients without being physically present because clients are connected to a system that beams television and other signals to the provider's office. In 2000, the United States Food and Drug Administration approved Eastman Kodak's LifeView Care Station for virtual house calls. The system consists of a video camera, monitor, thermometer, blood pressure cuff, and stethoscope. The nurse calls the client to connect to the system. The nurse receives real time images and data that can be stored electronically. This system provides client access to a home health nurse on a 24-hour-a-day basis (Reuters Health, 2000).

Telemedicine, although sometimes used interchangeably with telehealth, refers to the actual use of telehealth technology for disease diagnosis and treatment of a patient at a remote location by a physician. Telenursing refers to nursing care delivered to a client at a remote site. The term telemedicine first appeared in the literature in the 1960s, when telephone lines were used to transmit client information, such as laboratory test results and radiographic data using facsimile machines. Eventually, technology enabled transmission of electrocardiograph information using telephone lines. Now, a comprehensive telehealth system enables clients to interact in real time with health care providers with computer connections. In the process known as "store forward," images, photographs, and client records become digitalized for transmission from one location to another (Thede, 1999). With telehealth, health care professionals working in remote locations can participate in continuing education programs that occur in large urban health centers. They also can receive step-by-step instructions from specialists in how to perform complex surgical procedures in emergency situations.

## Robotics

With the impending nursing shortage, some nursing tasks may be safely accomplished by machines. **Robotics** is the design of machines to perform tasks usually done by humans. In the home, vacuum sweepers and lawn mowers are equipped with sensing devices to avoid bumping into and being stopped by environmental obstacles. Pharmacy robots have been in use for over a decade to perform mundane tasks associated with preparing and dispensing medications. In California, a robot equipped with television cameras allows nurses and physicians to see, hear, and talk to clients and staff through a wireless Internet connection. Some nursing tasks performed by robots (nursing bots) include meal tray delivery, filling water pitchers, making routine rounds, and taking vital signs (Jossi, 2004). In Canada, robots also can be used for surgery; the surgeon controls the robot that has better dexterity and eliminates human error when performing delicate dissections. Surgical costs are reduced as clients who need specialized surgery need not travel to a large metropolitan medical center, but rather have the surgery in a local hospital with a robot performing the surgery (Jossi, 2004).

### Research Brief 15-1

Bohnenkamp, S., McDonald, P., Lopez, A., Krupinski, E. L., & Blackett, A. (2004). Traditional versus telenursing outpatient management of patients with cancer with new ostomies. *Oncology Nursing Forum, 31*(5), 1005–1010.

The investigators sought to compare telenursing with traditional outpatient management of clients with new ostomies who had been diagnosed with cancer. Using a convenience sample of 28 clients, 14 clients were each assigned to be in one of two groups: traditional home health nursing visits or home health visits plus contact using telenursing. Persons in the telehealth group received the routine home health visits plus two telehealth encounters with the ostomy clinical nurse specialists between scheduled visits. Data were collected regarding number of traditional home health visits, number of telenursing encounters (telehealth group only), dates when clients could self-mange their ostomies, and amount of ostomy supplies used. Clients also completed an investigator satisfaction survey about each type of visit at the 6-week follow-up visit and Maklebust's (1985) Ostomy Adjustment Scale (OAS) at a 3-month interval.

Eleven participants had urostomies, and three participants had colostomies. The traditional home health group had a mean of 6.29 nursing visits and the telehealth group had a mean of 5.43 face-to-face visits and 3.57 telenursing encounters. The telenursing group could independently change their pouches 13.71 days after surgery and the home health visit group could do this in 15.07 days after surgery (no statistically significant difference). Client satisfaction was 12% higher in the telenursing group ($P < .01$). The telenursing group had one less face-to-face home nursing visit and telenursing encounters cost $44.10 less than home health visits. The telenursing group spent an average of $52.40 less on pouch supplies. However, the overall cost for each group was $444.52 for the home health visit only group and $444.81 for the combined home visit/telenursing group. No statistically significant score differences occurred on the OAS between the groups.

Implications for practice include that clients in this study seemed satisfied with telenursing, the telenursing group believed that the ostomy nurse who consulted using telenursing understood their problems better than the home health nurse did, and the telenursing group used fewer pouch changing supplies. Both groups achieved independent pouch changes within 2 days of each other. Because of the small sample, more research is needed to demonstrate comparability of services with telenursing and to see if cost savings would apply with larger groups and with persons with different health conditions and special needs. No information was collected on how home health nurse perceive telenursing, which is another area that could benefit from future investigation. Telenursing may be an answer to providing nursing services if the nursing shortage results in insufficient numbers of professional nurses employed in the specialty of home health nursing.

## Genomic Medicine

Complex technology also has enabled scientists to discover more about nature. Advances in science have profound implications for health care. More than any other scientific discovery, mapping the human genome means the transformation of health care delivery. Knowing the genetic sequence of organisms causing various infectious diseases enables scientists to develop new vaccines against them (Rappouli & Covacci, 2003). **Genomic medicine** applies knowledge generated from human, bacterial, and viral genomes to develop new medical treatments and determine specific regimens for clients based on their particular human genetic sequence. Vastly different approaches to health promotion and disease management surface as more becomes known about how human genes affect health. Wang, Brock, Herberich, and Schultz (2001) report that 20 common amino acids comprise the genetic code for all organisms. Initial publicized findings of the Human Genome Project revealed that humans have approximately 34,000 genes and that people are 99.5% identical. However, the 34,000 genes have the capability to make between 500,000 to 1 million proteins. Results indicate that genes do not cause disease, but proteins do. Implications for disease screening and therapy most likely lie with the study of proteomics (human proteins). Millennium Predictive Medicine has identified three dozen proteins that may serve as markers for ovarian cancer. However, in Alzheimer's disease research, six genes have been identified that increase the "risk" of this disease. The official diagnosis of Alzheimer's disease relies on the presence of beta amyloidal fragments that bear responsibility for the development of brain plaques. Researchers at Johns Hopkins University and Large Scale Proteomics Corporation have developed a list of human proteins responsible for the development of depression, schizophrenia, and bipolar disease (Check & Rogers, 2001). Stone (2001) reported that the mapping of the 3 million DNA base pairs of the human genome would have been impossible without the field of bioinformatics.

Estimates indicate that the amount of information generated by the Human Genome Project would take scientists centuries to decipher. Companies such as Informax in Bethesda, Maryland, and Lion Biosciences in Germany have developed software programs to facilitate data analysis. For costs as high as $100 million, these companies license software and offer consultation services to small laboratories and giant pharmaceutical companies. These software programs contain the capability to indicate if certain genes are active in certain kinds of tissue (such as malignant cells). Other computer giants, such as Compaq, IBM, and Oracle, are developing similar programs. These new tools can shorten the development process for new medications. Eventually, physicians may send a genetic sample from a patient and receive a medication designed specifically for the patient's illness. Newborns may be genetically tested and receive a lifetime plan (including when to begin taking medications designed for their genotypes) to prevent illness (Stone, 2001).

Discoveries in genetic research indicate that a variety of illnesses, including hypercholesterolemia (Garcia et al., 2001; Holden, 2003), obesity, type I and type II diabetes, multiple sclerosis, Alzheimer's, autism, schizophrenia, nicotine dependence, alcohol dependence (Merikangas & Risch, 2003), and some cancers (Merikegas & Risch; Offit, 1998), result from the presence of specific genes. Each year, an estimated 50,000 to 100,000 new cases of cancer in the United States have an inherited susceptibility (Offit, 1998). Health care professionals currently use information related to the inherited susceptibility of cancer. The cancers linked to inherited susceptibility include breast, ovarian, colon, prostate, and skin (Giarelli & Jacobs, 2001). Genetic testing already has altered protocols for breast cancer prevention. Two genes, breast cancer gene 1 (BRCA-1) and breast cancer gene 2 (BRCA-2), have been related to familial cases of breast cancer, representing approximately 5% to 10% of all breast cancers. Although both genes affect tumor suppressor genes, each has a somewhat different function. The BRCA-1 has also been associated with familial cases of ovarian cancer. A BRCA-2 presence in women is associated with a lower incidence of ovarian cancer. However, BRCA-2 has been associated with female and male cases of breast cancer. Estrogen-receptor positive breast cancer tends to develp in women with the genetic marker, BRCA-2. Exactly how these gene mutations lead to the development of breast cancer remains unknown (Couzin, 2003). However, benefits in identifying the presence of BRCA-1 and BRCA-2 include offering earlier and more frequent screening for breast cancer, chemoprevention therapy, or prophylactic mastectomy.

Along with predicting persons as risk for a particular disease, inherited metabolic flaws have been identified. Labeling of 20 medications warns persons who prescribe them of potentially fatal reactions based on genetically identifiable inherited metabolic disorders. Genetic differences in metabolism explain variations in therapeutic responses based on ancestral heritage (Holden, 2003; Marshall, 2003). Genetic differences have been identified to explain the lack of effectiveness of angiotensin-converting enzyme inhibitors in controlling blood pressure in some persons of African descent. Over millennia, persons from India have survived famines that resulted in a "thrifty gene" presentation in approximately one third of the Indian population. This gene is linked to the development of hypercholesteremia when Indians westernize their diets (Holden). Risky genes have been identified in persons who experience long QT syndrome after receiving specific medications (Marshall, 2003a). Currently, the cost of testing for a single gene that affects drug metabolism or identifying a person at risk for a disease ranges from $100 to $1,000 (Marshall, 2003). However, the day of genetically-tailored drug regimens for treating specific diseases, although possible, remains far away (Holden).

The use of genetic information and engineering triggers social responses. Health care professionals can identify persons at risk for specific illnesses and institute early health screenings. Genetic testing may be offered to persons at risk for a particular illness. However, personal behaviors and environmental factors also play a role in disease development. Once a genetic predisposition to an illness within a family is identified, the professional nurse sometimes becomes a resource for how to tell other family members they are at risk (Giarelli & Jacobs, 2001). Many professional nursing programs have incorporated course content into curricula, especially issues related to genetic testing for diseases, ownership of biomedical research samples, client confidentiality, and legislative initiatives. Finally, the Internet serves as a public resource for genetic information.

## Stem Cell Therapy and Research

Technology has given medical researchers the ability to grow body parts using embryonic or adult stem cells. Approximately 3,000 human illnesses could benefit from stem cell therapies (Lanza et al., 2001). **Stem cells** are immature human cells that have not yet committed to becoming a particular type of human cell. Patients with Parkinson's disease, hematologic disorders, and malignancies currently use stem cell therapies. Stem cells readily multiply and can be "coaxed into creating nearly any type of cell" (Gutterman, 2001, p. A19) developing into fat, bone, cartilage, or muscle. However, human progenitor cells could grow into any form of human tissue. With a research team, Charles Vacanti at the University of Massachusetts Medical School has discovered tiny cells (3 to 5 microns across) in human tissue that become activated to repair damaged tissue. Spore cells from human ears, livers, and lungs grow into healthy-looking tissue when implanted under the skin of mice (Gutterman, 2001). Lumelsky and colleagues (2001) have grown insulin-secreting structures similar to pancreatic islets in vitro using human stem cells. However, whether these body parts function effectively remains unknown. This exciting research potentially solves the problem of waiting lists for organ donation, eliminates the need for isolating adult stem cells for growing body parts, and bypasses the ethical issues related to use of embryonic stem cells for laboratory-grown tissue or skin (Gutterman, 2001).

Because of the advances in the treatment of certain diseases such as leukemia, parents of newborns need to have information related to the storage of stem cells from the placenta and umbilical cords. Some obstetricians present this information to women during pregnancy. However, most health insurance companies do not cover storage fees. Parents also have the option of donating stem cells to private or public stem cell banks. Cells stored in private stem cell banks are reserved only for use by the family that stores them. Some nurses collect umbilical stem cell blood for storage as part of their job as labor and delivery nurses. Ethical issues arise, such as equal access to stem cells as well as what is done with stored cells when they are no longer needed.

As technological capabilities increase, humans learn more about nature, generate more information, develop new ways to relay information, and create different work processes. Technological advances serve as the impetus and provide the means to alter professional nursing practice.

## Online Educational Options

Many clients use the Internet for health-related information before consulting a health care professional. Some information sources offer valid and reliable information; whereas, others present less than reputable information (especially websites that sell products). Persons suffering from chronic illnesses may know more about their disorder than the health care provider. When discussing the condition with clients, nurses can find useful sources of information. By visiting the websites clients visit for health-related information, nurses can assess the information for credibility.

Like clients, health care professionals receive educational information from the Internet. Many nursing organizations offer online continuing education programs. Along with specialty organizations, some nursing journals have websites that provide continuing education programs. Even some nursing specialty certification examinations are administered online.

Some nursing schools offer online courses. Perhaps the course that uses this text is an online course. Such courses provide students with distance education options. Some institutions charge higher fees for online courses (McHugh & Gibson, 2000). Access to distance education becomes available to anyone connected to the Internet. Each institution specifies required hardware and software for online courses and has vendor contracts for student discounts. Students also need to exercise care when selecting an Internet service provider (ISP) before enrolling in an online course. Some ISPs disconnect users after a specified time, especially during high network congestion (Short, 2000). Also, some web-based course materials (especially those with sound and complex graphics) require digital service line connections for complete downloading.

Before enrolling in an online course, a student must possess the skills for success and verify the quality of education. A self-assessment of computer skills reveals if a student has the ability to connect to the class, engage in online class discussions, download complex documents, manage files, and access help. A student should ask questions related to available technical assistance and provision of a backup computer if problems with technology occur (Mueller & Billings, 2000; Short, 2000). Asking questions about course content, the number of times the course has been offered online, and faculty experience with online education can lead to clues to the quality of the course and instruction. The following five indicators reflect similarity between on-campus and distance online education: (1) reasonable faculty electronic office hours, (2) online library resources, (3) alternative ways to interact with student colleagues beyond e-mail, (4) online secure examinations, and (5) course content that balances passive lecture with interactive teaching techniques. Two critical elements that distinguish online from on-campus education are asynchronous capability to access course content and tests so that students may set individualized class schedules and technical support availability during evenings and weekends (Short, 2000). However, some online courses require synchronous class meetings.

Because online courses differ from those taught in traditional classrooms, some students might not learn as well. If a student relies heavily on peer contact, isolation of home study may impede learning. Persons who need structure and strict deadlines to complete course requirements do not fare well with online education (Short, 2000).

Because most faculty-to-student and student-to-student interactions occur in written format, students with poorly developed writing skills may find online courses too burdensome (Mueller & Billings, 2000). Some students perceive that because they determine the time of instruction, there is less work associated with an online course. Online courses require completion of assignments similar to courses taught on campus. However, class discussions held using bulletin board software, especially with large numbers of students, sometimes consume lots of time (Mueller & Billings).

## ✦ CHALLENGES MANAGING HEALTH-RELATED INFORMATICS AND TECHNOLOGY

The rapid introduction of technology in clinical practice provides a challenge to professional nurses. Once a nurse becomes competent and confident with a new piece of patient care equipment, medical device manufacturers introduce a new generation of the device. Within a decade, I have had the pleasure of working with five versions of a peripheral blood glucose monitor. Changes in client care equipment may create distress for some nurses. However, new generations of client care equipment usually contain features that increase accuracy or efficiency.

The vast amount of health-related information can create confusion for health care professionals and consumers. Professional nurses, like any other consumer, use the Internet to find information. Health care service organizations often set up organizational computer networks. As integrated delivery systems emerge, information networks between organizations within a health system are developed.

### Confidentiality

When an individual has a positive result for certain genes, a breach of confidentiality with regard to those findings may result in discrimination in health or life insurance coverage and employment. Issues also surface related to genetic screening of other family members, childbearing, and rights of privacy. A positive finding for a breast cancer gene can cause psychological distress for some women. A negative test result may give the woman a false sense of security when all American women have a one in seven chance of experiencing breast cancer in their lifetimes (Houshmand, Campbell, Briggs, McFadden, & Al-Tweigeri, 2001).

Medical and pharmaceutical research centers rely on biologic material and data to develop new therapies for illnesses. Donors of human tissue and cells have a right to privacy but not a right to ownership, based on the Genetic Confidentiality and Non-Discriminatory Act of 1997. Medical researchers have the obligation of obtaining informed consent from persons who donate tissues and cells for biomedical research (Giarelli & Jacobs, 2001).

When confidential data are transmitted across communication lines, security issues arise. Before participating in any telehealth program, clients should be informed of the potential loss of the information. Clients also should have the right to determine who has access to their health-related information and the right to view information that is generated through telehealth proceedings (Thede, 1999). No computer connection offers complete security, and information can become lost in cyberspace.

Computerized or electronic records contain a lot of personal information. Institutions using computerized records in areas such as academe protect private data with passwords and firewalls (Foster, 2001). Likewise, client health data must be securely protected.

However, privacy experts sometimes fail to fully understand the capabilities of computer technology. Incidents resulting in privileged information falling into the wrong hands or being abused demonstrate the vulnerability of any electronic record. Computer hackers anywhere in the world have the capability of infiltrating any system that houses records containing private and personal information. Hackers can program denial-of-service messages in any system. When new software programs are tested within the health care system, transmission of private medical data to an outside computer server provides an opportunity for it to be viewed by unauthorized persons (Foster, 2001).

To combat these problems, tools have been created to promote confidentiality of health care records. Currently, most health care organizations protect electronic health records with computer passwords. Organizations providing health care also require employees and outside contractors to sign confidentiality agreements before being given computer access. Some institutions have written policies specifying penalties for persons who violate confidentiality agreements. Future protection for electronic health care records may be provided with more complex technology, including voice recognition systems and devices that scan a care provider's fingerprint or retina (Thede, 1999, 2003).

In February 2001, a new federal law went into effect to protect the privacy of personal health information (PHI). Documented consent from the health care consumer is required before health care providers can disclose PHI for treatment, payment, or other health care operations. This law provides health care consumers with the following four rights: to receive written notice related to PHI storage and use changes before they are implemented; to access one's health information; to obtain an account of how PHI has been disclosed; and to request a correction or amendment to PHI. Documentation permitting PHI disclosure must be kept for 6 years. Those breaking the law may be fined $25,000 to $250,000 and imprisoned for up to 10 years for unauthorized disclosure of PHI. Because of the consequences related to misuse of PHI, many health care providing organizations have a privacy officer to manage the integrity of client PHI (Huchenski, 2001).

## Ethics

Ethical debates surround stem cell research. The key issue centers on the definition of the beginning of human life. Many stem cells come from human embryos, which may be products of early abortions. Some abortion opponents view use of embryonic human cells as approval of abortions for convenient or therapeutic reasons. Proponents of stem cell research suggest that clinicians dispose of products of abortion and that using them for stem cell research provides societal benefits. If needed, researchers could grow human embryos and harvest stem cells in laboratories. In 2001, plans for federal support of human embryonic stem cell research were halted. Withdrawal of public support for these projects means that private organizations and overseas researchers will continue stem cell research efforts without comprehensive ethical oversight (Lanza et al., 2001).

Other ethical issues surrounding expensive procedures focus on access to services. If insurance companies do not cover the cost (for example storing umbilical cord stem cells and genetically designed medications), then only persons with personal financial resources reap the benefits of such technology. Thus in the future, the disparities over the quality of health care for the rich and poor may become more apparent.

## Evaluating the Quality of Information

In the 1990s, the Internet became a common source of health care information for consumers. Internet-based health care networks link caregivers with clients and persons who share health-related problems with each other. Consumers of health care access the latest research information and become educated about health promotion and illnesses (sometimes from unreliable sources), take health-screening surveys, and purchase health care products.

Not all of the information related to health and nursing falls under the careful watch of the informatics nurse specialists. The availability of information and access to it has greatly increased as more persons become connected to the Internet. Health care professionals working on similar research and practice projects can almost instantaneously share critical information with each other. Health care consumers can use the Internet as a source of health-related information, and many purchase medical equipment online. Health care professionals must become cognizant of the information available to consumers because sometimes a person with a rare health disorder may have more knowledge about the condition than his or her health care provider. Carty (2000) emphasizes that the explosion of information and easy access result in a change in the current delivery of health care. Carty (2000) also suggests that an information-driven system would provide consumers with a different way of receiving health care services. The information-driven system would provide an enterprise-based integrated delivery system that focuses on wellness, as well as illness. Consumer encounters with the systems would be comprehensive and occur across a lifetime, rather than in various episodic encounters. These consumer-focused systems would provide rapid worldwide access to health-related information and would generate individual longitudinal computerized medical records. Some clients would become experts about their individual health issues. However, not all clients have access to the Internet or the desire to seek health information. Clients have varying knowledge bases of health-related information, which professional nurses need to consider when working as partners with clients to promote health and manage illness.

The World Wide Web (the Web) serves as a major source of advertising for-profit and nonprofit organizations. Businesses frequently use the muscle of websites to lure customers into purchasing products (Akens, 1999). As a health care professional, nurses must be wary of all sources of health-related information with which they come into contact. Printed sources, such as professional books and journals, are subject to peer and editorial review before publication. However, anyone with computer access can publish information on the Internet. Caution must be exercised before using information from the Internet for professional use.

### Questions for Reflection 15-2

1. How do I manage the sea of information generated by computer technology?
2. Why is it important to stay abreast of health-related information on the Internet?
3. What strategies could I use to stay abreast of health-related information on the Internet?
4. How would the strategies affect my professional practice and personal life?

## Data Security

The potential loss of data is the biggest concern when using individual electronic health records. Loss of health data may occur with hardware failures and system programming errors. Through the processes of acquisition, storage, and processing, some data may be lost. Routine data backups and off-site storage protects information against natural disasters (Thede, 2003). Recent evidence reveals that long-term storage of computerized data appears unstable, especially for data stored on older, single-density floppy disks. In addition, computer drives capable of reading such disks have disappeared. Recent observations indicate that data stored on CD-ROMs may begin to disintegrate after 5 years. Files and disks can become corrupt at any time.

Computer systems sometimes quit for no apparent reason. They also must rely on quality information entry by humans. Bad information input results in poor use of technology. Computers cannot catch many of these mistakes but are capable of performing complex mathematical operations and making complex decisions provided humans enter information correctly (Thede, 1999, 2003). Finally, computers rely on a power source (electricity or battery) to work. When the power source is severed, the computer stops. Many clinical practice settings that use computer systems require nurses to print hard copies of documents for client medical records.

Some quick link programs take information from personal computers and send it to data banks that companies use to market products. The fine print in consumer agreements specifies that information may be generated for managing and targeting advertisements. Information sent over secure links that use encryption technology remains private (Levy, 2001). However, all computer systems used by businesses have tracking devices that could be monitored by specific information management personnel. Even the most complex password systems and strongest firewalls fail to provide complete protection from hackers (Foster, 2001).

To safeguard clients from unauthorized access and use of confidential health information, most organizations use audit trails that can trace who accesses the information and when it was accessed. Many organizations limit employee access to client data to those who need to know based on job descriptions. Organizations routinely conduct security audits consisting of impostor (nonemployee) use of the system; unattended confidential on-screen or printed client information; visitors sitting unattended at a computer station; and visitor or impostor accessing or receiving printed copies of confidential health information to verify proper use of confidential health information (Thede, 2003). In some cases, employees may be terminated for violation of policies related to the unauthorized use of client confidential information.

Along with insider misuse of confidential information, health care organizations protect client information from outside intruders. Firewalls offer some protection. Firewalls may be software programs or part of computer hardware. They require constant maintenance and updating to assure no penetration from creative computer hackers. Some agencies hire outside hackers to see if they can penetrate the system (Thede, 2003).

## Struggling to Stay Abreast of New Technologies

The success of high-technology client care devices depends on the ability of the nurse (or consumer) to operate them. If a device is shown to promote client comfort or save time, professional nurses tend to adopt them readily as part of routine client care. New devices are more readily accepted by nurses if nurses contributed to the decision-making process regarding which of the competing products are adopted for organizational use.

Of all the disadvantages, the inclination of nurses to focus on the machinery, rather than the client, is the most dangerous for professional nursing. Sometimes, nurses attend to machinery alarms before client observation. By doing this, professional nurses develop the reputation of being cold and aloof to clients and their significant others. No machine can replace the warmth of a genuine, caring human interaction.

Advances in technology create challenges for professional nurses. Recent predictions suggest that information and technological advancements will expand exponentially during the next five years. With the vast amount of information required for effective client care, professional nurses frequently experience information overload. Complex information related to disease prevention and treatment makes it impossible for nurses to be effective generalists. Nurse subspecialties in identified areas of nursing practice have begun to surface. To provide effective client care, nurses must stay abreast of new developments in health care and technology while keeping focused on the importance of interacting with clients with authentic caring.

## Computer Networks

Nurses use clinical care devices and computers in a variety of ways. When two or more computers connect, they form a network. The advantages of networking include enabling employees to work away from the office, sharing information and equipment (such as a printer), and eliminating a courier or service to carry information from one computer to another. A local area network denotes computers that are connected to each other in the same building or in several buildings within a given locale, such as a college campus. Wide area networks (WAN) consist of computers that are connected to each other across a wide geographical distance, such as a city or country (Akens, 1999). Currently, health delivery organizations (or systems) with locations across town or state lines use WAN. Most network systems protect their system by using a firewall, which is special software or hardware to protect it from unauthorized use (Maran, 1998). A network administrator manages the network and verifies that it runs smoothly. The Internet is a global computer network in which computers from all over the world are connected by telephone lines or radio waves (Akens).

To get connected to the Internet, the computer user must have a computer, an ISP, and some form of connecting device, such as a telephone or cable modem or a digital subscriber line. Satellite and television Internet access also are available. Most persons pay a monthly fee for a service provider, satellite dish, or television cable connection. Along with the required hardware, browser software must be purchased to have the tools needed to navigate the Web. Most ISPs include the software as part of the package. To receive electronic mail, the computer must have an electronic mail (e-mail) program loaded (Nicoll, 2001).

Group e-mail lists are called list servers (Listserv). Usually, there is no charge for Listserv membership. Discussions occur asynchronously, and they may address professional or personal concerns. Before being able to participate in list discussions, the user must subscribe to the service. Because of the number of participants in a group e-mail list, computer users face an enormous amount of information for reading and processing. Nicoll (2001) recommends requesting a digest of the online discussion to avoid receiving hundreds of e-mail messages.

Along with Listserv groups, electronic publications are available using Internet access. Electronic publishing provides an alternative to printed books and magazines. Blumenstyk (2001) reported that, according to Forrester Research, by 2003, 14% of all textbook sales will be electronic books (e-textbooks). Such books contain built-in multimedia elements that provide moving pictures to explain concepts. Electronic publishing reduces the costs for consumers. However, despite such books being designed to be used on a personal computer, users find several disadvantages to them, including having to scroll down the screen instead of turning pages; having to be connected to the Internet by a cable or wireless technology; having to use a large notebook computer; and the need for compact disk versions to be downloaded into a personal computer. Readers are limited to where they can read e-textbooks (Blumenstyk). Electronic libraries provide access to many books for a weekly, monthly, or annual fee. Providers gain complete access to holdings at any time, even if another patron is using the holding. Many libraries refrain from purchasing a needed book only in e-textbook form because the electronic library company may remove the book from the online collection.

Along with electronic books, some libraries subscribe to journals published in electronic format. Several online nursing journals offer articles in abstracted or full text form. Most of these journals require a fee for viewing an entire article unless accessed from a library with a specialized subscription. When readers subscribe to an online journal, they pay a fee for access to all items published in the journal.

Persons spend lots of money for hardware, software, and Internet services. Computer prices continue to decrease, and machines have increasing capabilities (Akens, 1999). The speed with which technology improves increases daily. Often, as soon as a consumer purchases computer hardware, manufacturers have released the next model, which has even more capacity. Most major software producers also update programs every 2 to 3 years. New editions of a software program read documents developed on previous versions, but the old version usually does not read documents produced with the later version. When purchasing programs for home use, one must be cognizant of this problem because older software may be available at work, making transfer of work produced at home difficult or even impossible. Some nurses work in organizations that provide remote access to mainframe computer systems. Nurses employed in these settings must have compatible software programs loaded on their home computers. In addition, organizations and nurses must exercise the utmost care to preserve information confidentially when allowing nurses to work with the computer system from remote sites.

## Accessing Information

The United States Armed Forces started the Internet in the late 1960s. Today the Internet is the largest global computer network. Subscribers include scientists, researchers, businesses, schools, libraries, and individuals (Maran, 1998). Contrary to popular belief, the Web and the Internet are different. The Internet is a worldwide computer network that uses transmission control protocol/Internet protocol. Small personal computers and large supercomputers are connected to the Internet. A network of collected websites uses hypertext transfer protocol as the procedure for sharing information. All Web addresses have the same letters and symbols to begin their address (http://), and this is automatically inserted when a computer user enters a universal resource locater (Maran, 1998; Nicoll, 2001). Internet sites not connected to the Web require that the user type in the complete address, including a transfer protocol abbreviation. The Internet must be accessed through a server (or large computer that provides services to other computers), also known as an ISP. Of all the Internet services, e-mail is the most popular, followed by talkathons (chat groups, bulletin boards, net news). Electronic mail addresses typically start with a user's name, followed by the symbol @ (to denote "at"), the provider of service, and the type of organization. For example the author's business e-mail address is lucyhood@sbcglobal.net. In contrast, a Web address starts with the letters www, then the name of the organization or person, followed by the type of organization. For example, the website address of the publisher of this book is www.lww.com. When inputting an e-mail or website address, there is no margin for error; the address must be entered accurately for a successful link to occur (Akens, 1999).

A website is a collection of pages posted on the Internet (Akens, 1999). A home page is the beginning point of a website, where a browser enters the site and usually views content within the website. Most home pages contain text, graphics, sound, animation, and other interactive features (Akens). In the United States, the following six domains are used to designate the type of server that hosts a website: (1) commercial = .com; (2) educational = .edu; (3) network = .net; (4) nonprofit organization = .org; (5) governmental = .gov; (6). military = .mil (Nicoll, 2001; Thede, 1999, 2003).

If a person can type and use a mouse, accessing information on the Internet is a simple task. Many information searches start with the use of a search engine. All Internet software programs contain a search engine, with which the computer user inputs a topic of interest, then hits a key to command the computer to find matches. Sometimes a computer search can retrieve hundreds of thousands of matches on a single topic.

Nurses also can find Internet sites by using publishing guides, reading journal articles, and using bibliographies. Millions of websites exist. Many have long lives, but some become obsolete when organizations merge. Once a site has been accessed and found to be useful, the computer user can file it by using a bookmark or a list of favorites, thereby eliminating the need to again enter the complex website address.

Newsgroups and chat rooms connect persons with similar interests. Information can be exchanged through synchronous or asynchronous postings. Participants in a newsgroup can receive thousands of e-mail messages (also called articles) daily (Maran, 1998). Some groups feature a summary of messages for members. Software can be purchased to read and post messages to newsgroups. Some newsgroups charge a fee for participation, and others are free. Some newsgroups are moderated and rely on volunteers to read each message and decide if it should be posted. Messages can be sent to the author of the posted message, to the entire newsgroup, or both (Maran, 1998).

Chatting enables instant communication with persons around the world. Persons send messages back and forth to chat. Most chatting is text-based. Persons can participate in group conversations. Participation in chat rooms enables persons to keep in touch with friends, colleagues, and relatives who reside in a wide geographical area without paying long-distance telephone fees. When participating in a chat room with unfamiliar persons, chatters tend to use a nickname for personal protection. Forms of chatting include Internet relay chat, instant messaging, web-based chat, and multimedia chat (Maran, 1998). Some nurses use chat rooms as a means for professional networking. Chat rooms enable nurses to identify problems within professional practice that occur across care delivery settings, serve as a means for offering each other moral support, and provide a means for seeing how other nurses have solved practice problems.

The Internet also lets you browse through files stored on computers around the world by using the file transfer protocol (FTP), which also allows users to download files. Private FTP sites require member registration and password entry before file access can occur. Anonymous FTP sites grant access without password entry. Types of files found on FTP sites include text, images, sound, video, and computer programs. Large files from FTP sites are compressed to increase the speed of travel over the Internet. These files must be decompressed using a decompression program (Maran, 1998).

## Optical Technology

With traditional electronic technology, transmission of a three-dimensional computed tomography scan would take almost 55 years. **Optical technology** uses light waves to transmit signals. Pure optical networks would enable all forms of data (print, photographs, voice, video) to be transported at the speed of light. Optical technology has transformed the way consumers store information. In the 1980s, most computer users stored information and used programs using floppy disks. Now, compact and digital videodisks are widely used. However, optical data transmission requires data routers with increased processing capability. Researchers at the University of California have fabricated wavelength converters from inexpensive semiconductor materials. Optical routers have the capability of receiving and sending data from multiple cables simultaneously. Optical cables have the capacity to carry thousands of wavelengths, and each wavelength has the ability to accommodate enormous amounts of traffic. Current research efforts focus on using optical technology to further enhance the speed of telecommunications; redefine materials used for telecommunications to withstand ambient temperatures and variations in electrical currents; improve wireless transmissions; detect minute traces of environmental biohazards; improve the quality of lasers for medical therapies; develop diagnostic tests to determine specific genetic mutations and abnormal actions of enzymes, co-enzymes, and proteins in biologic membranes; and improve the accuracy of forensic tests (United States Department of Commerce, 2004).

## Cyberstalking

Along with information insecurity, computer users connected to the Internet may fall victim to **cyberstalking**. Cyberstalking has three primary forms: harassment, spamming, and phishing. Institutions that provide employee e-mail addresses and office telephone numbers place them at risk for cyberstalking. Harassment includes receiving unwanted ads, pornographic material, and threatening messages (Foster, 2001). Spamming, another form of receiving unwanted information, occurs when a person distributes a piece of advertising to members of a large distribution list. Nurses and others using e-mail sometimes receive hundreds of messages daily, and much time is spent reading or deleting spam. Internet criminals use phishing to attempt to access personal information about Internet uses that is later used to steal identities or drain bank accounts. In addition, some legitimate businesses attach spyware programs to computers when consumers complete product registration forms online (Hartman, 2005). Hartman offers the following suggestions as ways to protect against cyberstalking: (1) use a nonsense password and change it frequently; (2) never post personal information on a website; (3) if female, use computer sign-on entries that prevent identification as a female user; (4) check websites that collect information about people and request that personal information be removed from them; (5) never use a credit card for a purchase in a nonsecure environment; (6) read and understand security policies before making Internet purchases from any company; (7) report any spam to the system administrator of the person who received the spam and the person who sent the spam; (8) report any Internet abuse to CyberSnitch, a network that automatically files reports to appropriate law enforcement agencies; (9) use e-mail filtering programs; (10) invest and use firewalls, virus protection, and other computer safety programs.

### Questions for Reflection 15-3

1. Have I ever been a victim of cyberstalking?
2. What safeguards do I have on my home and work computers to prevent cyberstalking?

## Balancing Technology with Life

Personal responses to computers range from curiosity and excitement to fear and dread. Computers alone or the introduction of a new computer application may cause anxiety for nurses (Simpson & Kerrick, 1997; Thede, 1999, 2003). Because nurses are people, computers may become an impediment to leading a balanced life. Some nurses have become enthralled with computers and purchase each new device when it hits the market. They spend hours engaged in computer chat rooms and surfing the Internet. Small handheld devices enable persons to be constantly connected to the Internet. Using technology may become an addiction or serve as an excuse for not interacting with other persons.

Some persons rely heavily on personal pagers and cell phones. Having nearly instantaneous information related to medical emergencies and community health hazards enables nurses (especially those working in emergency department or community health settings) to act swiftly, save lives, and prepare for victims of a disaster. However, the need to respond to them immediately sometimes impedes a person's ability to engage in deep, meaningful, face-to-face conversations. Display 15-1 presents signs that perhaps, someone has too much technology in one's life.

### Questions for Reflection 15-4

1. How do I balance high tech with high touch in my personal and professional lives?
2. Why is it important to strike a balance between high tech and high touch in client care?
3. Why is it important to strike a balance between technology and other personal life aspects?

---

**Signs of Too Much Technology**

DISPLAY 15-1 ◆

1. You have a device on your body that beeps, buzzes, or vibrates when you sit to eat a meal or while you watch a movie.
2. You would rather spend time talking with persons from computer or tech support than with your family or friends.
3. You navigate the Internet with ease but get lost in the mall or supermarket.
4. You cannot remember the names of your children, siblings, nieces, or nephews, but you have pet names for all your gadgets.
5. You have more telephone lines at home that are linked to machines that communicate with each other than with the outside.
6. You are less concerned with miles per gallon than bytes per second.
7. You spend hours on the computer and have no time to eat, sleep, or interact with family or friends.
8. You remember to turn off the computer, but leave the coffee maker, oven, or other appliances operating when you leave home.
9. You carry your cell phone, beeper, or Palm Pilot with you at all times and immediately attend to its signals, no matter where you are or what you are doing.
10. You must have the latest electronic personal gadget as soon as it hits the market.
11. You have lost the ability to engage in personal conversation with people, but you maintain relationships with others mainly through electronic communications such as e-mails and chat rooms.
12. You start your computer as soon as you awaken.
13. You experience severe emotional distress if you do not use a computer or personal electronic gadget within a 24-hour time frame or you lose one of them.

---

◆ **SUMMARY AND SIGNIFICANCE TO PRACTICE**

Nurses must develop competence in managing the complex technology used for health care delivery. With the vast amount of information available to anyone with computer access, nurses face many challenges. They must stay abreast of the latest scientific developments related to health care, work with clients who have become experts in many health issues and diseases, and manage enormous volumes of information. Nurses must be familiar with sophisticated technological equipment and balance the demands of technology with a human touch.

In the future, telehealth could replace one-on-one human interaction for delivery of health care. Computer technology could be used to replace nurses who deliver care to clients in homes, schools, and rural clinics. Eventually, homebound clients could use telehealth to contact health care providers and eliminate the need for office or home visits. School secretaries could use computer technology to consult physician offices or emergency departments when students become ill or injured. People in rural areas could use technology to connect to physician offices to receive primary health care and use the Internet to answer health-related questions.

In addition to the benefits to nursing, computer systems save health care institutions time and money. Information systems provide billing information when tests and procedures are entered using computers. Information systems streamline quality improvement, infection control, and risk management programs. Managers and staff save time by using computer programs to create staffing schedules. Acquisition of new diagnostic and interventional technology serves as a marketing tool. Computerized examinations streamline the process of validating staff competencies for institutional accreditation. Information systems also facilitate financial and institutional recordkeeping.

Technology has revolutionized health care. Complex computerized machinery enables accurate diagnoses of medical problems. Some diagnostic equipment machines have eliminated the need for invasive and painful procedures. Pharmaceutical companies have been able to find many new medications for the treatment and prevention of illness. Surgical procedures that once required large incisions now are performed with scopes. Microsurgical techniques also provide surgeons with improved visualization of operating fields. Some health care organizations use docking stations to track the accuracy of point-of-service (bedside) laboratory testing. The test results are downloaded into a laboratory computer, where client identification is verified, and the bill for the test is sent directly to the business office. Integration of point-of-service tests to a mainframe computer also can generate data for quality improvement.

Finally, technology has improved the delivery of nursing care. Nurses use computerized machines to save time and reduce errors in client care delivery. Sometimes, assessment data collection and recording occur simultaneously when computerized systems are used in practice. Machines regulate intravenous drip rates with improved accuracy and alert nurses to potential problems with infusions. When used for documentation, computer systems save time by preventing duplicated entries and the need for long handwritten notes. Even stocked client care supplies can be ordered simultaneously as the last one is used. The ability to handle technology and informatics is an integral part of a nurse's responsibilities.

## FROM THEORY TO PRACTICE

1. Re-read the vignette in the chapter opener. Based on your current use of computers and technology in clinical practice, what information would you share if you were part of the discussion?
2. Outline a plan to introduce a computerized documentation system to a group of nurses who have never used computers as a routine part of their clinical practice. Justify each portion of the orientation program.
3. What are the advantages of using computers and technology in clinical practice for nurses? What are the disadvantages of using them in clinical practice for nurses?
4. What are the advantages of using computers and technology in the delivery of health care for consumers? What are the disadvantages of using them?

## WWW INTERNET EXERCISES

1. Create your own personal website for free by visiting one of the following sites: GeoCities, www.geocities.com or Tripod, www.tripod.com. You also can use any web software provided by your ISP. Have your colleagues view and critique your website for ease of access, content quality, and visual appeal.
2. Select a topic that interests you as a professional nurse. Using any search engine (www.metacrawler.com; www.yahoo.com; or whatever search capability is offered by your ISP) enter the topic. Identify the number of potential websites to visit. Select two or three of these websites and compare and contrast them in terms of the type of website, the fees required to use the site information (if they are selling something), when the web page was last updated, and if the information presented is credible.

3. To learn about nursing specialty certification opportunities, visit the American Nurses Association website at www.ana.org/ancc/certification/catalogs.html. Select a nursing specialty area of interest and write out the professional qualifications, test plan topics, dates of examination, and certification fees.

4. Complete the questionnaire, "Are Telecourses for You?" found at the Public Broadcasting Services website (www.pbs.org/adultlearning/als/college/quiz.htm). This survey identifies how well distance education courses fit learner needs.

## INTERNET RESOURCES

Visit the American Nurses Association website at: www.nursingworld.org to find information related to clinical practice, specialty certification, and political issues that affect the practice of professional nursing.

Nursing Informatics Association: http://www.ania.org.

For the practical implications of telehealth on nursing practice, visit http://telehealth. hrsa.gov. Click on the "What's new" icon for updates on legislation, privacy issues, and current guidelines.

For information about federal guidelines related to genetically engineered crops, visit the United States Department of Agriculture site: www.usda.gov and the Environmental Protection Agency site: www.epa.gov.

For information related to human genetics, visit the International Society of Nurses in Genetics site: http://www.isong.org; the Cancer Genetics Genome Project site: www.ncbi.nlm.nih.gov/ncicgap/; The National Human Genome Research Institute: www.genome.gov; and the Human Genome Project Information Guide: www.ncbi.nlm.nih.gov/genome/guide/.

To report an incident of Internet Abuse: CyberSnitch, http://wwww.cybersnitch.net.

## REFERENCES

Akens, D. S. (1999). *Computers in plain English*. Huntsville, AL: PC Press Inc.

American Association of Colleges of Nursing. (1998). *The essentials of baccalaureate education for professional nursing practice*. Washington, DC: Author.

American Nurses Association. (1994). *Standards of practice for nursing informatics*. Washington, DC: American Nurses Publishing, NP-100 7.5M 3/95.

American Nurses Credentialing Center. (2000). Informatics certification catalog [Online]. Washington DC: American Nurses Credentialing Center. Available at: www.ana.org/ancc/certification/catalogs/html Accessed July 9, 2005.

Ammenwerth, E., & Haux, R. (2000). A compendium of information processing functions in nursing: Development and pilot study. *Computers in Nursing, 18*, 189–196.

Begley, S., Check, E., & Rogers, A. (2001). Solving the next genome puzzle. *Newsweek, 137*, 52–53.

Blumenstyk, G. (2001). Publishers promote E-textbooks, but many students and professors are skeptical. *The Chronicle of Higher Education, 47*, A35–A36.

Bohnenkamp, S., McDonald, P., Lopez, A., Krupinski, E. L., & Blackett, A. (2004). Traditional versus telenursing outpatient management of patients with cancer with new ostomies. *Oncology Nursing Forum, 31*, 1005–1010.

Carty. B. (2000). Nursing informatics: Preparing nurses for an evolving role. In B. Carty (Ed.), *Nursing informatics: Education for practice* (pp. 1–16). New York: Springer Publishing.

Couzin, J. (2003). The twist and turns in BRCA's path. *Science, 302,* 591–593.

Dickenson-Hazard, N. (Ed.). (2001). Palm Pilots may aid clinical decisions. *Reflections on Nursing Leadership, 27*(2), 41.

Foster, A. L. (2001). The struggle to preserve privacy. *The Chronicle of Higher Education, 47*, A37–A39.

Garcia, C., Wilund, K., Arca, M., Zuliani, G., Fellin, R., Maioli, M., Calandra, S., Bertolini, S., Cossu, F., Grishin, N., Barnes, R., Cohen, J., & Hobbs, H. (2001). Autosomal recessive hypercholesterolemia caused by mutations in a putative LDL receptor adaptor protein. *Science, 292*, 1394–1398.

Giarelli, E., & Jacobs, L. (2001). Issues related to the use of genetic material and information. *Oncology Nursing Forum, 27*, 459–467.

Gutterman, L. (2001). How to make a kidney, an ear, or even a heart. *Chronicle of Higher Education*, XLVII, (34) A19.

Hartman, R. (2005). Cyberstalking and internet safety FAQ. Available at: http://www.sfwa.org/gateway/stalking.htm. Accessed July 8, 2005.

Hassert, M. (1999). Information systems. In L. Q. Thede (Ed.), *Computers in Nursing: Bridges to the Future*. pp. 237–247. Philadelphia: J. B. Lippincott.

Holden, C. (2003). Race and medicine. *Science, 302*, 594–596.

Houshmand, S. L., Campbell, C. T., Briggs, S. E., McFadden, A. W. J., Al-Tweigeri, T. (2000). Prophylactic mastectomy and genetic testing: An update. *Oncology Nursing Forum, 27*, 1537–1547.

Huchenski, J. (2001). New federal rule protects individual healthcare information privacy. *Computers in Nursing, 19*, 41, 43–44, 46.

International Medical Informatics Association, (1999). The standards for health care informatics. Available at: http://www.imia.org. Accessed July 8, 2005.

Jossi, F. (2004). Robostaff. *Healthcare Informatics Online*. Available at: http://www.healthcare-informatics.comissues/2004/04 04/jossi.htm. Accessed July 8, 2005.

Lanza, R., Ciebelli, J., West, M., Dorff, E., Tauer, C., & Green, R. (2001). The ethical reasons for stem cell research. *Science, 292*, 1299.

Levy, S. (2001, February 19). Is it software? Or spyware? *Newsweek*, 54.

Lumelsky, N., Blondel, O., Laeng, P., Velasco, I., Ravin, R., & McKay, R. (2001). Differentiation of embryonic stem cells to insulin-secreting structures similar to pancreatic islets. *Science, 292*, 1389–1394.

Maran, R. (1998). *Teach yourself computers and the Internet visually* (2nd ed.). Foster City, CA: IDG Books Worldwide Inc.

Marshall, E. (2003). Preventing toxicity with a gene test. *Science, 302*, 588–590.

Marshall, E. (2003a). First check my genome, doctor. *Science, 302*, 589.

McConnell, E. A. (2001). Open the lines of communication. *Nursing Management, 32*, 45.

McHugh, M. L., & Gibson, G. (2000). Teaching a web-based course: Lessons from the front. In J. Novotny (Ed.), *Distance education in nursing* (pp. 23–42). New York: Springer Publishing.

Merikangas, K., & Risch, N. (2003). Genomic priorities and public health. *Science, 302*, 599–601.

*Merriam-Webster's collegiate dictionary* (10th ed.). (1994). Springfield, MA: Merriam-Webster.

Mueller, C. L., & Billings, D. M. (2000). Focus on the learner. In J. Novotny (Ed.), *Distance education in nursing* (pp. 65–84). New York: Springer Publishing.

Nelson, L. (2001). Point of care testing: Is it right for everyone? *Nursing Management, 32*, 50.

Nicoll, L. H. (2001). *Nurses' guide to the Internet* (3rd ed.). Philadelphia: Lippincott Williams & Wilkins.

Offit, K. (1997). *Clinical cancer genetics: Risk counseling and management*. New York: John Wiley.

Olsen, F. (2001). Optical networks hold the promise of incredible speed and efficiency. *The Chronicle of Higher Education, 47*, A31–A32.

Platt, A., & Reed, B. (2001). Meet new pain standards with new technology. *Nursing Management, 32*, 40–43.

Rappouli, R. & Covacci, A. (2003). Reverse vaccinology and genomics. *Science, 302*, 602.

Rauch, J. (2001). The new old economy: Oil, computers and reinvention of the earth. *The Atlantic Monthly, 287*, 35–49.

Reuters Health. (2000). FDA approves system for virtual house calls [Online]. Available at: www.phschool.com/atschool/health/health update/spring2000.pdf.

Short, N. (2000). Online learning: Ready, set, click. *RN, 63*, 28–32.

Simpson, G., & Kerrick, M. (1997). Nurses' attitudes toward computerization in clinical practice in a British general hospital. *Computers in Nursing, 15*, 37–42.

Staggers, N., & Gassert, C. (2000). Competencies for nursing informatics. In B. Carty (Ed.), *Nursing informatics: Education for practice* (pp. 17–34). New York: Springer Publishing.

Stone, B. (2001). Wanted: Hot industry seeks supergeeks. *Newsweek, 137*, 54–55, 58.

Thede, L. Q. (1999). *Computers in nursing: Bridges to the future*. Philadelphia: Lippincott Williams & Wilkins.

Thede, L. (2003). *Informatics and nursing: Opportunities & challenges* (2nd ed.). Philadelphia: Lippincott Williams & Wilkins.

Turley, J. P. (2000). Informatics and education: The start of a discussion. In B. Carty (Ed.), *Nursing informatics: Education for practice* (pp. 271–294). New York: Springer Publishing.

United States Department of Commerce (2004). *Strategic Plan for Optical Technology*. Available at: http://physics.nist.gov/Divisions/Div844/publications/Strategicplan04.pdf. Accessed July 9, 2005.

United States Department of Labor Bureau of Labor Statistics. (2000). *The 10 occupations with the largest job growth 1998–2008*. Available at: http://www.recruitmilitary.com/careercenter/occupation2.asp. Accessed July 9, 2005.

Wang, L., Brock, A., Hereberich, B., & Schultz, P. G. (2001). Expanding the genetic code of *Escherichia coli*. *Science, 292,* 498–500.

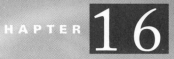

# The Professional Nurse's Role in Public Policy

## KEY TERMS AND CONCEPTS

Responsible Citizenship
Grassroots Effort
Policy
Politics
Laws
Policies
Lobbying
Legislative Agenda
Lobbying Strategies
Federal Legislative Path
Coalition
Political Action Committee
Mutual Recognition State Compact Licensure

## LEARNING OUTCOMES

By the end of this chapter, the learner will be able to:

1 Define public policy, politics, political competence lobbyist, and political action committee.

2 Differentiate between the roles of lobbyists and political action committees.

3 List strategies used to lobby elected officials.

4 Distinguish direct lobbying from indirect lobbying techniques.

5 Discuss key elements of effectively written letters to elected officials.

6 Outline a plan for a personal visit with an elected official.

7 Discuss ways for nurses to become involved in politics and public policy development.

8 Specify strategies to stay abreast of current legislative and public policy issues.

## VIGNETTE

As a result of budget cuts, school districts in a state no longer have resources to provide registered nurses (RNs) for health screening, medication administration, and health teaching for their students. State law specifies that a licensed practical nurse (LPN) may develop health promotion classes and health programs for a school district. Since enactment of the budgetary cut, lack of preventive health care services has resulted in the increase of the following adolescent health problems: ethanol abuse, drug abuse, sexually transmitted diseases, teenage pregnancy, and immunization noncompliance.

Nurses with children in school band together to work to overturn state policy. By assuming the roles of client advocates and change agents, the nurses approach members of the state legislature and the governor to see if they would propose legislation mandating "a registered nurse in every school."

Working to lower the speed limit on a busy stretch of highway; petitioning city legislators to limit traffic in a residential neighborhood; writing or visiting an elected official to persuade him or her to support limited use of unlicensed assistive personnel (UAP) in acute health care institutions; organizing a group of nurses to develop a legislative agenda; visiting formally or informally with an elected official; protesting legislation aimed at limiting health care access for the poor; lobbying for a bill aimed at increasing governmental funding for breast cancer research, nursing education, or nurse run health centers; these are a few examples of how professional nurses can influence governmental and institutional policies. Governmental and institutional policies greatly affect nursing practice and health care delivery in the United States.

This chapter provides an overview of public policies, various levels of governmental influence on the development and implementation of public policies, and the roles assumed by professional nurses concerning public policies. It offers strategies for professional nurses to use while influencing public policy development, implementation, and revision. Finally, it presents examples of nurses who have influenced public policy development and strategies for nurses to learn the art and science of political action.

## ⬤ THE NURSE'S ROLE IN INFLUENCING PUBLIC POLICY

Many nurses have lots of knowledge about health and the delivery of health care. Practicing nurses frequently identify flaws in the health care delivery system. However, nurses represent the largest health professional group in the United States, but have failed in playing a proportionate role in shaping health policies for Americans at the national, state, and local levels of government (Bissonette, 2004). According to Wakefield (2004), nursing lacks the financial resources prevalent in more highly influential groups such as organized medicine, insurance corporations, pharmaceutical firms, and other organized businesses. In the United States (and elsewhere in the world), money frequently equates with political power and influence.

### The Nurse's Role as a Responsible Citizen

The United States Constitution ensures the right of American citizens to have a voice in the government. Americans have the freedom to ask questions, offer suggestions, and debate the effects of public policies. Nurses have a history of political activism. During the women's suffrage movement of the early 1900s, the American Federation of Nursing (now the American Nurses Association) joined forces with other women's groups to work successfully in attaining the right for women to vote. Nurses educated other women about health promotion and disease prevention once women achieved voting privileges as citizens. Nurses quickly discovered that they could affect public policy by working independently and with other women to exert pressure on elected officials to develop policies that supported health promotion and disease prevention (Feldman & Lewenson, 2000).

The degree of political action varies from nurse to nurse. In 1996, Cohen, Mason, Kovner, Leavitt, Pulcini, and Sochalski outlined four stages of political activism in nursing that still apply today.

1. Buying in: Nurses become aware of the importance of political activism to attain professional goals, and they use the political system to have input into public policy development.
2. Self-interest: Nurses continue to use the political system to the sole advance of intraprofessional agendas.
3. Political sophistication: Nurses engage in complex political activity, such as building coalitions and running for political office.
4. Leading the way: Nurses serve as influential persons by holding key governmental positions and in the process select the course for public policy changes.

Professional nurses participate in public policy formation in a variety of ways. However, most nurses tend to be in the first stage of political activism. Casting an informed vote during an election is the first level of responsible citizenship in a democracy. **Responsible citizenship** consists of being an active participant in the governing process. The second level of responsible citizenship is engaging in the process of affecting governmental policies. Once they are successful in affecting public policy by providing input, some nurses progress to higher levels of political activism.

Feldman and Lewenson (2000) identify how being involved in politics and the political process fits with the goals of professional nursing to benefit society. The public perceives nurses as being trustworthy and credible. Nurses advocate for large groups of clients when they use their specialized knowledge of wellness, health, illness, and delivery of health services to influence policy makers to create new and fund public health programs. Nurses also have well-refined communication and assessment skills that enhance the ability to determine what types of health programs are needed (and wanted). Because of the ability to understand nursing and health-related research, nurses can present strong cases based on solid evidence to document needs for new programs and to continue present ones. Politically active nurses frequently use nursing process to guide their thinking for public policy development and evaluation.

Along with using professional nursing expertise to influence public policy, some nurses have held political offices. Feldman and Lewenson (2000) note that some nurses begin political careers because of grassroots efforts to accomplish a particular public policy goal. **Grassroots efforts** start at the basic unit of society (local community or special interest group) and expand to reach more centralized areas of influence (Mish, 1994). Grassroots efforts frequently start as action to improve a local community that snowballs into bigger action. Grassroot activities involve building coalitions, writing letters, and telephoning officials, visiting personally with elected officials, and testifying before governmental committees. When nurses successfully attain political action goals, they directly affect public policy (Feldman & Lewenson; Milstead, 1999). Successful action in grassroots efforts builds the nurse's self-confidence, a reputation that he or she can be trusted to get the job done, and public support to run for political office (Milstead).

## Research Brief 16-1

Itzhaky, H., Gerber, P., & Dekel, R. (2004). Empowerment skills and values: A comparative study of nurses and social workers. *International Journal of Nursing Studies, 41,* 447–456.

The investigators sought to discover the differences of nurses and social workers on perceptions and reported action on the skills and values of the concept of empowerment.

Two-hundred thirteen social workers and 152 RNs participated in the study that employed a cross-sectional survey design. Participants completed the Frans's Social Worker Empowerment Scale, Alperin and Richie's Social Service Skills Scale, and Schwartz's The Values Scale.

Differences were analyzed using multiple analysis of variance techniques. The following differences were identified:

1. The nurses scored higher in knowledge, self-concept, critical awareness, and propensity to act than the social workers who scored higher on the scale measuring collective identity.
2. Nurses also scored higher on therapeutic communication skills than the social workers.
3. Social workers were ranked higher in social action skills (including finding government resources, lobbying and contacting elected officials) than the nurses, but they scored lower in collective identity than nurses.
4. Nurses reported having more emphasis on spiritual and material values than social workers.
5. Social workers had higher levels of political activity than nurses.

The significance of these findings reveal that nurses and social workers, even though they both are helping professions, have distinct differences. The investigators suggested that the differences could have arisen because nurses consistently use therapeutic communication when working with clients and families and see results of interventions quickly, which may build perceived competence and self-confidence. Results also reveal that nurses tended to think of themselves as individuals rather than as a collective group. Results of this study must be interpreted with caution because the study was conducted in Israel. However, the study points to the need to increase nurse awareness of the political process and how they could influence public policy. More research is needed to see how all members of the interdisciplinary health team perceive empowerment and how they use their influence in helping to shape public policy and health care delivery.

To be aware of current legislation and policies, the professional nurse must have access to information. Many nurses read newspapers, newsmagazines, and professional journals that contain information about current legislative issues and societal needs. The Internet also serves as a source of legislative information. The second stage of political action is that of self-interest. An analysis of the current American government reveals that many times small groups of people expend great resources and much energy to have their agendas approved (especially when competing for a piece of the federal budget). The final stage of political action involves working with other groups to attain what is best for all. During this stage, individuals and groups collaborate and reach consensus about how to best use available resources to better society (Feldman & Lewenson, 2000).

A **policy** is an established course of action determined to achieve a desired outcome. Governments and institutions create policies to achieve their missions. However, policy development and implementation are not limited to governments and institutions. Any health care–providing agency, professional organization, nonprofit organization, or family may make policies for members to follow. When health care policies are developed and revised, nurses bring special expertise to issues. This expertise brings a holistic approach that helps to protect the health and safety of the public.

### Questions for Reflection 16-1

1. In which stage of political activism do I fit?
2. What are the current barriers to my participation in the political process?
3. Do I want to be more politically active? Why or why not?
4. What current behaviors do I need to change to become more politically active?

## Key Definitions for Understanding Politics

Politics plays a key role in policy development. *Merriam-Webster's Collegiate Dictionary* (Mish, 1994, p. 901) defines **politics** as "the art or science concerned with guiding or influencing governmental policy" and "the art or science of winning and holding control over a government." When the specified course of action is to develop or revise a policy, persons use political activities to influence policy development and implementation. Some policies may evolve into law. **Laws** are a set of established rules that create a system of privileges and process for persons to solve problems with minimal force. Laws outline and govern the relationships of individuals to other individuals, organizations, and their government. In addition, laws outline and govern the relationships of the government to its citizens. In democratic societies, citizens use political action to influence the legislative process required for law enactment.

Once laws become established, polices must be developed to ensure consistency in procedures to uniformly enforce the laws. **Policies** are formalized procedures that are followed by persons responsible for delivering governmental or institutional services (Stanhope, 1996). In most cases, the government acts as the ultimate authority within society for policy enforcement (except in cases of rebellions or coups). Most laws are public policies. However, not all public policies are laws.

## Governmental Role in Public Policy Development

The federal and most state governments are organized using three branches: the legislative, executive, and judicial. The legislative branch develops and approves legislation for executive branch consideration. The executive branch approves legislative acts and administers and regulates governmental policies. Once laws are passed, the government must develop policies to enact them. The judicial branch interprets laws and the meaning of approved policies.

Legal bases for legislative action in health care are found in Article I, Section 8 of the United States Constitution, which states that the government bears the responsibility to provide for the general welfare of its citizens, regulate interstate commerce, fund the military, and provide funds for governmental operations. Each state bears the responsibility to enforce national policies while protecting the safety, health, and welfare of its citizens. State and national governments award grants for funding programs that enhance citizen safety, health, and welfare. Local governments implement national programs and develop laws, regulations, and policies to ensure public health.

## The Nurse's Role in Public Policy Development

Because laws govern professional nursing practice, nurses have a stake in public policy legislation and enforcement. Legislators pass laws and provide funding for health care programs, access, professional education, and research. Nurses might react to proposed legislation by writing their elected officials to influence their action during the legislative process. Some nurses engage in proactive political action by proposing legislation, persuading an elected official in the legislature to introduce a bill, devising public relations campaigns around their proposal, **lobbying** (attempting to sway an elected official to take a desired action) to get the bill passed by both houses of Congress, and influencing the head of the executive branch to sign it. Nurses participate in national, state, and local legislative efforts. A national or statewide effort to pass legislation requires the participation of many for success. However, once legislation becomes law, some nurses continue to work with state or federal agencies responsible for devising the regulations to implement the law.

### Nursing's Legislative Agenda

The American Nurses Association (ANA) develops an annual legislative agenda. A **legislative agenda** outlines the goals and actions of an organization to exert its influence on passing bills and developing governmental policies. Legislative goals are developed and approved by the ANA board. Once approved, the organization publicizes its agenda. Its membership bears the responsibility for supporting the agenda, whereas the ANA staff advances it. State nurses associations (SNAs) and the ANA hire professional lobbyists to promote legislation that favorably affects the practice of professional nursing (deVries & Vanderbilt, 1992). The current legislative agenda approved by the ANA outlines the following legislative and regulatory goals: (1) maintain control of nursing practice; (2) influence health care policy development and reform; (3) advocate on the behalf of health care consumers; and (4) initiate workplace reforms.

The first step in publicizing a legislative agenda is the development of position papers on the legislative goals. A position paper is a one-page paper that specifies a goal. A position paper forces clear, concise communication of the rationale behind the agenda based on solid facts and persuasive arguments.

During preparation of the position paper, some effort should be spent exploring the opposition's viewpoints on the issue. Time spent here prepares the organization to anticipate arguments that will be used when confronted by the opposition. Supportive data, including documents, articles, and statistics, may be attached. Printing the paper on an organizational letterhead adds to its credibility. Elements of the position paper include the background, position, rationale, group name, and contact person (name, address, and telephone number) (deVries & Vanderbilt, 1992).

### The Art of Lobbying

The world of politics moves quickly. Sometimes a piece of legislation changes in less than an hour. To stay abreast of proposed legislation and its changes, nursing organizations hire lobbyists. The ANA has lobbyists for federal legislation. Most SNAs hire a lobbyist for state legislation. Lobbyists visit with elected officials in the hopes of influencing action on a piece of pending legislation. In addition, lobbyists are responsible for keeping their organizational membership informed of proposed changes to a piece of legislation. At the local level, nurses attend city council and other community organizational meetings.

In addition to hiring lobbyists, the ANA and SNAs offer the Nurses Strategic Action Team (N-STAT), a coordinated effort to ensure that nurses' voices are heard at the federal and state governmental levels. Nurses use **lobbying strategies**, activities aimed to get an elected official to take a desired action. When presenting information on a legislative or local issue, nurses and lobbyists must do their homework to develop expertise on the impending issue.

Before briefing an elected official on an issue, it is mandatory to develop expertise on it. Having facts and statistics related to an issue provides a solid foundation for the art of persuasion. Effective use of statistics involves: (1) putting the numbers in human terms; (2) reporting the statistics in simple terms while avoiding the use of percentages; (3) including practical and statistical significance when reporting numbers; (4) using national, state, and local statistics (legislators concern themselves with the local impact of an issue); and (5) citing the source of information (deVries & Vanderbilt, 1992).

Besides statistics, personal stories may be used effectively to influence elected officials. Effective use of personal stories involves (1) using a personal story about a citizen who resides in the elected official's district; (2) telling the true story in clear, concise, declarative, strong, and simple terms; (3) requesting a specific action by the legislator; and (4) emphasizing the importance of the issue (deVries & Vanderbilt, 1992).

A clear, concise, precise, and persuasive presentation is mandatory to provide information to elected officials because they deal with many issues that multiply daily.

Before effective lobbying can occur, nurses must be aware of current changes in proposed legislation. Staying abreast of constant changes in issues surrounding a piece of legislation is an important, never-ending challenge. Nurses can find information related to pending legislation by reading daily newspapers, watching television news reports, listening to radio news broadcasts, reading current professional journals and newsletters, and accessing legislative websites. The United States Library of Congress has an electronic information site (http://thomas.loc.gov/) to link citizens to federal legislative information. This Internet site has the following information available for downloading, printing, or studying: pending legislation, committee hearing transcripts, e-mail addresses of senators and representatives, and the *Federal Register*.

Professional nursing associations post legislative issue information on websites. Some associations post information for all nurses to view; whereas, others reserve information for members only. The American Nurses Association (http://www.nursingworld.org/gova) and the Canadian Nurses Association (www.cna-nurses.ca) websites also contain information about pending national legislation affecting health care and professional nursing practice. The American Nurses Association offers an online *Capitol Update* and opportunities for its membership to participate in *N-Stat*, a nursing grassroots lobbying group. Availability of information regarding state issues depends on the state or provincial nursing association. Several state nursing associations (SNAs) reserve information on current state legislative issues for their members.

Elected legislators frequently provide constituents with periodic reports during the legislative session. Reports may be delivered to constituents via e-mail or the postal service.

Reports sent to constituents before the end of the legislative session usually ask for voter opinions on pending legislative issues. When nurses return questionnaires addressing pending legislation, they participate in the legislative process and staff members usually add their names to a list to receive future information from the legislator.

### The Federal Legislative Path

Because of the complex process set forth by the authors of the Constitution, the path of legislation provides ample opportunity for citizen input. **The federal legislative path** outlines each step of the process by which an idea becomes a law. A member of the House of Representatives or the Senate must introduce a bill before it can be considered. Once a bill is introduced, it goes to a committee, where it may be referred (passed to another committee), become the topic of a hearing, marked up (rewritten and amended), or reported out (sent to the House or Senate for floor action).

The chair of the committee considering the bill decides on its action. This person possesses much power because he or she may delay presentation of the bill to the committee (deVries & Vanderbilt, 1992). During this phase of the legislative process, nurses may brief the committee chair to attempt to influence scheduling of the bill for committee discussion or action on the floor.

Once either chamber passes a bill, it goes to the other chamber and is subjected to the entire legislative process again. After the second chamber approves the bill, it is submitted to a conference committee that consists of members from both chambers. The conference committee negotiates differences between the two bill versions, adopts the conference bill, and submits (reports) the bill to both chambers for adoption or rejection. If both chambers adopt the conference bill, it becomes an Act of Congress.

Each Congressional Act (also known as an enrolled bill) is referred to the president (or governor in state legislatures), who signs or vetoes it. If the bill is signed, it becomes law. If the bill is vetoed, the House and Senate may override the veto by a two-thirds majority vote, and the bill becomes public law. If the veto is sustained, the bill dies (deVries & Vanderbilt, 1992).

During the legislative process, nurses must communicate with their legislators to ensure that no bill adversely affects health care recipients and professional nursing practice. Nurses may lobby for a specific action on a piece of legislation during any step of the legislative process.

The United States Constitution provides the president 10 days (excluding Sundays) to act on an enrolled bill. The president has four possible options. The bill may be approved; approved by inaction (i.e., the president takes no action within 10 days, an option used when it is considered unnecessary or politically unwise to sign a bill, or if there are questions regarding its constitutionality); pocket veto (used at the end of a legislative session when Congress adjourns before the 10-day expiration date); or veto (the president refuses to sign the bill, and presents both bodies of Congress a message stating his or her objections to it) (deVries & Vanderbilt, 1992). When the enrolled bill is submitted for executive approval, nurses should contact the president (for federal legislation) or governor (for state legislation) via a telephone call, fax, or letter (electronic or postal) to voice support for approval or other desired action.

### Lobbying Strategies

Lobbying techniques are classified into two types: direct and indirect. Direct lobbying involves personal contact with elected officials. Indirect lobbying involves influencing

TABLE 16-1

## Lobbying Strategies

| Direct Strategies: Through a Legislative Body | Indirect Strategies: Through Public Opinion |
| --- | --- |
| Participate in party platform development | Publicize nursing organizational agendas |
| Contribute time and money to political campaigns | Use the media, especially television broadcasts, to further the agenda |
| Influence legislative committees by personally visiting or writing committee members | Write editorial pieces for written media, such as the newspaper or news magazines |
| Contact agency regulators in writing or by personal visits | Seek public opinion by polling members of the public and publishing the results |
| Engage in direct lobbying by visiting or writing elected officials or hiring a professional lobbyist | Use paid media advertisements: television, radio, and printed media |
| Attend social events at which elected officials appear | Print and distribute books or pamphlets |
| Develop an understanding of elected officials' key positions on issues | Develop and execute educational campaigns |

Source: deVries, C., & Vanderbilt, M. (1992). *The grassroots lobbying handbook: Empowering nurses through legislative and political action.* Washington, DC: American Nurses Association.

public opinion on a particular issue. Table 16-1 outlines direct and indirect lobbying strategies.

Before implementing lobbying strategies, nurses should outline a working plan that includes a chronological record of accomplishments. By keeping records of reactions and responses from elected officials, nurses may use this information in future interactions. Appointment of a spokesperson helps to maintain a consistent lobbying approach and enhances public recognition of a particular issue viewpoint.

Constituent pressure is perhaps the most effective weapon for the lobbyist. Mobilization of a group of individuals for collective action involves educating nurses, other health team members, and the public. Letter-writing campaigns are effective when a bill is pending in Congress or in a state legislative body. A well-written letter received from a constituent may appear in the Congressional Record. Because the elected official relies on voter support for reelection, each letter and personal contact counts. Follow-up letters of appreciation for action on an issue enhance relationships among elected officials and their constituents. See Display 16-1 for characteristics of an effective letter to an official.

Using e-mail to lobby an elected official has advantages and disadvantages. It is economical and quick. Use of this technology enables users to send messages at any time. The message is not dependent on postal delivery or a receptionist relaying the message to the official. Some legislators, especially younger ones, may prefer e-mail messages rather than formal letters (Yates, personal communication, February 16, 2004).

However, e-mail also has distinct disadvantages. The quality of messages sent depends on the software used to create them and the ability of the nurse to individualize the message. Some software programs feature ways to emphasize specific message points. These programs cost more than other programs, and users may find mastery of these features difficult. Thus, the intended strength of the desired message may be

---

## Characteristics of an Effective Letter to an Official — DISPLAY 16-1 ⬥

1. Limit the letter to one page.
2. Correctly address the letter, referring to the elected official as The Honorable (first name followed by surname).
3. Greet the official according to title (e.g., Dear Senator _____, Dear Representative _____, Dear Congressman/ Congresswoman _____, Dear Mr. Chairman or Madam Chairwoman _____, or Dear Mr./Madam Speaker _____).
4. Identify yourself as a constituent, health care expert, member of a large organization, and a credible source on the issue within the first paragraph.
5. Refer to the specific piece of legislation by title (H.R. [number] for a House bill; S. [number] for a Senate bill) in the first paragraph if the letter pertains to a specific legislative proposal.
6. Emphasize the local importance of the proposed issue.
7. Be brief and specific and include key information.
8. Handwrite the letter because computers can print many seemingly personalized letters in a matter of minutes.
9. Use a professional letterhead if possible.
10. Verify that the letter is neat and free of spelling, grammatical, or typographical errors (if typewritten).
11. Be specific about the desired action on the part of the elected official.
12. Offer personal assistance or the organization's assistance in the closing.
13. Thank the official for his or her action.

*Source:* deVries & Vanderbilt, 1992.

---

impossible to achieve. Reading messages on the screen is not as easy as reading printed material. Recent software improvements have improved the appearance of printed e-mail messages, but they may lack the professional look of a typed letter on letterhead stationery (Skaggs, 1997). Some special interest groups bombard legislators with e-mail messages, many of which may be written identically. Because many elected officials receive large volumes of e-mail, some rely on staff members to read e-mail messages because it may be impossible for them to read each message received (Yates, personal communication, February 16, 2004).

Because members tend to hear exclusively from dissatisfied constituents, they may be led to believe falsely that large numbers of their constituents disagree with a pending issue. A bill may be introduced for years before it is passed. "Persistence and patience are two key factors in lobbying" (deVries & Vanderbilt, 1992, p. 59). When nurses stay in regular contact with elected officials, the officials are more likely to remember them and work to help support nursing's agenda.

Lobbying techniques other than writing personal letters may be used. Mailing a form letter is superior to sending nothing. If a nurse has no idea how to begin writing a letter, professional nursing organizations and nursing issue textbooks offer sample letters. If a specific piece of legislation is supported by a nursing organization, the organization may have a sample letter drafted for membership use.

A telephone call offers a way to deliver a brief and quick message to an elected official. A legislator's staff members frequently keep a tally of how many calls support and how many calls disapprove of pending legislation. Many nurses calling officials find it beneficial to have the desired message scripted for reading when relaying messages to an elected official. All national elected officials have offices located in Washington, DC, and in the state or district where they reside. Telegrams and e-mail messages are effective

---

**Steps for Facilitating a Personal Visit with an Elected Official**

1. Confirm the appointment and arrive on time.
2. Provide the official with a business card after greeting him or her with a firm handshake and a personal introduction.
3. Open the meeting by informing the official of an established tie between you.
4. Inform the official of the mission and how the visit represents it. Refer to pending legislation by bill number and title.
5. Present statistics and personal stories when appropriate, while emphasizing the issue's importance to the local community.

6. Request the name of the staff member who handles the issue and request follow-up.
7. Be concise and focus totally on the issue of the meeting.
8. Leave a one- or two-page fact sheet summarizing the issue and your position on it.
9. Conclude the meeting by thanking the official for spending time with you.
10. Write a thank you letter after the meeting.

*Source:* deVries & Vanderbilt, 1992.

---

tools to send quick messages requesting prompt action. Petitions containing large numbers of signatures usually are effective only for public relations because it is difficult for staff to verify whether all signatures on the document represent constituents.

In addition to written communication, a personal visit is a very effective method of lobbying. Constituents are invited to meet with elected officials in the local or governmental offices. A personal visit lays the foundation for future contacts. A scheduled appointment usually ensures a personal meeting with an elected official. Frequently, visits are limited to 15 to 30 minutes. Because of legislative emergencies, appointments may be canceled, especially if a floor vote is scheduled during the planned meeting. See Display 16-2 for suggestions that will facilitate a personal visit with an elected official.

Once reliable relationships are established with elected officials, nurses may be invited to testify at legislative committee hearings. When this happens, careful preparation is required, and a technical expert or attorney may accompany a witness. DeVries and Vanderbilt's *The Grassroots Lobbying Handbook* (1992), published by the ANA, outlines strategies to follow when testifying before Congress. The ANA president frequently testifies at committee hearings when issues regarding professional nursing practice are debated. Rich sources of evidence for testimony include the Agency for Health Care Policy and Research (www.ahcpr.gov), Center for Telemedicine Law (www.ctl.org), the National Council of State Boards of Nursing (www.ncsbn.org), and the Department of Health and Human Services (www.hhs.gov).

Writing letters and visiting legislators are the best-known lobbying techniques. Traditionally, persons lobby officials they have elected into office while ignoring powerful legislators, such as party leaders and committee chairpersons. Different lobbying strategies work more effectively during different phases of the legislative process. Table 16-2 outlines specific lobbying strategies recommended for use during each phase of the legislative and regulatory processes.

## Obstacles to Effective Lobbying

Major obstacles encountered by nurses include not knowing whom to lobby, where to contact officials, and the best time for contact. Some do not know the names of their

TABLE 16-2

## The Legislative Process: Steps and Suggested Lobbying Strategies

| Legislative Process: Steps | Suggested Lobbying Strategy |
|---|---|
| Legislation introduction | Hold a technical expert meeting to map out a strategy.<br>Form a coalition of persons and organizations with the same goal.<br>Identify a legislator in each chamber of Congress who would be likely to introduce the proposal.<br>Schedule a staff meeting with the legislators staff members.<br>Initiate a letter-writing campaign to other congressional members who may wish to co-sponsor the bill. |
| Immediately following introduction before committee assignment | Meet with interest groups to map out additional lobbying strategies.<br>Create a one-page fact sheet to distribute to interested parties.<br>Initiate a letter-writing campaign to elected officials to urge bill co-sponsorship.<br>Draft proposed amendments to bill. |
| Committee consideration | Write letters to all committee members to emphasize the need for a public hearing.<br>Enlist letter-writing campaign by members of other interested organizations.<br>Submit written information about oral or written testimony if a hearing is to occur.<br>Have someone monitor the mark-up session and share information with letter writers.<br>Conduct a letter-writing campaign to committee members either supporting or disagreeing with bill amendments added in committee.<br>Conduct a letter-writing campaign to elected officials from local district outlining support or disapproval of the revised bill, or to enlist their support by contacting committee members or testifying at a committee meeting.<br>Call a meeting of interested persons to verify whether or not new amendments are tolerable.<br>Work with committee staff in drafting the final draft of the bill.<br>Notify the press about the bill. |
| Rules Committee action | Work with Rules Committee members to determine if amendments can be made while the bill is debated on the floor of either chamber. |
| Legislation on the floor of a chamber | Send short messages to all members of the chamber in great quantities (postcards, telegrams, e-mail messages, and telephone calls).<br>Develop a swing list of officials.<br>Initiate personal visits to officials on undecided, leaning no, and leaning yes lists. |
| Conference Committee action | Meet with other interested persons to verify which version (House or Senate) is to be supported.<br>Write, visit, or call district officials and members of the Conference Committee. |
| Return to both chambers for approval | No lobby strategies needed if work has been consistent.<br>Write or call elected officials from district. |
| Presidential or gubernatorial signature | Call the White House or governor's staff, leaving a message for veto or signature. |
| Veto override | Write or call locally elected official.<br>Intensify lobbying efforts at those who appeared on the leaning yes list. |

*Source:* deVries, C., & Vanderbilt, M. (1992). *The grassroots lobbying handbook: Empowering nurses through legislative and political action.* Washington, DC: American Nurses Association.

elected officials. Before contacting elected officials, nurses should find out about their personal biographies, committee memberships, voting records, and introduced or cosponsored legislative activity. In addition to this information, knowledge of their personal causes or pet projects may be useful.

All members of the national legislative chambers maintain a Washington office and a local one in their district. Many have fax machines and e-mail systems that are connected to both offices. Nurses can save much time and money by visiting elected officials while they are visiting their home districts when the legislature is out of session.

## Legislative Staff Members

Because of their enormous responsibilities, all elected officials have staff. (Elected officials work with thousands of pieces of legislation during one legislative session.) Staff members routinely handle much of the elected official's work. Good relationships with congressional staff at the national and local offices provide invaluable contacts and advantages when engaging in lobbying activities.

An elected official's personal staff may include an administrative assistant, a legislative director, legislative assistants, legislative correspondents, a press secretary, caseworkers, a secretary, an office manager, and a receptionist. Nurses may be members of the staff. Staff members are responsible for scheduling appointments and activities. More importantly, officials fill staff posts with highly qualified persons who assist them in making decisions. For example, Sheila Burke, RN, MPA, FAAN, served as chief of staff for Bob Dole when he was the Senate majority leader (Goldwater & Zusy, 1990). During his tenure as majority leader, Burke advised Senator Dole on health care reform and other issues affecting public health, while directing all public activities of the Senator and his staff.

When nurses serve as staff members, they bring their expertise on health and safety issues to the team. To become a staff member, nurses should get to know political candidates, join political parties, donate time to work for election campaigns, contribute funds to campaigns, and market nursing expertise on issues related to health care and health promotion.

When lobbying for specific action on an issue, inviting an elected official for a personal tour of a local hospital or to participate in a local community service event may assist in advancing the cause. These activities increase the official's visibility and provide an opportunity for interaction with constituents. Because this may be viewed as an opportunity for press coverage, special attention to the press secretary at this time may increase the chances of future access to the elected official (deVries & Vanderbilt, 1992).

## Maintaining a Working Relationship

Expressing appreciation frequently is an overlooked step in the lobbying process. Elected officials should be acknowledged for introducing and supporting legislation that enhances the practice of professional nurses. Some SNAs bestow honors on elected officials who have developed records for supporting "nursing-friendly" legislation. A thank you letter that includes a statement about informing other nurses living in the district about an official's action in supporting legislation increases support for an official running for reelection.

Honesty is perhaps the most important factor contributing to effective lobbying. When lobbying, nurses must be willing to spend the time to explore the issues and collect valid and reliable data surrounding them. When encountering questions that cannot be answered accurately with complete certainty, nurses should refer the question to another expert or offer to find the desired information and present it to the official at a later date. Attempts to "wing it" or inadvertently share untrue information could sabotage the personal relationships established with officials (deVries & Vanderbilt, 1992).

There are multiple ways to cultivate a working relationship with an elected official. Wakefield (2004) suggests that working for an election (or re-election) campaign, and joining and becoming a member of a political party fosters networking with elected officials. Attendance at events where legislators are scheduled to speak or fund raise serves as other opportunities for access. Some SNAs offer programs to meet political candidates at district meetings. A political campaign contribution offers a token of appreciation (Wakefield, 2004). Taking time to listen to candidates running for office when they canvass neighborhoods enables nurses to meet candidates. Sometimes, the elected official may just happen to live in the nurse's neighborhood.

Without nurses' active participation in the legislative end election processes, public policy may not remain friendly to the nursing profession or health care consumers. In the United States, public policy development and implementation is affected by money, power, and societal position. To maintain their position and power, elected officials frequently strive for reelection. Because officials acknowledge the importance of pleasing their constituents, their acts are aimed at protecting and serving their voters. Politically astute persons acknowledge the importance of building **coalitions** (forming a larger group from smaller groups of people with similar goals and interests) and contributing resources to a political campaign to get their candidate elected to office.

### Questions for Reflection 16-2

1. Do I know the number of the congressional district in which I reside at the national and state government levels?
2. Who are the Senators serving in the US Senate from my State?
3. Who is my House of Representatives member from my congressional district?
4. Who are my representatives in the State legislature?
5. Which of the lobbying strategies is most appealing to me? Why?

### Coalition Building

Although difficult to establish and maintain, coalitions unite diverse groups, organizations, and people for a common specific purpose. Coalitions operate under the assumption that "there is strength in numbers." Many coalitions begin with an informal structure that formalizes as the coalition evolves and becomes more active. Once formal structure has been established, employees may be needed to accomplish the coalition's goals. Before extending an invitation for membership, a background check verifies any strengths or weaknesses individuals or organizations bring to the coalition. The goal of building a coalition is to capitalize on all members' strengths (Skaggs, 1997). Usually, the organization that started the coalition becomes its leader. However, if a goal is viewed as being self-serving for nurses, a member of another group should be designated as the coalition's official spokesperson. When the ANA and American Medical Association (AMA) work together to support a piece of legislation, they build a coalition of health care providers.

### Political Action Committees

**Political action committees** (PACs) are created by existing organizations for the purpose of financing campaigns for political office. Federal election guidelines prohibit non-profit groups from contributing to political campaigns. Funding for PACs is independent of its founding organization's funding.

Federal election guidelines mandate that PAC donations may be solicited from an organization's membership only for candidates for public office. However, general organizational funds may finance a political education program for members of the PAC's founding organization. Sometimes candidates for office receive political contributions from the PAC. However, some candidates may request only a public endorsement of their campaigns.

The ANA PAC, founded in 1972, is the sixth largest health care PAC in the United States and supports political candidates with "nursing-friendly" agendas. The AMA PAC is the largest health care PAC, followed by the American Psychological Association PAC. The American Hospital Association PAC ranks fourth in size (ANA, 2001).

The ANA PAC raised close to $1 million for each national election since 1992 and raises similar amounts in most election years. Before the ANA PAC endorses a candidate during an election, he or she must meet the following criteria: (1) good potential to win the election; (2) expressed support of nursing issues; (3) track record of being a friend of nursing (acted favorably on nursing issues at the local, state, and national levels of government); (4) seeking an office that has specific ANA or SNA interest; (5) member of a local SNA if the candidate is a registered nurse (ANA, 2001).

Of the congressional candidates the ANA PAC supported during the 2004 election cycle, 82% became members of the 109th Congress Membership of the 109th Congressional Session in the United States House of Representatives session including the following nurses:

- Eddie Bernice Johnson, RN, the Democratic representative from the 30th congressional district of Texas.
- Carolyn McCarthy, LPN, the Democratic representative from the 4th congressional district of New York.
- Lois Capps, RN, the Democratic representative from the 22nd congressional district of California (ANA, 2004).

## ● CURRENT POLITICAL AND LEGISLATIVE ISSUES AFFECTING PROFESSIONAL NURSING PRACTICE AND HEALTH CARE

Laws regulate nursing practice and health care delivery. Each state regulates nursing practice by its Nurse Practice Act. Federal and state governments regulate health care access and indigent health care service reimbursement. Many issues confronting legislators affect citizen safety, health care policy, and the control of nursing practice.

Hundreds of bills addressing health care are introduced into Congress and state legislatures annually. If a bill is not passed during the session of Congress when it was introduced, it dies. However, the bill may be introduced during each successive session of Congress until it passes. Issues that are current at the time of the writing of this chapter may become tomorrow's history. Through lobbying efforts and by serving as elected officials, nurses influence the future of health care delivery, public safety, and nursing practice. In the recent past, nurses have been successful in influencing the passage of legislation related to patient safety, nursing and health care research funding, human immunodeficiency virus programs, family leave, tobacco settlements, abuse programs, advanced practice nurse reimbursement through Medicare, and nursing education funding. Many times a particular issue surfaces over several legislative sessions before legislative action is finalized. For example, health care reform has remained on the legislative table for decades. Funding for government programs requires passage of legislation from legislative bodies followed by a signature of approval by the executive branch (Sultz & Young, 2004). The following section discusses pending legislative issues that may be of interest to professional nurses.

## Improving Access and Funding of Health Care

Access to and paying for health care for all in America remains a consistent problem. Approximately 44 million persons have no health insurance coverage in the United States (Feldman & Lewenson, 2004; Wakefield, 2004a). Two key factors contribute to recent increases in the uninsured: the rising cost of insurance and low incomes of workers. Companies who provide health insurance to employees pass on increased rates to them. Workers with low wages cannot afford to purchase employer-offered benefits (Sultz & Young, 2004).

Twenty-five percent of all health care expenditures in the United States are spent on 1% of the population; 5% of the population consumes more than half of the funds spent on health care services (Wakefield, 2002). The federal government develops a budget for all expenditures annually. During budget formation and negotiation, before approving the budget annually by the end of October, nurses need to be aware of funding of established health-related, nursing research, and nursing education programs (Wakefield, 2004).

Costs for programs can be astounding. The 2003 Medicare Prescription Drug Improvement and Modernization Act may cost the federal government between $1 to 2 trillion for 2014 to 2023. Feldstein (2004) reports that Americans spent $250 billion to fund Medicare in 2002. Despite a cash surplus, the program should enter deficit spending by 2016 (this was before funding of the 2003 Prescription Drug Program) (Sultz & Young, 2004). The Medicare program must be revised to maintain financial solvency.

Recent state budgetary problems have resulted in the deterioration of the Medicaid program. The Medicaid program covers vulnerable populations such as the elderly residents of long-term care facilities, pregnant women, and poverty-stricken children. Nurses working in community care clinics see many of these clients and know about their problems (Wakefield, 2004). States rely on the federal government to reimburse providers who deliver health care to the uninsured.

## Improving the Quality of Health Care

The American government spends billions of dollars to monitor and improve quality of health care services. The federal government funds the Agency for Healthcare Research and Quality (AHRQ) Policy and Research, the National Institutes of Health, The Centers for Disease Control and Prevention, the Food and Drug Administration, the Health Care Financing Administration, and the Health Resources and Services Administration. Without adequate funding, the quality of health and health care in the United States would suffer.

The AHRQ mission is to "support research designed to improve the quality, safety, efficiency and effectiveness of health care for all Americans." Fiscal year funding for the AHRQ for 2005 was $303,695,000. The goal of the agency is to provide evidence-based data on outcomes, quality, use, access, and costs of health care in the United States. AHRQ disseminates research findings to persons who make decisions in public policy development, health care systems, and clinical practice. Legislation in 1999 reauthorized AHRQ to improve health care quality, promote patient safety, reduce medical errors, foster the use of technology for patient care, quality improvement, and study national outcome data. The agency initiated its Translating Research into Practice Program to promote the use of best practices for health care across the nation. The AHRQ is only one of the many government agencies that promote quality of life and health care (AHRQ, 2001; Wakefield, 2002).

### The Safe Nursing and Patient Care Act

In 2003, the 108th United States Congress considered H.R. 745/S. 373, The Safe Nursing and Patient Care Act of 2003. This piece of legislation would prohibit mandatory overtime for RNs and other licensed members of the interdisciplinary care team, but would not set limits on voluntary overtime. Neither version of this bill moved out of committees of both legislative bodies despite support from the ANA and the AMA (Institute of Medicine, 2004).

### The Quality Nursing Care Act

In 2004, H.R. 3656, the Quality Nursing Care Act of 2004, was introduced in the house. The bill had a companion bill in the Senate (S. 881 the RN Safe Staffing Act of 2003). If passed, RNs involved in direct client care must be involved in the development of safe staffing systems. The bill would also offer whistle-blower protection for nurses who speak out about unsafe client care situations and issues (ANA Government Affairs, 2004). Similar legislation has been introduced into the U.S. House and Senate in previous years, but has never progressed beyond committee hearings.

## Nursing Workforce

In 2004, the U.S. Department of Health and Human Services reported a shortage of close to 139,000 RNs in the United Sates. By 2012, the figure is expected to rise to over 400,000 (Horrigan, 2004). To meet the need for RNs and to keep RNs active in the workforce, federal and state governments have introduced legislation. Some pieces of legislation have been addressed earlier because they relate to the quality of client care. Other pieces of legislation attempt to increase funding for nursing education. However, not all recent pieces of enacted legislation promote keeping current nurses in the workforce.

### Revised Department of Labor Overtime Rules

In August, 2004, new Department of Labor overtime regulations became effective. Part 541 of the rule redefines salaried professional, administrative managers and executives as being exempt from receiving overtime. Other workers can also be exempt if job qualification and duties involve supervision and/or management responsibilities and if they earn more than $455 per week. The regulations lack clear and concise language about persons with supervisory responsibilities and could provide an opportunity for hospitals and other health care organizations to exempt RNs from being eligible for overtime pay (Donnellan, 2004).

## State Legislative Initiatives

States frequently address similar health care issues in legislative bodies. To track state legislative initiatives, SNAs monitor pending legislation that affects health care and professional practice. Some of the issues that are active in various state legislatures include the prohibition of mandatory overtime, minimum nurse–patient ratios, malpractice tort reform, whistle-blower protection for nurses, public reporting of data collected on nursing quality indicators, mandatory development and use of valid and reliable nursing staffing systems for acute and long-term care facilities, collection of nursing work force data, funding for nursing work force studies, and state funding for nursing education.

### Mutual Recognition State Compact Legislation

Within the past few years, the National Council of State Boards of Nursing (NCSBN) developed a system with which professional nurses wishing to practice across state lines do not have to secure individual state licenses; this is known as **mutual recognition state compact licensure**. Under this provision, the registered nurse holds a professional nursing license in the state of his or her primary residence. When practicing in another state, the professional nurse is held accountable to the Nurse Practice Act of the state in which he or she practices professional nursing. This licensure alternative seems quite attractive to nurses who live close to state lines and those who are employed by traveling nurse agencies (NCSBN, 2001).

Each state regulates professional nursing practice within its borders. For a state to participate in the mutual recognition program, the state legislature must adopt the Mutual Recognition Nurse Licensure Compact. In some states, such as Kansas, participation in a multistate compact violates the state constitution and will require a constitutional change (NCSBN, 2001). Some SNAs, such as the Missouri Nurses Association (MONA), failed to support the mutual recognition compact legislation against the desires of the Missouri State Board of Nursing. Reasons for the lack of support included projected higher professional nursing licensure fees, loss of local control of professional nursing practice, and failure of the State Board of Nursing to consult MONA.

### Questions for Reflection 16-3

1. What are my views on some of the current legislative issues?
2. Do my views match those of nursing professional organizations to which I belong?
3. Do positions of nursing organizations prevent me from becoming a member? Why or why not?

# ● EXAMPLES OF NURSES INFLUENCING PUBLIC POLICY

Although politics frequently is equated with corruption and abuse of power, the combination of political activity and professional nursing does not create cognitive dissonance. Nurses bring a caring perspective to the political process. Health care delivery and access are greatly affected by the political process. Becoming politically active is one way to assume the professional nursing roles of client advocate and change agent. The following examples provide evidence that nurses have fulfilled these roles by becoming politically active.

The ANA PAC endorses candidates at the state and national levels. Before candidates are endorsed, the ANA PAC Board of Trustees reviews the candidates' records and considers recommendations from SNA members. The SNA PAC presents checks to state political candidates (deVries & Vanderbilt, 1992). During the 1996 presidential election, the ANA PAC sent surveys to the Clinton and Dole campaigns to discover where each candidate stood on health care issues. The Dole campaign failed to respond. Considering the information received from the Clinton campaign and the legislative records of both candidates, the ANA PAC endorsed the re-election of President Clinton. The ANA endorsed Al Gore during the 2000 presidential election; Gore lost to George W. Bush by a narrow margin. In 2004, ANA endorsed John Kerry for the U.S. Presidency, but he lost his bid to George W. Bush (ANA, 2004).

In addition to influencing legislation, nurses have assumed responsibility in the legislative process by becoming members of legislative bodies. The right to run for and hold public office is guaranteed by the First Amendment of the United States Constitution (Tammelleo, 1990).

Elected to Congress with 74% of the popular vote from her district in 1992, Representative Eddie Bernice Johnson, RN (D-TX) serves as the Democratic deputy whip and holds membership on the House Committee on Transportation and Infrastructure, the House Committee on Science, and House subcommittees on surface transportation, public buildings and economic development, technology, and the environment. These committees and subcommittees frequently address issues related to public health, including transportation, roadways, and environmental safety. The US Committee on Science frequently drafts legislation regarding funding for scientific research. In addition to these appointments, Johnson also serves as the secretary of the Congressional Black Caucus. In Congress, passage of legislation frequently relies on members voting along party or special group positions.

Carolyn McCarthy, LPN, represents the fourth congressional district of New York. Although she had no previous political experience, she ran as a Democrat and won her election in a predominantly Republican district. McCarthy was spurred to challenge a Republican incumbent who supported the repeal of a ban on assault weapons after McCarthy's husband was killed and her son seriously injured in the 1993 Long Island Railroad massacre. McCarthy serves on the Education in the Workforce and the Small Business Congressional committees.

Lois Capps, RN, became a member of the House of Representatives in 1998 after winning a special election to succeed Congressman Walter Capps, her late husband. She represents the citizens of the 22nd congressional district in California. Capps serves on the Committee on Energy and Commerce and the subcommittees on Health, Commerce, Trade and Consumer Protection, and Environment and Hazardous Materials. Before being elected to Congress, Capps worked as a nurse and health advocate for the Santa Barbara School District and directed Santa Barbara County's Teenage Pregnancy and Parenting Project and the Parent and Child Enrichment Center. She uses her extensive health care background as the co-chair of the following Congressional groups: the Congressional Heart and Stroke Coalition, the House Democratic Task Force on Health, and the bipartisan Congressional School Health and Safety Caucus. She also participates as a member of the bipartisan Campaign Finance Reform Task Force, the Budget Task Force, the Congressional Task Force on Tobacco & Health, the Prescription Drug Task Force, the Diabetes Caucus, and the Congressional Caucus for the Arts (Capps, 2003). Capps has introduced and co-sponsored bills related to nurse staffing issues, whistle-blower protection, and mandatory overtime.

Many nurses have testified before congressional committees. The president of the ANA frequently shares nursing expertise before Congress. Barbara Blakeney provided testimony regarding the current nursing shortage (ANA, 2004a). Mary Foley, RN, MS, provided congressional testimony on the topics of medical records privacy and confidentiality and ergonomic standards for nurses (ANA, 2001a). Diane Baker, RN, BSN; Kathryn Hall, RN, MS; and Anne O'Sullivan, RN, MSN, provided congressional testimony on the current nursing shortage in 2001 (ANA, 2001). Jane Aiken, RN, PhD testified about the impact of RNs on prevention and early detection of complications encountered by hospitalized patients (ANA, 2004a). Theresa Valiga, RN, PhD provided testimony to Congress regarding the current and worsening shortage of nursing faculty (Murray & Corcoran, 2004).

Along with the 69 nurses and former nurses serving in state public offices (ANA, 2001b), individual nurses have an impact on public policy. In Ohio, Ann Hamilton, RN, and Ron Hamilton, RN, brought attention to the plight of professional nursing as hospitals in Ohio engaged in work redesign. They had bumper stickers made with the statement "Nurses. You'll miss us when we're gone," and after being deluged with requests, buttons made using a black ribbon design similar to the red ribbon symbol of AIDS awareness. The two also founded the Concerned Nurse Coalition, an organization of nurses concerned about recent changes in professional nursing positions and their effects on patient care. Their actions resulted in a Cincinnati City Health Commission formal investigation of local hospital use of UAP. The Cincinnati City Council passed a resolution publicly denouncing RN replacement with UAP in hospitals, an action that helped support the introduction of the Patient Safety Act of 1997 at the federal level.

Nurses also can influence government reimbursements for health care. Linda Aiken, PhD, RN, FAAN, has served on the White House Physician Payment Review Commission that was created to make recommendations about provider payments under Medicare and Medicaid. Carolyne K. Davis, RN, PhD, served as the administrator of the Health Care Financing Administration. She credited her appointment to her direct political involvement in Michigan politics (Goldwater & Zusy, 1990). The Kansas State Nurses Association successfully lobbied for the addition of an RN position to the Health Care Data Governing Board in Kansas. The board's mission is to promote the availability of and access to health care data and to guide the use of such data. This board develops policies and procedures for the Kansas health care database administered by the Kansas secretary of health and environment (Irwin, 1997).

## ● OPPORTUNITIES TO LEARN THE ART OF INFLUENCING PUBLIC POLICY

There are many ways to learn the art of influencing public policy development and legislative activity. Kathleen Schumacher (personal communication May 12, 1997) suggests that ANA membership and involvement provides an avenue to learn how to play the political game. The ANA has four political action specialists who educate nurses about the political process, communicate directly with elected officials about pending legislation, collect information about elected officials' voting records, identify politicians who are friends of nursing, and advise the ANA PAC Board on potential candidates for ANA endorsement (Kathleen Schumacher, personal communication, May 12, 1997). In addition to active involvement in national politics, SNAs offer daylong or week-long internships in the art and science of influencing public policies.

Fellowships and internships also offer nurses an opportunity to learn the process of public policy development through actual experience. Fellowships and internships inform participants about the complexities of health care policy and legislative priorities and provide knowledge and skills to function in the public policy arena. Nurses may participate in formal fellowships and internships or create their own Washington internship. Some colleges and university graduate programs offer college credit to students who complete the Capitol Hill practicum. Internships offer nurses the ability to network professionally with members of Congress and congressional staff. In addition, personal experience working with the organizational structure and the legislative process demystifies the political and legislative processes. An internship may start a long-term relationship with a legislator or an influential staff member. In addition, the internship may instill the nurse with political passion.

Informal internships can be set up by sending a brief letter and résumé to an elected official. The letter should be sent to the member's administrative assistant or chief of staff. Formal public policy fellowships are offered by a number of groups (Display 16-3). Information about fellowship opportunities can be found at the local public library or obtained by writing to the foundations.

---

**Groups Offering Formal Public Policy Fellowships**   DISPLAY 16-3 ●

The Robert Wood Johnson Foundation

The W.K. Kellogg Foundation

The Congressional Black Caucus Foundation

The White House Commission

The Women's Research and Education Institute

The Coro Foundation

The American Association of University Women Educational Foundation

The Business and Professional Women's Foundation

The Everett McKinley Dirksen Congressional Leadership Research Center

The Supreme Court of the United States

The Woodrow Wilson National Fellowship Foundation

The Employee Benefit Research Institute

The Office of Technology Assessment of the United States Congress

*Source:* Sharp, Biggs, & Wakefield, 1999.

## ⊕ SUMMARY AND SIGNIFICANCE TO PRACTICE

Each nurse brings to the profession different talents that can be used for political action. Speaking out on unfair issues or writing elected officials takes time and courage. Nurses must make their voices heard in the political arena to ensure public safety in and access to health care delivery. Health care policies are developed through the legislative process at the national, state, and local levels. Developing expertise in influencing public policy requires dedication, time, practice, and a willingness to work with others. Issues affecting personal and public health are too important to be left to the politicians. Political involvement is a means to influence and control public policy while demonstrating ethical caring for all citizens in a democratic society.

### FROM THEORY TO PRACTICE

1. Do you think that all schools within a state should have a RN on the premises at all times during school hours?
2. List the benefits of having a RN on school premises during school hours.
3. What impact would having a RN on school premises during school hours have on students? Faculty? School staff and administration? Parents? Taxpayers?
4. Find a piece of legislation that you think may affect your nursing practice or client care delivery. Write a one- to two-page position paper on the pending piece of legislation using research and other evidence to support your position. Give the paper to a colleague and have them critique it in terms of clarity, conciseness, and strength of your position argument. Revise the paper based on your colleague's critique.

### WWW INTERNET EXERCISES

#### Exercise 1

1. Visit the following governmental websites: www.senate.gov and www.house.gov.
2. Visit the home pages of your two state senators and your representative to the United States House of Representatives. If you do not know their names, you can use your state name to discover the names of your two state senators. To identify your House representative, you can either search for him or her by using your home zip code, clicking your home location on a map, or typing in the number of your legislative district found on your voter registration card.
3. Search for current legislation affecting nursing and health care delivery by performing a topic search or typing in key words. You can read the full bill text or bill summaries.
4. Send an e-mail correspondence to your senators and House representative using strategies for composing letters and messages found in this chapter.
5. Find your state legislature by typing in (your state's name) Legislature. Most state legislative sites have search capabilities. Type in nursing and health care delivery as key words to find information about current legislative efforts affecting professional nursing in your state.

## Exercise 2

Visit the ANA website at http://www.nursingworld.org.

1. Find on the menu bar the following words: "Nursing Issues and Programs."
2. With your mouse on "Nursing Issues and Programs," a menu drops down. Click on the words "Government Affairs."
3. On the Government Affairs page, see if the ANA has issued any Action Alerts. If so, click on one of them and on the next page, find the menu and click on "Track Legislation."
4. After reading information tracking action on current legislative initiatives, hit the Back button on your toolbar twice to get to the Government Affairs page.
5. On the Government Affairs page, click on "Nursing's Legislative and Regulatory Initiatives for the 109th Congress" (the number of the Congress will change to 110 after the 2006 Federal Election).
6. On the next page, scroll down and find a topic of interest. Summarize the topic and bring it to class for discussion.

## Exercise 3

Visit the National Council of State Boards of Nursing website at http://www.ncsbn.org.

1. On the home page, find the words "Nurse Licensure Compact" and click them.
2. View the Nurse Licensure Compact: FAQ. What are the benefits of participation in the compact for states and nurses?
3. Hit the Back button. View the Nurse Licensure Compact Map. What states participate in the compact? Does your state participate in the interstate nursing licensure compact?
4. Scroll down the page to view a table of states that have introduced or passed this piece of legislation and see the enactment dates. As you scroll down, you can see a map of the United States of legislative action on the Mutual Recognition Compact.
5. Make a list of states that recognize the Mutual Recognition Compact.

## WWW INTERNET RESOURCES

The United States Government Legislative Website: http://thomas.loc.gov.
American Nurses Association: http://www.nursingworld.org.
Canadian Nurses Association: http://www.cna-nurses.ca.
Occupational Safety and Health Organization: http://www.osha.gov.
American Organization of Nurse Executives: http://www.aone.org.
American Hospital Association: http://www.aha.org.
For a database with more than 1.5 million US government web pages, see:
    http://firstgov.gov.

## REFERENCES

Agency for Healthcare Research and Quality (2001). AHRQ Profile, Advancing excellence in health care. Available at: http://www.ahrq.gov/about/profile.htm.
American Nurses Association (ANA). (2001). *2001* Nurse state legislators and state administrative leaders. Available at: http://nursingworld.org/gova/state/nurseleg#2.htm. Accessed July 10, 2005.

American Nurses Association (ANA). (2001a). American Nurses Association: selected testimony. Available at: http://www.nursingworld.org/gova/federal/legis/testimon/index/htm. Accessed July 10, 2005.

American Nurses Association (ANA). (2004). Saying goodbye to old friends and saying hello to new ones. *The American Nurse, 36*(6), 12.

American Nurses Association (2004a). *ANA & you: The house of nursing. The 2003 annual stakeholder's report*. Washington, DC: Author.

American Nurses Association Government Affairs (2004). HR 3656: Quality Nursing Care Act of 2004. Available at: http://vocusgr.vocus.com/grconvert1/wepub/ana/ProfileBill.asp?BillID=5970&SL=Priority.htm. Accessed January, 2005.

Bissonnette, T. (2004). Passion, engagement, and political action. *Michigan Nurse, 77,* 1.

Capps, L. (2003). *Congresswoman Capps' biography*. Available at: http://www.house.gov/capps/aboutlois.shtml. Accessed July 10, 2005.

Cohen, S. S., Mason, D. J., Kovner, C., Leavitt, J. K., Pulcini, J., & Sochalski, J. (1996). Stages of nursing's political development: Where we've been and where we ought to go. *Nursing Outlook, 44,* 259–266.

deVries, C., & Vanderbilt, M. (1992). *The grassroots lobbying handbook: Empowering nurses through legislative and political action*. Washington, DC: American Nurses Association.

Donnellan, C. (2004). DOL overtime rules take effect. *Capitol Update, 2,* 1.

Feldman, J. R., & Lewenson, S. B. (Eds.). (2000). *Nurses in the political arena*. New York: Springer Publishing.

Feldstein, P. J. (2004). *Health policy issues: An economic perspective* (3rd ed.). Chicago: Health Administration Press.

Goldwater, M., & Zusy, M. (1990). *Prescription for nurses: Effective political action*. St. Louis: Mosby.

Horrigan, M. (2004). Employment projections to 2012: Concepts and context. *Monthly Labor Review 127,* 3–22.

Institute of Medicine (2004). *Keeping patients safe, transforming the work environment of nurses*. Washington, DC: The National Academies Press.

Irwin, L. (Ed.). (1997, April 21). On the board: Nurse will be appointed to state health care post. *Kansas City Nursing News*, pp. 1, 4.

Itzhaky, H., Gerber, P., & Dekel, R. (2004). Empowerment skills and values: A comparative study of nurses and social workers. *International Journal of Nursing Studies, 41,* 447–456.

Milstead, J. A. (Ed.) (1999). *Health policy and politics: A nurse's guide*. Gaithersburg, MD: Aspen.

Mish, F. (Ed.) (1994). *Merriam-Webster's Collegiate Dictionary,* (10th ed.). Springfield, MA: Merriam-Webster.

Murray, J. & Corcoran, R. (2004). *The National League for Nursing Executive Report, October 2003-September 2004*. New York: National League for Nursing.

National Council of State Boards of Nursing (NCSBN). (2001). Mutual recognition information. Available at: http://www.ncsbn.org/mutual_compact.pdf. Accessed January 12, 2002.

Sharp, N., Biggs, S., & Wakefield, M. (1999). Public policies: New opportunities for nurses. *Nursing & Health Care, 12,* 16–22.

Skaggs, B. (1997). Political action in nursing. In J. Zerwekh, & J. Claborn (Eds.), *Nursing today, transitions and trends* (2nd ed.). Philadelphia: W. B. Saunders.

Stanhope, M. (1996). Policy, politics, and the law: Influences on the practice of community health nursing. In M. Stanhope, & J. Lancaster (Eds.), *Community health nursing: Promoting health of aggregates, families, and individuals* (4th ed.). St. Louis: Mosby.

Sultz, H., & Young, K. (2004). *Health care USA: Understanding its organization and delivery* (4th ed.). Sudbury, MA: Jones and Bartlett.

Tammelleo, A. D. (1990). Nurse terminated for election to public office. *The Regan Report on Nursing Law, 31,* 1.

Wakefield, M. (2004). A call to political arms. *Nursing Economic$, 33,* 166–167.

Wakefield, M. (2004a). 2004: A federal and state health odyssey. *Nursing Economic$, 22,* 47–48.

Wakefield, M. (2002). Health services research: A threatened foundation for the work of nurse executives. *Nursing Economic$, 20,* 142–144.

Professional nurses assume a variety of nursing roles as they engage in clinical practice. Frequently, professional nurses assume multiple roles simultaneously while providing nursing services. They consciously choose the roles to be assumed based on the nature of the client system, specific client needs, and the interdisciplinary team's efforts. Because nurses cannot be all things to all client systems, they work with other members of interdisciplinary health care teams. Professional nurses aspire to provide the best quality of health care to all persons and play key roles in monitoring and improving health care.

# Professional Nursing Roles

# CHAPTER 17

# Nursing Approaches to Client Systems

## KEY TERMS AND CONCEPTS

Human Systems

Clients

Change/Growth View of Change

Persistence View of Change

Change/Growth Model

Change/Stability Model

Family

Family as Client

Family System

Family Functions

Community

Community as Client

Health Promotion

Risk

Disease Prevention

Primary Prevention

Secondary Prevention

Tertiary Prevention

## LEARNING OUTCOMES

By the end of this chapter, the learner will be able to:

1  Define individual, family, and community as nursing clients.

2  Outline how various nursing conceptual models differentiate client systems in professional nursing.

3  Explain why nurses will be ineffective in nursing processes if they attempt to limit their view of the client system to individuals within the contexts of family and community.

4  Compare and contrast nursing approaches in the realms of family nursing using the change/growth view, and the change/stability view.

5  Explain the differences in viewing communities as aggregates of people, human systems, and human field/environmental field process.

6  Identify key gaps that exist in information that assists nurses to use nursing models in their practice with families and communities as clients.

Lisa is a teenage girl who prides herself on her skill in gymnastics, ballet, and academics. She strives for perfection in all her endeavors because she knows that her parents make great sacrifices so she can pursue her interests. Her ballet teacher has been encouraging her to lose 20 pounds because she carries 125 pounds on her 5-foot 7-inch frame. Today, Gina, a friend of Lisa's who also takes ballet lessons, collapsed during physical education class while running a relay race. Gina had recently lost the 20 pounds as requested by the ballet teacher and secured a starring role in a local ballet production.

Upon hearing the news about Gina, Lisa has come to the Health Room complaining of dizziness. Her friend Cindy helps her to the Health Room. Nancy notices that Cindy also appears to be extremely thin and has sunken eyes. Nancy, an experienced school nurse, gives Lisa and Cindy some orange juice. Nancy suspects that the girls have eating disorders. When she asks Cindy and Lisa about their eating habits, they both say they can eat anything they want without gaining weight. Both girls fail to make eye contact with Nancy when responding to her questions.

Nancy notices that both girls are wearing clothes similar to those worn by the cover model on a magazine. Nancy, concerned for the health of both girls, realizes that families play a key role in eating disorders and that peer pressure sometimes makes teenagers do foolish things. Nancy realizes that this as an opportunity in nursing practice to help individual clients, their families, and the school community.

**Human systems** are living systems open to interactions with other systems. Interacting systems are characterized by mutual change; that is, each human system can effect change in another and at the same time is influenced (changed) by that other system. Nurses involved in professional practice interact with client systems and the health care delivery system. The nursing profession defines **clients** as the recipients of nursing care. Besides being passive recipients of care, clients assume the important role of active participants, or partners, with nurses when they seek the services of professional nurses. This chapter explores the professional nurse's role with client systems. It presents a beginning in differentiation of the client systems—individuals, families, and communities.

Traditionally, nurses have cared for individuals; conceptual models of nursing have developed their views of "the person" (individual); and nurses have practiced with families and communities. The traditional practice with families and communities usually has been practice with individuals in a collective setting; thus, family and community actually have been treated as contexts of the identified client. The major questions for the professional nurse are: How do I implement processes of nursing with the whole human being, the individual client? With the whole family unit, the family as client? With the community as client?

## Questions for Reflection 17-1

1. Have I ever encountered a nursing situation that required more than caring for the individual as client?
2. How did I handle the situation?
3. Does consulting with family breach client confidentiality? Why or why not?
4. How does a nurse know when a health-related issue involves more than an individual or family system?

Change in human beings is lifelong, natural, and evolutionary. As human beings move through their lives, they establish themselves as integral elements of larger and more complex systems. The individual synthesizes the concept of "me" with "my family" and "my community." At times, nurses effectively and appropriately work with "me" in professional relationships. In other instances, the nurse must consider that working with "the family" may be more effective. Finally, nurses sometimes have to work with "the community," especially when the health of a large group of persons may be affected.

According to the paradigm selected for application in this book—the growth or persistence views of change (Fawcett, 1989)—it is the client–environment relationship that is most important. In the **change/growth view of change,** growth serves as the outcome of change. In the **persistence view of change,** the outcome is stability. The way individual nurses think about change determines how they view the client. In the **change/growth model,** nurses see clients with the ability for continuous growth, and nurses facilitate the change process by focusing the client on the client's strengths and abilities. In the **change/stability model,** nurses see clients as potentially capable of stability, and they facilitate the process by identifying and assisting with plans for resolving client problems.

When all of the conceptual models of nursing originally were developed, the nursing scholars equated "person" with the individual client. The developers of some models and other thinkers in nursing have attempted to explain how the models can be applied to family and community as client. Some nurse leaders believe that "person" has been redefined in the models to include families as clients, the recipients of care (Anderson & Tomlinson, 1992). Hanchett (1988) declares that community also can be defined as client; thus, "community" replaces "person" as the human being in some conceptual models.

## ● THE INDIVIDUAL AS CLIENT

The philosophy inherent in this book is that a person progresses through life. This progression is characterized by unique evolving patterns of interaction between the person and the environment. Such patterns of interaction determine the person's health. In general, the changes that occur in the developing human being are characterized by higher abilities to organize interactions and deal with more complex levels of interaction. The person's patterns are unique and are continuously evolving from earlier life experiences, including biologic, genetic, cultural, interpersonal, and social influences, as well as current interactions and conception of the future.

Because the conceptual models of nursing were developed with persons defined as the client, professional nurses derive directives for nursing practice from the discussion of nursing processes according to both the integration and interaction nursing models. The following section reflects our efforts to differentiate the professional nursing care of families and communities from that of individuals.

## ● FAMILY AS CLIENT

Who is defined as family? This question has evoked many definitions of family, from the conjugal or nuclear family (the family of marriage, parenthood, or procreation) to the extended family (the kinships of biologically related persons—grandparents, aunts, uncles, and cousins). Such definitions have limited applicability and usefulness in today's society. Thus, the definition of **family** that is accepted is "two or more individuals who depend on one another for emotional, physical, and/or economic support. The members of the family are self-defined" (Hanson, 1996 p. 6).

How is family nursing care viewed today? Some call it family-centered care; some call it family-based care; others call it family-focused care; and others call it simply family nursing. These different terms reflect confusion about whether the family is the client (the recipient of care) or is the context of care (in which the individual family member is the recipient of care). Gilliss (1991) says that family nursing care traditionally has been offered from the perspective of the family as context.

According to Wright and Leahey (1988, p. 30), there is a trend toward the family as the unit of care (family systems care) in which the nurse focuses on interaction: "It is becoming more natural for nurses to accept the interaction between illness, the individual, and the family," and that interaction can be addressed at all levels of the system, "from the micro level of fluid and electrolytes to the macro level of the family and the community." The **family as client** approach means that the entire family rather than individuals become the recipient of nursing services. For example, in the vignette, the presenting problem is the teenage girl, Lisa, who is complaining of dizziness. If the nurse focuses on the unit of care as the individual, nursing interventions would address only specific interventions for Lisa. However, because of Lisa's age and the nature of eating disorders, a more appropriate unit of care would be the family.

What are the indices and phenomena that represent the family as a holistic unit upon which the professional nurse must focus if the family is to be the client system? One approach is to view the family as a system interacting with subsystems and suprasystems. Artinian (1994) indicates that some of the assumptions of the family systems perspective are:

- A **family system** is an organized whole; individuals within the family are parts of the system and are interdependent.
- The family system is greater than and different from the sum of its parts.
- There are logical relationships (connectedness patterns) between the subsystems. In some families, the connectedness patterns may reflect rigid and fixed structures and relationships. In other families, the patterns of connectedness may reflect highly flexible structures and relationships.
- Using feedback from the environment, the family system responds (adapts) to change in ways that reduce strain and maintain a dynamic balance.

In the systems approach, the phenomena of interest are wholeness, relationships, belief systems, family rules, family needs, roles, and the tensions between individuation and togetherness. Two family theories that are congruent with the family systems model are the Calgary family assessment model (Hanson, 1996; Wright & Leahey, 1994) and the framework of systemic organization (Friedmann, 1995). A summary of the family systems model is presented in Display 17-1.

Another approach to family as client focuses on the family as a structural–functional social system (Artinian, 1994). The focus is the family structure and its effectiveness in performing its functions. Friedman (1992) identifies seven **family functions**: (1) affective support (meeting the emotional needs of family members); (2) socialization and

---

## The Family Systems Model

DISPLAY 17-1 ✦

**Overview:** Focuses on interaction between members of the family system and on the family system with other systems. A change in one member of the family system influences the entire system.

**Concepts:** Subsystems, boundaries, openness, energy, negentropy (energy that promotes order), entropy (energy promoting chaos), feedback, adaptation, homeostasis, input, output, internal system processes.

**Assumptions:** Family system is greater than the sum of its parts. Subsystems are related and interact with one another, and the whole family system interacts with other systems. Family systems have homeostatic features and strive to maintain a dynamic balance.

**Clinical Application:** Assess, diagnose, and intervene with family according to major concepts.

*Sample Assessment Questions*
- How did change caused by the critical illness event affect all the members of the family?
- How are members of the family system relating with one another?
- How is the family system relating to the critical care environment?
- What is the "input" into the family system?
- Is the family system internally processing the input? What is the family system output?
- How open is the family system? Does the family system have homeostasis?
- Determine how family behavior affects the patient.

- Determine how the patient's behavior affects the family.

*Interventions*
- Encourage nurse–family interactions through establishing trust and using communication skills to check for discrepancies between nurse and family expectations.
- Establish a mechanism for providing family with information about the patient on a regular basis.
- Foster the family's ability to get information.
- Listen to the family's feelings, concerns, and questions.
- Orient the family to the critical care environment.
- Answer family questions or assist them to get answers.
- Discuss strategies for normalizing family life with family members.
- Provide mechanisms for the patient and other family members to interact with one another through pictures, videos, audiotapes, or open visiting.
- Monitor family relationships.
- Facilitate open communication among family members.
- Collaborate with the family in problem solving.
- Provide necessary knowledge that will help the family make decisions.

*Source:* Artinian, N. T. (1994). Selecting a model to guide family assessment. *Dimensions of Critical Care Nursing, 14,* 6. Used with permission of the publisher.

---

social placement (socializing children and making them productive members of society); (3) reproduction (producing new members for society); (4) family coping (maintaining order and stability); (5) economic (providing sufficient economic resources and allocating resources effectively); (6) providing physical necessities (food, clothing, shelter); and (7) health care (maintaining health).

The Friedman family assessment model (Friedman, 1992; Hanson, 1996) appears congruent with a combination of the structural–functional model and the family systems model. Friedman designates that nurses must view the family in two ways when implementing family nursing: as each individual within the family context and the family as the unit of care. A summary of the structural–functional model is presented in Display 17-2.

A third approach to family as client is the family stress model. Artinian (1994) lists the following assumptions of this model: (1) the family is a system, (2) unexpected or unplanned events usually are perceived as more stressful than expected events, (3) events

---

## The Structural–Functional Model

**Overview:** Focuses on family structure and family function and how well family structure performs its functions.

**Concepts:** Structural areas include family form, roles, values, communication patterns, power structure, or support network. Functional areas include affective, socialization, reproductive, coping, economic, physical care, and health care functions.

**Assumptions:** Family is a system and a small group that exists to perform certain functions.

**Clinical Application:** Assess, diagnose, and intervene with family according to major concepts.

### Sample Assessment Questions

- What impact did the critical illness event have on family structure and function?
- How did the critical illness alter the family structure?
- What family roles were changed? What family functions have been affected?
- What are family members' physical responses to the illness event?

### Interventions

- Assist the family to modify its organization so that role responsibilities can be redistributed.
- Respect and encourage adaptive coping skills used by the family.
- Counsel family members on additional effective coping skills for their own use.
- Identify typical family coping mechanisms.
- Tell the family it is safe and acceptable to use typical expressions of affection.
- Provide privacy for the family to allow for family expression of affection.
- Provide for family visitation.
- Encourage family members to recognize their own health needs.
- Help family members find ways to meet their health needs while helping them feel their concern for the patient has not diminished.
- Assist the family to use existing support structure.

*Source:* Artinian, N. T. (1994). Selecting a model to guide family assessment. *Dimensions of Critical Care Nursing, 14,* 6. Used with permission of the publisher.

---

within the family that are defined as stressful are more disruptive than events outside the family, (4) lack of experience with a stressor leads to greater perceived stressfulness, (5) ambiguous stressor events are more stressful than unambiguous ones. Artinian (1994) indicates that client assessment should include family resources; the meaning of the situation to the family (e.g., is it viewed as a threat or a challenge?); the level of crisis the family is experiencing; and coping mechanisms.

Patterson (1999) presents a postmodern view of a family and provides an ecological perspective that requires nurses to think in layers with the smallest unit, the person, being in the center, with larger units extending outward until it comprises the entire cosmos. In this model, the family is an integral part of an ecosystem, and many variations in family form exist. Children receive support and protection from family members (parents, grandparents, siblings, and other relatives). The family serves as a unit of the community that encompasses schools, child-care providers, churches, health care providers, workplaces, locally supportive services (police, fire, city and county services), neighborhoods, and friends. The community is part of society, which is composed of the military, government, multinational corporations, technology, prisons, research institutions, courts, banks, insurers, multinational corporations, transportation systems, media, and welfare systems. Patterson (1999) designates the following four family functions.

- Family formation and membership: to provide a sense of belonging, personal and social identity, and meaning and direction for life.

- Economic support: to provide basic shelter, food, clothing, and other things to facilitate and enhance human development.
- Nurturance and socialization: to provide holistic development and support of members while instilling social values and norms.
- Protection of vulnerable members: to provide care for the young, disabled, ill, or aging members incapable of self-care or at risk for harm.

Patterson also proposes that each family develops specific functioning patterns that include consistent ways a family displays affection, shows anger, copes with stress, deals with conflict, accomplishes daily routines, disciplines children, seeks health care, and celebrates special occasions. The family alters these patterns as the family experiences developmental transitions (birth, raising children, departing children, aging, and death). Because the familial experience is multidimensional, Patterson suggests that limiting assessment to completing family questionnaires limits data collected by health care providers. Health care professionals should consider observing family interactions when families enter the health care system. Because a family is a system, the conceptualization of family health requires consideration of the individual health status of each member and the health of the family's functioning patterns (Patterson, 1999). Alteration in the health of one member usually results in altered family functioning patterns.

Two theories that are congruent with a combination of the family stress model and the family systems model are the family assessment and intervention model (Hanson, 1996; Mischke & Hanson, 1995) and the resiliency model (McCubbin & McCubbin, 1993). A summary of the family stress model is presented in Display 17-3.

Anderson and Tomlinson (1992, p. 61) identify five realms of family experience that represent elements of the approaches identified and that direct professional practice.

1. Interactive processes: (a) family relationships, (b) communication, (c) nurturance, (d) intimacy, and (e) social support
2. Developmental processes: (a) family transitions and (b) dynamic interactions between stages of family development and individual developmental tasks
3. Coping processes: (a) management of resources, (b) problem-solving, and (c) adaptation to stressors and crisis
4. Integrity processes: (a) shared meanings of experiences, (b) family identity and commitment, (c) family history, (d) family values, (e) boundary maintenance, and (f) family rituals
5. Health processes: (a) family health beliefs, (b) health status, (c) health responses and practices, (d) lifestyle practices, and (e) health care provision during wellness and illness

Therefore, nurses need to implement the nursing process in a way that facilitates exploration of all the family realms listed rather than focusing exclusively on health processes. In all the conceptual nursing models, the client system is viewed holistically; thus, the professional nurse cannot extricate the health processes from the other processes (integrity, coping, development, and interaction).

Family nursing interventions depend on the clinical practice context. For example, early discharge planning requires that nurses teach and counsel families as they anticipate taking clients home from inpatient settings. Nurses listen to families as they express concerns about the changes in the family's previous lifestyle. They teach families knowledge and skills so that they can safely provide care, anticipate potential complications, and

---

## The Family Stress Model

DISPLAY 17-3

**Overview:** Focuses on stressors, resources, and perceptions to explain the amount of family disruption caused by a stressful event.

**Concepts:** "A"—stressful event with associated hardships; "B"—physical, psychological, material, social, spiritual, informational resources of family; "C"—family's subjective definition of the stressful event; "X"—crisis, the amount of disruption or incapacitation within the family caused by the stressful event.

**Assumptions:** Family is a system. Unexpected and ambiguous illness events are more stressful. Stressful events within the family are more disruptive than stressor events that occur outside the family. Lack of experience with a stressor event leads to increased perceptions of stressfulness.

**Clinical Application:** Assess, diagnose, and intervene with family according to major concepts.

*Sample Assessment Questions*
- Identify the family's understanding and beliefs about the situation.
- What family hardships are associated with the critical illness event?
- What are other situational stressors for the family?
- Did the family have time to prepare for the event?

- Has the family had experience with the event?
- What resources are available to the family?
- Are the resources sufficient to meet the demands of the event?
- What are the family's perceptions of the event?
- Do they perceive the event to be a threat or a challenge?
- Does the family blame themselves for the event?
- How incapacitated is family functioning?

*Interventions*
- Help the family to cope with imposed hardships.
- If appropriate, provide spiritual or informational resources for the family.
- Introduce the family to others undergoing similar experiences.
- Discuss existing social support resources for the family.
- Assist the family in capitalizing on its strengths.
- Assist the family to resolve feelings of guilt.
- Help the family visualize successfully handling all the hardships associated with the situation.
- If possible, encourage the family to focus on the positive aspects of the situation or cognitively reappraise the situation as positive.

*Source:* Artinian, N. T. (1994). Selecting a model to guide family assessment. *Dimensions of Critical Care Nursing, 14,* 7. Used with permission of the publisher.

---

know what to do in case they occur. In inpatient settings, families frequently find the ability to room-in with their loved one most beneficial. Nurses also assess family dynamics as families interact in all nursing care settings. Nurses collaborate with families in all nursing care settings to design family nursing care plans when needed (Li, Melnyk, & McAnn, 2004). Sometimes nurses can use creative arts as an innovation to reduce stress and lower anxiety in family caregivers (Walsh, Martin, & Schmidt, 2004).

## Research Brief 17-1

Walsh, S., Martin, S., Schmidt, L. (2004). Testing the efficacy of a creative-arts intervention with family caregivers of patients with cancer. *Journal of Nursing Scholarship, 36,* 214–219.

The investigators sought to determine the effects of using an art cart (ArtKart) on family caregiver mood, anxiety, and affect while a family member received outpatient chemotherapy. The family caregiver selected a simple art project, was visited by a nurse-artist intervention team every 15 to 30 minutes as they worked on the art project designed to take 60 minutes. Family caregivers completed the Mini Profile of Mood States (Mini-POMS), Beck Anxiety Inventory (BAI), and Derogatis Affects Balance

Scale (DABS) before starting and after completing art projects. Forty caregivers engaged in the study for 6 months.

Paired $t$ tests were used to analyze differences on the Mini-POMS, BAI, and DABS. Large effects were noted in improvement of caregiver stress, anxiety, and positive emotion scores ($P < .001$). Therefore, creative activities for the 40 caregivers in this study improved caregiver mood, anxiety, and affect. Field notes revealed that works of creativity provided the caregiver with feelings of accomplishment, enabled them to control choices (selection of art project), and enabled them to express humor more freely.

Results of this study are consistent with those of other studies using art activities to improve client and caregiver moods. Because of the small sample size, caution should be exercised before making practice changes. Nursing implication for this and other studies demonstrate that use of the creative arts may be an effective intervention in improving client and caregiver mood, anxiety, and affect. However, more studies of this nature need to be performed across settings to support the use of creative arts routinely as a nursing intervention.

Sometimes, practice barriers prevent nurses from addressing the relevant realms when the family is the client. Situations such as decreased length of stay in inpatient settings, inadequate staffing, poor coordination of services across the health care setting continuum, lack of coordinated inpatient and outpatient services, less than optimal communication among interdisciplinary health providers, lack of nurse education regarding family structure and processes, and overwhelming complexity of family needs serve as reasons for ineffective family nursing care. In addition, many health care settings emphasize medical care over nursing care (Rose, Mallinson & Walton-Moss, 2004).

**Questions for Reflection 17-2**

1. How do I define family?
2. What ideas related to health and health care have I gotten from my family?
3. Where and when did I seek health care services as a child?
4. Do I still use the same approach to health care services? Why or why not?
5. What obstacles to working with family as client have I experienced in my current clinical practice setting? How can I create a clinical practice environment that supports family care?

How would nurse theorists explain the family as the client and the application of nursing to the nurse–family relationship? Following is a discussion of how the family may be understood in nursing models within the change/growth paradigm (Orem, 1983; Watson, 1996; Peplau, 1952; Rogers, 1983; Parse, 1996, 1998; and Newman, 1983) and those nursing models within the change/stability paradigm (King, 1983; Neuman, 1983; Roy, 1983).

## The Family in the Change/Growth Models of Nursing

When nurses use the change/growth models of nursing, they acknowledge that families experience growth when confronted with change. Like the individual, the family possesses great potential to develop in ways to maximize health for all members. The following section outlines professional considerations for nurses using the change/growth models of nursing.

### Orem's Self-Care Deficit Model

According to Taylor and Renpenning (1995, p. 356), Orem views family as a multiperson care system, which is:

those courses and sequences of action which are performed by the persons in multiperson units for the purpose of meeting the self-care requisites and the development and exercise of self-care agency of all members of the group and to maintain or establish the welfare of the unit . . . . The sub-systems of the multiperson system are the self-care systems of the individuals.

Whall and Fawcett (1991, p. 20) indicate that Orem's self-care conceptual framework primarily "views the family as only a backdrop for individuals." In her own words, Orem (1983, p. 368) directs the nurse to "first, accept the system of family living, the physical and social environment of the family, and the family's culture as basic conditioning factors for all the family members." She stresses that the family support system needs to be explored and "adjusted as needed and then incorporated into the system of family living" (Orem, p. 368).

Family is context in self-care, in which family members take actions to create conditions essential for human functioning and development, and for dependent care, in situations when family members need their care provided by others. Both self-care and dependent care are directed toward creating and maintaining conditions that support life and integrated functions and promote human growth. Self-care and dependent care "are forms of deliberate action, learned behaviors, learned within the family and other social units within which individuals live and move" (Orem, 1983, p. 209). However, Orem also considers the family to be a unit, "a complex entity which can be regarded as a whole" (Taylor & Renpenning, 1995, p. 350). Thus, there is concern with the quality of interaction and the outcomes of those interactions on the family as a whole.

Two realms of family can be readily implemented in Orem's self-care model: the interactive processes, particularly the social support systems in the family, and the developmental processes, particularly in the understanding of dependent care needs at various life stages. "Conditions which justify identifying the multi-person unit include a need for protection and prevention, regulation of a hazard, need for environmental regulation, [and] need for resources" (Taylor & Renpenning, 1995, p. 366).

Lapp, Diemert, and Enestredt (1991) stress the concept of the family as a partner in health care decision making. In keeping with the self-care perspective, they see "the primary responsibility for health and life choices as ultimately resting with the client family" (Lapp et al., p. 306). They further suggest that the main responsibility of the nurse is "ensuring that those choices were made on the basis of the most complete information possible while facilitating self-discovery of strengths and resources already existing for a family" (Lapp et al., p. 306).

Chevannes (1997) specifies that Orem's three levels of care enable nurses and family to develop caring partnership. The nurse and family collaborate to determine the care level needed to fulfill the needs of the incapacitated member. In the wholly compensatory level of care, the nurse provides care to the incapacitated person while beginning to teach family members. The nurse assesses family needs for nursing care or provides episodic care in the home when the family requires partly compensatory nursing care. Finally, when families assume full care responsibilities, the nurse provides support and education as needs arise.

If the nurse in the vignette practiced nursing according to Orem's self-care deficit theory, the nurse would assess Lisa and her family for their ability to access physical and mental health services independently and offer her assistance if the family could not access required services independently; discuss treatment options for Lisa (and the family); and help them select specific services and treatment plans. Once the family obtained the help they needed, the nurse would offer education and support to them.

## Watson's Human Science and Human Care Model

Watson's caring model lends itself to a view of the family as client if the nurse redefines the phenomenal field to be the family within the family system's environment. The nurse assesses family values by exploring the five realms of family experience (Anderson & Tomlinson, 1992)—namely, the integrity processes—through the family's shared meanings of experiences; its members' identity and commitment to that family identity; the family history; members' shared values and rituals; and their strategies for maintaining family boundaries.

Nurses identify family needs for information and problem-solving abilities by identifying the family's coping processes, such as how members obtain and manage resources and how the group solves problems. Nurses evaluate developmental conflicts by studying the family's developmental processes, which are the transitions of the family and the interaction of the family's stage of development with the individual developmental tasks. Losses and feelings about the human predicament can be analyzed through exploring the interaction processes, focusing on relationships and the family's communication patterns, patterns of nurturance, expressions of intimacy, and support networks. In the model of caring, nurses relate all of these processes that occur in the family to the health processes, clarifying with the family specific health beliefs, responses, practices, and the patterns of caring for each other during times of wellness and illness.

If the nurse in the vignette used Watson's approach to professional practice, she would offer education about eating disorders, help to access required resources, and provide support during the treatment process. However, she would also pay more attention to the deep meaning of the experience for them, their family health beliefs, and their patterns of caring for each other.

## Peplau's Interpersonal Relations Model

Because Peplau based her nursing model on the central concepts of growth and development facilitated by relationships with significant others, the model provides the foundation for the nurse to focus on the family as the unit of care if the patterns of interaction within the family, and the family developmental processes, replace individual needs as the central area of concern. Forchuk and Dorsay (1995, p. 114) stated that Peplau's model and family systems nursing "both share a common focus on interactions, patterns and interpersonal relationships."

Perhaps Peplau's greatest contribution to the family nursing process is the enumeration of the stages of the nurse–client relationship. According to Friedman (1992, p. 42), "trust and rapport-building set the stage for and are the cornerstones of effective family nursing care." In the orientation stage, if the nurse and the family are to have an effective relationship, each member of the family must be able to share his or her concerns so that the nurse and other family members may more fully understand the whole family and the meaning of its experience together. In the planning stage, mutual goal setting—that is, jointly formulated among family members and the nurse—and ways to meet commonly derived goals are directed toward reframing the need for help in the professional relationship to be a learning and growth experience.

It is proposed that, in the intervention stage (called the exploitation stage by Peplau) with families, Peplau's role behaviors originally designated as professional nursing roles could be developed as strategies for the entire family. Family needs replace individual needs, and the roles of resource person, teacher, leader, counselor, and surrogate may be played by both the nurse and various family members. Each role performance in the family should be fully explored in a way that the family learns about its interactive processes and the effect of those interactive processes on health processes.

If the nurse in the vignette used Peplau as a framework for professional practice, the nurse would work to build trust and rapport with the family unit, explore all family members concerns, work with the family to understand the total experience, and collaborate with the family to set goals. The nurse would primarily assume the roles of teacher and counselor/teacher as the family learns about the daughter's eating disorder, what it means, and treatment options. Emphasis would be placed on how the disorder and treatment regimens would affect performance of family roles and how the overall interactive processes would affect the health of each family member and the family as a unit.

## Rogers's Science of Unitary Human Beings

Various analysts agree that Rogers's conceptual model of nursing science lends itself readily to the family as the recipient of nursing care—the client system. As Friedman (1992, p. 62) says, "Rogers's legacy is clearly associated with general systems theory, and because of this orientation there is a good fit between Rogerian nursing theory and family nursing." Rogers herself says that the family system is an energy field that serves as the focus of study and interaction. She asserts that family fields and their respective environmental fields are engaged in a continuously evolving mutual process and that patterns identify this ongoing process (Rogers, 1983, p. 226). Some patterns may represent togetherness, others may represent activity/rest, and still others may represent rhythmicities in the family experience.

Whall and Fawcett (1991, p. 22) suggest that, in the Rogerian model, the family is "viewed as an irreducible whole that is not understood by knowledge of individual family members." Newman, Sime, and Corcoran-Perry (1991, p. 4) point out that, from the unitary–transformative perspective (the perspective first described by Rogers), a phenomenon (any client system) is "viewed as a unitary, self-organizing field embedded in a larger self-organizing field . . . [and] identified by pattern and by interaction with the larger whole." Given this perspective, the family represents a unitary phenomenon embedded in the larger environmental field and a phenomenon that has patterns of energy exchange within its field and within its interactions with the larger environment.

Whall (1986) suggests that, despite Rogers not being completely clear about what assessment strategies are used in the unitary model, she deserves credit for the idea that the nurse providing care must assess the family as a whole. Other nurses have developed some of the tools needed for assessing the whole family. For example, Smoyak developed the idea of using genograms and the identification of family rules of organization as approaches in the nursing process (Whall, 1986). The genogram records information about family members and their relationships over at least three generations. It involves mapping the family structure, recording family information, and delineating family relationships. According to McGoldrick and Gerson (1985, p. 1), genograms "display family information graphically in a way that provides a quick gestalt of complex family patterns and a rich source of hypotheses about how a clinical problem may be connected to the family context and the evolution of problem and context over time."

The genogram is one of nursing's most useful tools for studying family patterns because it maps relationships and patterns of functioning and thus "may help clinicians think systemically about how events and relationships in their clients' lives are related to patterns of health and illness" (McGoldrick & Gerson, 1985, p. 2). Using the historic data obtained by completing the genogram, the nurse assesses previous life cycle transitions. This assessment helps the nurse to "picture the important connections between the family and the world" (Wright & Leahey, 1994, p. 49). Readers are referred to McGoldrick and Gerson, and Wright and Leahey, for additional details on constructing and interpreting the genogram as a tool for nursing assessment of the family.

All of the family realms described by Anderson and Tomlinson (1992) and discussed earlier in this chapter represent patterns of the family as a unitary phenomenon. Thus, these realms could be used as a basis for assessment, planning, intervention, and evaluation by nurses practicing on the basis of a Rogerian philosophy of nursing.

If the nurse in the vignette used Rogers's Science of Unitary Human Beings to guide practice, she would see that the health status of both girls in her office was a manifestation of the pattern of the whole. The nurse would focus on understanding all mechanisms that affect the life process of the girls, one of which is the family.

## Parse's Human Becoming Model

The nursing models of Parse and Newman may be considered Rogerian-based. Thus, the nurse practicing within any of these models would incorporate Rogerian concepts in the care giving process with the family.

For Parse, "since the abstract term 'human' includes all human phenomena, it encompasses family phenomena as inherent in being human" (Cody, 1995, p. 11). Parse, who views the person as an open being always in the process of becoming, probably would describe the family as open and always in the process of becoming. "Family health is co-created by persons as they live family process" (Cody, p. 14). Nurses would direct nursing care most likely at structuring meaning, co-creating rhythmic patterns of relating, and co-transcending with the possibles through the interpersonal processes occurring among family members and the nurse for the purpose of improving the quality of life for the family.

"For each participant family, a multiplicity of views co-creates the reality of the family situation as lived by each person" (Cody, 1995, p. 23). Clearly, the family realms (Anderson & Tomlinson, 1992) that characterize Parse's model are the interactive processes (family relationships, communication, nurturance, intimacy, and social support) and the integrity processes (shared meanings of experiences, family identity and commitment, family history, family values, boundary maintenance, and family rituals).

If the nurse in the vignette used Parse's Human Becoming Model as a framework for professional practice, the approach would be similar to Rogers's Science of Unitary

Human Beings. However, the nurse would expend more energy to uncover the meaning that underlies the behaviors associated with the eating disorders. To discover the true meanings, the nurse would be truly present with the family as they expressed concerns that would ultimately reveal the meaning of thoughts, feelings, values, and changes that may have potentially contributed to Lisa's problems. The nurse would also provide a relationship so that the family can express these things as they engage in the treatment process and recover once treatment is completed.

## Newman's Theory of Health as Expanding Consciousness

Newman, who views the individual as a center of energy, views the family the same way—a center of energy in constant interaction with the environment. Newman (1983) makes five assumptions about families.

1. Health encompasses family situations in which one or more family members may be diagnosed as ill.
2. The illness of family members can be considered a manifestation of the pattern of the family interaction.
3. Elimination of the disease condition in the identified ill family member will not change the overall pattern of the family.
4. If one person's becoming ill is the only way the family can become conscious of its pattern, then that is health (in process) for that family.
5. Health is the expansion of consciousness of the family. Consciousness has been defined as the informational capacity of the system, a factor that can be observed in the quantity and quality of responses to stimuli.

The nature of nursing with the family would be the repatterning of partnerships between the family and the environment that promote higher levels of consciousness. Newman (1983) says that the purpose of nursing with the family is to facilitate the development of an increased range of responses of family members to each other and to the world outside the family and to facilitate the refinement of those responses (quality). She suggests that the first task is to assess the patterns of movement, space, time, and consciousness in the family. The nurse would consider the following factors to assess movement through observation: (1) the coordinated movement of language between speaker and listener; (2) other coordinated movements (such as dancing, lovemaking, and sports); (3) the freedom of individual movement within the family; and (4) the movement outside the family.

Time is assessed for the quantity and quality of private time, coordinated time, and shared time. Space is assessed for territoriality, shared space, and distancing. Finally, consciousness is assessed by collecting data on the informational capacity of the family system, the quantity and quality of interaction within the family, and the quantity and quality of the interaction of the family with the community.

By completing these assessments, the nurse providing care for the family would be able to analyze the patterns of energy exchange between the family and the environment, and the transforming potential and life patterns of the family. These patterns will identify where the family energy is flowing and where it is blocked, depleted, or diffused and will determine whether there is overload or build-up of energy in the family. Newman (1983, p. 173) says that as these patterns emerge, the family's informational capacity will be increased in the nurse–client relationship. Assessment of these patterns also will reveal the family's evolving capacities, diversity, and complexity. If the nurse in the vignette used Newman's Health as Expanding Consciousness, she would intervene to facilitate repatterning the family into a higher level of consciousness.

Consistent with the models of Rogers, Parse, and Newman is the fact that the family functions as a unitary, open system integrated with its environment. Family functions may be organized around Anderson and Tomlinson's (1992) five realms of family experience; thus, the assessment, planning, implementation, and evaluation of the family as client by nurses practicing from any of the change/growth nursing models should reflect interactive, developmental, coping, integrity, and health processes and the relationship among all of these processes.

## The Family in the Change/Stability Models of Nursing

When nurses use change/stability models of nursing, they acknowledge that nursing roles focus on assisting families in solving problems. This section presents a brief discussion of how the family may be viewed as the recipient of care in the nursing models in which the changes are directed toward restabilizing the client system.

### King's Systems Interaction Model

King (1983, p. 179) views the family as "a social system that is seen as a group of interacting individuals." Thus, the family is an interpersonal system. In King's model, a theory of goal attainment in the family emphasizes interaction between the family members.

The major concepts in this theory of goal attainment are self, role, perception, communication, transaction, stress, growth and development, time, space, and interaction. Each of these concepts is assessed in the nursing process between the nurse and the family. Communication is the interrelating factor among these concepts. Nurses and families make transactions to attain goals. King says that family movement through space and time may be social (called vertical movement) or physical (called geographic mobility). She also states that family roles are related to growth and development and stress in the family.

To summarize King's perception of the family as client, the nurse assesses the family situation to identify real or potential problems. The nurse "assist[s] family members in setting goals to resolve problems [and] provide[s] relevant information to help families make decisions about those factors that detract from or enhance healthy living" (King, 1983, p. 183). If the nurse in the vignette used King's approach to professional practice, the nurse would assess the family to identify factors contributing to the suspected eating disorders, and help families identify actual and potential issues and concerns regarding having a family member with an eating disorder.

### Neuman's Health Care Systems Model

A stress/adaptation-based conceptual model for family nursing is Neuman's health care systems model. The nurse practicing with this model can modify assessment strategies to plan, implement, and evaluate primary, secondary, and tertiary interventions with families.

According to Neuman (1983, p. 241), "the concept of family as a system can be viewed as individual family members harmonious in their relationships—a cluster of related meanings and values that govern the family and keep it viable in a constantly changing environment." Stability is considered to represent the wellness state, instability the illness state, and transition the mixed wellness–illness state. The role of the nurse is "to control vigorously factors affecting the family, with special goal-directed activities toward facilitating stability within the system" (Neuman, p. 243). To understand influences on the stability of the family system, Neuman proposes the following points.

1. The nurse must deal with the needs of each family member in terms of his or her developmental age, developmental state, individual differences (strengths and weaknesses), and environmental influences according to his or her perceptions of events.
2. The nurse must determine the structure and process of the family by studying the values and interaction patterns. The significant values and interaction patterns are the decision-making process (how power is distributed); coping style (how differences are negotiated in relation to stress); role relationships (the controlling or facilitating effects of roles in meeting individual and family needs); communication styles and interaction patterns (congruence of verbal and nonverbal messages and the effects of situational or entrenched defense mechanisms in the family); goals (the sharing and supporting of concerns and feelings between members); boundaries (rules that define the type of behaviors that are acceptable or unacceptable to the family); socialization process (the adequacy of resources to support cultural and structural factors in meeting family needs); individuation (the quality of individuality of each family member that defines the wellness or stability of the unit); and sharing (an index for family stability).
3. The nurse must facilitate the meeting of family needs by intervening in the intrafamily stressors (all things occurring within the family unit), the interfamily stressors (all things occurring between the family and the immediate environment), and extrafamily stressors (all things occurring between the family and distal or indirect external environment). These interventions occur as primary prevention, secondary prevention, or tertiary prevention.

Tomlinson and Anderson (1995) described five areas of interface between Neuman's systems model and a general family health system paradigm.

1. Complexity of the system: The "need to consider not only the individual stressor response in relation to the family but also the family's response relative to lines of defense and resistance" (pp. 138–139).
2. Conceptualization of the core of the family: "The core of the family is composed of its individual members, and assessment of the family is done in relation to the dynamics of individual member contributions to the whole within their environmental interactive context...[in comparison] the core of the family systems is viewed as the interface of its members in interaction with the environment" (p. 139).
3. Goal of family health: "Neuman's central concern is to facilitate optimal client system stability or wellness in the face of change . . . [in comparison] from a family health system perspective, it is most desirable to facilitate family system wellness using strengths to reduce stressor effects and enhance family growth toward positive transformation" (p. 140).

4. Entry point in caring for families: The family becomes partners in health care. "According to Neuman, nursing functions to conserve system energy" (p. 140).
5. Nursing interaction: In the Neuman model, "the nurse role creates an explicit cooperative alliance with the client . . . [in comparison] based on a family systems perspective . . . in the family caregiving situation there may be considerable boundary ambiguity" (p. 141).

The nurse's prevention activities are the heart of Neuman's model of care. Primary preventions are the activities aimed at preventing stressors from invading the family. Secondary preventions are the protective activities that follow stressor invasion. Tertiary preventions are the activities during the family's reconstitution from stressors. All of these preventions are aimed at re-establishing stability within the family. If the school nurse in the vignette used the Neuman systems model as a foundation for practice, she would assess the family for stressors using five variables (physiologic, psychological, sociocultural, developmental, and spiritual). She would look for ways to minimize the impact of stressors associated with living with a family member with an eating disorder as well as the stressors associated with treatment.

## Roy's Adaptation Model

Roy's adaptation model can be used by the nurse dealing with the family as client. Roy (1983) believes that the family as an adaptive system can be analyzed and that interventions can be organized around enhancing stimuli to the family.

Inputs for family include individual needs and changes within members and among members, and external changes in the environment. These inputs serve as focal stimuli for the family system. Processes handling the inputs are the control and feedback mechanisms. The control mechanisms—supporting, nurturing, and socializing—serve as contextual and residual stimuli to the family system. The feedback mechanisms are the transactional patterns and member control.

Outputs of the family system are the behaviors manifested. Roy (1983) has chosen three goals as proposed output of the adaptive family system: (1) survival, (2) continuity (role function), and (3) growth (the system's self-concept). At the current stage of development, Roy (1983, p. 275) simply says that "family behavior can be observed as it relates to the general family goals of survival, continuity, and growth."

The nurse observes for the outputs of survival, continuity, and growth and for the transactional and member controls that serve as feedback to the family to signal the need to adjust the behavior of a member or the group. Nursing practice emerges from the assessment of the previously described family factors. The nursing process continues to (1) identify and validate with family members the factor that is most immediately affecting their behavior; (2) identify individual family member needs as focal stimuli; (3) make nursing diagnoses and set goals; and (4) intervene to enhance stimuli configuration in the family.

Friedman (1992, p. 61) supports Roy's suggestion that "nursing problems involve ineffective coping mechanisms, which cause ineffective responses, disrupting the integrity of the person" and suggests that "this notion could easily be broadened to the family unit, where ineffective family coping patterns lead to family functioning problems." Whall and Fawcett (1991, p. 24) acknowledge the potential contribution of Roy's model of nursing care to care of the family as an adaptive system but notes that "theories of family adaptation and nursing practice theories of family need to be generated and tested."

Family adaptation theories need to be elaborated by identifying specific and concrete inputs, processes, and outputs of the family system.

It can be clearly seen that the family as client, rather than context, is a significant new conceptual basis for nursing. Although the attribution "of wellness and illness to the family unit is a recent phenomenon" (Gilliss, Highley, Roberts, & Martinson, 1989, p. 5), it is anticipated that an eclectic view of family incorporating both the nursing conceptual models and other social systems approaches will continue to be refined.

Nurses frequently integrate family approaches to clinical situations. Family theory and nursing models provide solid foundations for professional practice. Many family assessment tools exist. Most inpatient admission databases collect data surrounding family life. Although family models and theories are not specific to a particular nurse theorist, they compliment many current nursing models and theories. In some cases such as the structure provided by Anderson and Tomlinson (1992), cited earlier in this chapter, provides an eclectic approach when working with families as clients. The family plays a key role in its own health and the health of individual members. Current family health practices evolve from previous health practices. When a family unit forms, the health practices of the new family frequently blend health patterns that the family heads learned as children. Women tend to assume primary responsibility for family health, family members have specific health routines, and community and cultural context affect family health (Andrews & Boyle, 1999; Denham, 1999; Lundy & Janes, 2001).

## ● THE COMMUNITY AS CLIENT

In this book, the emerging philosophy defines community as a social system with open communication networks between structural and functional subsystems and the greater societal systems. Vertical bureaucratic relationships tie the community to the larger society. A **community** always has a sense of common identification, even if it does not exist as a common geographic location. Thus, the boundaries of a community can be determined in terms of role relationships as well as geography. As with all open systems, the nurse influences change in the community. The change is directed toward higher levels of wellness in the system.

Several concepts from community health nursing are basic to the care of the **community as client** (Capuzzi, 1996, p. 358):

- **Health promotion**—improving the well-being of the community.
- **Risk**—probability that the community will be affected by a health problem.
- **Disease prevention**—protection of the population from diseases and disabilities and their consequences.
- **Primary prevention**—preventing the occurrence of health problems.
- **Secondary prevention**—activities to identify and treat health problems early.
- **Tertiary prevention**—activities to correct health problems and prevent further deterioration.

### Definitions of Community

Because community has been thought of primarily as a setting for care, nurses need to explore the various definitions of community to determine how they may view the community as a client for nursing services. Shamansky and Pesznecker (1991) identify no less than 100 definitions for the term "community." Clark (1999, p. 6) defines a community as a "group of people who share some type of bond, who interact with each other, and who function collectively regarding common concerns." From a nursing perspective, Hanchett (1988, p. 7) says that community can be considered as an aggregate, a system, or as a human–environmental field: "As an aggregate, the individual is the basic unit of the community; that is, the community is a number of separate individuals." As a system, one must consider the "relationships among the individuals or groups who constitute the community" (Hanchett, p. 8). As a human–environment field, the community represents a human field integral with its environment and "manifesting correlates of the patterning of that field process" (Hanchett, p. 8).

If the nurse views the community as an aggregate, nursing really is organized around the concept of the community serving as a context for individuals. Clark (1999, p. 56) defines community health nursing as "a synthesis of nursing knowledge and practice and the science and practice of public health, implemented via systematic use of the nursing process and other processes, designed to promote health and prevent illness in population groups. The focus of care is the aggregate." Clark indicates that community health nursing is characterized by the following attributes:

1. Health orientation—health promotion and prevention of disease, rather than cure of illness.
2. Population focus—emphasis on aggregates, rather than individuals or families.
3. Autonomy—greater control of health care decisions.
4. Continuity—providing continuing, comprehensive care, rather than care on a short-term, episodic basis.
5. Collaboration—nurse and client interacting as equals.
6. Interactivity—awareness of interaction of a variety of factors with health.
7. Public accountability—accountability to society for public health.
8. Sphere of intimacy—greater awareness of the reality of client lives and situations.

Nurses can select from a variety of community nursing and community health models to follow when working with the community as client. Christensen and Kenney (1990) proposed a comprehensive model for implementing the nursing process focusing on the aggregate within the context of a geopolitical environment.

Zotti, Brown, and Stotts (1996, p. 211) differentiate between community-based nursing and community health nursing; community-based nursing "means a philosophy of nursing that guides nursing care provided for individuals, families, and groups wherever they are, including where they live, work, play, or go to school." In contrast, community health nursing "represents a systematic process of delivering nursing care to improve the health of an entire community" (Zotti et al., 1996, p. 212). Characteristics of community-based nursing and community health nursing are compared in Table 17-1.

Bullough and Bullough (1990, p. 19) prefer to use the term "community health nursing" for preventive services, and the term "home health nursing care" for the work of nurses providing direct care to individual clients in their homes. They define community health nursing as the delivery of nursing services to population groups, families, and individuals in the community setting. The population groups are aggregates of people who share a common identity or have common interests.

TABLE 17-1

## Community-Based Nursing Compared with Community Health Nursing

| Component | Community-Based Nursing | Community Health Nursing |
| --- | --- | --- |
| Goals | Manage acute or chronic conditions<br>Promote self-care | Preserve/protect health<br>Promote self-care |
| Client | Individual and family | Community |
| Underlying philosophy | Human ecological model | Primary health care |
| Autonomy | Individual and family autonomy | Community autonomy<br>Individual rights may be sacrificed for good of the community |
| Client character | Across the life span | Across the life span, with emphasis on high-risk aggregates |
| Cultural diversity | Culturally appropriate care of individual and families | Collaboration with and mobilization of diverse groups and communities |
| Type of service | Direct | Direct and indirect |
| Home visiting | Home visitor | Home visitor |
| Service focus | Local community | Local, state, federal, and international |

From Zotti, M. E., Brown, P., & Slotts, R. C. (1996). Community-based nursing versus community health nursing: What does it all mean? *Nursing Outlook, 44,* 212. Used with permission of the publisher.

If nurses view the community as a system, then they seek to introduce changes in the community systems and base interventions on their understanding of the impact of these changes on system functioning (Spradley, 1990). Christensen and Kenney (1990) also proposed a general systems assessment model for directing the nursing process with families. Considerable work on viewing the community as a system that is the recipient of nursing care has emerged from Neuman's conceptual model of nursing. This model is discussed later in this chapter. Hanchett (1988) postulates that Roy's adaptation model of nursing and King's general system framework also offer the nurse the opportunity to practice nursing with the community as a client system, in which the focus is on the pattern of relationships among the elements of the system.

Following are brief discussions of (1) a systems model of community as client based on Neuman's conceptual model, in which change is directed toward restoring stability to the system; and (2) a human field/environment model of community as client based on Rogerian nursing science, in which change is directed toward increasing capacities and evolving growth. In both models, the emphasis is on health promotion and the characteristics of space, interaction, and population (McCarthy, 1990, p. 134). The community has geographic and interactional aspects in both models.

When the school nurse in the vignette operates from a community as client perspective, her focus on eating disorders shifts. Once, she intervened with individual students affected by the problem. Now, she considers how the problem affects the entire school community. She plans and executes educational programs for students, faculty, staff, and administration on the detection and prevention of eating disorders. Along with education, she offers her time and attention to listen to concerns and counsels all persons affected by the declining health of students with eating disorders.

## A Systems Model of Viewing the Community as Client

Anderson and McFarlane (2000) adapt the Neuman health care systems model in an effort to provide a way for nurses to conceive of the community as the recipient of care. This effort synthesizes public health with nursing. In this systems approach, the community has eight subsystems: (1) recreation, (2) safety and transportation, (3) communication, (4) education, (5) health and social services, (6) economics, (7) politics and government, and (8) the physical environment.

The boundaries of a community are generally geopolitical. The interactive nature of these eight subsystems results in a whole that is more than the sum of its parts. Other nurse leaders have expanded views on this model in terms of the nursing process (Christensen & Kenney, 1990). For example, Beddome (1995) stresses the need to clearly define the client system that is the target of data collection and nursing intervention (geopolitical or aggregate).

The application of Neuman's model to the development of the nursing process with the community as the recipient of care is built around the redefinition of person, environment, health, and nursing. Community nursing scholars describe communities as groups of persons who share common characteristics, such as language or culture, who may or may not live in a specific geographical area (Anderson and McFarlane, 2000; Lundy and Janes, 2001). They redefine the environment to include all conditions, circumstances, and influences that affect the development of the community. Health is equated with competence to function and "a definable state of equilibrium in which subsystems are in harmony so that the whole can perform at its maximum potential" (Saucier, 1991, p. 59).

Nurses participate in the care of the community by participating in community assessment, identifying and diagnosing problems amenable to nursing interventions, planning for and implementing interventions that enhance the interacting forces within the system, and evaluating the outcomes of the interventions on the community's health.

The systems model focuses on prevention. Primary prevention strategies for the professional nurse include (Saucier, 1991): (1) increasing the public's awareness of health problems; (2) increasing the public's knowledge of the available community resources and services to resolve the problems; (3) preparing the public to self-refer to appropriate resources; and (4) preparing the public to become involved in preventing the factors that lead to the problem.

Secondary prevention strategies include facilitating people to do self-screening and referral to appropriate community resources. Tertiary prevention strategies include lobbying for adequate services and resources to meet the particular community health problems. An example is "health care reform by rethinking health policy and writing new health legislation at many levels of government" (Beddome, 1995, p. 571). The systems model presents a comprehensive approach when nurses serve the community as client. However, the systems approach uses the change as stability perspective.

## A Human Field/Environment Model of Viewing Community as Client

From the paradigm of nursing in which change is directed toward growth, the following brief discussion uses the Rogerian framework for viewing the community as client.

Hanchett (1988, p. 128) says that, in this view, the community is seen as an energy field in process with the environmental energy field, and health is viewed as the dynamic well-being of the community–environmental process. Manifestations of these energy fields in process may be reflected in visible expressions such as motion, rhythms of quiet and activity, and the togetherness of the community people in participating in change.

For example, motion that is observable by the nurse is the speed of persons and traffic in daily life. Rhythms of quiet and activity may be seen in the sleep–wake patterns of the community. Everyone has heard about how the streets are "rolled up at night" in some communities. Gatherings of people in community settings can be observed to analyze togetherness. Other pattern manifestations of this energy process include the "number of cultural and ethnic groups of the community, the variety of lifestyles and ideas that flourish, and the pragmatic, imaginative, and visionary approaches to change evidenced by the community" (Hanchett, 1988, p. 129).

The goal of nursing is to help the community achieve maximum well-being. According to Hanchett (1988), this is done by the nurse participating in the process of change, assisting community groups to move toward well-being. Rogers's definition of health as "dynamic well-being" means that the community must become more aware of factors that maximize well-being and minimize conditions that limit actualization or realization of full potential.

This view of health directs the actions of the nurse in this model. These actions all center on facilitating persons to become more aware of their patterns of energy exchange with the environment and the evolving outcomes of these exchanges. Manifestations of field patterning include "diversity, rhythms, motion, the experience of time, sleep–wake and beyond-waking states, and pragmatic, imaginative, and visionary approaches to conscious participation in change" (Hanchett, 1988, p. 128). The nurse attempts to facilitate evolutionary change in the human field/environmental field process from lesser diversity, longer rhythms, slower motion, experiencing time as slower, pragmatic foci, and longer sleeping, to greater diversity, rhythms that seem continuous, motion that seems continuous, experiencing time as timelessness, visionary foci, and longer waking, perhaps even beyond waking, respectively (Hanchett, 1988).

The essence of this model for community nursing is that the community as a group/environmental field process determines the health of the community. In each community, the process unfolds at a unique pace and in unique patterns. The community's health is an expression of the mutually evolving process. Nursing's approaches to enhance the well-being of people/environment speak of community well-being. Influencing public policies to provide improved shelter, food, and clothing for all people are examples of approaches to improve community well-being. Nursing is "the science that the art of nursing uses in the conscious participation in the human–environmental field process toward the goal of maximum well-being" (Hanchett, 1988, p. 132).

In the Rogerian model of nursing, the community field/environmental field process integrates all other definitions of community; that is, it validates the community as a social system, as a place (space), and as a people. The resultant health of the client system (community) is more than the sum of these identified parts. Well-being is an integral process in which human beings/environment evolve toward greater awareness of their being. Respect for both diversity and sameness in patterns of energy exchange is essential for the professional nurse to operate out of this conceptual model of nursing.

It is evident from the general nature of the discussion of this model that much research is needed to assist further development of the Rogerian model. Determining manifestations of patterning of life, identifying patterns that maximize health, and developing strategies that focus on the community field/environmental field process are necessary for fuller implementation of this model in community nursing practice in which the community is the recipient of the care.

To learn how to care for communities as clients, nurses may benefit most from participating in service-learning projects or clinical experiences in community agencies. Community-based nursing experiences enable nurses to appreciate the value of being an engaged citizen in a community while learning how to provide nursing services to larger groups of people. Community-based experiences offer situations where nurses give to the agency while they increase their repertoire of community nursing skills. When engaging in community nursing, nurses must expand their views to see how internal and external factors affect an agency while collaborating with community members to assure that they offer relevant services (Narsavage, Batchelor, Lindell & Chen, 2003). Nurses also work to build stronger communities as well as improving community health. Through role modeling, nurses can inspire community members to participate actively in the political process, increase participation in community activities, develop community goals, manage conflict effectively, attain consensus on goal priorities and how to reach them, use resources effectively, and obtain external resources for desired programs (Head, Aquilino, Johnson, Reed, Mass, & Moorehead, 2004). Finally, most importantly, nurses advocate for underprivileged community members so they gain access to health care and other basic services (McElmury, Park & Buseh, 2003).

### Questions for Reflection 17-3

1. What additional professional nursing skills do nurses need when the community is the client?
2. What are current health concerns within my local community?
3. What are current health concerns within my academic community?
4. What health concerns can I identify in my clinical practice community?
5. Why are these health concerns important for each community?

## ● SUMMARY AND SIGNIFICANCE TO PRACTICE

Conceptual models of the client–environment relationship provide frameworks to guide practice with family and community clients as well as individuals. Views of change reflected by the models underlie strategies to promote growth of the family or community or to facilitate return to stability. When working with the family or community as clients, nurses must develop an ability to think in multiple dimensions because more than one person becomes the client system. In most cases, the impact of an individual's health-related change affects a family system. The impact of a health change also may have implications for the entire community. As health care professionals, nurses must look beyond individual clients and develop strategies to care for families and communities.

## FROM THEORY TO PRACTICE

Review the vignette at the start of the chapter and answer the following questions:

1. List the individual as client, family as client, and community as client in the out-lined school nursing situation.
2. Why is it important to expand the definition of client to include the family and community in this situation?
3. What do you think is the top priority in the vignette? Why do you think this issue should be addressed first?
4. What other issues do you see that need to be addressed? Why are these important?

## WWW INTERNET EXERCISES

1. Visit the National Clearinghouse on Child Abuse and Neglect website at http://nccanch.acf.hhs.gov. Click on the words "General Resources." On the next screen, click on the underlined words "State Statute Search." Complete Step 1 by identifying your state. Complete Step 2 by clicking on the following words to check the boxes for Mandatory Reporters, Reporting Laws, Reporting Penalties, and Reporting Procedures. Complete Step 3 by scrolling to the bottom of the page and clicking the word "Go!" Read to find out if professional nurses in your state are legally required to report child abuse and neglect. Read the laws and find out if any provisions are made for immunity for reporters in your state. Share your thoughts with your colleagues.
2. Visit the Centers for Disease Control website at http://www.cdc.gov/nip/. Read information about this year's influenza season and national immunization guidelines.
3. Visit the *Healthy People 2010* website at http://healthypeoplegov. Click on "Leading Health Indicators." On the next screen, click on the words. "What are the Leading Health Indicators?" Assess your family, academic community, clinical practice community, and neighborhood to see where improvements to health could be made. Outline a plan to assist family and community members to make improvements in one of the identified areas.

## WWW INTERNET RESOURCES

### For Family as Client
Children's Institute International: http://www.childrensinstitute.org.
National Clearinghouse on Child Abuse and Neglect: http://nccanch.acf.hhs.gov/.
The Hudson Institute: http://www.hudson.org/.
Center for Health Care Strategies: http://www.chcs.org/.
Children Now: http://www.childrennow.org.
Centers for Medicare & Medicaid Services: http://cms.hhs.gov.
American Academy of Pediatrics: http://www.aap.org.
March of Dimes: http://www.modimes.org/.

### For Community as Client
Healthy People 2010: http://healthypeople.gov.
Centers for Disease Control and National Immunization Program:
  http://www.cdc.gov/nip.

National Highway Traffic Safety Administration: http://www.nhtsa.dot.gov.
The Substance Abuse and Mental Health Services Administration: http://www.samhsa.gov/.

## REFERENCES

Anderson, E. T., & McFarlane, J. (2000). *Community as partner* (3rd ed.). Philadelphia: Lippincott Williams & Wilkins.

Anderson, K. H., & Tomlinson, P. S. (1992). The family health system as an emerging paradigmatic view for nursing. *Image, 24,* 57–63.

Andrews, M. & Boyle, J. (1999). *Transcultural concepts in nursing care* (3rd ed.). Philadelphia: Lippincott Williams & Wilkins.

Artinian, N. T. (1994). Selecting a model to guide family assessment. *Dimensions of Critical Care Nursing, 14,* 4–12.

Beddome, G. (1995). Community-as-client assessment. A Neuman-based guide for education and practice. In B. Neuman (Ed.), *The Neuman systems model* (3rd ed., pp. 567–579). East Norwalk, CT: Appleton & Lange.

Bullough, B., & Bullough, V. (1990). *Nursing in the community.* St. Louis: Mosby.

Capuzzi, C. (1996). Families and community health nursing. In S. M. H. Hanson & S. T. Boyd (Eds.), *Family health care nursing: Theory, practice, and research* (pp. 351–368). Philadelphia: F. A. Davis.

Chevannes, M. (1997). Nursing caring for families: Issues in a multiracial society. *Journal of Clinical Nursing, 6,* 161–167.

Christensen, P. J., & Kenney, J. W. (1990). *Nursing process: Application of conceptual models* (3rd ed.). St. Louis: Mosby.

Clark, M. J. (1999). *Nursing in the community* (3rd ed.). Stamford, CT: Appleton & Lange.

Cody, W. K. (1995). The view of family within the human becoming theory. In R. R. Parse (Ed.), *Illuminations: The human becoming theory in practice and research* (pp. 9–26). New York: National League for Nursing.

Denham, S. A. (1999). Part I: The definition and practice of family health. *Journal of Family Nursing, 5,* 133–159.

Fawcett, J. (1989). *Analysis and evaluation of conceptual models* (2nd ed.). Philadelphia: F. A. Davis.

Forchuk, C., & Dorsay, J. P. (1995). Hildegard Peplau meets family systems nursing: Innovation in theory-based practice. *Journal of Advanced Nursing, 21,* 110–115.

Friedemann, M. L. (1995). *The framework of systemic organization.* Thousand Oaks, CA: Sage.

Friedman, M. M. (1992). *Family nursing: Theory and practice* (3rd ed.). East Norwalk, CT: Appleton & Lange.

Gilliss, C. L. (1991). Family nursing research, theory and practice. *Image, 23,* 19–22.

Gilliss, C. L., Highley, B. L., Roberts, B. M., & Martinson, I. M. (1988). *Toward a science of family nursing.* Reading, MA: Addison-Wesley.

Hanchett, E. S. (1988). *Nursing frameworks and community as client.* East Norwalk, CT: Appleton & Lange.

Hanson, S. (1996). Family assessment and interventions. In S. Hanson & S. Boyd (Eds.). *Family care nursing: Theory, practice and research* (pp. 147–172). Philadelphia: F. A. Davis.

Head, B., Aquilino, M., Johnson, M., Reed, D., Maas, M., & Moorehead, S. (2004). Content validity and nursing sensitive community-level outcomes from the nursing outcomes classification (NOC). *Journal of Nursing Scholarship, 36,* 251–259.

King, I. M. (1983). King's theory of nursing. In I. W. Clements, & F. B. Roberts (Eds.), *Family health: A theoretical approach to nursing care* (pp. 147–155). New York: Wiley.

Lapp, C. A., Diemert, C. A., & Enestredt, R. (1991). Family-based practice. In K. A. Saucier (Ed.), *Perspectives in family and community health* (pp. 305–310). St. Louis: Mosby-Year Book.

Li, H., Melnyk, B., & McCann, R. (2004). Review of intervention studies of families with hospitalized elderly relatives. *Journal of Nursing Scholarship, 36,* 54–59.

Lundy, K., & Janes, S. (2001). *Community health nursing caring for the public's health.* Sudbury, MA: Jones and Bartlett.

McCarthy, N. C. (1990). Health promotion and the community. In C. L. Edelman & C. L. Mandle (Eds.), *Health promotion throughout the lifespan* (2nd ed.), 521–550. St. Louis: Mosby.

McCubbin, M. A., & McCubbin, H. I. (1993). Families coping with illness: The resiliency model of family stress, adjustment, and adaptation. In C. B. Danielson, B. Hamel-Bissell, & P. Winstead-Fry (Eds.), *Families, health, and illness: Perspectives on coping and intervention* (pp. 21–63). St. Louis: Mosby.

McElmurry, B., Park, C., & Buseh, A. (2003). The nurse-community health advocate team for urban immigrant primary health care. *Journal of Nursing Scholarship, 35,* 275–281.

McGoldrick, M., & Gerson, R. (1985). *Genograms in family assessment.* New York: Norton.

Mischke, K. M., & Hanson, S. M. H. (1995). Family health assessment and intervention. In P. J. Bomar (Ed.), *Nurses and family health promotion: Concepts, assessment, and interventions* (2nd ed., pp. 38–51). Philadelphia: Saunders.

Narsavage, G., Batchelor, H., Lindell, D., & Chen, Y. (2003). Developing personal and community learning in graduate nursing education through community engagement. *Nursing Education Perspectives, 24,* 300–305.

Neuman, B. (1983). Family interventions using the Betty Neuman health care systems model. In I. W. Clements & F. B. Roberts (Eds.), *Family health: A theoretical approach to nursing care* (pp. 218–230). New York: Wiley.

Newman, M. A. (1983). Newman's health theory. In I. W. Clements & F. B. Roberts (Eds.), *Family health: A theoretical approach to nursing care* (pp. 231–254). New York: Wiley.

Newman, M. A., Sime, A. M., & Corcoran-Perry, S. A. (1991). The focus of the discipline of nursing. *Advances in Nursing Science, 14,* 1–6.

Orem, D. E. (1983). The self-care deficit theory of nursing: A general theory. In I. W. Clements & F. B. Roberts (Eds.), *Family health: A theoretical approach to nursing care* (pp. 193–217). New York: Wiley.

Parse, R. R. (1996). The human becoming theory: Challenges in practice and research. *Nursing Science Quarterly, 9,* 55–60.

Parse, R. R. (1998). *The human becoming school of thought.* Thousand Oaks, CA: Sage.

Patterson, J. M. (1999). Healthy American families in a postmodern society: An ecological perspective. In H. M. Wallace, G. Green, K. J. Jaros, L. L. Paine, & M. Story (Eds.), *Health and welfare for families in the 21st century* (pp. 31–52). Sudbury, MA: Jones and Bartlett.

Peplau, H. (1952). *Interpersonal relations in nursing.* New York: G. P. Putnam's Sons.

Rogers, M. E. (1983). Science of unitary human beings: A paradigm for nursing. In I. W. Clements & F. B. Roberts (Eds.), *Family health: A theoretical approach to nursing care* (pp. 293–316). New York: Wiley.

Rose, L., Mallinson, K., Walton-Moss, B. (2004). Barriers to family care in psychiatric settings. *Journal of Nursing Scholarship, 36,* 39–47.

Roy, C. (1983). Roy adaptation model. In I. W. Clements & F. B. Roberts (Eds.), *Family health: A theoretical approach to nursing care* (pp. 255–278). New York: Wiley.

Saucier, K. A. (Ed.). (1991). *Perspectives in family and community health.* St. Louis: Mosby-Year Book.

Shamansky, S. L., & Pesznecker, B. (1991). A community is . . . . In B. W. Spradley (Ed.), *Readings in community health nursing* (4th ed., pp. 52–89). Philadelphia: J. B. Lippincott.

Spradley, B. W. (1990). *Community health nursing: Concepts and practice* (3rd ed.). Glenview, IL: Scott, Foresman/Little Brown Higher Education.

Taylor, S. G., & Renpenning, K. M. (1995). The practice of nursing in multiperson situations, family and community. In D. E. Orem (Ed.), *Nursing: Concepts of practice* (5th ed., pp. 348–367). St. Louis: Mosby.

Tomlinson, P. S., & Anderson, K. H. (1995). Family health and the Neuman systems model. In B. Neuman (Ed.), *The Neuman systems model* (3rd ed., pp. 133–144). East Norwalk, CT: Appleton & Lange.

Walsh, S.; Martin, S. & Schmidt, L. (2004). Testing the efficacy of a creative-arts intervention with family caregivers of patients with cancer. *Journal of Nursing Scholarship, 36,* 214–219.

Watson, J. (1996). Watson's theory of transpersonal caring. In P. H. Walker & B. Neuman (Eds.), *Blueprint for use of nursing models: Education, research, practice and administration* (pp. 141–184). New York: National League for Nursing.

Whall, A. L. (1986). *Family therapy theory for nursing: Four approaches.* East Norwalk, CT: Appleton-Century-Crofts.

Whall, A. L., & Fawcett, J. (1991). *Family theory development in nursing: State of the science and art.* Philadelphia: F. A. Davis.

Wright, L. M., & Leahey, M. (1988). Family nursing trends in academic and clinical settings. Paper presented at International Family Nursing Conference, Convention Centre, Calgary, Alberta, Canada, May 24–27, 1988, Conference Proceedings, pp. 29–37.

Zotti, M. E., Brown, P., & Stotts, R. C. (1996). Community-based nursing versus community health nursing: What does it all mean? *Nursing Outlook, 44,* 211–217.

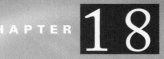

# The Professional Nurse's Role in Teaching and Learning

## KEY TERMS AND CONCEPTS

Teaching

Product

Learning

Process

Patient Education

Experts

Readiness for Learning

Validation

Feedback

Participant-Focused Teaching

Motivation

## LEARNING OUTCOMES

By the end of this chapter, the learner will be able to:

1 Provide the rationale for identifying clients and nurses as "experts" in the client education process.

2 List the three main communication concepts that facilitate teaching–learning.

3 Explain how mutuality enhances client learning.

4 Outline the steps of the traditional teaching–learning process.

5 Describe each step of the traditional teaching–learning process.

6 Outline key strategies for effective client education.

7 Specify ways to validate client learning.

## VIGNETTE

Lillian works as a staff nurse in a small rural community hospital. Frequently, she takes care of persons with poorly controlled diabetes, cancer, chronic obstructive pulmonary disease, back injuries, and a variety of conditions corrected with surgery. During her last performance evaluation, the nurse manager suggested that Lillian improve her patient teaching skills. Lillian acknowledges that her performance in client teaching could be improved. However, Lillian feels that client education is very time-consuming and that she must concentrate on providing safe, effective nursing care to clients who are physically unstable. Her heavy workload and unanticipated dismissals prevent Lillian from spending as much time teaching clients and families. She knows that improved client education may prevent recurrent hospital admissions and promote the general health of clients and families. She wonders how she can deliver effective education to clients and families while frequently being the only registered nurse on her unit.

Teaching has been accepted as a leadership role for professional nurses for decades, even before the development of nursing models on which nurses could base their practices. **Teaching** is a process of imparting or sharing knowledge with another. Teaching involves instructing, coaching, and guiding another through unfamiliar content or procedures. In 1918, the National League for Nursing Education issued a statement that expressed the need to educate professional nurses to assume teaching tasks. In earlier times and sometimes today, nurses base practice on knowledge borrowed from other disciplines, such as the medical, biologic, and social sciences. Nurses acknowledge the importance of sharing information with clients about their medical conditions, their medications, and ways to carry out their prescribed medical regimens when they are discharged from the hospital, sent home from outpatient diagnostic and surgical centers, and leave clinics and offices. Historically, patient teaching was "centered on a rather rigidly defined goal of compliance with the medical regimen" (Redman & Thomas, 1992, p. 304).

Nurses agree that clients need information from them; however, some professional nurses have learned that the content of their teaching emerges from a mutually determined process between nurse and client and that it focuses on the health of the client, rather than on the medical diagnosis. Whereas, other nurses simply follow standardized client teaching outlines found on client clinical paths or computer programs. Schlotfeldt (1988, p. 18) says that one specific function of a scholarly nursing practitioner is "teaching and guiding persons toward pursuit of their own health goals, stimulating and sometimes inspiring them toward knowledgeable pursuit of optimal health and recovery."

Teaching–learning also has been considered to be a public duty of all the professions. For example: lawyers inform clients about the law; physicians teach clients about diseases; physical therapists teach clients how to ambulate safely; social workers educate clients about available community resources; and pharmacists teach clients about medications. Like other health team members, nursing has an obligation to present educational programs and lead public discussions on issues related to health. Professional responsibility goes beyond individual professional–client teaching–learning relationships. Nursing as a professional entity has the opportunity and obligation to educate the larger client system (the public) about the relationships between quality of life and health and to influence the mission of health care delivery institutions regarding the social ends they should serve. Listening and learning from the public, the professional nurse grows in the ability to provide information that promotes health.

Likewise, many health care consumers want and need health education. Needs and wants vary according to clients. Some clients want to learn how to best promote personal health and to avoid illnesses. Other clients may not see the value of health information until they find themselves ill and in need of health care services (Rankin, Stallings, & London, 2005). When confronted with a health issue that involves early detection, some clients want to know the latest diagnostic techniques (Herzlinger, 2004). Clients also need to be aware of treatment options for health problems so they can make informed choices (Herzlinger; Rankin, Stallings, & London). Health care consumers also need to know about the complex health care delivery systems, health insurance options, available community resources, and how to ask questions of health care providers to get desired information (Herzlinger). In many cases, clients need health care information to take medications safely, comply with complex treatment regimens, avoid potential complications of prescribed therapies, and know when to consult health care providers (Herzlinger; Rankin, Stallings, & London).

Because the length of stay in inpatient client care settings has decreased, client education becomes more important in assuring client safety and to reduce the incidence of hospital readmissions (Herzlinger, 2004).

# ● PHILOSOPHICAL ASSUMPTIONS ABOUT TEACHING AND LEARNING

The description of teaching–learning as a leadership function for professional nurses is based on the beliefs that teaching–learning is a process, not a **product** (or result); the process is implemented in a relationship between experts; and communication is the essential element of the process. Clients are experts in how health issues affect them and nurses frequently have information that help clients to adjust to health alterations.

## Process—Not Product

Believing in the significance of interpersonal relationships, the nurse must consider the possibility that the health of a person is determined to a large extent by the quality of the person's relationships with other people. Through relationships, growth can occur; that is, the person integrates new functions that lead to a more satisfying life. Thus, the nurse needs to provide the client with educative experiences that increase the integration of behaviors and attitudes that improve health. Teaching–learning in the nurse–client relationship is directed toward such growth.

Defined as development to a more complex form (*The American Heritage Dictionary of the English Language*, 1992, p. 801), growth includes the development of capacity for healthy behaviors. This development of capacity occurs in teaching–learning relationships between nurses and clients. "**Learning** is a process that is dependent on an interchange between the learning individual and the environment" (Babcock & Miller, 1994, p. 22). Learning may involve skills and performance (psychomotor), feelings or beliefs (affective), or thinking (cognitive) and usually is associated with a change in behavior.

Such operations cannot occur in the client if nurses simply offer information as a product of their profession. Rather, such operations require that teaching–learning be viewed as a **process** in which the nurse offers the client information and educational experiences to learn self-care and personal growth strategies. Client education culminates with the client receiving validation from the nurse that new knowledge, ideas, or skills have developed effectively. Teaching–learning is an interpersonal process in which both the teacher and the learner acquire new information, experience new relatedness, and behave in new ways as a result of the relationship.

**Patient education** is "a process of helping someone to learn through planned sequences of teaching, supportive activity, and directed practice and reinforcement" (Redman & Thomas, 1992, p. 304). Clients are encouraged to assume responsibility for improving their health and self-care. Argyris (1982, p. 94), who believes that human beings are "self-governing and personally responsible," says that people have the ability to bring about certain consequences, have ideas about how to accomplish their intentions, and feel success or failure on the basis of their achievement or nonachievement of their intentions.

When professional nurses believe that clients have these abilities, nurses view learning as far more than discovery by the client. They define their educator role as focusing on "learning that leads to new action and new problem-solving, which enable individuals and systems to continue to learn" (Argyris, 1982, p. 160). Thus, teaching–learning becomes an ongoing dynamic process.

If learning is not the passive acceptance by the learner of information from the teacher, then nurses must commit themselves to collaborative relationships with clients to fulfill their teaching–learning role functions. This means that the teaching enables clients to participate, to define their own strengths and problems, and to construct their own meanings. Thus, teaching–learning is a collaborative process that is most effective when nurses fully engage clients as participatory learners.

## Relationship Between Experts

Teaching–learning can be viewed as a relationship between experts. **Experts** are persons who have special knowledge and skills about a particular subject (Mish, 1994). In the professional nursing process, we view nurses as the experts on health and clients as the experts on their experience of health and the circumstances of their life. In the teaching–learning process, sometimes clients and professional nurses view nurses as the experts on knowledge about health and the information that enables people to achieve health, and clients as experts on the context of their life and the need for information and experiences to achieve their intentions to maximize health.

### Nurse: Information and Knowledge Expert

Teaching–learning may be seen as a part of the healing process. Nurses who have reported that they believed their interventions made a difference in their clients' progress described several steps in that healing relationship (Benner, 1984, p. 49): mobilizing hope for the nurse as well as for the client; finding an acceptable interpretation or understanding of the illness, pain, fear, anxiety, or other stressful emotion; and assisting the client to use social, emotional, or spiritual support.

Viewing teaching as a coaching function, Benner (1984) proposes that "nurses become experts in coaching a patient through an illness. They take what is foreign and fearful to the patient and make it familiar and thus less frightening," (p. 77). The teacher also needs to have expertise in helping. Helping the learner become aware of learning and thinking processes and helping the person understand the nature of the problems may be equally as important as providing information.

To be an expert in the teaching–learning process, the nurse also must be an enabler. Learning is facilitated when teachers treat learners as responsible people. In addition, learning empowers clients to take action and assume responsibility for their health (Rankin, Stallings, & London, 2005).

In addition to coach and enabler, several other roles have been proposed for the nurse–teacher, including (Forbes, 1995, p. 99): (1) learning facilitator, who breaks down barriers to learning by listening, probing, and being aware of feelings; (2) authority, who sets up a teaching structure and rules; (3) ego ideal, who serves as a role model for the client's "altered existence"; (4) socializing agent, who acknowledges concerns and fears for the future; and (5) person, who relates to clients as people on the basis of much more than a disease diagnosis.

### Client: Context and Need Expert

No one knows better the meaning of his or her life, individual health status, and full circumstances integral to life experiences than does the client. Thus, clients serve as the experts on the context in which they will be attempting to implement new health behaviors. They are the experts on individualized needs for information, support, and relatedness. When nurses appreciate their professional expertise and the personal expertise of the client, the teaching–learning process can truly be implemented as a mutual responsibility.

## Questions for Reflection 18-1

1. How do I involve my clients and families during health teaching?
2. How frequently do I teach clients/families/communities about things that promote health?
3. What types of education strategies do I tend to use when providing client/family/community education?
4. What factors in my current working environment support my role as a client teacher?
5. What factors in my current practice environment prevent me from providing effective client education?

The Joint Commission on Accreditation of Healthcare Organizations (JCAHO) has developed standards for client and family education as an essential element of nursing. According to JCAHO (1996), the purpose of patient education is to convey knowledge and understanding, create a different perspective or attitude, build self-care skills, and change behavior. Standards for education set by JCAHO (1996, 1998, and 1999, 1999a) include the following:

1. Comprehensive learner assessment before education occurs (ability, readiness, literacy, preferences, cultural or language obstacles, physical or mental limitations).
2. Age and academic level appropriate teaching.
3. Education on safe and effective use of medications, medical equipment, potential food–drug medication interactions, therapeutic diets, and rehabilitation techniques.
4. Information on available community resources and how to obtain additional treatment (if needed).
5. Education on client and family responsibilities for ongoing health care needs and the knowledge and skills on how to fulfill these responsibilities.
6. Education on basic personal hygiene when needed with due respect for client privacy.
7. Educational strategies that are interactive, provide detailed instructions, and present available resources for future use.
8. Use of collaborative educational approaches involving interdisciplinary health care team members and the client and family.

JCAHO standards provide a framework for nurses to follow as they plan and execute client educational activities. When providing clients with printed materials, nurses should consider client ability to read. Frequently, published printed and posted Internet educational materials are written above the average reading level of Americans (Anhang, Goodman, Goldie, 2004; Murphy, Chesson, Berman, Arnold, Galloway, 2001; Singh, 2000; Singh, 2003).

### Research Brief 18-1

Singh, J. (2003). Reading grade level and readability of printed cancer education material. *Oncology Nursing Forum, 30,* 867.

The investigator analyzed ten cancer educational brochures targeted to inform the public from the American Cancer Society, The Association for Brain Tumor Research, Channing Bete Company, Leukemia and Lymphoma Society of America, and the National Institutes of Health. Using the Simple Measure of Gobbledygook (SMOG) and the Readability Assessment Instrument (RAIN), the researcher found that the brochures were written between the ninth- and fifteenth-grade reading levels. The current average reading ability of Americans is at the eighth-grade level.

Results of this study reveal that persons reading cancer brochures may need help from others to understand them. Nurses may need to simplify language and sentence structure of printed cancer brochures if given as part of client education. Because of the low number of cancer brochures that were analyzed, nurses cannot assume that all published cancer educational materials are too difficult for clients to comprehend. However, other studies analyzing printed materials and those posted on the Internet related to various disease processes tend to suggest that many client educational materials are indeed too difficult for clients to understand. More research is needed to determine if most cancer publications are written at too high of a reading level and what interventions may be useful in alleviating the problem or assisting clients to understand material contained in them.

Because JCAHO accreditation is required for federal reimbursement to organizations for delivered care, documentation of client education becomes very important. In addition to documenting client education for reimbursement purposes, the professional nurse provides solid evidence of nursing's contributions to the interdisciplinary client care efforts. Documentation of education also may provide useful information regarding specific communication strategies that work well with individual clients and families.

## Communication: The Condition for Teaching–Learning

The nurse who displays empathy, respect, mutuality, and genuineness while teaching is likely to set the stage for effective teaching–learning sessions. The nurse needs empathy to understand the client's situation and to take full advantage of the expertise the client brings to the relationship. The client needs empathy to perceive that the nurse is sensitive to the client's human needs and to reinforce that the client is able to act as a full human being.

If the teaching–learning process is to be accepted by both the nurse and the client as a mutual responsibility, respect must be experienced in the communication between the two. The perception of self-worth is based on this respect, and an enhanced sense of self-worth facilitates both teaching and learning.

Full exploration and analysis of the health concerns and information needed to change behaviors cannot occur unless both the nurse and the client perceive each other as real, as genuinely human, open, honest, and caring in their responses to each other. The nurse must provide the client with accurate health-related information, and the client must perceive that the nurse has information to facilitate health promotion, maintenance, or restoration. The client must display an authentic interest in what information will be shared with him or her by the nurse. The client determines if and when information received in a nurse–client educational encounter will be used.

Nurses empower clients to have control over their lives when they give them information or teach them skills to care for themselves. Rankin, Stallings, and London (2005) outline the following four-step counseling model for empowering individual clients: (1) identify the problem or issue (past), (2) explore feelings and meanings (present), (3) identify goals and choices (plan for the future), and (4) commit to action (future) (p. 75).

To identify the problem or issue and its impact on the client, the nurse uses holistic assessment skills. Once the issue or problem has been identified, the nurse uses the nursing process step of planning to specify goals and strategies to resolve the problem or issue in collaboration with the client. Once the client has committed to action, the change process begins.

## ● THE TRADITIONAL TEACHING–LEARNING PROCESS

The traditional process for organizing teaching–learning into a specific framework that has been accepted as both workable and traditional is presented first, followed by a discussion of other approaches implied in advocacy and change theory. The activities in this process are assessment, planning, implementation, evaluation, and documentation. The synthesis of the process in practice is diagrammed in Figure 18-1.

The first activity on the part of the nurse–teacher is assessment: to gather facts and information that will help the nurse meet the client's or the family's needs for learning. Rankin, Stallings, and London (2005) indicate that there are four steps in the assessment process: (1) selecting the areas to be assessed; (2) gathering the data; (3) sorting and categorizing the data; and (4) writing a summary statement (nursing diagnosis). Purposes of assessment can be found in Display 18-1 (Rankin, Stallings, & London, 2005; Redman, 1993).

The assessment may be conducted by using the following behaviors: listening and questioning, observing, reviewing records, collaborating with the health care team, and

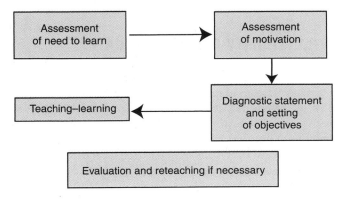

**Figure 18-1**
The process of teaching (from Redman, B. K. [1993]. *The process of patient education* [7th ed., p. 12]. St. Louis: Mosby–Year Book. Used with permission of the publisher.)

| Purposes of Client Assessment for Education | DISPLAY 18-1 ● |
|---|---|

1. Identify what the client wants to learn.
2. Identify what information the client needs.
3. Establish a point of reference for learning (relate new information to preexisting knowledge).
4. Identify incorrect information and assumptions.
5. Determine what factors in the environment may pose barriers.
6. Identify potential client barrier to learning (language, cultural, educational level, cognitive or physical limitations).

7. Identify what will need to be evaluated.
8. Build trust and rapport.
9. Provide for involvement of family.
10. Set priorities for the needs and problems.

*Source:* Rankin, Stallings, & London, 2005; Redman, 1993.

integrating the client's verbal description with the nurse's observation. To fully understand the impact of the issue to be addressed in the educational process, the nurse must engage in active listening and validate perceptions with the client.

After determining the learning needs in the assessment stage, the nurse develops a plan that contains objectives for the client's learning that have been established together with the client and the family. These objectives clarify what is to be taught, what is to be learned, what and how to evaluate, and what to document. An objective must be singular to be specific, inclusive of all elements of content necessary to be understood, measurable, and realistic to the extent that it can be attained by the client.

After objectives are clarified and validated in the plan, implementation of the learning objectives is done by analyzing the information to be presented and selecting a method of presentation that maximizes the involvement of the client's senses. The nurse often can complement the presentation of information by using supplemental materials, such as audiovisual aids. Another major function of the nurse in the implementation phase is to observe the client's reaction to the teaching–learning.

In evaluation, the next activity in the teaching–learning process, the nurse and client determine whether or not the client has achieved the objectives. The criteria used in evaluation are the specifications of what the client will do and the particular behavior that the client will demonstrate, which are stated in each objective. The outcomes must be recorded on the client's official record. Using the objectives as a basis, the nurse should record client achievements and note client reactions on the record.

## ● TEACHING–LEARNING AS A RESPONSIBILITY OF THE ADVOCATE

The belief in advocacy as an appropriate role of the nurse has evolved in harmony with a larger social movement characterized by consumerism, self-care, justice and human rights, equal opportunity for all, and individual accountability for health. People no longer believe that illness is an event over which the person has no control. Given these values, nurses today readily accept the obligation to act as advocates in their relationships with clients. One of the most significant activities of the nurse advocate is to provide informational support to assist the client to make the wisest possible decisions in the pursuit of well-being.

## The Purpose of Teaching–Learning

The search for meaning in the nursing process should be focused on the client's perception of his health situation. The phenomenologic model of curriculum proposed by Diekelmann (1988) fits the role conception of the nurse as an advocate for the client. In this model, "the central concern is the communicative understandings of meanings given by people who live within the situation" (Diekelmann, p. 142). Thus, the purpose for teaching–learning is to provide the opportunity for the nurse and the client to explore together the importance and meaning of the client's experience.

Applying Diekelmann's proposition, the essential aspect of the process is not transmitting or acquiring facts; rather, it is "making meaning and giving meaning . . . through the initiation and maintenance of dialogue" (Diekelmann, 1988, p. 143). In addition, Diekelmann (p. 143) proposes that the teacher's role is to "link the contextual and conceptual worlds of students," who are, in this discussion, clients participating in the nursing process. In this kind of dialogue, clients retain the authority and responsibility for their decisions and health behaviors.

According to Babcock and Miller (1994), if nurses expect clients to take interdependent and independent responsibilities for decision making, they need nurses who can identify central issues, recognize underlying assumptions, recognize evidence of bias and emotion, solve problems, and think creatively.

The development of these abilities appears in definitions of critical thinking, an essential skill for effective professional nursing practice. In client education situations, nurses guide the client to master knowledge and skills that are needed to make decisions. As clients begin to make informed choices for health and health care–related decisions, they look to professional nurses for support.

## Functions of the Advocate in the Teaching–Learning Process

Providing the opportunity for dialogue to fully explore health concerns is the major function of the nurse acting as an advocate for clients, whether they are experiencing high or low levels of wellness. Within this exploration, nurses use their expertise to "not only offer information [but also] offer ways of being, ways of coping, and even new possibilities" for the clients (Benner, 1984, p. 78).

Benner (1984) proposes that teaching–learning transactions take on new dimensions when the learner (client) is ill. She cites the following competencies necessary for the nurse to assume the teaching–coaching function with a client who is ill:

1. Carefully time the interventions to capture the client's readiness to learn.
2. Help the client integrate the implications of the illness and recovery into the client's lifestyle.
3. Elicit and respect the client's interpretation of the illness.
4. Respond fully and cogently to the client's request for explanation of what is happening (within the limits of both the client's and the nurse's own understanding).
5. Make approachable and understandable any culturally avoided or uncharted aspects of an illness by exploring ways of being and coping for the client and the family and by identifying new possibilities.

Growth through learning is maximized if the nurse fulfills these functions with the client.

### Mutuality in the Teaching–Learning Process

One of the primary characteristics of an advocate–client relationship is mutuality. Watson (1988, p. 4), supporting the concept of mutuality, stresses that nurses must "shift from oppressive interactions to liberating interactions." In her view, both the teacher and the student should be learners, rather than simply "givers of information" (Watson, p. 4). Learning should be mutual, characterized by anticipatory–participatory behaviors, shared power, and the absence of separation of "doing from knowing and being" (Watson, p. 2). Watson's model of nursing is cited as one example of a model that mandates mutuality in the nursing process and places high priority on teaching–learning as a significant intervention mode in a reciprocal nurse–client relationship.

Mutuality can be defined as "a connection with or understanding of another that facilitates a dynamic process of joint exchange between people. The process of being mutual is characterized by a sense of unfolding action that is shared in common, a sense of moving toward a common goal, and a sense of satisfaction for all involved" (Henson, 1997, p. 80). Mutuality balances power and respect, encourages accountability, and "facilitates active involvement of both nurses and clients in effectively working toward mutually identified goals" (Henson, p. 77). Mutuality is consistent with any learning theory used to guide the teaching–learning process.

**Questions for Reflection 18-2**

1. Have I ever learned anything from a client, client family, or community? If so, what did I learn?
2. How do I feel when a client or family members learn a new skill or finally grasps key information regarding self-care for the first time?
3. How do I promote active participation by clients, families and communities in the client education process?
4. Why is active participation important in the teaching–learning process?

##  LEARNING THEORIES

The process by which learning occurs has been described in several different ways. Learning theories and models explain how people learn. When nurses use models and theories to guide the client education process, they can use principles to structure meaningful client educational experiences, prevent overloading clients with information, and understand reasons for unsuccessful client education encounters. In client education, educational effort should be focused on learners (client, families, significant other, communities).

### Learning Models

Bruner (1986) cites five popular models of how the learner learns: empiricism, hypothesis generator, nativism, constructivism, and novice-to-expert. Empiricism is considered the oldest model. It is based on the premise that "one learns from experience" and that "such order as there is in the mind is a reflection of the order that exists in the world" (Bruner, p. 199). People need life experience for success in educational situations based on empiricism.

Unlike the rather passive view of the empiricism model, the hypothesis generator models include a major premise of intentionality. "The learner, rather than being the creature of experience, selects that which is to enter" (Bruner, 1986, p. 199). The characteristic of the learner is "active curiosity guided by self-directed projects" (Bruner, p. 199). A person is a successful learner in this model if the person has a good theory from which hypotheses are generated.

The nativism model proposes that the mind is innately shaped by "a set of underlying categories, hypotheses," both forms of organizing experiences (Bruner, p. 199). The task of the learner in this model is to develop a way of organizing perceived reality. Using the innate powers of the mind is the formula for successful learning in this model.

The constructivism model was developed primarily by Piaget, who, according to Bruner (1986, p. 199), states that "the world is not found, but made, and according to a set of structural rules that are imposed on the flow of experience." These structural rules provide boundaries for learning. The learner goes through stage-like progressions characterized by tension between previously assimilated structural rules and changes in the rules that come in later stage development. In accommodating these new rules, the learner is successful if his or her learning structure changes by moving to higher systems that subsume earlier structures.

The newest of the learner models, according to Bruner (1986), is the novice-to-expert model. It "begins with the premise that if you want to find out about learning, ask first about what is to be learned, find an expert who does it well, and then look at the novice and figure out how he or she can get there" (Bruner, p. 199). In this model, the formula for success is to be specific and explicit in taking the steps to attain expertise.

Bruner (1986, p. 200) suggests that there is not just one kind of learning and that we would be better served if we understood that "the model of the learner is not fixed but various." When nurses appreciate the diversity in learner models, teaching–learning becomes "more than a scripted exercise in cultural rigidity" (Bruner, p. 200). In many health care organizations, nurses use standardized teaching guides and frequently documentation consists of checking off items on a list. Nurses who use Bruner's learner models individualize client education, thereby maximizing client mastery of desired outcomes.

## Types of Learning

Bevis (1988, p. 40) offers a helpful differentiation of six types of learning that may be useful in the teaching–learning process (see Display 18-2). Bevis suggests that different educational approaches work best for different types of learning.

Bevis (1988, p. 45) suggests that syntactic learning, contextual learning, and inquiry learning are necessary for change that can truly maximize the client's abilities to gain the best control of his or her health. Syntactic, contextual, and inquiry learning incorporate personal meaning, cultural considerations, and discovery in the client education process rather than approaching learning as an exercise in mastery of relationships, rules, and logic.

## Types of Learning

DISPLAY 18-2

1. Item learning: simple relationships between separate pieces of information, as seen in mechanistic and ritualistic lists and procedures
2. Directive learning: rules, injunctions, and exceptions, as seen in safety requirements
3. Rational learning: use of theory to buttress action, enabling logical decision making and logical judgments
4. Syntactic learning: seeing meaningful wholes, relationships, and patterns "addresses the lived moment and the relationships that ideas, concepts, have with each other" and enables the learner to develop insights and find meaning
5. Contextual learning: acceptance of culture, mores, folkways, rites, and rituals as ways of being; these learning transactions are "caring, compassionate, and positive"
6. Inquiry learning: investigating, categorizing, and theorizing in a way to generate ideas and develop a vision

*Source:* Bevis, 1988, p. 40.

### Principles of Learning

Principles identified by Babcock and Miller (1994) are considered useful in any of these learner models or types of learning. These principles to guide the nurse in the teaching–learning process are listed in Display 18-3.

## Principles to Guide in the Teaching–Learning Process

DISPLAY 18-3

1. Focusing intensifies learning.
2. Repetition enhances learning.
3. Learner control increases learning.
4. Active participation is necessary for learning.
5. Learning styles vary.
6. Organization promotes learning.
7. Association is necessary to learning.
8. Imitation is a method of learning.
9. Motivation strengthens learning.
10. Spacing new material facilitates learning.
11. Recency influences retention.
12. Primacy affects retention.
13. Arousal influences attention.
14. Accurate and prompt feedback enhances learning.
15. Application of new learning in a variety of contexts broadens the generalization of that learning.
16. The learner's biologic, psychological, sociologic, and cultural realities shape the learner's perception of the learning experience.

*Source:* Babcock & Miller, 1994, pp. 45–48.

In addition, because clients vary in individual learning preferences, the professional nurse needs to understand the multiple models and types of learning to personalize the teaching–learning process effectively. Effectiveness is measured by the success the nurse and client experience in changing the client's health behaviors in a positive direction.

### Questions for Reflection 18-3

1. How do I assess clients for preferred learning styles?
2. How do I learn best? Why is it important for me to know my preferred learning style?

# ● IMPLICATIONS OF CHANGE THEORY ON TEACHING–LEARNING

Growth is inherent in the definition of learning. Growth implies that change occurs. Because change is about the only thing that occurs constantly, change, growth, and learning happen continuously throughout life. Desired outcomes of education are changes in behavior, attitude, and psychomotor abilities (Bloom, 1974).

## Change as a Goal of Teaching: Growth

The mutually determined goal of the nurse and the client who are participating in the teaching–learning process is "becoming different than before" (Douglass, 1988, p. 226). Douglass notes that forces that influence change can be external or internal. The nurse is an intentional external force assisting the client to demonstrate different and better health behaviors.

In a series of sequential steps that are consistent with planned change theory, the nurse in the teaching–learning relationship needs to follow the list shown in Display 18-4 (Douglass, 1988). The sequential steps mirror nursing process because the initial step is exploring and identifying factors for the change (assessment), determining specific knowledge gaps (diagnosis), selecting an educational strategy (planning), executing the strategy (implementation), and determining the overall results (evaluation).

## Outcomes of Knowledge Acquisition

The outcome of knowledge acquisition in the teaching–learning process may not always be satisfying to the nurse and client. Harmony within the human system results when the newly acquired information is congruent with previously integrated functions. However, if the new information is incompatible with previously integrated functions, clients and nurses may perceive disharmony in the human system. Feelings of being

---

### Sequential Steps Consistent with Planned Change Theory

DISPLAY 18-4 ●

1. Explore the client's perceived need for change.
2. Identify the forces for change with the client.
3. Help the client state health concerns.
4. Identify constraints and opportunities in the situation.
5. Provide the information needed to analyze both the change needs and the potential strategies to achieve the desired change.
6. Critique each of the possible change strategies on the basis of both the information understood and the situational factors.
7. Select the change strategy to be attempted in the effort to achieve a different and better health behavior.

8. Plan the implementation, filling in all of the informational gaps perceived by the nurse and the client.
9. Design an evaluation process to determine success in changing health behavior.
10. Client: Implement the planned behavioral activities.
    Nurse: Offer feedback and facilitate opportunities in the delivery system environment to promote success of the client.
11. Evaluate the overall results of the teaching–learning interaction and the specific health behavior changes on the part of the client.

*Source:* Douglass, 1988, pp. 226–232.

unsettled, restless, and uncertain frequently accompany periods of growth. Nurses often need to help clients understand that change may not be a painless process.

O'Connor (1986, p. 52) advises that the nurse and the client should analyze the "situational context of a proposed change," taking into account "the individuals involved, the institutional climate, and societal trends." She also suggests that the nurse and client need to analyze their motivation to work on the planned change in terms of "potential threats to or fulfillment of basic human needs" (O'Connor, p. 54). Both the situational context and the motivational aspects of planned change play a significant role in the client's ability to integrate information and develop new behaviors. The quality of the integration of new functions from the new information is affected by the perceived harmony or disharmony in the system.

For example, a single, working mother with newly diagnosed diabetes has many learning needs. In today's fast-paced society, eating regularly scheduled meals, making appointments for follow-up, securing insulin administration supplies, performing blood sugar checks, and performing special foot care may be difficult as she juggles multiple roles. Unless the client understands the benefits of controlling glucose levels, she may put taking care of herself behind caring for her children. The nurse needs to fully assess all learning needs for the client while considering the impact of lifestyle changes for optimal management of diabetes.

## Readiness for Learning

A central issue for professional nurses in implementing the teaching–learning process as a strategy for changing behaviors is the client's **readiness for learning**. Benner (1984, p. 79) notes that teaching–learning interventions often are dictated by schedules in the health care delivery environment: "Assessing where a patient is, how open he is to information, deciding when to go ahead even when the patient does not appear ready, are key aspects of effective patient teaching."

Nurses frequently find themselves pressured to implement client teaching, especially in inpatient settings when they become aware of an unanticipated client dismissal. In the case of the woman with newly diagnosed diabetes, the nurse must decide where to begin and how to give the woman all the information she needs to know to test her blood sugar; administer insulin; know the significance of hyperglycemia and hypoglycemia; realize the complications of poor glucose control, and understand the role of diet, exercise, and medication on glucose control (Hurxthal, 1988). The dilemma is that the client needs the information to safely control her blood sugar at home, yet in the current, acute situation she is overwhelmed and unlikely to absorb more than a limited amount of information. Quick assessment needs to be done to determine how simple or complex the teaching can be. Priorities have to be made, such as always keeping in mind that the client "must be safe until he can learn to be proficient [and that] meal timing is more important than meal content" (Hurxthal, p. 1099).

Most persons undergoing surgery and receiving new diagnoses frequently experience anxiety. Thus, learning readiness must be evaluated in terms of the degree of anxiety the client expresses. Minimal anxiety serves as a positive force for attention, alertness, or awareness, all of which are necessary for learning and integration of function to occur. Moderate anxiety usually is associated with selective inattention and decreasing awareness; extreme anxiety is associated with lack of attention and loss of awareness.

Moderate or extreme anxiety usually is an indicator of the client's lack of readiness for learning. In these two anxiety states, the nurse's focus needs to be on reducing anxiety to enable the client to regain a sense of security and repossess the energy required for attention and awareness, which are prerequisites for learning (Rankin, Stallings, & London, 2005).

## Validating Learning: Feedback

Validation is a necessary element of teaching–learning. **Validation** is a process of confirmation. In client education, validation means that the client understands the educational material, has mastered a particular health care skill, or uses the new information or skill effectively. For a behavioral change to become well integrated, it must be validated by persons significant to the client. Throughout life, a person requires validation through feedback from significant others to maintain the integrity of his or her self-system. Nurses frequently play a significant role in clients' lives. As teachers, nurses share their knowledge and expertise with clients. Learners appreciate feedback from teachers (Milde, 1988). **Feedback** is the transmission of information regarding how well learning outcomes are being met by learners. Frequently, constructive feedback stimulates learners to want to learn more. In client education, nurse feedback provides clients (and families) with specific information on how well they have learned information and skills to care for themselves (Rankin, Stallings, & London, 2005).

Through research, Milde (1988) found that groups who received both verbal and visual feedback on prescribed performance in a teaching–learning situation achieved at a higher level than did those who received only verbal feedback. Although the subjects in this study were student nurses, nurses in practice might find value in replicating this study to determine the value of visual feedback on client integration of new and desired health behaviors.

## ● STRATEGIES FOR EFFECTIVE TEACHING AND LEARNING

Nurses use many strategies and resources for effective client education. When nurses tailor the strategy to fit client-preferred learning styles, teaching is more effective. The subsequent discussion presents some (not all) strategies that may be used in planning and executing client education.

## Focus on the Participants

In today's fast-paced delivery of health care, nurses frequently use standardized teaching plans. However, **participant-focused teaching** focuses on individual client learning needs and preferences. Client education works better when nurses and clients involved in the teaching–learning process know about each other. What does the nurse (teacher) need to know about the client (learner)? Fine (1988, p. 70), drawing from recommendations from a consumer health policy group, suggests that nurses individually and collectively provide "their standards of education and training, standards of practice, licensure standards, . . . anticipated treatment outcomes of health providers, as well as the varied classifications of health care providers." She specifically advises that "each primary care nurse should present the patient or patient's family with a professional card that has appropriate concise information, stating his or her professional degrees, certification, and scope of practice" (Fine, p. 70). In addition to providing these credentials to the client, the nurse should communicate clearly her intentions in the teaching–learning process, share a clear plan of the times she will commit to the client, and establish how additional contact can be established if the client feels the need to do so.

For effective instruction, the professional should know the following information about clients involved in the education process: (1) how the client perceives the health situation; (2) what limits or opportunities may be expected on the nurse's activities with the client in terms of other providers' plans for the client or other providers' assessment of the client's health status that may not be clear to the client; (3) what the client's conscious intentions and desires are regarding health behaviors; and (4) what information the client perceives that is needed to achieve the client's health goals. With this basic information, nurses and clients should be able to engage fully in the teaching–learning process.

## Motivational Strategies

There are many teaching strategies to enhance the client's **motivation** (stimulus) to participate in learning, only a few of which are mentioned in this chapter. Additional motivational teaching strategies may be found in books devoted to teaching strategies.

In 1995, Theis and Johnson synthesized the existing research examining teaching strategies and found "66% of subjects receiving planned teaching had better outcomes than did control group subjects receiving routine care" (p. 100). The literature review revealed that structured approaches, reinforcement, independent study, and multiple strategies appeared to be the most effective teaching strategies. Other teaching strategies are included in Display 18-5 (Babcock & Miller, 1994; Rankin, Stallings, & London, 2005; Redman, 1993).

Motivation for learning is enhanced if the student and the teacher trust and respect each other; the teacher assumes and expects that the student can learn; the teacher is sensitive to the student's individual needs; and both the student and the teacher feel free to learn and make mistakes in their own unique styles. Boswell, Pichert, Lorenz, and Schlundt (1990) reinforce the idea that active participation in learning is a strong motivator. Display 18-6 gives effective motivating strategies for learning, as defined by Bevis (1988, p. 45).

---

**Other Teaching Strategies**                          DISPLAY 18-5 ⬤

1. Computer-based instruction materials
2. Observation and assessment scales
3. Demonstration
4. Lecture/discussion
5. Modeling
6. Programmed instruction
7. Role playing

8. Group activities
9. Use of media (posters, flip charts, overhead projections, videotapes, audiotapes, film)
10. Games and simulations

*Source:* Babcock & Miller, 1994; Rankin, Stallings & London, 2005; Redman, 1993.

---

**Effective Motivating Strategies for Learning**　　　　**DISPLAY 18-6** ●

1. Engaging the learner in active analysis
2. Raising questions
3. Nurturing
4. Finding ways to make the learning meaningful and significant for the learner
5. Following the ethical ideal in giving clients all the information they need to make sound choices
6. Displaying a caring attitude
7. Using and encouraging creativity in the teaching–learning process
8. Encouraging curiosity and the search for satisfying ideas
9. Being assertive
10. Desiring to engage in and to seek dialogue

*Source:* Bevis, 1988, p. 45.

---

### Contextual Constraints and Opportunities

Some contextual constraints, such as the dilemma of insufficient time and great need on the part of the client, have been mentioned. To attempt to control the environmental constraints that might be imposed on the teaching–learning process, the nurse should keep the following teaching strategies in mind: (1) try to arrange learning experiences when the learner feels relatively healthy; (2) provide time for learning at a comfortable pace; (3) have sufficient grasp of the subject matter to translate concepts into different terms for different learners; and (4) make sure expectations and standards are clear.

Bruner (1986, p. 198) suggests that educators need to assist learners to perceive the value of the rich diversity in the world. He encourages them to view the learner as "equipped to discriminate and deal differentially with a wide variety of possible worlds exhibiting different conditions, yet worlds in which one can cope." The nurse should perhaps heed this advice and have confidence in the client's ability to mutually participate in teaching–learning and to succeed in a diverse world, rather than trying to control all the contextual constraints that might interfere with learning. Power sharing would be more likely by nurses with this confidence in clients. Perceived abilities and learning are more likely in such relationships.

### ● SPECIFIC CLIENT EDUCATION ACTIVITIES

Many routine nursing activities involve client (and family) education. When clients enter a health care institution, they frequently need instructions related to their expected role responsibilities. Health care professionals cannot deliver effective care unless clients are willing to provide them with information related to health problems and educational needs. During an initial client encounter, the professional nurse may learn more about the client needs and concerns, and the client actually assumes the role of teacher. To plan effective nursing care, the nurse needs to understand the client's perspective of the health problem or illness. Additional information related to specific care needs (special adaptive devices, cultural concerns) usually also surface during the initial encounter.

Nurses also assume the role of educator when they inform clients and families of the purposes behind nursing interventions and rationale for administered medications. Educational efforts such as these enable clients to understand the reasons behind care activities and learn why they must comply with the ordered medical regimen. Most teaching related to medication administration reinforces information clients have received from physicians. However, sometimes, as in the case of a client with newly diagnosed diabetes, the physician delegates the task of teaching insulin administration to a professional nurse or certified diabetic educator (who usually is a professional nurse). Educating families of unconscious or dysphagic patients to not attempt to give them food or fluids by mouth can help prevent the problem of aspiration pneumonia.

Sometimes the roles of educator and client advocate become intertwined. As a client advocate, the professional nurse frequently verifies that patients understand procedures that are about to happen. Nurses frequently obtain signatures on consent forms before clients undergo invasive procedures. Informed consent requires that the client is competent, has had other treatment options disclosed to him or her, understands the treatment/test and its potential adverse effects, volunteers for the procedure without coercion, and consents to having the procedure performed (Beauchamp & Childress, 1994). Nursing process is used to determine the multiple elements of informed consent. When assessing for the elements required for informed consent, questions related to the procedure may arise. The nurse who answers them engages in the process of client education. However, if the nurse discovers that the client fails to fully understand the anticipated procedure, the role of educator ceases, and the nurse assumes the role of advocate informing the physician of an inability to obtain a signature on a consent form because the client fails to understand the risks and benefits of the invasive procedure.

Professional nurses also participate in community health education. Successful community education starts with the participation of community members. Professional nurses secure community input when planning community education programs by performing a needs assessment. In a manner similar to that used to identify individual client learning needs, the nurse asks community members to identify community learning needs. Methods for performing a needs assessment include individual interviews, informal polls, focus groups, or written surveys. Key community leaders must also be asked to identify group learning needs to assure successful program development and implementation. Once a learning need has been identified, professional nurses secure credible resources and financial support for the program. Financial support may be secured in the form of grants, corporate sponsorships, or from the community. Involvement of community members during the program planning process increases the chance that the program will appeal to community members. Teaching strategies that appeal to individual clients (videos, slides, flip charts) may be highly effective for community education. However, the teaching strategies must consider the projected number of persons who will attend the program (Rankin, Stallings, & London, 2005).

Not all client education occurs in a formalized setting, such as a health care organization or community agency. Professional nurses reside in neighborhoods and are members of families. Family members, neighbors, and friends frequently consult the professional nurse when health care concerns or questions about a health condition arise. Sometimes, the questions fall within the realm of the professional nurse's area of expertise; other times they do not. Directing family, friends, and acquaintances to credible resources sometimes poses a great challenge for the professional nurse. As more persons use the Internet as a source of health information, the professional nurse should become aware of various websites and be able to assess the quality of information posted on each site. Professional nurses have an obligation to share accurate health-related information or refer the question or concern to another health team member when unable to provide the requested information.

Rankin, Stallings, and London (2005) and Smeltzer (2005) outline several factors that distinguish credible from less reputable information for client education and care. Hallmarks of suitable and unsuitable information are outlined in Table 18-1. The process of peer review increases the credibility of the information because the information has been appraised by experts in the field. Before suggesting materials for client education, nurses must review them to verify accuracy, readability, and ease of use.

**TABLE 18-1**

## Determining Suitability of Information for Client Education

| Suitable Sources | Unsuitable Sources |
|---|---|
| Peer reviewed | Use secondary sources of information |
| Primary source of information | May use editorial ideas as facts |
| Known experts in a field | Advertise products or information for sale |
| Editorial ideas clearly documented as such | Websites not updated on a regular basis |
| Government and higher education sources | No review of content by medical experts |
| Recognized nonprofit organizations for disease processes (e.g., American Cancer Society, Multiple Sclerosis Society) | For-profit organizations |
| Professional nursing organizations | Nonprofit organizations displaying narrow viewpoints |
| Websites updated on a regular schedule | High reading level required |
| Clearly delineate editorials, and advertisements from objective information | For elderly and visually impaired: print smaller than 12-point font |
| Display biographical information of all content authors (academic and professional credentials) as well as relationship to the organization | Websites that are poorly designed or are directly linked to advertising firms (automatic pop-up ads come when site accessed) |
| Disclaimer present that sends clients to physicians or other health care providers for their specific use | No disclaimer statement to warn clients of the need to consult with a health care provider to meet specific needs |
| Open disclosures if funds from companies were used to develop the study or website | |
| Hyperlinks to reports of original studies or primary sources of information | |
| Website design easy to navigate in order to reach desired information (internal search engines very helpful) | |
| Options for persons who do not read English | |

*Source:* Rankin, S., Stallings, K., & London, F. (2005). *Patient education in health and illness.* (5th ed., pp. 280–282). Philadelphia: Lippincott Williams & Wilkins. Smeltzer, S. (2005). Is that information safe for patient care? *Nursing 2005, 35,* 54–55.

## CLIENT EDUCATION AS AN INTERDISCIPLINARY PROCESS

Along with nurses, other members of the health care team make significant contributions to client education. Because nurses tend to spend more time with clients than other providers, they have the opportunity to assess client learning needs and responses to health teaching implemented by other team members. The nurse also has the ability to determine if the client has the capability to absorb teaching from other disciplines. Thus, the nurse may suggest that other health team members (such as dietitians, physical therapists, social workers, or pharmacists) refrain from educational activities until clients are in physically stable condition and emotionally ready to benefit from detailed education for self-care.

In addition to determining the best times for client education, the nurse has the responsibility to coordinate educational activities and to verify that clients receive the same information from all health team members. Documentation of teaching by all disciplines (including nursing) serves as a key so that instructions from one discipline can be effectively reinforced. Documented teaching content also may eliminate duplicated teaching efforts and provide a detailed record to meet JCAHO standards for client education and for third-party reimbursement.

Within the past decade, nurses have participated in the development of client care paths. Care paths designate specific client educational activities so that client education does not occur haphazardly or at the last minute when the physician writes a dismissal order. Some institutions have formed multidisciplinary educational committees to develop guidelines for client education and identify continuing educational needs for the entire health care team.

## SUMMARY AND SIGNIFICANCE TO PRACTICE

Teaching–learning is presented as a process among experts, the teacher, and the learner, in which all acquire new information, experience new relatedness, and behave in new ways as a result of the interaction. The nurse–teacher is an expert on health, and the client–learner is an expert on the client's experience of health and life circumstances. Before recommending educational materials for clients, professional nurses must assess them for suitability. For teaching to be an empowering process for the client, the nurse must consider the clients as individuals with experiences and preferred learning styles that have implications for planning and implementing client-teaching activities.

Teaching is an essential role of the nurse as advocate. When the nurse acts as an advocate, mutuality characterizes the teaching–learning process. Frequently, nurses may learn from clients, even though nurses may be seen as the health care expert. Clients more readily assume responsibility for managing their health when they understand their health problems and learn ways to manage them. Because the nurse spends prolonged time with clients and families, the professional nurse assumes a leadership role in planning activities for and evaluating client and family responses to health education delivered by a multidisciplinary team. Effective listening and setting up an environment for meaningful dialogue enhances the teaching–learning process with individual clients or in the community.

## FROM THEORY TO PRACTICE

1. Reread the vignette at the front of the chapter. Using the information that you have read in the chapter, answer the following questions:
   a. What are the barriers encountered by Lillian to provide effective client education?
   b. What are the consequences when clients are dismissed without receiving detailed education about medications, diet, activity, and follow-up health care?
   c. What suggestions could Lillian make to the hospital to improve client education? What potential barriers might prevent Lillian's suggestions from being implemented? How would these suggestions be financed?
2. After reading this chapter, what ideas will you incorporate into your client education in clinical practice? Why are these ideas important?

## WWW INTERNET EXERCISES

1. Look up a health topic of your interest using a general search engine found in your Internet software program. Scan the first ten websites that you can view from the results of your search. How many of these sites are trying to sell a product or products? How many of the sites are nonprofit organizations? How many of the sites are sponsored by a national or local government agency? Compare the quality of each website. Which websites would you recommend to clients for health information? Why or why not? Which sites would you use for personal health information? Why or why not?
2. Visit one of the recommended Internet websites listed in Internet Resources. Which sites contain health-teaching materials in more than one language? Print out information that you would like to use for client teaching and bring it to class. Analyze the information according to the following criteria:
   • Readability
   • Visual appeal
   • Accuracy of information
   • Ability to sustain interest and actively engage the learner.
3. What types of policies does your current work setting have related to distribution of Internet resources for client education? Describe the materials for client education in your current work setting. Select a topic for which you frequently provide client/family education. Obtain your organization's teaching materials on this topic. Search the Internet to find teaching materials on the same topic. Compare and contrast the two resources.

# INTERNET RESOURCES

The Joint Commission on Accreditation of Healthcare Organizations: http://www.jcaho.org.

American Medical Association: http://www.ama-assn.org.

American Cancer Society: http://www.cancer.org.

American Academy of Family Practitioners: http://www.aafp.org

Lab Tests Online: http://www.labtestsonline.org.

NOAH: http://www.noah-health.org.

American Heart Association: http://www.americanheart.org.

National Institutes of Health: http://www.nih.gov.

Cancer Control Planet: http://www.cancercontrolplanet.cancer.gov

National Women's Health Information Center: http://www.4woman.gov/.

Office of Minority Health Resource Center: http://www.omhrc.gov.

Centers for Disease Control: http://www.cdc.gov.

Health Information Quality Assessment Tool: http://hitiweb.mitretek.org/iq/begguide.asp.

Canadian Women's Health Network: http://www.cwhn.ca/indexeng.html.

# REFERENCES

Anhang, R., Goodman, A., & Goldie, S. (2004). HPV Communication: Review of existing research and recommendations for patient education. *CA A Cancer Journal for Clinicians, 54,* 248–259.

Argyris, C. (1982). *Reasoning, learning, and action: Individual and organizational.* San Francisco: Jossey-Bass.

Babcock, D. E., & Miller. M. A. (1994). *Client education: Theory and practice.* St. Louis: Mosby-Year Book.

Beauchamp, T. L., & Childress, J. (1994). *Principles of biomedical ethics* (4th ed.). New York: Oxford.

Benner, P. (1984). *From novice to expert.* Menlo Park, CA: Addison-Wesley.

Bevis, E. O. (1988). New directions for a new age. In National League for Nursing, *Curriculum revolution: Mandate for change* (pp. 27–52). New York: National League for Nursing.

Bloom, B. (Ed.) (1974). *Taxonomy of educational objectives.* New York: D. McKay.

Boswell, E. J., Pichert, J. W., Lorenz, R. A., & Schlundt, D. G. (1990). Training health care professionals to enhance their patient teaching skills. *Journal of Nursing Staff Development, 6,* 233–239.

Bruner, J. (1986). Models of the learner. *Education Horizons, 64,* 197–200.

Diekelmann, N. (1988). Curriculum revolution: A theoretical and philosophical mandate for change. In National League for Nursing, *Curriculum revolution: Mandate for change* (pp. 137–158). New York: National League for Nursing.

Douglass, L. M. (1988). *The effective nurse: Leader and manager* (3rd ed.). St. Louis: Mosby.

Fine, R. B. (1988). Consumerism and information: Power and confusion. *Nursing Administration Quarterly, 12,* 66–73.

Forbes, K. E. (1995). Please, more than just the facts. *Clinical Nurse Specialist, 9,* 99.

Henson, R. H. (1997). Analysis of the concept of mutuality. *Image, 29,* 77–81.

Herzlinger, R. (2004). *Consumer-driven health care.* San Francisco: Jossey-Bass.

Hurxthal, K. (1988). Quick! Teach this patient about insulin. *American Journal of Nursing, 88,* 1097–1100.

Joint Commission on Accreditation of Healthcare Organizations (JCAHO). (1996). *Educating hospital patients and their families, examples of compliance.* Oakbrook Terrace, IL: Author.

Joint Commission on Accreditation of Healthcare Organizations (JCAHO). (1998). *Comprehensive accreditation manual for hospitals: The official handbook.* Oakbrook Terrace, IL: Author.

Joint Commission on Accreditation of Healthcare Organizations (JCAHO). (1999). *Assessing patient learning needs.* Oakbrook Terrace, IL: Author.

Joint Commission on Accreditation of Healthcare Organizations (JCAHO). (1999a). *Nursing: Hospital examples of compliance for patient-focused standards*. Oakbrook Terrace, IL: Author.

Milde, F. K. (1988). The function of feedback in psychomotor-skill learning. *Western Journal of Nursing Research, 10*, 425–434.

Mish, F. (Ed.) (1994). *Merriam Webster's Collegiate Dictionary* (10th ed.). Springfield, MA: Merriam-Webster.

Murphy, P. W., Chesson, A. L., Berman, S. A., Arnold, C. L., & Galloway, G. (2001). Neurology patient education materials: Do our educational aids fit our patients' needs? *Journal of Neuroscience Nursing, 33,* 99–104.

O'Connor, A. B. (1986). *Nursing staff development and continuing education*. Boston: Little, Brown.

Rankin, S., Stallings, K., & London, F. (2005). *Patient education in health and illness* (5th ed.). Philadelphia: Lippincott Williams & Wilkins.

Redman, B. K. (1993). *The process of patient education* (7th ed.). St. Louis: Mosby-Year Book.

Redman, B. K., & Thomas, S. A. (1992). Patient teaching. In G. M. Bulechek & J. C. McCloskey (Eds.), *Nursing interventions: Essential nursing treatments* (2nd ed., pp. 304–314). Philadelphia: WB Saunders.

Schlotfeldt, R. M. (1988). The scholarly nursing practitioner. In *Alternate conceptions of work and society: Implications for professional nursing* (pp. 15–30). Washington, DC: American Association of Colleges of Nursing.

Singh, J. (2000). Readability of HIV/AIDS educational materials. *AIDS Education and Prevention, 12,* 214–224.

Singh, J. (2003). Research briefs reading grade level and readability of printed cancer education materials. *Oncology Nursing Forum, 30,* 867–870.

Smeltzer, S. (2005). Is that information safe for patient care? *Nursing, 35*, 54–55.

*The American heritage dictionary of the English language* (3rd ed.). (1992). Boston: Houghton Mifflin.

Theis, S. L., & Johnson, J. H. (1995). Strategies for teaching patients: A meta-analysis. *Clinical Nurse Specialist, 9,* 100–105.

Watson, J. (1988). A case study: Curriculum in transition. In National League for Nursing, *Curriculum revolution: Mandate for change* (pp. 1–8). New York: National League for Nursing.

# CHAPTER 19

# Leadership and Management in Professional Nursing

## KEY TERMS AND CONCEPTS

Management
Leaders
Managers
Formal Leaders
Informal Leaders
Leadership and Management Skills
Leadership
Transformational Leadership
Interpersonal Leadership
Empowerment
Leadership Development
Empowered Caring
Strategic Plan
Budgeting
Staffing
Marketing
Change
Change Agent
Habits of Effective Leaders
Criteria for Evaluating Leadership

## LEARNING OUTCOMES

By the end of this chapter, the learner will be able to:

1 Explain contemporary thoughts about the concepts of leadership and management.

2 Compare and contrast the concepts of leadership and management.

3 Identify the essential habits of effective leaders.

4 Outline the strengths of a feminine approach to leadership.

5 Discuss methods the nurse leaders and managers can use to balance task accomplishments with interpersonal relationships.

6 Specify the value of empowering others and oneself in professional nursing relationships.

7 Specify how nurses use leadership and management skills as they assume various professional nursing roles.

8 Explain how professional nurses can become effective leaders and managers.

9 Outline criteria to evaluate leadership effectiveness.

Alice is a registered nurse who works in a hospital as a staff nurse. While attending a Parent/Teacher Association (PTA) meeting at her daughter's school, she learned that the school does not have a nurse on the premises during school hours. At the last meeting, many parents voiced numerous complaints related to the current school policies regarding student health care and the current curriculum addressing personal health and hygiene. The PTA forms a task force. Because Alice is a registered nurse (even though she graduated from school a year ago), the task force elects Alice to serve as the chairperson. Uncomfortable with her new community leadership position, Alice decides that she needs to read about principles of leadership. Fortunately, she finds her nursing leadership textbook that she used in her undergraduate-nursing program on her bookshelf.

### Questions for Reflection 19-1

1. How would I feel if I were in Alice's position?
2. Do you think that the task force made a wise decision in selecting Alice as their leader? Why or why not?
3. Why do you think that the task force wanted Alice to spearhead their efforts?
4. What would you do if you found yourself in a similar situation?

Distinguishing leadership and management is difficult because, in the business literature, the terms are used interchangeably. The concepts of leadership and management have evolved. Leaders are persons who have the ability to influence others. The concepts of leader and manager overlap. **Leaders** influence others. Effective leaders view things more globally, create visions of what might be, inspire others, tolerate chaos and ambiguity, do not fear taking risks, and work with others in a more connected way. **Managers** receive their title usually because they have a position within an organization. Managers tend to focus energy and efforts to assure smooth workflow and efficient use of resources to meet the objectives of the organization. Relationships between managers and subordinates are usually defined by organizational culture or administrative policies. Effective managers and leaders possess expertise in working with people, understanding organizations as being authentic, and pursuing work with passion (Covey, 2004). Ineffective managers usually tend toward using power to control subordinates, make independent decisions, and tend to emphasize getting the work done with the least possible expense. **Formal leaders** are persons who hold a position of power (either in an organization or workplace). **Informal leaders** are persons who do not hold a recognized position within an organization (or workplace) but influence others to act in a certain manner (Donnelly, 2003). In the vignette, Alice became the chair of the task force because the PTA members elected her to assume to a formal leadership position.

This chapter explores various perspectives of leadership and management. All professional nurses are leaders because they influence others. Nurses influence clients and other members of the health care team as they assume the roles of caregiver, colleague, client advocate, counselor–teacher, critical thinker, change agent, and coordinator.

A strong knowledge base of **leadership and management skills** enhances the ability of professional nurses to influence clients to make optimal choices regarding health and other members of the interdisciplinary health care team to provide the best client care.

## ● CONCEPTUAL AND THEORETICAL APPROACHES TO NURSING LEADERSHIP AND MANAGEMENT

**Leadership** may be defined as a process of "influencing individuals or groups to take an active part in the process of achieving agreed-upon goals" (Epstein, 1982, p. 2). Transactional outcomes, "in which relationships with followers are based upon an exchange for some resource valued by the follower" (Trofino, 1995, p. 45), were emphasized in these definitions. **Transformational leadership** emphasizes the notion of inspiring and empowering others to create and work toward attaining what is possible (Burns, 1978). Bass (1998) describes transformational leaders as those who are admired and emulated by their followers, provide meaningful and challenging work, question assumptions when making decisions and drawing conclusion, and serve willingly as mentors to others.

### Perceptions of Power and Empowerment

The ideas of mutuality, empowerment, and transformation as key elements of leadership surfaced in the late 1970s (Burns, 1978). These ideas correspond to a feminist approach to leadership because more emphasis is placed on "power with" rather than "power over" a more masculine approach toward the world (Noddings, 1984). However, the widespread use of these ideas about leadership became popular in the 1990s. Table 19-1 presents some currently used leadership theories and classifies them according to their approach to the use of power. The theories provide an explanation for how persons in management and leadership positions act in given situations. In addition, persons in leadership positions can use them to determine the best methods to use for attainment of the mission (or goals). Leaders choose which theory to use based on their philosophical beliefs and the nature of a given situation. For example, Alice, the nurse in charge of the task force, may decide that she needs to analyze the situation and the followers before deciding what approaches may work best for the task force deliberations. Thus, she is more likely to use strategies from the contingency, path-goal, or situational theories.

### Questions for Reflection 19-2

1. Think of your current manager (or faculty member if unemployed). Which of the following leadership theories do you suppose they use to motivate workers (or students)? Why do you think that they use the identified leadership theory?
2. Identify a situation in which a masculine approach to power would best get the mission accomplished. Why would this approach be best in the identified situation?
3. List the pros and cons of masculine and feminine approaches to use of power. Which approach would best fit clinical practice situations? Why?

TABLE 19-1

## A Feminist or Masculine Approach: Contemporary Management and Leadership Theories

| Theory Name | Theory Creator(s) | Key Principles | Approach to Leadership/Management |
|---|---|---|---|
| Leadership styles | White, R. & Lippitt, R. (1960) | The style of the leader affects worker performance. Three basic leadership styles were identified: | |
| | | *Authoritarian:* Leader exercises great control to get the work done | Authoritarian: masculine |
| | | *Democratic:* Leader and group work together to get things accomplished | Democratic: more feminine than masculine |
| | | *Laissez-faire:* Leader abstains from leading and lets subordinates lead themselves | Laissez-faire: feminine to empower workers, but no attention paid to relationships |
| Theory X | McGregor, D. (1960) | The manager must control, direct, and motivate workers by offering rewards or threatening punishment <br> Workers avoid responsibility and seek security <br> Workers cannot be trusted | Masculine |
| Theory Y | McGregor, D. (1960) | Managers can trust workers to do the best possible job <br> Workers value their work, are motivated by rewards, contribute to the organization, and derive satisfaction from meeting goals. Workers can solve work-related problems with their own initiative and creativity <br> Managers can create an environment to increase worker commitment and self-direction | Feminine |
| Managerial grid model | Blake, R., & Morton, J. (1964) | Five basic leadership styles based on balancing concern for task and concern for people: | |
| | | *Impoverished: :* Low concern for task and persons | Impoverished uses neither. |
| | | *Produce or Perish*: High concern for tasks with low concern for persons | Produce or perish: masculine |
| | | *Country club*: High concern for persons with low concern for tasks | Country club: feminine |

*(continued)*

## A Feminist or Masculine Approach: Contemporary Management and Leadership Theories (Continued)

| Theory Name | Theory Creator(s) | Key Principles | Approach to Leadership/Management |
|---|---|---|---|
| Managerial grid model (continued) | Blake, R., & Morton, J. (1964) | *Middle of the road*: Balanced, but not high concern for persons or tasks<br>*Team:* High concern for persons and tasks | Middle of the road: poor use of both<br><br>Team: feminine |
| Be–know–do | The United States Army (2004) | Leaders influence other people by providing them with purpose, direction, and motivation while operating to achieve the mission and improve the organization. Effective performance is the result of transforming human potential<br>To be a leader means to have values and attributes of a leader (loyalty, duty, respect, selfless service, honor, integrity, and personal courage)<br>To know involves knowledge and mastery of interpersonal, conceptual, technical, and tactical skills<br>To do means to live out the values, use knowledge and skills to influence others to achieve the mission, and improving the organization by providing everyone with purpose, meaning, and motivation<br>High level of trust among soldiers and officers<br>Officers have a duty to protect their subordinates and subordinates have a duty to follow orders issued by officers | Masculine |
| Theory Z | Ouchi, W. (1981) | Leaders share responsibility with workers<br>Leaders match work with employee strengths<br>Work processes are designed and work problems are solved by using quality circles where workers and managers have equal status<br>Democracy and consensus building are the ways decisions are made. However, leaders consider the long-term effects to evaluate management decisions | Feminine |

## A Feminist or Masculine Approach: Contemporary Management and Leadership Theories (Continued)

| Theory Name | Theory Creator(s) | Key Principles | Approach to Leadership/Management |
|---|---|---|---|
| Contingency Leadership | Fieldler, F. (1967) | A leader selects a particular leadership style to best fit a given situation that includes the nature of staff–leader relationships, formal position of the leader, and the nature of the task | Masculine or feminine depending of the style of leadership selected by the leader to fit the specific situation. |
| Leader Participation Model | Vroom, V. & Yetton, P. (1973) | Leaders choose from the following three leadership styles: autocratic, consultative, or participative when needing to make decisions. The leader uses a list of questions to analyze the environmental contingencies that may affect the quality of the decision made | Autocratic: masculine<br>Consultative: primarily masculine<br>Participative: primarily feminine |
| Transformational Leadership | Burns, J. (1978) | Identifies two types of leaders: transactional leaders who maintain daily operations using rewards to motivate subordinates; transformational leaders who inspire and empower everyone with the vision of what could be possible. The transformational leader has a high level of trust, gets others to share common values and mission, shows a committed work ethic, defines reality, keeps the dream alive, examines effects of actions, and makes adjustments as needed | Transactional leaders use the masculine approach<br><br>Transformational leaders use the feminine approach |
| Path–goal theory | House, R. & Mitchell, T. (1974) | Leaders coach, guide, and reward staff to select the best paths to meet organizational goals. Achievement-oriented approaches are used to set challenging goals for competent followers<br>A directive style is used to set expectations and operational methods for followers<br>A participative style is used when the leader wants follower suggestions<br>A supportive style is used to build follower trust and confidence | Achievement-oriented and directive approaches use the masculine approach<br><br><br>The participative approach uses a more feminine approach<br>The supportive style blends the masculine and feminine approaches |

*(continued)*

## A Feminist or Masculine Approach: Contemporary Management and Leadership Theories (Continued)

| Theory Name | Theory Creator(s) | Key Principles | Approach to Leadership/Management |
|---|---|---|---|
| Situational Theory | Hershey, P. &, Blanchard, K. (1977) | The leader selects from four styles of leadership while considering the following three dimensions of a situation: (1) the amount of direction required, (2) specific factors about the situation, and (3) the maturity of followers | |
| | | Telling: High task/low relationship (leader needs to be in command in a situation with one correct response) | Telling: masculine |
| | | Selling: High task/high relationship (leader has most of the controls but assists followers to boost confidence) | Selling: masculine |
| | | Participating: High relationship/low task (leader and followers share decision making) | Participating: primarily feminine |
| | | Delegating: Low task/low relationship (leaders assume the follower are competent and are capable of assuming full responsibility for the decision or task) | Delegating: feminine |
| Transforming Leadership | Anderson, T. (1998) | "Transforming leadership is vision, planning, communication, and creative action that has a positive unifying effect on a group of people around a set of clear values and beliefs to accomplish a clear set of measurable goals. This transforming approach simultaneously impacts the personal development and corporate productivity of all involved" (p. 270). Transforming leadership anticipates future trends; develops new leaders; assesses, plans and implements organizational-wide leadership and self-leadership development programs; and creates a community within the | Primarily feminine |

## A Feminist or Masculine Approach: Contemporary Management and Leadership Theories (Continued)

| Theory Name | Theory Creator(s) | Key Principles | Approach to Leadership/Management |
|---|---|---|---|
| | | organization. The leader uses communication, counseling, and consulting to create the organizational community | |
| Authentic Leadership | George, B. (2003) | Leadership is not about style, but rather it is about authenticity. Five qualities of authentic leaders are "understanding their purpose, practicing solid values, leading with heart, establishing connected relationship, and demonstrating self-discipline" (p. 18). Leadership is more effective when the leader leads a balanced life with authenticity in each of life aspects | Feminine |
| Servant Leadership | Greenleaf, R. (1977) | Leaders use their values to empower workers by providing them with all the needed resources and an environment that enables each one to achieve their maximal potential. The top priority for the leader is to serve others (employees, customers, and the community) | Feminine |
| Quantum Leadership | Porter-O'Grady first presented the idea in 1997. Porter-O'Grady, T. & Malloch, K. (2003) | Leaders use systems thinking to thrive in a world of complexity that is constantly changing. The leader uses personal insight and skills to facilitate change. Leaders become vulnerable when they take risks and stretch themselves to attain new possibilities. The leader and group work together to attain a collective mindfulness where all have keen awareness of significant details, catch errors before they occur, and all have the freedom to use shared expertise to create a sustaining community | Feminine |
| Trait theories | Evolved in the early history of man | Leaders are born. They inherit characteristics that make them suitable as leaders | Either, depending on how the leader uses power |

Mutuality empowerment and transformation serve as hallmarks of contemporary leadership. Manfredi (1994, p. 51) describes leadership as "an interactive process directed toward mutual goal achievement of leader and follower." Taking issue with the term "follower" as being submissive and inactive, Rost (1994, p. 3) defines leadership as "an influence relationship among leaders and collaborators who intend real changes that reflect their mutual purposes." Gurka (1995) emphasizes change, innovation, and commitment to the growth of self and others. Covey (1996) proposes that today's leaders must combine personal values and visions to develop a strategic pathway, align organizational resources and processes to fulfill the mission and vision, and empower persons to attain the common vision and mission. Leaders create a vision that inspires commitment and empowers people by sharing authority. They are not satisfied with transactional outcomes; rather, they want to be transformational, thereby changing individuals, organizations, and societies.

According to Covey (1989, p. 222), the real test of **interpersonal leadership** is the leader's ability to permit others to validate their own lives and the ability to "bring most people to a realization that they will win more of what they want by going for what you both want." In transformational leadership, there is "mutual learning, mutual influence, mutual benefits" (Covey, p. 216). Donnelly (2003) notes that all definitions of leadership contain the following elements: "relationship, context, purpose and accountability" (p. 40).

For example, in the vignette, Alice has assumed a leadership position and as she works toward improving the health services and education offered to students in the school district (purpose), she will have to focus much of her efforts on relationship building, such as getting to know persons on the task force; understanding the relationships among task force members; and cultivate relationships with others who affect student health education and services (school board, school administrators, teachers responsible for health education, students, and parents).

Along with establishing and maintaining effective relationships with involved persons, Alice must identify the basic components of the context within which she and task force members will work. The PTA established the goal or mission for the group (to improve student health education and services). As chairperson, Alice needs to spend some time analyzing the subgroups that comprise the task force as well as assessing capabilities of individual task force members. After learning a bit about each task force member, she can better determine which members can assume various tasks, roles, and responsibilities. Based on her assessment, she may want to work on ways to empower each member to use specific knowledge and talents to change student health programs.

## Leadership as a Process of Empowerment

Perceptions of power and power relationships have changed markedly in recent years. Who will control changes in the future—who will have power—is being redefined (Toffler, 1990). Noting that the rules of the power game are changing and that the nature of power is being revolutionized, Toffler (pp. 7–8) declares that the heyday of physician dominance in health care is over, noting that physicians no longer can keep "a tight choke-hold on medical knowledge." No longer is the prescription written in a secret code (Latin); no longer are the medical journals and texts restricted to physicians alone; no longer is the information about health and medicine inaccessible to nonprofessional people. Rather, anyone can purchase the state-of-the-art information on drugs, the *Physician's Desk Reference* (either in book or computerized form); anyone can tune into video versions of material from the *Journal of the American Medical Association*; anyone can find information from medical journals (such as *The New England Journal of Medicine*) in the newspapers; and anyone with a personal computer and Internet access can access databases such as *Index Medicus* and obtain scientific papers on almost any topic. Clearly, "as knowledge is redistributed, so, too, is the power based on it" (Toffler, p. 8).

Porter-O'Grady and Malloch (2003) propose that power has conflicting connotations. People can think of power in terms of coercion and domination or influence and strength. They view that each person has power and that "the legitimate exercise of power is a right that belongs to everyone" (p.120). Instead of centralizing power to persons in administrative positions or decentralizing it to an elite group, Porter-O'Grady and Malloch suggest that power should be shared by all (decentralized) so that all persons can use their expertise in delivering client care. This power shift provides all nurses with a real opportunity to become full-fledged professionals. By sharing knowledge and expertise with others, nurses empower clients, families, and communities.

Blanchard, Carlos, and Randolph (1996) perceive **empowerment** as a releasing of the knowledge, experience, and motivation that people already possess, rather than giving power to them. They have identified three keys to empower persons within organizations. Sharing information with everyone is the first key. When people receive information, especially sensitive, privileged information, they feel they are trusted by administration. In addition, they feel compelled to act responsibly. The second key requires the creation of autonomy through boundaries. The following boundary areas create autonomy: organizational purpose, values, image, goals, roles, structure, and system. When this key is used, individuals within an organization translate the organizational vision into roles and goals that have personal meaning. Replacing the traditional organizational hierarchy with self-directed teams is the third and final key. Workers assume responsibility for entire work processes and products. This includes planning, performing, managing, and evaluating the work from beginning to end (Blanchard et al., 1996).

Empowering leadership gives energy to the work of nursing. This energy empowers the nurse and the client in the professional process. Thus, empowerment is an outcome of leadership. Bennis (1989, p. 23) says that empowerment is evident in the four themes (adapted for nursing) shown in Display 19-1.

---

## Empowerment Themes Related to Nursing Leadership    DISPLAY 19-1 ✦

1. People feel significant. All feel that they make a difference and that what they do has meaning and significance. In the nursing process, the nurse and the client are equal in significance; both have meaning and what they do together is mutually significant.

2. Learning and competence matter. The nurse and the client value learning and mastery. The nurse makes it clear that there is no failure, only mistakes that provide feedback and tell us what to do next.

3. People are part of a community. The nurse, the client, and other health care providers are experienced as a team, a family, a unit. A person does not have to like another to feel a sense of community (striving for a common goal).

4. Work is exciting. The nursing process is stimulating, challenging, and fun. The nurse "pulls," rather than "pushes," a client toward a goal. This pull style of influence energizes the client to "enroll in an exciting vision of the future....It motivates through identification, rather than through rewards and punishments" (Bennis, 1989, p. 23). The nurse articulates and embodies the ideals of health toward which both the nurse and the client strive.

Thus, the empowered nurse makes each person with whom they interact feel important. Along with making individuals feel important, nurses assume responsibility for maintaining professional competence and lifelong learning to stay abreast of changes within the health care arena. Professional nurse leaders also value the knowledge and skills that each person brings as part of the health care team. Finally, clients, nurses, and health team members collaborate to determine a common vision for the future, and everyone works together to attain the envisioned future.

## ⟡ LEADERSHIP DEVELOPMENT

When nurses envision themselves as leaders they embark on the journey of **leadership development**. Aspiring leaders need to realize that leadership does not automatically occur with the appointment to a managerial position, but rather leadership must be learned. Many seasoned leaders acknowledge that they went through a process before becoming effective (Barrett, 1998; Donnelly 2003; Dotlich, Noel, & Walker, 2004; Porter-O'Grady & Malloch, 2003; Van Velsor, Moxley, & Bunker, 2004). Table 19-2 outlines two different approaches for leadership development and includes examples of how a nurse might experience leadership development. Most of the approaches begin with establishing a personal mission to become a leader followed by self-analysis. Once the aspiring leaders envision the type of leader they want to become, then they engage in a process of mastering key leadership skills (or management skills if the person has assumed an administrative position within an organization).

McCauley and Van Velsor (2004) specify that leadership development occurs from a variety of experiences. Managers learn from challenging assignments, education, significant persons, hardship, and other unidentified situations. They propose that through leadership development programs, aspiring leaders learn self-management capabilities (increasing self-awareness, balancing conflicting demands, learning new skills and ideas, and developing a personal set of values for leadership). Along with personal capacity for development, novice leaders learn social capabilities (building and maintaining relationships, developing effective work groups, enhancing interpersonal communication skills, and learning how to develop other people). Finally, leaders develop work facilitation capacities by learning management skills, how to engage in strategic thought and action, increasing the ability for creative thinking, and learning how to imitate and implement change (McCauley & Van Velsor, 2004).

### Questions for Reflection 19-3

1. What steps have I taken to develop leadership in professional nursing practice?
2. Have I encountered any obstacles toward developing leadership? If I have what are they and how did I handle them?
3. What areas do I need to develop to improve my leadership abilities? Why are these areas important to develop?

TABLE 19-2

## Approaches to Leadership Development

| Barrett (1998) | Leadership Passages (Dotlich, Noel, & Walker (2004) | Professional Nurse Experience |
|---|---|---|
| Becoming a facilitator by focusing on physical, emotional, mental, and spiritual balance and aligning a personal mission, vision, and values with an organizational one | Joining an organization or company and learning the organizational culture | Finding a first nursing job, learning work expectations, and the culture of the particular nursing department as well as the culture of the larger organization the organizational culture |
| | Moving into a leadership role that results in losing one's personal identity, losing one's status as the upcoming star, and learning how to balance tasks and people | Realizing that some client care tasks particularly enjoyed must now be delegated to other persons in order to provide efficient client care |
| Becoming a collaborator by developing one's emotional intelligence; learning effective interpersonal skills; building collaboration and team spirit; accessing the intuition, creativity of others; empathizing with others; and giving and receiving effective feedback | Accepting the stretch assignment resulting in the need for overcoming feeling like a victim, coping with skepticism and hostility from others, and realizing what is not known and when to seek out other trustful team members | Accepting the position of "charge nurse" |
| | Assuming responsibility for actions by valuing the unfamiliar, displaying a resilient mentality despite setbacks, and accepting the paradoxical characteristics of the work | Taking responsibility for when the nursing unit fails to run smoothly, realizing that more tasks need to be delegated, deciding that more knowledge and practice is needed for managing coworkers effectively, and doing what is needed to improve job performance |
| Becoming a servant/ partner or wisdom/ visionary by increasing individual role awareness, understanding the role of the organization, creating a sustainable future, partnering, forming strategic alliances to attain long-lasting success, deepening and strengthening personal and professional growth as a leader | Dealing with significant failures for which one has caused or are responsible by examining decisions that resulted in the failure, sharing experience with a trusted boss, coach or advisor, reflecting on the failure and devising different actions for future situations, and rallying the energy needed for perseverance | Sharing personal frustrations with a trusted professional nurse with more experience; developing a mentoring relationship; generating alternative actions if similar situations are encountered in the future; and keeping oneself physically, emotionally and spiritually healthy to remain in professional nursing practice |

(continued)

## Approaches to Leadership Development (Continued)

| Barrett (1998) | Leadership Passages (Dotlich, Noel, and Walker (2004) | Professional Nurse Experience |
|---|---|---|
| | Coping with a bad boss or competitive coworkers by developing a strategy to manage the ineffective relationship, analyzing your reaction to the boss or peer as to what it tells you about yourself, and defining personal values | Finding effective strategies to manage an ineffective manager or jealous coworkers while learning their weaknesses mirror your own, and engaging in a process of clarifying one's personal values |
| | Losing a job or not getting an expected promotion by using the following strategies: not letting a job or event define you as a person, try to understand what occurred by contemplation, use a support network, devise a strategy to address "what next" | Engaging in conversations with other nurses who have survived similar circumstances, recognizing that professional nursing does not need to consume one's total being, and perhaps changing to a new area of professional practice (or leave the profession) |
| | Being part of an acquisition or merger | Learning new ways of working and learning a new organizational culture (this is true especially when a not-for-profit health care organization becomes part of a larger for-profit network) |
| | Living in a different country or culture | Learning alternative ways of living and working (some nurses may go on medical missions, travel abroad, relocate to a different area, or go to a different location to further their education) |
| | Finding and maintaining a meaningful balance between family and work | Achieving an effective balance between one's personal and professional lives |
| | Letting go of ambition by realizing that you do not have to be "the best" or "first," accepting that all persons cannot be the best forever, redirect energy to other things, and redefining a personal definition of achievement | Acknowledging that "perfection" in nursing is impossible, developing a meaningful professional practice, becoming more involved in things outside of nursing and realizing that others need to be educated to fill nursing positions as you and some of your colleagues consider retirement |
| | Facing personal upheaval by accepting tragedy as a means for humanization by revealing personal vulnerabilities to others, being authentic, and accepting fate and carrying on | Using personal losses and challenges to connect more effectively with clients, colleagues, and other health team members |
| | Losing faith in the system by finding meaning in one's life and current work, sponsor a protégé for a leadership position, finding fulfillment with a current project, achieving new skills, reconnecting with what originally lead you to your area of expertise | Being a mentor to a younger professional nurse, clarifying personal values, and finding joy and meaning with current professional work |

# ● KEY LEADERSHIP AND MANAGEMENT SKILLS FOR NURSES

Because of the nature of professional practice, all nurses need to develop leadership skills. Some nurse leaders hold management positions that require the development of managerial skills. Table 19-3 outlines key leadership and management skills for nurses. Nurses use many leadership skills even if they do not hold management positions. In many instances, the skills for leadership also apply to management situations. Nurses who hold informal leadership positions may not need to spend time mastering key management skills. Some of the skills that appear on the table require more attention than can be covered in this chapter. Therefore, consulting a textbook devoted to nursing leadership and management or a book devoted exclusively to one key skill might be helpful.

The subsequent discussion focuses on how leadership and management skills are used by nurses as they assume the various professional nursing roles.

# ● PROFESSIONAL NURSES AS LEADERS

Nurses use leadership and management skills to meet professional responsibilities. The professional nursing roles of critical thinker, caregiver, client advocate, change agent, counselor–teacher, coordinator, and colleague require use of many leadership and management skills. Usually, professional nurses assume more than one of the professional roles simultaneously as they engage in practice. Examples of key leadership and management skills are discussed with each presented nursing role.

## Leadership in the Role of Critical Thinker

Most nurses engage in critical thinking as they engage in all aspects of clinical practice. Critical thinking prevents nurses from blindly following physician orders and jumping to conclusions about client care situations. When nurses assume leadership positions, they use critical thinking to analyze situations, identify problems, set priorities, develop multiple possible approaches to a specific situation, and consider the consequences of a strategy before taking action. Therefore, nurses assume the role of critical thinker as they engage in each of the professional roles.

## Leadership in the Role of Caregiver

As an empowered professional nurse, the nurse assumes a leadership role as part of a collegial health team member. The professional nurse uses a holistic approach when working with client systems. To provide holistic health care, nurses use power to accomplish tasks and build relationships with others. Because client welfare serves as the main concern for professional nurses, they use power to assure that client care needs are met. Empowered nurses use power according to a feminine approach to empower clients to assume responsibility for managing their own care needs. When nurses understand levels of power, they use power more effectively. Rafael (1996) describes three levels of power as it is exercised in caring. The first level, power in ordered caring, has the following characteristics: uses a patriarchal (male supremacy) ideology; fosters separation,

TABLE 19-3

## Key Leadership and Management Skills for Nurses

| Leadership Skills | Skills for Leadership and Management | Management Skills |
| --- | --- | --- |
| Focused and intense approach to work | Expand one's self-awareness | Clarify organizational goals and expectations |
| Challenge others to expand thinking and actions | Maintain composure and a high energy level when encountering multiple competing demands (stress management) | Use established relationships to influence others in the organization |
| Deliver compelling messages | Learn from experience | Create a strong organizational culture |
| Take risks | Seek feedback from a variety of sources | Uses all incentives available to motivate others |
| Set personal goals | Find common ground with others | See that day-to-day operations are effectively executed |
| Deep, connected, and emotional involvement with followers | Demonstrate sincere empathy toward others | Set organizational goals |
| Strong concern and investment with ideas | Make self available to others | Low level of emotional involvement with employees to be fair |
| See the gestalt of situations | Ability to listen effectively | Concern with results |
| Inspire others | Express appreciation for the contributions of others toward goals | Strong investment with the organization |
| Tolerate ambiguity | Abide consistently and constantly to ethics and principles | Staff inpatient and outpatient departments |
| Tolerate diverse perspectives | Establish trust with all persons | Enhance productivity |
| | Establish and agree upon goals using collaboration | Budget to meet operations |
| | Use facts or evidence to clarify expectations rather than assumptions or rumors | Market the organization |
| | Identify rumors, clarify their truth, and dispel them if false | Reduce risks in the organization |
| | Display optimism in all situations | Write and deliver employee performance appraisals |
| | Analyze situations from multiple perspectives to identify issues and concerns | Follow organizational guidelines and procedures |
| | Network with others to identify issues and concerns that need to be addressed | |
| | Monitor the impact of change | |

## Key Leadership and Management Skills for Nurses (Continued)

| Leadership Skills | Skills for Leadership and Management | Management Skills |
|---|---|---|
| | Learn new things quickly | |
| | Set effective priorities | |
| | Generate multiple courses of action | |
| | Take decisive action but know when to change to a different course of action | |
| | Commit self to effective action plans | |
| | Attract others to assume leadership or management positions | |
| | Share power with followers/subordinates | |
| | Form alliances with key players in any given situation | |
| | Precise and consistent communication | |
| | Communicate in ways that are acceptable and clear to others | |
| | Manage resistance | |
| | Clarify roles of others and encourage them to assume a leadership role | |
| | Resolve conflicts | |
| | Motivates others to be their best | |
| | Manage the vast sea of information | |
| | Mastering computers and other high-tech equipment | |
| | Meet standards of professional nursing practice | |
| | Work to attain optimal client outcomes | |
| | Delegate tasks to others | |
| | Deconstruct 20th-century barriers and structures | |
| | Recognize future trends that will point to a need to change to meet the needs of the future | |
| | Celebrate all progress toward change to meet 21st-century health care demands | |

Adapted from Blank, W. (2001). *The 108 skills of natural born leaders*. New York: AMACOM; Donnelly, G. (2003). How leaders work: Myths and theories. In Steltzer, T. (Ed.). *Five keys to successful nursing management* (pp. 31–60). Philadelphia: Lippincott; Porter-O'Grady, T., & Malloch, K. (2003). *Quantum leadership: a textbook of new leadership*. Sudbury, MA: Jones and Barlett; McCauley, C., & Van Velsor, E. (2004). *The Center for Creative Leadership handbook of leadership development* (2nd ed.). San Francisco: Jossey-Bass.

strength, and control (esteemed properties of masculinity); relates to having control over others and nature; sustains organizational hierarchies; and is "vested in certain positions and legitimized as authority over nurses" (p. 8).

Examples include increased use of unlicensed personnel in acute care settings per the American Medical Association (AMA) recommendation for a new category of health workers known as "registered care technologists" and persistent lobbying efforts by the AMA opposing advanced practice nurses as independent primary health care providers (Rafael, 1996). Another example of ordered caring would be when nurses use behavior modification systems to reward clients for relinquishing unhealthy health habits. Unfortunately, use of power in this manner usually results in client changes only for a short duration.

At the second level, assimilated caring, power is gained through "access to male power through assimilation of male characteristics, practices, and values" (Rafael, 1996, p. 12). Assimilated caring is ethically based on "maelstrom ethics," with its emphasis on application of universal principles, such as self-determination, beneficence, and rights-based justice. As caregivers, nurses use this power level when manipulating the health care system in order to get clients access to needed services.

**Empowered caring**, the third level, has 12 characteristics, which are listed in Display 19-2. Nurses use empowered caring when they incorporate research results into daily clinical practice, share nursing knowledge with clients and other health team members, and treat clients as equal partners when planning and delivering nursing care.

When nurses use nursing process, change in client status serves as the focus for care.

Professional nurses cannot effectively promote change in client behavior if they wield power over clients. Behavioral changes emerging from such a "power" environment probably are rote, not well integrated, and exist for a short duration. Behavioral changes emerging from an "empowerment" experience are more likely to be realistic,

---

## Characteristics of Empowered Caring

**DISPLAY 19-2** ◉

1. Both sexes are publicly recognized as at least equal.
2. Credentials are a source of power. (Nurses' credentials must be equally valued and respected as those of members of other health care disciplines.)
3. Expertise is closely linked to research and credentials but also develops from practice.
4. Knowledge is distributed so that all may grow (rather than hoarding it to give a few the edge).
5. "Collegiality that values and respects the expertise and experience of other nurses" (p. 13, Rafael, 1996) and "nurturance of others in recognition that they are integral to one's own existence" (p. 14).
6. Power is based on respect for and connection with others and nature.

7. It "involves an awareness of and a commitment to change problematic social and cultural contexts" (p. 14).
8. It is not invested in a position.
9. Enabling power requires the active and equal participation of the nurse and the client in health care decisions.
10. It is "not consistent with deference to medical or administrative authority" (p. 15).
11. In a relational way of becoming, both the nurse and the client are transformed during the caring relationship (p. 15).
12. A relational ethics is contextual (i.e., may be guided by principles but is not driven by them).

*Source:* Rafael, 1996.

genuine, and well integrated (because the person has fully participated in the process), and may become habitual over an extended period.

The position has been taken that leadership in promoting change in client behavior is best accomplished through the appropriate use of authority and influence, emphasizing the empowerment of self, clients, and other providers. However, nurses also should assume power to exert professional leadership.

1. Power based on knowledge and expertise should be used to affect the organizational climate within which nurses work, using nursing knowledge to promote desirable change. For example, knowledge of Circadian rhythm theory and research on the effects of shift changes presents a strong rationale for changes in staffing patterns to avoid shift rotation. In the vignette, Alice was selected for leading the task force because of her nursing knowledge as to what children's health services should be offered.
2. Power based on legitimate right and authority should be used to affect the quality of the support systems available to the nurse in client care. For example, the staff nurse has a legitimate right to expect that administration will provide sufficient resources and assistance so that nurses' energies and time are not dissipated in activities not related to nursing.
3. Nurses can apply referent power (based on identification with the personal qualities of the nurse) to mobilize community resources in support of desired change. For example, Alice, the nurse in the vignette, has established rapport with the PTA, which turned to her to head the task force.

The professional nurse must be an activist in the work setting and in the community, setting an example of what it means to live a healthy lifestyle and be an advocate for health for all persons. When assuming the activist role, the professional nurse exercises all three power bases to improve the quality of and access to health care.

## Leadership in the Role of a Client Advocate

When assuming the role of client advocates, nurses use power on the client's behalf. The concept of client advocacy has many different meanings. To clarify the professional nursing role of client advocate, the concept of client advocacy must be explicated. The following discussion attempts to clarify the concept of client advocacy by explaining its key attributes of mutuality, facilitation, and protection.

### Meaning of Advocacy

If nurses believe that clients have a right to a nurse–client relationship based on mutuality, shared respect, consideration of information and feelings, and full participation in the problem solving related to their health and health care needs, they believe in advocacy. If nurses believe that it is their responsibility to ensure that clients have access to the health care delivery systems appropriate to their needs, they believe in advocacy. If nurses believe that clients are responsible for their health and that nurses are responsible for mobilizing and facilitating the strengths of clients in achieving the highest level of health possible, they believe in advocacy. An advocate "supports or defends someone or something and recommends or pleads in another's behalf...[and] works to change the power structure so that a situation will be improved" (Douglass, 1988, p. 259).

Nurses cannot be effective advocates unless they believe fully in their strengths and those of their peers or clients and hold themselves and their clients responsible for outcomes. Power is shared, and nurses serve as resource persons for clients or peers. Both the nurse and the client have authority and responsibility for advancing the client's health care. Because advocacy requires conviction, it is important for the nurse to overcome personal feelings and beliefs about nurses' "powerlessness" to take the first step in the process of empowerment (Richardson, 1992, p. 38).

### Key Attribute: Mutuality

Evidence is abundant that decisions made for persons by other persons without participation of those affected or those who have the expertise to make the most informed judgments are less likely to be understood or workable. Nurses have both the expertise in health and the ability to help people achieve health. Clients have the expertise in understanding and evaluating their situations; they have control of their lives and their health. It is entirely appropriate that decisions affecting health be made by the client, with full informational support, empathy, and respect from the nurse.

Mutuality means that the nurse and the client together fully describe the client's health situation, agree on the direction and nature of change that the client would like to make, explore alternative ways to achieve the mutually agreed-on goals, and work together as the client implements the changes. At this stage, the advocate makes sure that technical and informational supports are provided for the client and assist the client in gaining access to the health care services needed.

In almost every identifiable nurse–client situation, it is possible to focus on the client's strengths and to reasonably expect that the client be responsible. For example, in work with bereaved parents after the death of a child, nurses found the potential for positive growth in significant numbers (Miles & Crandall, 1983). The researchers pointed out that focusing on the growth potential in bereaved parents was in no way meant to minimize the pain of grief, but was to help them find meaning in their lives at the time.

How does emphasis on mutuality enter into this nursing situation? It is important because two essential elements of mutuality are respect and sharing. Respecting the client's right to make decisions about working on finding meaning, while emphasizing the client's ability to be responsible for him or herself, the nurse sets up a relationship based on mutuality. The nurse empathizes with the parents, showing understanding of the pain from loss, respects the strengths of the parents, and gives choices to the family as they mutually establish the goal of reducing the pain of grief and searching for meaning in their lives.

The communication process of empathy is important to understand in the advocate role because "empathy involves feelings of mutuality with another" (Olsen, 1991, p. 67). Olsen also says that "empathy can exist simply because both parties share humanity" and that "justification of another's humanity would make little sense in the way that justifications of another's actions or feelings do" (Olsen, p. 70). Thus, empathized humanity is the crux of the nurse–client relationship and the advocate's role.

The most important factor in mutuality is that the nurse and the client are seen as equally able and responsible for the outcomes of the nursing process. Their areas of expertise vary, but their authority and significance in the relationship are equal. Each person's potential can be more fully realized in a relationship characterized by mutuality.

### Key Attribute: Facilitation

The advocate assumes that every client has strengths and that the nurse's job is to help the client use those strengths to achieve the highest level of health possible. Several aspects of facilitation have been described.

Snowball (1996) suggests that emphasis on facilitation in the advocacy process requires that the advocate take responsibility to make sure the client has all the necessary information to make informed decisions and to support clients in the decisions they make. King (1984, p. 17) suggests that an effective way for the nurse to facilitate growth in self and others is through values clarification; that is, to help the client think through issues and develop a personal value system that aids decision making. Hames and Joseph (1980) suggest that facilitation is effected through helping clients understand the tasks before them; ensuring that they experience some success when they are trying to accomplish something; providing an environment that is conducive to learning (one of trust and respect); and offering information and emotional supports.

### Key Attribute: Protection

Client advocacy has been associated with an assumption that nurses have a responsibility to protect their clients. Commonly, nurses are called on to examine their roles in protecting the client's right to live or die. Bandman and Bandman (1995) report that nurses often are caught in an ethical dilemma between physicians and incurably ill or hopelessly disabled persons. The advocate must determine what actions to take in terms of protecting the client from forced treatments or withholding of treatments. Bandman and Bandman conclude that morality tends to support a client's right to live over letting others decide that the client's life is not worth living; that the welfare of others is not necessarily in conflict with a client's right to die; and that there are cases in which the nurse can legitimately decide to protect a client's wish to end life.

Perhaps the greatest need for the nurse to act as protector is the need to change a condition or situation in the health care delivery system in which the client is given inadequate care or the environment poses some hazard. Cassidy and Koroll (1994) indicate that in the current environment of cost containment, nurses may need to take the actions listed in Display 19-3. The nurse may have to take risks to fulfill these responsibilities, but risk taking is a skill associated with leadership.

However, recently it has been asked, "by what authority does the nurse assume the obligation of representing the patient's interests or preferences?" (Willard, 1996, p. 65). Also questioned is the "hero model," in which the nurse, possessing unusual strength and courage, is engaged in a socially visible struggle. This is the nurse who is described

---

**Nurses' Responsibilities in the Era of Cost Containment**    DISPLAY 19-3 ●

1. Promote access to health care
2. Protect an individual's right to make autonomous or independent life choices
3. Refrain from causing intentional injury
4. Prevent injury from occurring
5. Eliminate potential sources of injury
6. Monitor the quality of client care
7. Intervene in a nonadversarial way when harmful behaviors are observed in any health care worker

in the advocacy model, who defends patients' rights and seeks to elevate nurses' professional status in an adversarial struggle against the forces of institutional oppression (Bernal, 1992, p. 21).

Given the personal risks (Snowball, 1996) and the rigorous demands of the advocate role (Willard, 1996), it has been suggested that the client be represented by an independent advocate who is without conscious bias (Kirkpatrick, Hull, Katrabos, & Sherman, 1995).

### Challenges and Rewards of the Client Advocate Role

For nurses to effectively carry out the role of client advocate, the health care delivery system must be restructured in terms of where the nurse is placed in the total organization. In many delivery systems, advocacy efforts are challenged by the nurse's lack of equality in authority. Equality in responsibility is more likely to be evident among health care disciplines. There is agreement that each discipline assumes full responsibility and accountability for its own practice. However, as noted throughout this book, authority is more commonly dispensed in a hierarchical manner, in which nursing frequently occupies a position of disadvantage.

Thus, nurses attempting to operate as client advocates in a hierarchical system will be more effective if they learn to negotiate the hierarchy and to develop image-building strategies that promote the significance of their advocacy work. If the nurse perceives the need for equal authority to fulfill the advocate's role as important, he or she must demonstrate both the effectiveness of the advocacy work (such as improved client outcomes and the accomplishment of serving more persons at a more affordable cost) and the improvement in satisfaction and retention of nurses.

Emphasis should be placed on the knowledge and skills needed to assist clients to increase competence in assuming responsibility for their health. In such a restructured system, the nursing staff would be supported in the areas listed in Display 19-4.

Work would be viewed in terms of professional responsibilities implicit in the preceding categories. The challenge to professional nursing to restructure the work of the nurse as an advocate includes gaining acceptance of and placing emphasis on role behaviors for professional nurses. The professional nurse would be expected to perform

---

**Ways for Health Team to Promote Self-Care in Clients**　　DISPLAY 19-4 ●

1. Development of understanding of clients' responses to various threats to health and development of strategies to respond effectively to these responses
2. Refinement and further development of health promotion and illness prevention abilities, as well as restorative abilities
3. Re-evaluation of belief systems about the independent versus dependent role of clients and self
4. Assumption of collaborative responsibility for monitoring the effectiveness of the delivery system, as well as of independent responsibility for evaluating the effectiveness of the nursing interventions in responding to the client's health needs
5. Implementation of interdisciplinary dialogue, with all professional workers sharing equal responsibility and authority for meeting clients' health needs
6. Provision of opportunity for all members of the team to evaluate effectiveness in collaboration, thereby avoiding the establishment of adversary relationships

the duties listed in Display 19-5. Fulfillment of these work role behaviors reflects the professional nurse's commitment to client advocacy as a legitimate nursing role.

To restructure their working conditions, nurses must be advocates for professional colleagues and for themselves. Chapters 6 and 10 suggest that an effective method for gaining control over practice is to develop and use data as a basis for recommending changes. Data, rather than opinion, give strength. Advocacy for anyone is more effective if the advocate is working from a position of strength, armed with data and the belief that what one is trying to accomplish is not only worthwhile for oneself but is vital to the quality of care the nurse can deliver.

Public support cannot be underestimated. A public image of the nurse as competent and an appreciation of the nurse's advocacy efforts will build public support, which is one of the most powerful forces for change in society. Nursing can use the public's help to restructure the health care delivery system.

As nurses gain the respect of the public they serve, they are more likely to gain the respect of interdisciplinary peers. Such respect is necessary to change the position of nursing in the delivery system, to ensure full participation in decision making. To fulfill the responsibilities of a client advocate, the nurse must participate in decision making, which is achieved through cooperation and coalition building (Richardson, 1992) and through consensus formation and equality of participation by all involved parties. To

---

## Duties of Nurse Serving as an Advocate

DISPLAY 19-5 ●

1. Interact with the client in a manner and quantity that permits:
   a. Exploration of the client's personal responses to health or threats to health
   b. Evaluation of the environmental circumstances in which the client exists
   c. Identification of strengths and limitations
   d. Identification of resources perceived to be needed
   e. Clear allocation of responsibilities of client and nurse, which ensures the client's assumption of responsibility for health and the nurse's assumption of responsibility for the informational and interactional supports needed
2. Prepare for and implement teaching programs needed by the client
3. Update technical skills as new therapeutic techniques and equipment are made available for health care
4. Discuss beliefs about the client's abilities with professional peers in an effort to evaluate own values about independence and dependence in various states of health
5. Update nursing care plans in an effort to evaluate outcomes of nursing care

6. Participate in nursing research as a consumer and assist in nursing studies conducted in the health care setting
7. Identify all units of the delivery system that need to be involved in the client's care
8. Coordinate efforts of the multiple health care workers involved in the client's care
9. Assess the adequacy of efforts of all workers involved in care, according to the client's stated needs
10. Resolve conflicts that might occur in relation to advocacy efforts for the client by:
    a. Respecting the position of all involved
    b. Gathering data that describe the whole system of client–environment
    c. Promoting expression of conflicts
    d. Participating in the problem-solving process
    e. Allowing the client to make decisions based on data, rather than on advice from others
11. Recognize and show appreciation for the contributions of team members to the client's health care
12. Periodically discuss and evaluate the quality of the interactions of health care team members and evaluate own interpersonal effectiveness with the client and team members

summarize, as a client advocate, the nurse uses power on the client's behalf or to empower clients to make their own decisions about health.

## Leadership in the Role of Counselor-Teacher

Professional nurses provide emotional support and education to clients, which has been explained in Chapter 7 and Chapter 18.

Along with providing client support and education, nurse leaders teach and counsel colleagues. Most nurse practice acts contain a clause that states that professional nurses teach others in any basic nursing care activities. Professional nurses and institutions set basic standards for educating unlicensed care personnel. As direct supervisors, professional nurses assess educational needs of staff and design inservice education programs. Nurses serve as role models for all health team members as they work at keeping the client at the center of health care delivery. When nurses diligently follow care standards and take time with clients, other team members may see the benefits of these behaviors and incorporate them into their clinical practice.

As a member of a nursing care team, professional nurses frequently find other members of the team experiencing distress. Nurses who spend time listening to the concerns of team members offer support to them. Because of their professional knowledge and therapeutic communication skills, some nurses informally counsel coworkers and refer them to community health resources as indicated. The following example illustrates how nurses can use the role of counselor–teacher with a coworker.

Jane, a registered nurse, finds Trina, a licensed practical nurse, crying in the staff lounge. After inquiring about what is wrong, Trina tells Jane that she has found a lump in one of her breasts and is terrified. Jane provides Trina with information about the various types of breast tumors. Trina dries her eyes and asks Jane for a referral to a surgeon. Jane gives her the name of a surgeon and offers to accompany Trina to the appointment. Trina immediately makes the appointment, has her best friend accompany her, and learns that her tumor is benign.

## Leadership in the Role of Coordinator

Nurses frequently find themselves in the role of coordinator. Nurses coordinate the efforts of others to provide safe, effective client care. Nurses assume responsibility for delivering basic client care, and executing physician orders. When competing demands are placed on the client's time, nurses frequently make decisions as to which activity has priority over another.

The role of coordinator becomes more apparent when professional nurses assume management or administrative positions. Managers assume responsibility for using people, supplies, money, and systems to provide high-quality, cost-effective care. They coordinate the efforts of others so that the job is performed efficiently. To meet the challenges of management, nurse managers use a variety of skills. Key skills used by nurse managers are people skills, budgeting and financing skills, information technology skills (see Chapter 15), and quality management skills (Chapter 20). The following discussion focuses on interpersonal, budgeting, and financial skills for effective coordination of resources for client care.

## Interpersonal Skills for Nursing Management and Supervision

Nurse managers need to set expectations for their departments and then communicate them effectively to others. Effective managers strive to bring out the best in their employees. In addition, nurse managers must provide the staff with resources and support to effectively care for clients. Besides effectively communicating with staff, nurse managers must also interact with administrators, other department managers, and physicians. Strategies for developing helpful and healing relationships outlined in Chapter 7 serve as the basis for developing effective communication with staff and all members of the interdisciplinary health care team (including clients).

In most organizations, the nurse managers have the responsibility to hire and manage qualified competent staff to fulfill an organization's mission (purpose). Nurses providing client care follow professional nursing standards of care as well as organizationally approved protocols. Nurses also monitor their peers and have an obligation to report unsafe colleagues. As members of the health care team (although not a health care provider), clients (or the client's significant others) assume some responsibilities. They must provide consent to specific procedures, abide by safety rules, and communicate their needs and concerns to health care providers (including complaints of perceived substandard nursing care). Nursing administrators, managers, and supervisors need effective interpersonal skills to assure that the best possible care is given to clients by their staff.

### Empowering Team Members: Decisions by Consensus

When decisions need to be made related to problems or changes in practice, decisions by consensus rather than those made by an individual tend to work better. A major tenet of transformational leadership is to inspire and empower others to achieve the best possible future state (Burns, 1978). Professional nurses have power to empower others. When nurses use their positions to influence others to make their own decisions, nurses empower clients and other health team members. In any clinical situation, the client, client's family (or significant others), nurse, unlicensed care provider, and other professional health team members possess a unique perspective and a specific skill set that may be used to facilitate optimal client outcomes. Sharing power and responsibility for outcomes is facilitated when all stakeholders (persons who are affected by a decision) participate in the process.

Participatory decision making is successful to the extent that adequate information is available and the persons involved do not become prematurely concerned with implementing the decision. Conley and Mariano (1991, p. 5) note that the "selective use or withholding of information influences the possessors' success in persuading the group to select one alternative even though that choice may not be the most effective or appropriate for the identified problem." Such manipulation of information usually represents a conflict over power. Thus, successful participatory decision making depends on genuine respect between the partners in the relationship and a willingness to share all that is known about the concern on which they are working.

The goal in participatory decision making is to reach the decision by consensus. Although reaching consensus takes more time than other decision-making processes, persons making the decision have a commitment to execute it (Porter-O'Grady & Malloch, 2003; Burns, 1978; McCauley & Van Velsor, 2004). In most situations, generating several options for action may be more effective than generating an exhaustive list.

Singular solutions are rare in human health concerns or in work situations. To enable the client to make the wisest choice, the choice that best fits the client's personal situation, the nurse and the client must responsibly and fully explore the client's situation and all of the options available.

For example, in the nursing process between the professional nurse and the client with newly diagnosed early stage breast cancer, consensus is obtained when both the nurse and the client together have sorted and processed all the relevant data, have weighed the risks and benefits of various options, understand fully the impact of the various options on functioning, and reach a choice together that is perceived to be the most helpful in the situation (Knobf, 1990). In consensus building, the commonalities and the connectedness of varying ideas are identified. It is this sense of connectedness that enables the nurse and the client to feel empowered and to take action.

Connections and feeling connected underlie the process of consensus. When a team works together for a common goal (in health care optimal client outcomes), team cohesion is enhanced when decisions are made by consensus. Consensus means that everyone will try and implement the decision even though each person may not agree fully with it. All persons participating in the process feel that they played a significant role in decision making, especially if participants engaged in meaningful dialogue (Wesorick & Shiparski, 1997). When persons engage in meaningful conversations with each other, each person listens intently to the other and focuses completely on what is being said, clarifies if ideas are not fully understood, and ignores all distractions.

Clearly, interdependence characterizes the relationships. The nurse's value is not more important than the client's, or other members of the health care team. Even though clients are the center of health care delivery, the client's value is not more important than the value of all health care providers. In a nursing situation, the nurse and client both have a presence; both have something to say, both inspire each other, and both are respected by the other (Ahern, 1992). Both equally share accountability and responsibility for the quality of the decisions made. The nurse brings expertise in health and health care to the relationship, and the client brings expertise in his or her abilities and the context of his or her health concerns. To reach effective consensus in decision making, all of these areas of expertise must be fully explored. Although some studies indicate that both nurses (mostly women) and physicians (mostly men) use command styles, rather than participatory styles, in attempting to influence decision making by clients (Taylor, Pickens, & Geden, 1989), some researchers predict that women are more likely to use empowerment and consensus building as major strategies in helping and work relationships. Common themes and meaning between the characteristics of transformational leaders and the attributes of women who are constructed knowers are described in Table 19-4. Barker and Young indicate that constructed knowers participate in a network or web that includes caring, moral responsibility, positive self-esteem, and use of intuition and logic. Both transformational leaders and women seek to establish an environment that generates empowerment in self and/or others (1994, p. 20). Many times decisions result in change(s). Decisions made through consensus result in commitment by all parties who made the decisions to execute them. As a change agent, the professional nurse works with the client to identify when and what change is needed and helps to facilitate the desired change to promote better health and positive work environments.

**TABLE 19-4**

## Transformational Leadership and Feminine Attributes

| Transformational Leaders | Constructed Female Attributes |
|---|---|
| Relationships engaged | Relationships networked |
| Individual consideration | Caring |
| Leader as moral agent: values and needs | Moral responsibility |
| Mutual dependence/trust | Reciprocity and cooperation |
| Communication | Integration of voices |
| Builder of self-esteem | Positive self-esteem |
| Listens to intuition, balances with analysis | Use of intuition and logic |
| Empowerment | Empowerment |

*Source:* Barker, A. M., & Young, C. E. (1994). Transformational leadership: The feminist connection in postmodern organizations. *Holistic Nursing Practice, 9,* 20. Used with permission of the publisher.

### Team Building Skills

Positive work environments are enhanced when all workers display commitment to the work and work together as a cohesive team (Porter-O'Grady & Malloch, 2003; Wesorick & Shiparski, 1997). Effective teamwork enables all team members to use their skills. Effective teams have members who collaborate to set visions and goals while identifying how they will work together to attain them. Effective teamwork balances unity with diversity. If a group is too unified, new ideas and divergent thinking may become stifled. If a group has too much diversity, conflicts may impede progress toward attaining the organizational (departmental) mission (McCauley & Van Velsor, 2004)

### Strategic Planning

A **strategic plan** provides a road map for ensuring the future of an organization. Organizations must constantly change to keep pace with the ever-changing world. Fogg (1999) outlines the key elements of a strategic plan as "(1) a direction statement, (2) strategic objectives, and (3) strategic priority issues" (p. 4). Table 19-5 outlines factors within each element. Once the priority issues are identified, action plans are created to guide organizational change. Some organizations involve employee participation in the strategic planning process. Whereas, other organizations have administrative and managerial staff develop the plan and then communicate it to workers. Some organizations opt to embed departmental strategic plans into the organizational strategic plans (Fog, 1999). In health care organizations, nursing service department strategic plans become part of the overall strategic plan.

Strategic plans work best when organizations hold individuals accountable for successful implementation. To track progress toward meeting objectives outlined in a strategic plan, a means to evaluate progress must be devised. Some organizations opt for the use of interlocking scorecards to assure that strategic objectives are accomplished by all departments. Scorecards are completed at the organizational, departmental and

TABLE 19-5

## Components of the Key Elements of a Strategic Plan

| Direction Statement | Strategic Objectives | Strategic Priority Issues |
|---|---|---|
| Mission statement: purpose and why | Statements used to measure performance on the direction statements | Broad issues that should be addressed to meet a desired future state |
| Vision statement: desired future state | Scorecard that measures success on meeting intentions | Internal changes to continue to hold a competitive advantage over competitors |
| Business definition: clear and concise presentation of products, offered services, target consumers, technology, distribution of products, and service and geographical area served | Frequently addresses performance on profitability, shareholder value (if a for-profit), market position, services, quality, and innovations | Target areas upon which to develop measurable action plans |
| Competitive advantage: what makes you better than other organizations offering the same or similar services | | |
| Core competencies: key systems, assets, intellectual prowess, programs, and special skills to enhance the competitive advantage | | |
| Values/beliefs: Philosophy and values that guide organizational behavior and processes | | |

Adapted from Fogg, C. D. (1999). *Implementing your strategic plan.* New York: AMACOM.

individual levels. Components of a scorecard include the key strategic measurement methods, and annual action steps. When the annual action steps do not happen, the organization holds persons responsible for their implementation. Managers hold individual employees responsible and the organization holds the manager responsible for departmental progress. In some instances, managers have faced demotion (or termination) and employees have been terminated for failing to take actions outlined by a strategic plan (Fogg, 1999).

### Budgeting Skills

To implement a personal or organizational mission, resources must be acquired, mobilized, and used. Human and material resources are required to provide health care services. In addition, clients must come to a facility or providers must go to clients. Viability of a health care organization (large medical center to the smallest office or clinic) relies on effective use of human and material resources.

**Budgeting** serves a process to plan for operations required to attain an organizational (or personal) mission. For example, acquiring the resources needed to go to school required planning, determining the amount of money needed to finance educational costs, and developing a plan to verify that all personal responsibilities could be met. Likewise, an organization must be certain that it has the capital and people to meet its mission effectively. The planning phase of the budgeting process is not an exact science, but rather a process in which nurses in management positions look at the current direction of health care, anticipate what future services may be needed, and make decisions based on sound business principles and education. The staffing budget projects the amount of money and the number of nursing personnel needed to provide safe, effective client care. Nurse managers use critical thinking skills when developing departmental budgets. The budget for staff includes staff salaries and fringe benefits. To assure that needed equipment is available to execute client care, nurse managers also submit capital expenditure and supply budgets (Hunt, 2003). Capital expenditures include material resources that are expensive and have a projected lifespan (e.g., cardiac monitors, intravenous [IV] pumps, computers). The supply budget consists of inexpensive items that are used for a short time (e.g., IV tubing, syringes, dressings, Foley catheters, paper, pens, etc.).

Once the budget is approved by a governing body (e.g., Board of Directors), nurse managers compare actual spending to the projected amounts outlined in budget reports. Periodic review of reports enables nurse managers to control excessive spending. Nurse managers must account for budgeting variances. For example, more money was spent on nurses' salaries than projected on a cardiac unit. The nurse manager must discover why this occurred and then justify the reason for the variance (Hunt, 2003). The nurse manager must identify the reasons for the increase in expenditures for staff salaries (e.g., increased number of cardiac procedures requiring overnight hospitalization, new cardiologist on the medical staff) and submit an action plan if the reasons fall into the realm of things that can be controlled at the unit level (abuse of employee sick time, employees working too slowly, or nurses not effectively delegating tasks to unlicensed personnel).

### Staffing

Seeing that enough nurses are available to deliver client care seems to be one of the most challenging tasks for nurse managers. The **staffing** process involves finding qualified persons to fill positions, and proving to the finance department how many persons are needed to provide quality nursing care. Many staffing plans use the full-time equivalent (FTE) model to develop staffing plans. A FTE is defined as a person who would work 2,080 hours annually (if no vacations, holidays, or sick days were taken). The following formula is used to determine the number of FTEs:

$$\frac{\text{Number of hours worked per shift} \times \text{Number of shifts worked/week}}{40 \text{ hours}}$$

When nurses work less than 40 hours per week, the nurse manager finds that they do not fit the definition of a FTE. Therefore, additional nurses must be hired to fill the gap in inpatient settings because nursing services are needed 24 hours a day, 7 days a week. Along with productive employee hours (hours actually spent working), managers must budget for nonproductive hours such as vacation, jury duty, holidays, education time, and other benefits (Hunt, 2003).

To determine the daily staffing requirements, the nurse manager must consider client census, client acuity, and the number of nursing care hours needed for each client. To accomplish staffing projections, nurses calculate the nursing hours per patient day (NHPPD). The number of NHPPD varies across nursing units with intensive care nursing units having more required hours of nursing care than a short-stay surgical unit. To determine daily staffing needs, the unit manager multiplies the average daily census times the NHPPD. With daily census fluctuations, some nurse managers prefer to use a staffing matrix, which is a staffing plan based on the number of clients needing nursing care. The matrix also presents a ratio of registered nurses, licensed practical/vocational nurses, unlicensed care providers, and unit secretary/clerk for each shift (Hunt, 2003).

Because nursing care needs cannot always be effectively predicted, nurse managers build overtime expenses into the staffing budget. Prudent nurse managers realize that in health care settings (especially acute care hospitals) staff workloads and the timing of essential nursing tasks cannot be predicted. The following examples describe the unpredictable nature of acute care nursing and result in overtime: (a) a client may have a cardiac or respiratory arrest as nurses are changing shifts; (b) a nursing unit could receive multiple admissions from the emergency department within a short time; (c) a staff member may need to leave because of a family emergency; or (d) a nurse could sustain an injury when providing client care. The amount of overtime to include in the staffing budget varies across institutions (Hunt, 2003).

### Marketing Skills

Many nurse leaders find themselves **marketing** the facility (advertising and bringing clients to the facility) in which they work and/or marketing the profession. Goals of marketing include increasing volume, maximizing client satisfaction, and improving the quality of life for the community. The steps of the market process mirror the steps of nursing process with assessing the current situation. Considerations for a marketing assessment include listing services offered, and assessing the community served by the facility. The next step is selecting strategies to inform potential clients about the organization and its services. Sometimes, health care organizations have marketing budgets that nurses can use. Marketing strategies are outlined in Table 19-6. Of all the strategies outlined in the table, personal recommendation tends to be the most effective (Hunt, 2003a).

## Leadership in the Role of Change Agent

One constant in the natural world is **change**. Change frequently affects persons holistically. Some persons find moving from a current, comfortable state (or process) distressing, whereas others find it exciting. The natural aging process affects the physical, psychological, sociocultural, and spiritual existence for many persons. The professional nurse, like her clients, confronts change on a daily basis. Learning how to cope with change and assisting others in coping with and adapting to change becomes a major professional nursing role.

**TABLE 19-6**

## Marketing Strategies for Nurses

| Strategy | Description | Expense |
|---|---|---|
| Personal recommendation | Word of mouth compliment | None |
| Newspaper advertisement | Print ad | Rates depend on circulation of the newspaper |
| Radio or television advertisement | Broadcast message | Free for a public service announcement; charge rates vary |
| Printed materials | Brochures, fact sheets, catalogs | Printing costs<br>Free distribution if volunteer time<br>Mailing costs<br>Fee for distribution racks housed in hotels, restaurants or businesses |
| Community outreach | Speaking engagements, health screenings at health fairs or contact agencies where potential customers may be | Free if services volunteered<br>Work release time for employees<br>Cost for health screening supplies, props, and printed materials |
| Introductory offers | Health promotion classes on a trial basis<br>Reduced cost for a new service | Costs of running program and delivering services |
| Traditional sales call | Sell health-related services to other companies | Salesperson salary, supplies, and fringe benefits |

Adapted from Hunt (2003a). Marketing your facility. In T. Stelzer (ed.). *Five keys to successful nursing management* (pp. 276–286). Philadelphia: Lippincott Williams & Wilkins.

"Resources and energy from within individuals are necessary to help accomplish [organizational] change" (Perlman & Takacs, 1990, p. 33). Change has an emotional meaning for people and often is associated with feelings of loss or pain (Davis, 1991). Based on the Kübler-Ross model of death and dying, Perlman and Takacs (1990) propose a ten-stage model to explain the psychological problems associated with change, the signs and symptoms of each stage, and nursing interventions to help others grow during the change process (Table 19-7).

In another model, Carnall (1990, pp. 141–146) proposes five steps in coping with change.

Stage 1: Denial of the validity of new ideas.
Stage 2: Defense (experiencing depression and frustration).
Stage 3: Discarding (acknowledging change as inevitable or necessary).
Stage 4: Adaptation (feeling anger).
Stage 5: Internalization.

Bridges (1980) approaches change from the perspective of psychological adaptation. He acknowledges that during any change, people enter a period of uncertainty (the neutral

TABLE 19-7

## Growing with Change: The Emotional Voyage of the Change Process

### Charted Summary

| Phase | Characteristics/Symptoms | Interventions |
|---|---|---|
| 1. Equilibrium | High energy level; state of emotional and intellectual balance; sense of inner peace with personal and professional goals in sync | Make employees aware of changes in the environment that will have impact on the status quo |
| 2. Denial | Energy is drained by the defense mechanism of rationalizing a denial of the reality of the change. Employees experience negative changes in physical health, emotional balance, logical thinking patterns, and normal behavior patterns | Employ active listening skills (e.g., being empathic, nonjudgmental, using reflective listening techniques). Nurturing behavior, avoiding isolation, and offering stress management workshops also will help |
| 3. Anger | Energy is used to ward off and actively resist the change by blaming others. Frustration, anger, rage, envy, and resentment become visible | Recognize the symptoms, legitimize employees' feelings and verbal expressions of anger, rage, envy, and resentment. Active listening, assertiveness, and problem-solving skills are needed by managers. Employees need to probe within for the source of their anger |
| 4. Bargaining | Energy is used in an attempt to eliminate the change. Talk is about "if only" Others try to solve the problem "Bargains" are unrealistic and designed to compromise the change out of existence | Search for real needs/problems and bring them into the open. Explore ways of achieving desired changes through conflict management skills and win-win negotiation skills |
| 5. Chaos | Diffused energy, feeling of powerlessness, insecurity, sense of disorientation; loss of identity and direction; no sense of grounding or meaning; breakdown of value system and belief; defense mechanisms begin to lose usefulness and meaning | Quiet time for reflection; listening skills; inner search for both employee and organization identity and meaning; approval for being in state of flux |
| 6. Depression | No energy left to produce results. Former defense mechanisms no longer operable. Self-pity, remembering past, expressions of sorrow, feeling nothingness, and emptiness | Provide necessary information in a timely fashion. Allow sorrow and pain to be expressed openly. Exhibit long-term patience; take one step at a time as employees learn to let go |
| 7. Resignation | Energy expended in passively accepting change; lack of enthusiasm | Expect employees to be accountable for reactions to behavior. Allow them to move at their own pace |
| 8. Openness | Availability to renewed energy; willingness to expend energy on what has been assigned to individual | Patiently explain again, in detail, the desired change |

## Growing with Change: The Emotional Voyage of the Change Process (Continued)

### Charted Summary

| Phase | Characteristics/Symptoms | Interventions |
|---|---|---|
| 9. Readiness | Willingness to expend energy in exploring new events; reunification of intellect and emotions begins | Assume a directive management style: assign tasks, monitor tasks and results so as to provide direction and guidelines |
| 10. Re-emergence | Rechanneled energy produces feelings of empowerment, and employees become more proactive. Growth and commitment are reborn. Employee initiates projects and ideas. Career questions are answered | Mutual answering of questions; redefinition of career, mission, and culture; mutual understanding of role and identity; employee's action based on own decisions |

From Perlman, D., & Takacs, G. J. (1990, April). The ten stages of change. *Nursing Management, 21,* 34. Used with permission of the publisher.

zone) when they fail to understand fully the meaning of and their role in implementing the change.

The Perlman and Takacs, Carnall, and Bridges models of change models are compared in Table 19-8. The models address various psychological responses experienced by persons when confronted with change. Before change can be internalized, persons tend to progress through various stages of acceptance. Pritchett and Pound (1995) suggest that, as persons progress through the various stages of acceptance of changes, they frequently make several mistakes when coping with organizational change (Display 19-6).

Pritchett and Pound acknowledge that change for some persons creates distress, and that these mistakes prevent a successful transition to new ways of doing things within an organization and even increase psychological distress. They emphasize the importance of individual workers assuming an active role in adapting to change. In today's health care arena, change seems to be the only thing that remains constant. Thus, professional nurses must learn how to adapt to change effectively.

### Team Roles in the Change Process
#### Roles of the Professional Nurse Change Agent
Based on a comparative analysis of the literature, Wooten and White (1989) identified five basic change roles: (1) educator/trainer, (2) model, (3) researcher/theoretician, (4) technical

## Mistakes Made When Coping with Organizational Change          DISPLAY 19-6

1. Assuming that the role of management is to keep them comfortable
2. Expecting another or others to reduce their stress
3. Aiming for a low-stress work setting
4. Attempting to control the uncontrollable factors
5. Refusing to abandon the expendable
6. Facing the future with fear
7. Choosing the wrong battles to fight
8. Unplugging psychologically from their jobs
9. Avoiding acceptance of new assignments

TABLE 19-8

## Comparison of Theoretical Stages in Coping with Change

| Perlman & Takacs | Carnall | Bridges |
| --- | --- | --- |
| Equilibrium | | *Endings* <br> Disengagement <br> Disidentification <br> Disenchantment |
| Denial | Denial | *The Neutral Zone* <br> Disequilibrium |
| Anger | Defense | Disidentification |
| Bargaining | | |
| Chaos | | |
| Depression | | |
| Resignation | Discarding | |
| Openness | Adaptation | *New Beginnings* <br> Re-engagement |
| Readiness | | Realignment |
| Re-emergence | Internalization | Reidentification |

expert, and (5) resource linker. The role of educator/trainer "is the focal point for the change process" (Wooten & White, p. 655). The **change agent** (the person who brings about a change) must model appropriate behaviors in an atmosphere of trust and openness, accept responsibility for getting data in an appropriate manner, provide skills and expertise, and link needed resources in ways that make the intervention effective. The selection and timing of particular roles depends on the specific needs of the situation.

### Roles of the Client System

Effective change depends on the client system assuming various roles. Wooten and White (1989) also describe four basic roles of the client system: (1) resource provider, (2) supporter/advocate, (3) information supplier, and (4) participant. The client system provides effort, time, and money resources; advocates the change; provides information involving self and others; and participates in the change process. It is crucial that the change agent and the client collaborate to promote effective change.

### Mutual Roles

Wooten and White (1989, p. 657) indicate, "mutual role enactment is at the heart of the change process." The mutual roles include (1) problem solver, (2) diagnostician, (3) learner, and (4) monitor. Instead of investing the change agent alone with the responsibility for the entire change process, this model focuses on joint responsibility and action.

Problem solving involves identifying a problem, generating alternatives, and testing assumptions. Diagnosis necessitates sensitivity to issues in the relationship. Learning includes knowledge, skills, or new attitudes, and monitoring involves "remain[ing] aware of alternatives, ascertain[ing] the consequences of action, gaug[ing] the effectiveness of the change effort and relationship at each stage of the intervention" (Wooten & White, 1989, p. 657). Each role can be adopted independently, as well as at the same time as other roles.

## Research Brief 19-1

Dalton, C., & Gottlieb, L. (2003). The concept of readiness to change. *Journal of Advanced Nursing, 42,* 108–117.

The investigator sought to examine indicators of client readiness to change as they adjusted to chronic illness and disability. Five persons newly diagnosed with multiple sclerosis (MS) participated in the study. After attaining Institutional Review Board approval for the study, the investigators made 42 contacts with the participants (28 face-to-face and 14 telephone calls).

One hundred twenty instances of change were identified and analyzed using Chinn and Kramer's (1995) concept analysis framework. Along with identifying change instances, clients were asked about their thoughts and feelings related to the change, their perceived readiness to embrace the change, and consequences of being ready or not ready to tackle the change.

The investigators created a concept map outlining trigger, process of readiness, and nursing strategies that were developed using the data. Triggers leading to the conclusion that clients needed to change were "importance of the health concern, availability of support, concurrent stressor, physical condition and energy level" (p. 111). They identified the process of readiness as the realization of what needed to be changed, weighing the costs and benefits to change, and planning for the change action.

Persons with low readiness for change pushed limits, discovered the costs, found themselves watching life and others from afar, hung onto old goals, waited for directions from others, had limited backup resources, and waited for others to rescue them.

Persons with ambivalence to change were described as those who reached the limit, and looked for benefits for changing. Actions taken by these persons included "becoming curious, modifying the plan, trying things outs, waiting for backup and testing the water" (p. 111).

Persons with high readiness for change were found to shift gears and discover the benefits of change. Persons with high readiness took action through discovery, creation of new goals, rehearsals, creation of a back-up plan, and taking steps to plunge into the new way of doing things.

The investigators identified several nursing strategies to help when clients expressed various levels of readiness to change (a state and process). For persons with high readiness for change, nurses should acknowledge client awareness, knowledge of benefits, efforts to change while offering support as needed while working with clients collaboratively. For clients ambivalent about or not ready to change, nursing interventions include exploring change obstacles or barriers, cost/benefit ratios, and support systems (such as persons and community resources). Along with these strategies, persons with the least amount of readiness to change may need to be confronted about their focus on the negative aspects of change. Because of various energy levels in persons with MS, the nurse may intervene in controlling the pace (amount and speed) of lifestyle changes.

Results of this study may not apply to all nursing situations in which clients need to change. The investigators identified that their conclusions were drawn from participants with MS who may have different needs than persons needing to make changes. More study on the concept of readiness to change, the levels of readiness for change, and nursing interventions to use while helping clients change is needed. Additional study needs to be done before extrapolating these findings to situations involving organizational change.

## Selecting a Change Strategy

As change agents, professional nurses select specific change strategies to use in practice situations. Change strategies are classified into the following six categories: empirical–rational, normative–re-educative, power–coercive, facilitative, re-educative, and persuasive and power. The following discussion defines each major category and supplies the reader with examples of how they are used in professional nursing practice when working with clients or other health team members.

### Empirical–Rational Strategies

The empirical–rational category assumes that persons will act in a way that is rational and in their own self-interest. These strategies are aimed at educating a person about the available options, assuming that the individual will change behavior because he or she knows that the new behavior will be desirable.

For example, inservice education may include a demonstration of the latest techniques available for a particular task, with the expectation that nurses will apply that knowledge to improve their care of clients. Recent research findings related to practice in flushing peripherally inserted venous catheters suggests that using a pulsing technique reduces the incidence of catheter occlusion. Nurses who attend an inservice demonstrating this technique may incorporate this technique when caring for these lines. However, they also may decide not to use this technique because it takes a few seconds longer than pushing the saline with one motion. Because persons do not always act rationally, these strategies often are not successful in facilitating a lasting change when used alone (Haffer, 1986).

### Normative–Re-educative Strategies

The normative–re-educative category assumes that sociocultural norms are fundamental to a person's behavior. In addition to rationality and intelligence, change must involve modification of attitudes, values, skills, and significant relationships. This is the basis for the belief that the change process must be based on mutuality and collaboration between the client and the change agent. This allows for the problem solving and personal growth believed necessary to promote effective change. According to Haffer (1986, p. 20), "if beliefs, attitudes, and values are the target of the needed change, then these strategies should be used."

For example, a young woman who needs to have surgery for a malignant ovarian tumor refuses to have it because she believes that the purpose of a woman's life is to bear children. When listening to the client, the professional nurse discovers that the client's mother had a sister who never had children and received the undivided attention of her husband. The client's aunt had a lavish lifestyle, was showered with gifts from her husband, and was considered to be spoiled and selfish by the other family members. After the aunt's husband died, the aunt became very demanding of other family members. The client expresses fear that she will become like her childless aunt because she cannot have her own children. The nurse and client engage in several meaningful dialogues about the purpose of life and alternative ways to create a family. The young woman's attitude changes, and she consents to having the gynecological surgery.

### Power–Coercive Strategies

The third category, power–coercive strategies, is based on the use of power. It is believed that despite the need for knowledge and for modification of attitudes and values, change will occur only when it is supported by power. This rationale is the basis for much political action, and it may imply the use of legitimate channels of authority or violent, non-sanctioned methods (Chin, 1976). This strategy effects change more quickly than do other strategies, but the change that results usually is not lasting (Haffer, 1986).

For example, a professional nurse working with an unlicensed assistive care provider (UAP) notices that every time they work together, the UAP fails to get postoperative clients out of bed during a 12-hour shift. Because the professional nurse supervises the UAP, the nurse initiates the first step of a progressive discipline process, which is documenting the conversation held with the UAP about not fulfilling job responsibilities. For a month, the UAP follows postoperative instructions to get clients out of bed, but returns to previous habits thereafter.

### Facilitative Strategies

Facilitative strategies are used to make clients aware of the availability of help in sufficient detail and clarity so that they know exactly what is available and where and how assistance may be obtained. Facilitative strategies are appropriate when there is openness to change, but they are relatively ineffective when resistance is expected. Examples of this type of strategy are (1) simplifying data, providing feedback, and providing other necessary tools to help the client to recognize a problem; (2) providing multiple potential solutions to the problem; and (3) involving the client and others in the decision-making process. These strategies produce greater commitment to change, but the agent must be sure that there are sufficient resources, commitment, and capability to maintain the change after the agent has withdrawn from the process. For example, a teaching hospital in a metropolitan area holds a medical clinic every Tuesday with a focus on monitoring persons receiving oral anticoagulant therapy on a weekly basis. Mrs. Jones, an elderly woman who lives alone, has missed her last three appointments. When the nurse calls Mrs. Jones, she asks why Mrs. Jones has missed her appointments. Mrs. Jones replies, "You know, I am just so busy that I forget about my appointments, and I also like to have my daughter with me during doctors' appointments because I just hate driving in the horrible city traffic." The nurse explains the reasons behind weekly bleeding time measurements and offers a variety of options to get Mrs. Jones to keep her scheduled appointments. They both decide that the nurse will call Mrs. Jones every Friday before her appointment and see if transportation needs to be arranged. With these resources in place, Mrs. Jones never misses another appointment.

### Re-educative Strategies

Re-educative strategies are based on empirical–rational theory. Relatively unbiased presentation of fact is assumed to provide a rational justification for action. This type of strategy is necessary when effective use of an advocated change requires skills and knowledge that the client does not possess. It also is desirable when resistance is prevalent and based on inaccurate information and when the change involved is a radical departure from past practices and there is a great deal of uncertainty about the ability to successfully perform the new practices. However, in themselves, re-educative strategies are inadequate to bring about change, unless there is a strongly felt need and a strong motivation to satisfy that need.

Re-educative strategies work slowly, so they are feasible only when time is not a pressing factor. Examples of re-educative strategies are creating awareness that a problem exists by indicating how much better off the client could be, connecting symptoms with causes to aid in problem identification, and demonstrating alternative possible solutions to an identified problem. Re-educative strategies work well when persons receive a new diagnosis of a chronic illness, such as diabetes or renal or cardiovascular diseases. Re-educative strategies heighten awareness of a problem and possible solutions, but they do not heighten the need or motivation to change. This requires persuasive strategies.

### Persuasive Strategies

Persuasive strategies attempt to bring about change partly through bias in the manner in which a message is structured and presented. Reasoning, urging, and inducement through incentives are examples of this type of strategy.

Persuasive strategies are more effective for those who are less open to change, and they can be used to increase attitudinal and behavioral commitment. Knowledge about the client can help the change agent be more persuasive, especially in combating resistance to change. A persuasive strategy is indicated when the proposed change is risky, not amenable to limited or small-scale trial, is technically complex, has no clear relative advantage, and must be implemented in a short time. These strategies are especially useful in situations in which the change agent has limited resources with which to initiate and sustain a change.

### Power Strategies

Power strategies imply the use of coercion. They typically result in compliance, which indicates a low level of commitment to the change but leads to adoption of the induced behavior because the person expects to gain specific rewards and avoid punishment by conforming. Power strategies may be necessary if the client or target group has limited resources and is generally unwilling to allocate available resources to the continued implementation of a change. However, forced compliance requires surveillance to maintain the change. This is not an appropriate approach if the goal is to produce a self-sustaining change.

For example, the Joint Commission on Accreditation of Healthcare Organizations (JCAHO) invites health care organizations to become accredited. An organization that is not accredited by JCAHO becomes ineligible to receive federally-based reimbursement for services. JCAHO routinely visits organizations for re-accreditation to verify that the organization meets all criteria and standards for maintaining an accreditation status.

## Benefits of Change Strategies

Professional nurses who have knowledge of the basic types of change strategies may select the best way to proceed when change is needed. Different persons vary in responses to the different classifications of change strategies. Sometimes the power–coercive strategy may be met with lots of resistance, and other times it may be very successful. The professional nurse also must assess the ability of individuals to cope with change and how many changes are occurring simultaneously. When one strategy fails, the professional nurse can try another one to bring about the desired change. Sometimes, the professional nurse must determine which change is the most important for the client, health care team, or organization to avoid extreme psychological distress in persons confronting multiple changes.

# Leadership in the Role of Colleague

Whether working with individual clients, client groups, other health team members, or across the organization, the professional nurse must establish collegial partnerships with others. Collegial partnerships enable equality among all persons involved in an interaction. Over time, health team members develop collegial partnerships with each other in which each person acknowledges the contributions and skills that the other members bring to client service. The professional nurse frequently uses holistic assessment skills and documents findings to substantiate the need for practice changes or modifications to the client plan of care. The pharmacist brings detailed knowledge about medications, including interactions of medications with other medications and food. The physician serves as the expert related to the physical dimension of the client. Rehabilitation therapists assess the potential for and guide the client toward attainment of independence in activities of daily living. Case managers (sometimes nurses) track client progress toward improved health across the continuum of care (e.g., acute care setting to home) by looking at the whole picture. To capitalize on the strengths of each other, the development of collegial partnerships must occur.

A collegial partnership is a relationship in which all persons view each other as providing equal contributions to a mutually defined outcome. Collaboration serves as the foundation for professional partnerships in health care. Collaboration begins when individuals realize they need others to attain an envisioned goal (Porter-O'Grady & Malloch, 2003; Wesorick & Shiparski, 1997; Wilson & Porter-O'Grady, 1999). Collegial partnerships may occur between nurses and clients, nurses and unlicensed assistive personnel, nurses and other nurses, nurses and physicians, nurses and other health team members, and even nurses and a community group. Partnerships may be short-lived or last for an extended time. When working in partnership with others, various partners assume leadership when an issue arises that falls within the realm of his/her expertise. The development of clinical paths or client care maps within health care organizations represents one outcome of interdisciplinary collegial partnerships.

Kreuger-Wilson and Porter-O'Grady identify potential barriers to effective collaboration among health care partners. Experience with a health care provider may create difficulties or even threaten the collegial relationship. Old animosities, such as perceived physician superiority, sometimes prevent the ability of the nurse or client to trust and relate effectively to the physician. Incongruence of philosophy related to the partnership also may create tension among partners. However, when these philosophical differences are acknowledged and a new common ground is found, professional partnerships may flourish. Competitive behavior also limits the ability to form effective collegial partnerships. Some physicians may view advanced practice nurses as competitors for clients. Social status also interferes with the development of partnerships. Information linkages also must be in place for successful collaboration. Information systems must be designed so that all partners have access to the same information so that responsible decisions and behaviors can occur. Finally, sometimes partners equate collaboration with total agreement on every issue, and processes must be in place for ways to negotiate differences between and among partners when disagreements arise (Wilson & Porter-O'Grady, 1999).

Professional nurses bear lots of responsibility for the development and maintenance of collegial partnerships. As client care coordinators, nurses must make certain that clients receive ordered treatments and tests as scheduled. This requires collegial partnerships with unlicensed care providers and professional health care team members. As client advocates, professional nurses must establish rapport and take time to listen to client concerns so that referrals can be made to address them. As change agents, professional nurses use nursing knowledge to generate changes in work processes while working with physicians, administrators, and nursing colleagues.

The current goal of health care is to provide the best possible outcome for clients while conserving precious health care resources. Recent efforts at an interdisciplinary team approach to client care have resulted in improved outcomes and have contained health care costs for consumers. In addition, the development of collegial partnerships among health team members has created a more congenial environment for health care providers.

## ⬥ LEADERSHIP EFFECTIVENESS

Professional nurses assume leadership in a variety of ways. As health experts, they offer knowledge and skills to clients. In many health care organizations, professional nurses hold leadership positions, lead others as they deliver client care, and participate in developing organizational policies, strategic plans, and other work processes. Nurses develop therapeutic relationships with clients to lead them toward improved health. Nurses collaborate with other health team members to assure that health care interventions remained focused on optimal client outcomes. When clients and health team members share a vision for health care outcomes, they work together to transform the vision into reality. Success in this endeavor requires open communication based on mutual trust.

The sharing of power, rather than the wielding of power, characterizes the transformational relationship of the nurse and client; in this way, both participants influence each other. Yukl (1981) describes different forms of influence (Display 19-7) that have been adapted to the nurse–client relationship. These forms of influence may also apply when the nurse works with unlicensed care providers (UCPs). For example, nurses make

---

**Forms of Influence Within the Nurse–Client Relationship**  **DISPLAY 19-7** ⬥

1. Legitimate request: responding to legitimate power; the client complies with the nurse's request because he recognizes her right to make such a request. The client's compliance represents internalized values of obedience, cooperation, courtesy, respect for tradition, and loyalty to the organization.
2. Instrumental compliance: responding to reward power; the client complies because the nurse has made an explicit or implicit promise to ensure some tangible outcome that the client desires.
3. Coercion: responding to the threat of aversive outcomes, such as economic loss, embarrassment, or expulsion. Because the influence is motivated by fear, it is most effective when it is credible.
4. Rational persuasion: responding to a logical argument. The client is convinced that the

nurse's suggested behavior is the best way to satisfy needs or attain objectives.
5. Rational faith: acting out of faith in the nurse's expertise and credibility. Such a response is based on expert power.
6. Inspirational appeal: responding to expressions of values and ideals without any tangible reward. The client acts from obedience to authority figures, reverence for tradition, self-sacrifice, and so forth.
7. Situational engineering: responding to manipulation of relevant aspects of the physical and social situation. The nurse must have control, and the client must accept the situation.
8. Personal identification: responding to referent power. The client imitates the behavior of an admired nurse.
9. Decision identification: responding to involvement in decision making.

legitimate requests to UCPs when delegating tasks to them within the realm of organizational job descriptions. As supervisors, nurses use coercion or rational persuasion to get UCPs to perform the delegated tasks. With time, UCPs may recognize nurses as experts, internalize some of the values of nurses they respect, relinquish control of independence to comply with nurse requests, participate actively in client care decisions, and begin to imitate nurses whom they admire.

In transformational leadership, rational persuasion and decision identification are the most valid forms of influence because they reflect empowerment through information and the sharing of power in relationships characterized by mutuality and respect. The nurse assumes leadership by initiating, facilitating, and successfully terminating professional influence in the process. The competencies a nurse needs to be a transformational leader are discussed subsequently.

## Transformational Leadership Competencies

Effective leadership requires that the leader display confidence and competence in working with and through other persons. Individual personality qualities facilitate the development of leadership. Some persons may seem to be natural born leaders, whereas others have to learn to develop leadership qualities and skills.

Gurka (1995, p. 170), synthesizing research findings, has identified three qualities of the transformational leader.

1. Individual consideration—exhibited by promoting others' growth, recognizing and supporting others' needs and feelings, and giving positive feedback and recognition.
2. Charisma—exhibited by inspiring and motivating, demonstrating enthusiasm, and communicating in a positive manner.
3. Intellectual stimulation—exhibited by creating a questioning environment, acting as a mentor, and challenging others to grow and learn.

Gurka (1995, p. 170) also identifies three qualities of the transformational leader that have been proposed experientially.

1. Vulnerability—exhibited by communicating authentically and openly, expressing emotions as well as ideas, and sharing the self with others.
2. Knowledge, concern, and courage—exhibited by seeking knowledge through study and experience, showing concern and caring for others, and being willing to take risks.
3. Feminine attributes—exhibited by maintaining accessibility, paying attention to process as well as outcomes, and practicing balance in lifestyle.

Based on transformational leadership concepts (Bennis & Nanus, 1985), the proposed actions listed in Display 19-8 reflect competence in leadership. These actions become part of the nurse's character, called habits. Because habits are powerful forces in determining health, professional nurses focus extensively on health habits. Leadership habits of the nurse also determine the effectiveness of the nurse in practice. The next section presents a brief discussion of the seven habits of leadership as envisioned by Covey (1989). When developed by a professional nurse, these habits should enhance the ability to be a transformational leader.

---

## Leadership Competencies                              DISPLAY 19-8 ◆

Acknowledging and using the inner wisdom of self and others
Setting goals and working to achieve them
Working with others to achieve a common vision and mission
Recognizing the interconnection of everyone on everything
Abandoning the hierarchical approach to leadership
Recognizing that persons performing the work are specialists
Engaging in systems thinking
Recognizing patterns
Synthesizing new ideas and processes
Committing to lifelong continuous learning
Adapting to and accepting chaos
Facilitating each team member's involvement and accountability

Empowering others
Being receptive to new ideas and the ideas of others
Facilitating group meetings and participation of everyone in organizational processes (especially decision making)
Coaching
Acting with immediacy and equality
Displaying technical expertise (organizational culture and design, financial management, economics, business ethics, evaluation methods, health care jurisprudence, information technology and strategic planning for the long term)
Practicing knowledge of relationship dynamics
Sharing administrative functions
Favoring collaboration over competition
Mentoring others to assume leadership

---

### Covey's Habits of the Effective Leader

Defined as the intersection of knowledge, skill, and desire (Covey, 1989, p. 47), a habit has great power in a person's life. Covey (p. 47) describes knowledge as the theoretical paradigm, the "what to do" and the "why"; skills as the "how to do"; and desire as the motivation, the "want to do." He warns that even if a person knows something (e.g., that people need to listen) and has developed the necessary skills (e.g., to listen intently), this is not enough to form an effective habit. Unless the person wants to listen, listening will not become a habit.

**Habits of effective leaders** are the internalized principles and patterns of behavior that reflect the three interrelated factors of knowledge, skills, and desire. All the habits that Covey (1989) designates for effective leadership are based on the theoretical premise of sequential growth moving people from dependence to independence and finally to interdependence, the phase in which true mutuality can occur.

Covey (2004) added another habit of great leaders. The eighth habit involves hearing one's own voice and inspiring others to find theirs. Finding one's own voice means periodic analysis of values and beliefs and finding quiet time to listen to oneself. Once found, the voice must be expressed by developing a personal vision, practicing discipline, showing passion in action, and not doing anything against one's conscience. Inspiring others means being a trim-tab (a small rudder that turns the large rudder of a ship), modeling character and competence, instilling trust, and blending voices to develop shared vision. Once others have discovered their voices, the great leader aligns goals and systems to achieve desired results (the shared vision) while empowering others to use their talents and live out passions. Covey identifies the four roles of leadership as modeling (inspiring trust), path finding (creating order), aligning (nourishing vision and empowerment), and empowering (getting others to internally unleash their human potential). Great leaders use their influence to serve others. The eight habits identified by Covey (1989; 2004) are listed in Display 19-9 and briefly described in terms of nursing leadership.

## Covey's Eight Habits, Adapted for the Nurse

1. Be proactive. Nurses need to set a goal and work to achieve it. They commit themselves to the client's perceptions and serve as a model for health, not a critic of those with expressed concerns. They accept their own ability to be "response-able" in dealing with clients' whole human responses to their health concerns. They believe that "it's not what happens to us, but our response to what happens to us that hurts us" (Covey, 1989, p. 73).

2. Begin with the end in mind. The nurse should identify what is really important and try to do what really matters the most every day. The nurse also must differentiate management from leadership: management, representing the bottom line, focuses on how the nurse can best accomplish certain things with the client, and leadership, representing the top line, focuses on what the nurse wants to accomplish. "Management is efficiency in climbing the ladder of success; leadership determines whether the ladder is leaning against the right wall" (Covey, 1989, p. 101).

3. Put first things first. The formula for the nurse who wants to stay focused on the important business of nursing and give less energy to the unimportant is to set priorities, organize, and finally, perform. The challenge for the nurse is to manage time in such a way that most of the time is used for urgent important activities, such as crises, pressing problems, and deadline-driven projects, as well as the not urgent but important projects, such as health promotion/illness prevention, relationship building, recognizing new opportunities, planning, and recreation (Covey, 1989).

4. Think win-win or no deal. Interdependence is the most mature goal for any relationship; thus, in professional relationships, interdependence would emphasize mutual benefits. Activities would reflect a commitment to both parties' growth, development, and satisfaction. For example, a client benefits from being empowered by the professional nurse providing informational support, and the nurse benefits by having the interventions validated and the sense of presence with the client valued. When such mutuality is experienced, neither person in the relationship loses or feels powerless (Covey, 1989).

5. Seek first to understand, then to be understood. Empathy is the habit reflected in this principle. The ability to focus on the client's reality as he experiences is vital to positive communication. Empathy is discussed in detail in Chapter 19, Professional Communication to Establish Helping and Healing Relationships. Credibility problems, such as the client's feeling that "you just don't understand," are prevented to the extent that the nurse empathizes with the client (Covey, 1989).

6. Value differences and bring all perspectives together. Respect is the characteristic that enables the nurse to develop this habit. Respect is discussed further in Chapter 15, Client Systems. To the extent that the nurse facilitates respect for differing perspectives, the client is likely to feel more free to seek the best possible alternative. If the nurse also experiences respect for his or her perspectives, synergistic relationships are enhanced. Using the principle of synergy, the nurse and client multiply their individual talents and abilities, and the outcome of their efforts is greater than the sum of the parts (Covey, 1989).

7. Have a balanced, systematic program for self-renewal. Consistency in having a regularly planned and balanced program for self-renewal prevents weakening of the body, mechanization of the mind, exposure of raw emotions, and desensitization of the spirit. Clearly, nurses' leadership ability is enhanced if they consistently participate in activities that renew four aspects of the self: physical, mental, emotional–social, and moral being. Renewal energizes capabilities that are necessary for productive helping relationships in nursing (Covey, 1989).

8. Find your own voice and inspire others to find theirs. Being truly authentic towards one's personal life mission, and helping others find themselves, fosters the development of new leaders and promotes deep satisfaction with life and work. Others quickly detect lack of authenticity in a relationship, especially when nurses establish helping and healing relationships with clients and health team members.

Adapted from Covey, S. R. (1989). *The 7 habits of highly effective people*. New York: Simon & Schuster; Covey, S. R. (2004). *The 8th habit*. New York: Free Press.

In addition, Prestwood and Schumann (1997, p. 68) suggest that the personal growth and state of mind needed for leadership require an understanding of the following principles.

1. Know who you are—what you know and do not know about yourself, resistance and tolerance for change, fears, preferences, and skills and abilities.
2. Let go of what you have hold of—discover chains that bind you to the past.
3. Learn your purpose—based on values, unfolding through a lifelong process of learning.
4. Live in the question—understand relationships, be open to the potential of the unknown, and avoid the quick fix.
5. Learn the art of "barn raising"—the need to work with and through others, shared purpose.
6. Give "it" away—ennoble, enable, empower, and encourage yourself and others.
7. Let the magic happen—let go of the demands of the ego.

Habits represent the integrated principles of the professional nurse. They also provide consistency in action. When leaders practice effective leadership habits, they earn the trust of their followers.

## EVALUATING LEADERSHIP EFFECTIVENESS

As a professional, the nurse engages in the process of self-evaluation and looks for ways to improve performance as a leader. Unfortunately, not all leaders are effective. Competing demands force leaders (especially managers) to make difficult decisions, which may result in win-lose situations. Ineffective leadership takes many forms, including the person who assumes a leadership position without proper qualification, one who bides his or her time until retirement, or the person who received a leadership appointment because of success in a previous appointment. Frequently, personal insecurity of persons in charge may result in dysfunctional leadership (Fitzpatrick, 2004). Poor nursing leadership also may occur when the well-respected, competent, professional nurse gets forced into accepting a leadership position. The quality of leadership suffers when the person assuming the leadership position would rather be doing something different. When nurses know themselves as persons and have a clear idea of life passions, they can thwart the influences of others before assuming a leadership position that they really do not wish to assume.

Signs of dysfunctional leadership vary and ways to manage ineffective leadership must fit the situation. Table 19-9 presents signs of dysfunctional leadership and offers suggestions for followers to manage them. Fitzpatrick (2004) proposes that the best way to confront a dysfunctional leader (or boss) is to discuss concerns directly because when bosses feel isolated, the symptoms may worsen because isolation fuels the insecurity and paranoia. Sometimes, professional nurses must take the risk to confront a dysfunctional leader especially when the health and well being of others are threatened. Frequently, dysfunctional leaders have no awareness of their weaknesses.

McCauley and Velsor (2004) propose that when persons assume a leadership position, they should conduct periodic evaluations of their performance. They suggest self-reflection and eliciting information from followers to provide a complete, accurate picture of one's

TABLE 19-9

## Dysfunctional Leadership Behaviors and Intervention Strategies

| Dysfunctional Leadership Behavior | Etiology | Signs and Symptoms | Consequences | Intervention Strategies |
|---|---|---|---|---|
| Micromanagement | Insecurity Lack of trust in followers Failure of ability to let go of previous responsibilities | Doing the work of all team members Inability to seek input from others for decisions Constantly supervising every single task | Follower frustration Feelings of being undervalued and incompetent Loss of motivation Staff turnover | Direct discussion with the leader about all the consequences, needing space to perform work, and clarify role expectations |
| Poor communication | Inability to confront issues directly Inability to provide direct feedback Insufficient education in effective communication | Pleasant during face-to-face interactions followed by unpleasant written communication messages Jump to conclusions Threaten followers with some form of punishment for failing to be accountable for required actions of which they are unaware Inconsistent moods when approaching persons | Staff uneasiness Confusion about work expectations Staff turnover | Keep records of inconsistent messages to take when you calmly discuss issues with the leader in person Suggest additional education in effective communication Confront leader when behavior is inconsistent |
| Using messengers to deliver bad news or do the "dirty work" | Inability to manage conflict Failure to assume responsibility | Inner circle of confidantes selected to work on "special" projects that may create team conflict and deliver messages to team members | Distrust among team members Staff turnover | Calm, direct discussions with persons involved to clarify information and expectations |
| Sabotage | High need to control others | Use of lies, slander, or other ethical breaches to get rid of a team member or prevent a subordinate from succeeding | Staff uneasiness Staff turnover | Keep written records of occurrences Direct confrontation of the leader |

*(continued)*

## Dysfunctional Leadership Behaviors and Intervention Strategies (Continued)

| Dysfunctional Leadership Behavior | Etiology | Signs and Symptoms | Consequences | Intervention Strategies |
|---|---|---|---|---|
| Sabotage (continued) | High need to control others | Withhold vital information<br>Passive-aggressive behavior<br>Treated like a best friend one time then like a worst enemy at another time | | |
| Petty jealousy | Envy of other persons achieving things that cannot be achieved | Dysfunctional communication<br>Personalizes success of others as a personal failure<br>Denial that issue exists | Staff uneasiness<br>Loss of motivation<br>Staff turnover | |
| Narcissism | Need to be admired<br>Delusional<br>Emotional isolation<br>Major security issues<br>Intense drive to attain power and glory<br>Inability to achieve intimate relationships | Behaviors that make others question the ability to trust them<br>Preoccupation with self<br>Grandiose<br>Self-involved<br>Abrasive interactions with followers<br>Calls followers anytime day or night<br>Inability to listen to others<br>Unable to empathize with others<br>Dominating behaviors<br>Becomes defensive and sometimes cries when confronted<br>Retaliation against persons who question them | Unsupported staff<br>Staff uneasiness<br>If combined with using messengers, distrust among all team members<br>Lack of basic trust in leader's ability to lead<br>Staff turnover<br>Deterioration of the organization | Give the leader ideas and let him/her take credit for them<br>Disagree only when you can convince the leader of benefits of an alternative action<br>Seek employment elsewhere |

## Dysfunctional Leadership Behaviors and Intervention Strategies (Continued)

| Dysfunctional Leadership Behavior | Etiology | Signs and Symptoms | Consequences | Intervention Strategies |
|---|---|---|---|---|
| | | May be very charismatic, skilled, and visionary Mentors others only to create an extension of oneself | | |

Adapted from Fitzpatrick, M. (2004). Facing challenges. In Holmes, N. (Ed.). *Five keys to successful nursing management* (pp. 162–191). Philadelphia: Lippincott Williams & Wilkins.

leadership. Some pertinent questions to use as **criteria for evaluating leadership** are listed in Display 19-10. Periodic evaluation of one's leadership provides information for future learning and professional development.

## ● SUMMARY AND SIGNIFICANCE TO PRACTICE

Effective nursing leadership is critical when working with individual clients, client groups, other health providers, and the health care system. When nurses use expert and ethical leadership processes, all members of the health care team (including clients) become empowered and receive support to attain goals for improved health and health care systems. Periodic self-evaluations of one's leadership enable the nurse to see areas of future professional growth.

---

### Criteria for Evaluating Nursing Leadership

DISPLAY 19-10

1. Can the leader be trusted?
2. Does the leader use effective verbal and non-verbal communication skills?
3. Is the leader accessible?
4. Is the leader aware of issues encountered by nurses engaged in client care activities?
5. Does the nurse leader support staff when problems arise?
6. Can the leader initiate, maintain, and terminate effective relationships?
7. Does the leader demonstrate sensitivity to the impact of self on others, leading to effective use of self?
8. Can the leader effectively modify his or her behavior and that of others?
9. Does the leader effectively delegate tasks to others or does he or she micromanage everything?
10. Does the leader provide the needed resources to provide quality nursing services?
11. Does the leader set high standards and hold others and self accountable for them?
12. Is the leader willing to help others grow as professional nurses?

Adapted from McCauley, C., & Van Velsor, (2004) *The center for creative leadership handbook of leadership development* (2nd ed.). San Francisco: Jossey-Bass.

## FROM THEORY TO PRACTICE

Reread the vignette at the beginning of the chapter and answer the following questions.

1. Which of the leadership theories would be most useful to Alice as she leads the group of parent volunteers to determine how to get a registered nurse in every school? Why do you think the selected theory would work best?
2. Outline the consequences of having a registered nurse in every school for the following groups of people:
   a. Students
   b. Faculty
   c. School administration
   d. School board
   e. Taxpayers of the school district.
   What obstacles do you think Alice and the task force might encounter from achieving the goal of a nurse in every school?
3. How will Alice evaluate her leadership as the task force leader? What suggestions would you give Alice for her to use to evaluate her leadership? Why did you make these suggestions?

## **WWW** INTERNET EXERCISES

1. Visit the International Council of Nurses website "site map" www.icn.ch/. Click on the words "site map." Click on the words in the yellow oval labeled "Leadership for Change." Read this information and answer the following questions:
   How can nurses contribute to global health care reform?
   What perceptions about nurses held by others prevent nurses from assuming leadership roles in global health care reform?
   How can the nursing profession dispel the negative perceptions of others?
   What do you think about the vision and mission statements for the Leadership for Change Initiative?
   How would you like to change health care delivery in your locale?

## **WWW** INTERNET RESOURCES

University of Connecticut Archives of Nursing Leadership (learn about nursing history and nursing leadership in the historical archive collection):
http://www.lib.uconn.edu/online/research/speclib/ASC/nursing/nursbroc.htm.
American Academy of Nursing: http://www.aannet.org/.
A national forum on nursing leadership (an article by Jo Anne Klein on the Nursing Network): http://nursingnetwork.com/leader.htm. Article title is *Leadership in Nursing*.
American Organization of Nurse Executives: http://www.aone.org.
American Nurses Association: http://www.nursingworld.org.
Transformational Leadership and Leader Effectiveness from Human Assets Limited in London, England: http://changingminds.org/disciplines/leadership/styles/transformational_leadership.htm.

Sigma Theta Tau International: http://www.nursingsociety.org.

International Council of Nurses: http://www.icn.ch.

Center for Innovative Leadership: http://www.cfil.com.

The Leadership Institute: http://www.leadership.org.

Leadership Communications: http://www.tolead.com.

Warren Bennis "Thoughts on Leadership," http://leader-values.com/Guests/Lead23.htm.

## REFERENCES

Ahern, J. (1992). Your presence is requested. *Revolution: The Journal of Nurse Empowerment, 2,* 80–82.

Anderson, T. (1998). *Transforming Leadership* (2nd ed.). Boston: St. Lucie Press.

Bandman, E. L., & Bandman, B. (1995). *Nursing ethics through the life span* (3rd ed.). East Norwalk, CT: Appleton & Lange.

Barker, A. M., & Young, C. E. (1994). Transformational leadership: The feminist connection in post-modern organizations. *Holistic Nursing Practice, 9,* 16–25.

Barrett, R. (1998). *Liberating the corporate soul: Building a visionary organization.* Boston: Butterworth- Heinemann.

Bass, B. M. (1998). *Transformational leadership: Industry, military and educational impact.* Mahwah, NJ: Lawrence Erlbaum Associates.

Bennis, W. (1989). *Why leaders can't lead: The unconscious conspiracy continues.* San Francisco: Jossey-Bass.

Bennis, W., & Nanus, B. (1985). *Leaders: The strategies for taking charge.* New York: Harper & Row.

Bernal, E. W. (1992). The nurse as patient advocate. *Hastings Center Report, 22,* 18–23.

Blake, R. & Morton, J. (1964). *The managerial grid: Key orientations for achieving production through people.* Houston: Gulf Publishing.

Blanchard, K., Carlos, J. P., & Randolph, A. (1996). *Empowerment takes more than a minute.* San Francisco CA: Berrett-Koehler Publishers.

Blank, W. (2001). *The 108 Skills of Natural Born Leaders.* New York: AMACOM

Bridges, W. (1980). *Transitions: Strategies for coping with the difficult, painful and confusing times in your life.* Reading, MA: Perseus.

Burns, J. M. (1978). *Leadership.* New York: Harper & Row Books.

Carnall, C. A. (1990). *Managing change in organizations.* Upper Saddle River, NJ: Prentice Hall.

Cassidy, V. R., & Koroll, C. J. (1994). Ethical aspects of transformational leadership. *Holistic Nursing Practice, 9,* 41–47.

Chin, R. (1976). The utility of systems models and developmental models for practitioners. In W. G. Bennis, K. D. Benne, & R. Chin (Eds.), *The planning of change* (3rd ed., pp. 90–122). New York: Holt, Rinehart, & Winston.

Chinn, P. L., & Kramer, M. K., (1995). *Theory and nursing: Integrated knowledge development* (4th ed.). St. Louis: Mosby.

Conley, A., & Mariano, C. (1991). Participatory decision making: Issues and guidelines. *Journal of the New York State Nurses Association, 22,* 4–8.

Covey, S. R. (1989). *The 7 habits of highly effective people.* New York: Simon & Schuster.

Covey, S. R. (1996). Three roles of the leader in the new paradigm. In F. Hesselbein, M. Goldsmith, & R. Beckhard (Eds.). *The leader of the future: New visions, strategies, and practices for the next era* (pp. 149–160). San Francisco: Jossey-Bass.

Covey, S. R. (2004). *The 8th habit.* New York: Free Press.

Dalton, C., & Gottlieb, L. (2003). The concept of readiness to change. *Journal of Advanced Nursing, 42,* 108–117.

Davis, P. S. (1991). The meaning of change to individuals within a college of nurse education. *Journal of Advanced Nursing, 16,* 108–115.

Donnelly, G. (2003). Why leadership is important to nursing. In T. Stelzer (Ed.). *Five keys to successful nursing management* (pp. 2–30). Philadelphia: Lippincott Williams & Wilkins.

Dotlich, D., Noel, J., & Walker, N. (2004). *Leadership passages.* San Francisco: Jossey-Bass.

Douglass, L. M. (1988). *The effective nurse: Leader and manager* (3rd ed.). St. Louis: Mosby.

Epstein, C. (1982). *The nurse leader: Philosophy and practice.* Reston, VA: Reston Publishing.

Fieldler, F. (1967). *A theory of leadership effectiveness.* New York: McGraw-Hill.

Fitzpatrick, M. (2004). Facing challenges. In N. Holmes (Ed.). *Five keys to successful nursing management* (pp. 162–191). Philadelphia: Lippincott Williams & Wilkins.

Fogg, C. D. (1999). *Implementing your strategic plan.* New York: AMACOM.

George, B. (2003). *Authentic leadership.* San Francisco: Jossey-Bass.

Greenleaf, R. (1977). Servant leadership: A journey into the nature of legitimate power and greatness. Mahweh: Paulist Press.

Gurka, A. M. (1995). Transformational leadership: Qualities and strategies for the CNS. *Clinical Nurse Specialist, 9,* 169–174.

Haffer, A. (1986, April). Facilitating change: Choosing the appropriate strategy. *Journal of Nursing Administration, 16,* 18–22.

Hames, C. C., & Joseph, D. H. (1980). *Basic concepts of helping—a wholistic approach.* New York: Appleton-Century-Crofts.

Hershey, P. & Blanchard, K. (1977). *Management of organizational behavior: Leading human resources* (3rd. ed.). Upper Saddle River, NJ: Prentice Hall.

House, R. & Mitchell, T. (1974). Path-Goal Theory of Leadership. *Journal of Contemporary Business, 3,* 81–97.

Hunt, P. (2003). Staffing for inpatient care. In T. Stelzer (ed.). *Five keys to successful nursing management* (pp. 202–235). Philadelphia: Lippincott Williams & Wilkins.

Hunt, P. (2003a). Marketing your facility. In T. Stelzer (ed.). *Five keys to successful nursing management* (pp. 276–286). Philadelphia: Lippincott Williams & Wilkins.

King, E. C. (1984). *Affective education in nursing.* Rockville, MD: Aspen Systems.

Kirkpatrick, M. K., Hull, A., Katrabos, S., & Sherman, C. (1995). Patient representative: More than an advocate. *Nursing Management, 26,* 92–94.

Knobf, M. T. (1990). Early-stage breast cancer: The options. *American Journal of Nursing, 90,* 28–30.

Krueger-Wilson, C., & Porter-O'Grady, T. (1999). *Leading the revolution in health care: Advancing systems, igniting performance* (2nd ed.). Gaithersburg, MD: Aspen.

Manfredi, C. M. (1994). The art of legendary leadership. *Nursing Leadership Forum, 1,* 62–64.

McCauley, C., & Van Velsor, E. (2004). *The center for creative leadership handbook of leadership development* (2nd ed.). San Francisco: Jossey-Bass.

McGregor, D. (1960). *The Human Side of Enterprise.* New York: McGraw-Hill.

Miles, M. S., & Crandall, E. K. (1983). The search for meaning and its potential for affecting growth in bereaved parents. *Health Values: Achieving High Level Wellness, 7,* 19–23.

Noddings, N. (1984). *Caring: a feminine approach to ethics & moral education.* Berkeley, CA: University of California Press.

Olsen, D. P. (1991). Empathy as an ethical and philosophical basis for nursing. *Advances in Nursing Science, 14,* 62–75.

Ouchi, W. (1981). Theory Z: How American business can meet the Japanese challenge. Reading, MA: Addison-Wesley-Longman.

Perlman, D., & Takacs, G. J. (1990). The 10 stages of change. *Nursing Management, 21,* 33–38.

Porter-O'Grady, T., & Malloch, K. (2003). *Quantum Leadership, a textbook of new leadership.* Sudbury, MA: Jones and Bartlett.

Prestwood, D. C. L., & Schumann, P. A. (1997). Seven new principles on leadership. *The Futurist, 31,* 68.

Pritchett, R., & Pound, R. (1995). *A survival guide to the stress of organizational change.* Dallas: Pritchett & Associates.

Rafael, A. R. (1996). Power and caring: A dialectic in nursing. *Advances in Nursing Science, 19,* 3–17.

Richardson, P. (1992, Spring). Hospital practices that erode nursing power by promoting job dissatisfaction. *Revolution: The Journal of Nurse Empowerment, 2,* 34–39.

Rost, J. C. (1994). Leadership: A new conception. *Holistic Nursing Practice, 9,* 1–8.

Snowball, J. (1996). Asking nurses about advocating for patients: 'Reactive' and 'proactive' accounts. *Journal of Advanced Nursing, 24,* 67–75.

Taylor, S. G., Pickens, J. M., & Geden, E. A. (1989). Interactional styles of nurse practitioners and physicians regarding patient decision making. *Nursing Research, 38,* 50–55.

The United States Army (2004). *Be-know-do: Leadership the army way*. San Francisco: Jossey-Bass.

Toffler, A. (1990). *Powershift: Knowledge, wealth, and violence at the edge of the 21st century*. New York: Bantam Books.

Trofino, J. (1995). Transformational leadership in health care. *Nursing Management, 26,* 42–49.

Van Velsor, E., Moxley, R., & Bunker, K. (2004). The leadership development process. In C. McCauley, & E. Van Velsor (eds.). *The center for creative leadership handbook of leadership development* (2nd ed., pp. 204–233). San Francisco: Jossey-Bass.

Vroom,V., & Yetton, P. (1973). *Leadership and decision making*. Pittsburgh: University of Pittsburgh Press.

Wesorick, B., & Shiparski, L. (1997). *Can the human being thrive in the work place? Dialogue as a strategy of hope*. Grand Rapids, MI: Practice Field Publishing.

White, R., & Lippitt R. (1960). *Autocracy & democracy: An experimental inquiry*. New York: Harper & Row (Published after Lewin's death).

Willard, C. (1996). The nurse's role as patient advocate: Obligation or imposition? *Journal of Advanced Nursing, 24,* 60–66.

Wilson, C. K, & Porter-O'Grady, T. (1999). *Leading the revolution in health care* (2nd ed.). Gaithersburg, MD: Aspen.

Wooten, K. C., & White, L. P. (1989). Toward a theory of change role efficacy. *Human Relations, 42,* 651–669.

Yukl, G. A. (1981). *Leadership in organizations*. Englewood Cliffs, NJ: Prentice Hall.

# Quality Improvement and Professional Nursing

## KEY TERMS AND CONCEPTS

Quality

Total Quality Management

Continuous Quality Improvement

Joint Commission on Accreditation of Healthcare Organizations

Quality Assurance

Plan, Do, Check, Act

Internal Customers

External Customers

Lean

Six Sigma

Benchmarking

Baldrige National Quality Award

Total Quality Improvement

Nursing-Sensitive Outcomes

## LEARNING OUTCOMES

By the end of this chapter, the learner will be able to:

1  Define the term quality.

2  Compare and contrast quality assurance, total quality management, and continuous quality improvement.

3  Explain the plan, do, check, act (PDCA) cycle used in quality improvement programs.

4  Identify internal and external customers in health care settings.

5  Explain Six Sigma and how it could be used to improve health care quality.

6  Describe the process of benchmarking.

7  Specify nursing-sensitive outcomes for clients and health care organizations.

## VIGNETTE

Laura is a nurse working on a busy cardiac care unit. This evening, she has admitted two persons with chest pain, and transferred another one of her assigned clients to the intensive care unit. As she charts all of the medications that were routinely ordered on her assigned clients, she notices that she administered the wrong doses of warfarin to two of her assigned clients who were roommates. She completes an incident report on herself after reporting the mistake to the physician, who yells at her. Because she is new to the unit, she wonders how the nurse manager and her colleagues will react to her mistake.

## Questions for Reflection 20-1

1. How does the organization in which I practice nursing handle medication errors?
2. Am I afraid to complete incident reports? Why or why not?
3. Who is at fault when a nurse makes an error?

When analyzing **quality** in health care, the term quality means "a degree of excellence" (Mish, 1994, p. 955). Different approaches can be used to measure quality of health care. Quality in health care means different things depending upon individual perspectives. Consumers look at different aspects to rate the quality of health care providers. According to the Institute of Medicine (2000), as many as 98,000 hospitalized Americans may die each year as a result of errors in care delivery. Errors occur when health care providers fail to complete planned actions as intended or when a wrong plan is used. Many errors result in adverse events or injuries sustained by clients as a direct result of the unintended intervention. Not all errors cause adverse events; however, other errors may cause permanent or temporary harm (Institute of Medicine, 2004). Quality health care means more than error-free health care. Quality health care means providing appropriate health care services, achieving optimal client outcomes, and using resources effectively.

## Questions for Reflection 20-2

1. What do I consider elements of quality of care when I receive health care services?
2. What do I consider elements of quality of care as a professional nurse?
3. How well do the lists of quality of care match?
4. What are the elements found in each list? Why are they important?
5. What elements are important to health care consumers that may not be important to health care providers? Why are these important to consumers?

Companies that manufacture products would be out of business if they had as many errors that occur in the health care arena. Quality management became popular in business and industry after American manufacturers lost market share to Japanese competitors (Ouchi, 1981). The terms **total quality management (TQM)** and **continuous quality improvement (CQI)** are used synonymously in the business and health care–related literature. For years, health care providers and organizations rationalized higher margins of error. After all, the outcome of life and death situations could not always be predicted. Historically, death remained an undesirable outcome (Duffy & Hoskins, 2003).

## ● HISTORY OF QUALITY IMPROVEMENT IN HEALTH CARE

Perhaps, Florence Nightingale can be considered the first nurse who engaged in quality improvement (QI) activities. During the Crimean War, Nightingale's work at the Barrack Hospital demonstrated the effects of nursing care on wounded and infirm soldiers. The mortality rate at Barrack Hospital was 60% when Nightingale arrived. It fell to just a fraction over 1% when she departed. Nightingale kept detailed records that included statistics about the effects of cleanliness, good nutrition, and fresh air on the survival of the soldiers (Kalisch & Kalisch, 2004). Her diligent attention to detailed records and continuous analysis of data provided evidence that nursing care by women could reduce mortality. She reported her success to the British government and documented her work in three books: *Notes on Matters Affecting the Health, Efficiency and Hospital Administration of the British Army* (1858); *Notes on Hospitals* (1858); and *Notes on Nursing* (1859) (Kalisch & Kalisch).

A group of surgeons concerned about the quality of care in American Hospitals formed the American College of Surgeons (ACS) in 1913. By 1918, work of the ACS led to the implementation of the Hospital Standardization Program (HSP). The HSP evolved into an accreditation process that designated minimum standards for credentialing, privileging and monitoring functions for medical staff. The HSP also developed minimal standards for medical equipment. To create a standardized system for record keeping, the HSP determined standards for health care recipient medical records (Koch & Fairly, 1993; Des Harnais & McLaughlin, 1999).

In 1951, the HSP evolved into the Joint Commission on Accreditation of Hospitals (JCAH), a private, nonprofit, voluntary agency that used ACS standards for accrediting hospitals. JCAH eventually expanded accreditation standards to include hospital administrative issues. Concerned about the quality of care received by subscribers during hospitalizations, Blue Cross required that participating hospitals be accredited for JCAH. Eventually, JCAH accreditation became a requirement for hospitals to receive payment under the federal Medicare program (Des Harnais & McLaughlin, 1999; Koch & Fairly, 1993; Sultz & Young, 2004).

Hospitals began to develop health systems that also included primary care services for consumers. In 1987, JCAH changed its name to **Joint Commission on Accreditation of Healthcare Organizations** (JCAHO) (Koch & Fairly, 1993). Along with its name change, JCAHO produced a new definition of health care quality that used quantitative approaches that emphasized patient outcomes. JCAHO currently accredits nearly 16,000 health care organizations that include hospitals, home health agencies, laboratories, and extended care and outpatient facilities. JCAHO uses standards, performance outcomes, and consumer perception of rendered services as criteria for accreditation (JCAHO, 2004).

Quality assurance programs became part of the hospital accreditation process in the 1970s. JCAHO standards require that health care organizations (especially hospitals) regularly review the following data in quality assurance programs: (1) mortality rates by department or service, (2) hospital-acquired infections, (3) patient falls, (4) adverse drug reactions, (5) unplanned returns to surgeries, and (6) hospital-incurred trauma (Sultz & Young, 2004, p. 108).

Along with assuring quality of services to health care consumers, JCAHO accreditation standards address efficacy of health care interventions and appropriateness of services delivered. JCAHO also looks at how well services are delivered to consumers. Aspects for quality services include the following: (1) availability of the needed health care intervention, (2) timeliness of services, (3) effectiveness of health care interventions, (4) continuity of health care services across various health care settings, (5) safety of patient and others, (6) efficiencies of provided care and services, and (7) respect given to consumers and caring with which services are rendered (DesHarnais & McLaughlin, 1999; Sultz & Young, 2004).

More recent JCAHO standards emphasize the importance of CQI or TQM. Success in CQI and TQM is based on the premise that if staff members who are closest to the point of service delivery are empowered and educated on the process of incremental change, the quality and efficiency of client care will improve (Sultz & Young, 2004). QI differs from **quality assurance (QA)** in that QA programs tend to be reactive in nature, and focus on correction of specific identified causes of problems with limited responsibility using authoritative problem solving. In contrast, QI is a proactive program aimed at correcting common system problems, holds everyone involved in a process responsible, leaders actively lead, and actual and potential problems are identified and solved by all employees (Koch & Fairly, 2003). In the literature QI, CQI, and TQM all basically mean the same thing. The concepts all mean processes used to improve all aspects of goods and services that are offered to consumers. QI, CQI, and TQM work constantly and continuously to improve consumer goods and services. Table 20-1 outlines the differences between quality assurance and quality improvement programs.

JCAHO sets annual National Patient Safety Goals for hospitals. The goal of this program is to avert errors that compromise patient safety. For 2005, the following goals were set: to improve the accuracy of patient identification, effectiveness of communication among health team members, safety of medication use, safety of infusion pump use, and to reduce risk of infections resulting from health care, reconciliation of medications across the care continuum, and incidence of patient falls (JCAHO, 2004a).

To understand the TQM/CQI approach, an understanding of key concepts related to this process is discussed in the following section.

**TABLE 20-1**

## Comparison of Quality Assurance and Quality Improvement Programs (QI, CQI, TQM or TQI)

| Quality Assurance Program | Quality Improvement Program |
|---|---|
| Conformance focused | Improvement focused |
| Reactive in nature | Proactive in nature |
| Looks for special sources of variation within a system | Focuses on internal variations within a system |
| Variation results from actions of specific persons or work groups | Variation results from increased complexity of work processes or may be random in nature |

Adapted from McLaughlin, C., & Kaluzny, A. (1999). *Continuous quality improvement in health care.* Gaithersburg, MD: Aspen.

# ● QUALITY IMPROVEMENT APPROACHES

Quality improvement approaches to business and industry began after World War II. In health care, providers rated quality in terms of mortality and morbidity. Health care institutions held "Mortality and Morbidity Conferences" on a regular basis. Even today, hospitals hold regularly scheduled conferences to analyze precipitating factors and outcomes of rescue efforts following cases of respiratory and cardiac arrest. In many cases, some providers consider a death as an indicator of poor quality in health care service. However, TQM/CQI offers an alternative way to measure, analyze, and control quality in health care.

## W. Edwards Deming

Dr. W. Edwards Deming (a physicist, mathematician, and engineer) was responsible for postwar construction in Japan. In 1950, he presented a quality management workshop in Japan that emphasized the importance of statistical control for managers. To maintain a competitive edge, Deming proposed that dedication to quality and productivity was essential. Deming suggested that errors increased and productivity declined as a result of flawed work processes rather than from the results of individual actions. He also believed that productivity and quality would improve when workers became empowered to make decisions about work processes.

He developed a cycle, today known as the Deming cycle, to improve quality. The cycle is a continuous loop consisting of the following steps: **plan, do, check, and act (PDCA)**. When using the Deming cycle, organizations *plan* what improvements need to be made, *do* by implementing the plan, *check* results of plan implementation using statistical data, and finally *act* by correcting work processes to improve the quality of services or products.

Deming also emphasizes that a successful QI program requires total commitment and accountability for all workers (including management). He created the following 14 points that must be applied for successful QI processes:

1. Create a constancy of purpose for improvement of products and services.
2. Adopt the new philosophy that poor workmanship and services must not be tolerated.
3. Cease dependence on mass inspection by enlisting the workers to develop ways to improve production processes and have them make decisions during the production process whether to discard or rework a product.
4. End the practice of awarding business solely on the lowest cost.
5. Work constantly and endlessly to improve the systems of production and service.
6. Institute training for all workers.
7. Reconfigure leadership based on supervisors to help workers perform better.
8. Drive out fear in the workplace because fear prevents persons from asking questions or expressing ideas and perpetuates error in job performance.
9. Break down barriers between staff areas by bringing various departments together to work toward the common purpose and find more opportunities for improvement.

10. Eliminate slogans, exhortations, and targets for the workforces by having the workers write their own slogans and targets.
11. Eliminate numerical quotas as they create the perceptions that employment status is based only on meeting quotas rather than producing high quality goods and services.
12. Remove barriers to the pride of workmanship by providing workers with the best equipment and materials so that workers can improve offered products and services.
13. Institute a vigorous program of education and retraining so that all managers and workers understand statistical techniques and teamwork skills needed for an effective QI program.
14. Take action to accomplish the transformation by defining the action plan required to lead the quality mission with dedication (Walton, 1986).

Along with proposals for successful QI programs, Deming warned of the following seven deadly diseases and obstacles that could derail the process:

1. Lack of constancy of purpose (everyone works toward different goals and no strategic plan is developed to assure continuation of the organization).
2. Emphasis on short-term profits (quality and productivity may decline if quarterly data are used because if great improvement is noted in one quarter, workers or managers may scale back efforts).
3. Evaluation by performance, merit rating, or annual performance reviews (potential for destroying teamwork, instilling rivalry, creating despondency, and encouraging management mobility).
4. Mobility of management (management must understand the work, complete changes for improved productivity and quality, which means managers must be on the job long enough to accomplish these tasks).
5. Running a company solely on visible figures (the effects of a satisfied or dissatisfied customer remain unknown).
6. Excessive medical costs (reveal potential problems with work environment or that employees have no time for health promotion).
7. Excessive costs of warranty, fueled by lawyers working for contingency fees (high losses reveal that inferior goods or services are being provided to customers) (Walton, 1986).

Deming provided businesses with an innovative approach. He outlined strategies for success that empowered workers. In addition, his obstacles warned about potentially catastrophic effects arising from failure to develop strategic plans, relying on technology rather than people to solve problems, and generating excuses for less than optimal performance (Walton, 1986).

If Deming's principles are applied to clinical nursing practice, efforts would be made to streamline work processes related to direct client care. For example, nurses would not be blamed if errors occurred while taking care of clients. Each error that occurred would be fully analyzed to determine the contributing factors resulting in the error. Work processes would be changed to prevent the error's reoccurrence. Nurses would be empowered to make changes in clinical policies and procedures as well as assuming control over their clinical practice environments.

## Joseph Juran

Like Deming, Juran noted the importance of careful planning to generate product quality. In 1945, Juran took his concepts to Japan. Juran used statistical quality control as a management tool. He created the Juran Trilogy consisting of quality planning, quality control, and QI. The process of quality planning consisted of identifying specific customers and their needs, developing products to meet customer needs, developing processes to produce product features, and transferring production plans and product features to operating forces. Quality control consists of evaluating actual performance, comparing it to product goals and acting on the difference. QI consists of establishing an infrastructure, identifying specific improvement projects, establishing project teams, and providing the improvement teams with resources, training, education, and motivation. The QI team works to diagnose causes of less than desired quality, propose and simulate remedies to identified causes, and establish control systems to maintain the gains (Juran, 1989).

Juran (1989) also differentiated quality circles from QI project teams. Quality circles (QC) serve primarily to improve human relationship and secondarily to improve quality. QC usually occur within a single department where members volunteer to tackle many QI projects. Managers and workers hold equal status in QC. Whereas, QI project team membership crosses departmental boundaries, has a primary mission of improving quality, is run by a manager (or professional), and disbands once the project ends.

Juran (1989) outlined the following eight factors that distinguish institutions that have improved quality and reduced quality-related costs:

1. Upper managers led the quality process and served on quality councils (QI teams) as guides.
2. **Internal customers** (persons working within the organization) and **external customers** (persons outside the organization but received products or services) needs were concerned as QI processes were applied to businesses and usual operating processes.
3. Senior managers were given clear responsibility to adopt mandated, annual quality improvement with a defined infrastructure that identified opportunities for improvement and were held accountable for making the improvements.
4. Managers involved everyone who affects the plan in the QI process.
5. Managers used modern quality methodology rather than empiric methods in quality planning.
6. Senior managers trained all management team members in quality planning, quality control and quality improvement.
7. Managers trained all workers in how to participate actively in QI.
8. QI became a major feature in the strategic planning process.

Juran's approach to QI stressed the importance of planning.

## Phillip Crosby

Philip Crosby (1979) proposed that quality is free. He specifies that time, manpower, and resources cost money. Crosby advocated for doing things right the first time and that quality saves money, thereby increasing profits. He defined quality as "conformance to requirements" (p. 8). Crosby's emphasis on doing things right the first time holds very true to health care delivery because health care professionals usually get only one chance to deliver effective, safe client care (i.e., the nurse has only one chance to administer the right medication to a client). He proposed that organizations needed to create climates in which attitudes and controls could make error prevention possible.

Like Deming, Crosby (1979) saw the need for all within an organization to be committed to the QI process. However, Crosby (1979) viewed that "...management needs to understand their personal roles in implanting quality and engaging employees in the vision of the company" (p. 78). Crosby also identified 14 essential elements to a quality management program:

1. Management commitment to the QI process
2. QI teams to oversee actions
3. Measurement tools appropriate to specific activities going through the QI process
4. Considering costs of quality evaluation (using estimates as needed)
5. Quality awareness promotion from all involved
6. Corrective action as needed to correct measurement tools, and reducing costs associated with the QI process
7. Planning for zero deficits
8. Supervisory education and training for all management levels
9. Holding a zero defects day to celebrate the new standard of performance
10. Goal determination for individual workers and work teams
11. Worker, rather than management removal of causes of error after notification
12. Recognition of all involved once performance goals are attained
13. Quality circle sharing of ideas, experiences and problems
14. Constant repetition of all steps (after all, QI is a continuous, never-ending process).

Crosby's thesis of the importance of doing things right the first time has been recently expanded by Toyota's lean operations and Chowdhury's Six Sigma Design approach to quality management.

## Toyota's Lean Operations

Since the 1980s, Toyota automobiles have been known for their quality construction and performance. The Toyota Production System involves creation of a learning environment that uses the following four key practices:

1. How people work: Workers follow strict production specifications, are encouraged to identify changes in work processes, and then perform controlled trials of new work processes.
2. How workers connect: Workers across all levels of the organization interact directly following standardized methods. These practices reduce ambiguity, prevent key issues from losing attention, encourage requests for help (to which assistance is provided immediately), set deadlines for problem resolution, and foster trust among everyone in the organization.
3. How work is constructed: Work processes are designed to attain maximum reliability, eliminate repetition, and follow principles to promote worker health and well-being.

4. How work is improved and errors are reduced: All workers are trained in how to affect change, assume responsibility for making them, and use the scientific method to identify and propose changes to improve productivity, product quality, and reduce errors.

Toyota also uses **lean** operation techniques that advocate the use of desired, value-added activities while eliminating undesirable activities and waste in all work processes. Lean techniques eliminate waste by using visual controls, streamlined physical plant layouts, standardized work processes, and point-of-use storage. If a health care organization operated using lean principles, operations flowcharts outlining steps for delivering various services would be posted in departments. Nursing units and other ancillary departments would be designed to promote the flow of activities required for client care. Routine work processes would be standardized (many institutions already use standardized clinical care pathways for commonly encountered diseases, surgeries and invasive diagnostic and intervention procedures). Finally, supplies, equipment, information, and procedures would be housed in convenient locations where client services are delivered (Institute of Medicine, 2004).

The lean system outlines the following seven categories of waste: (1) poor utilization of resources, (2) excess motion, (3) unnecessary waiting, (4) transportation, (5) process inefficiency, (6) excess inventory, and (7) defects/quality control.

When nurses go searching for equipment needed for client care, hospitals practice poor utilization of resources, excess motion, unnecessary waiting, and process inefficiency. Many times clients wait for long periods after undergoing diagnostic tests because of unavailability of someone to return them to their rooms (waste from transportation, unnecessary waiting, and process inefficiency). Nurses may make medication errors because they engage in multitasking to meet client care needs (waste in terms of process inefficiency). Hospitals frequently buy supplies in bulk to reduce cost per unit resulting in a higher inventory of supplies than actually needed; some supplies may become outdated and have to be discarded (excess inventory) (Institute of Medicine, 2004).

## Six Sigma

In the late 1980s, Motorola developed the Six Sigma as a means to sharpen its focus on quality improvement and to help accelerate the pace of change in a highly competitive technological and telecommunications market (Pande, Neuman, & Cavanagh, 2000). The concept has been expanded by other companies including General Electric, Allied Signal, and Honeywell (Pande et al., 2000). Six Sigma has its basis in quality principles outlined by Deming, Juran, Crosby, and lean but takes quality to a new level. "In a nutshell, **Six Sigma** is a management philosophy focused on eliminating mistakes, waste, and rework" (Chowdhury, 2002, p. 4). Sigma (the Greek letter for deviation) measures variation within a process. The standard deviation of a process quantifies how far a process functions from its ideal. Instead of using percentages (based on a system of 100 performances), Six Sigma looks at "defects per million opportunities" (Pande et al., 2000; Chowdhury, 2002). Table 20-2 summarizes the levels of Six Sigma, translates the levels in terms of performance accuracy and presents health care based scenarios.

Six Sigma methodology strives to improve products and work processes during the design rather than the quality control stage. Like TQM, Six Sigma processes emphasize providing the highest possible quality of goods and services to consumers. Pande

TABLE 20-2

## Six Sigma Levels, Performance Accuracy, and Implications for Nursing

| Sigma Level | Performance Accuracy/Million | Defective Performance/ Million | Implication for Nursing Practice |
|---|---|---|---|
| 1 | 310,000 (30.9% accuracy) | 690,000 | 309 of 1,000 clients interactions made the clients feel that the nurse truly understood their concerns |
| 2 | 692,000 (69.2% accuracy) | 308,000 | 692 of 1,000 IVs are inserted successfully on the first attempt |
| 3 | 933,200 (93.3% accuracy) | 66,800 | 933 of 1,000 postoperative complications are detected and treated effectively |
| 4 | 993,790 (99.4% accuracy) | 6,210 | 994 of 1,000 medications are accurately administered |
| 5 | 999,680 (99.98% accuracy) | 320 | 4,999 of 5,000 physician orders are transcribed accurately |
| 6 | 999,996.6 (99.9997% accuracy) | 3.4 | Between three and four errors are made per million client care documentation entries on medical records |

Adapted from Pande, P., Neuman, R., & Cavanagh, R. (2000). *The Six Sigma way*. New York: McGraw-Hill.

and colleagues (2000), p. 68) identify a Six Sigma Roadmap consisting of the following five sequential steps: (1) identify core processes and key customers, (2) define customer requirements, (3) measure current performance, (4) prioritize, analyze, and implement improvements, and (5) expand and integrate the Six Sigma System.

The steps apply to situations related to business transformation, strategic improvement, and problem solving. When transforming business, Pande and colleagues suggest limiting the scope of change to one or two core processes. However, in health care, Six Sigma may best be used for strategic improvement (finding out what key customers need and want, followed by implementation of initiatives to fulfill customer expectations) and for problem solving (looking for ways to improve delivery of effective health care while reducing costs).

Six Sigma uses a process similar to the PDCA cycle. The cyclical process used in Six Sigma involves the following phases for improving processes:

1. Define: Identify the problem, determine requirements, and set goals.
2. Measure: Validate the problem or flawed process, refine problems or goals, and measure key steps and inputs.
3. Analyze: Develop causal hypotheses, identify the "vital few" root causes, and validate a causal hypothesis.
4. Improve: Develop ideas to eliminate root causes, test solutions, standardize to a single solution and measure results.

5. Control: Establish standard measurements to maintain performance and correct problems as needed.

An acronym DMAIC "(pronounced deh-MAY-ihk" [Pande et al., 2000, p. 37]) is frequently used as a shortcut to communicate these Six Sigma process improvement processes or process design/redesign processes. Six Sigma may be superior to TQM/CQI initiatives. Six sigma has one definition, "...a business system for achieving and sustaining success through customer focus, process management and improvement, and the wise use of facts and data" (Pande et al., p. 3). Six Sigma is tied to the bottom line of the organization because funding efforts for it are based more on fact than TQM funding which is based on faith (Chowdhury, 2002; Pande et al.). Six Sigma sets a no-nonsense, but ambitious goal of 3.4 defective parts per million opportunities (Chowdhury, 2002; Pande et al.) rather than using **benchmarking** (comparing outcomes or results with other similar organizations) systems as indicators for improvement. Six Sigma has the capability to detect incremental and exponential change. TQM/CQI initiatives focus on product quality, whereas Six Sigma solutions attend to all business processes. Six Sigma may hold the key to delighting both customers and nurses in health care environments (Morgan & Cooper, 2004).

## Questions for Reflection 20-3

1. What is the quality improvement approach used in my current clinical practice settings?
2. How have I participated in the quality improvement process in my current clinical practice setting?
3. Is it important for nurses to participate in the quality improvement process? Why or why not?

### Research Brief 20-1

Morgan, S., & Cooper, C. (2004). Shoulder work intensity with Six Sigma. *Nursing Management 35,* 28–32.

The investigators performed a pilot project designed to change the workload intensity for nurses working on a medical, progressive-care, and women and children's units. Data were collected using staff survey generated from information obtained with telephone interview with nursing staff and leaders, and registered nurse (RN) focus groups. Persons completing surveys were patient care staff members, prescribers who admitted patients to the units, and patient care staff family members.

Results of the survey revealed that the two key contributors to work dissatisfaction were work assignments and invariability of client care supplies and equipment. According to the family members of staff, arriving home late and a lack of satisfaction with daily accomplishments were major contributors to job dissatisfaction. The project also identified the following key drivers that prevented nurses from feeling closure with daily assignments: client room readiness, multiple attempts to start intravenous (IV) lines, issues with phlebotomy, inability to find equipment, missing medication, delays with equipment repair, unavailability of supplies, client transportation, and no time for breaks.

The drivers then served as the basis for a work group to develop a workload data collection instrument in which RNs and licensed practical nurses collected data for daily (24-hour time frame) for 1 week. A baseline score was obtained. After focusing on missing medications, phlebotomy skills, IV line starting skills; standardizing location for supplies and equipment; and using color-coded tags for supply bins, data were recollected using the workload data collection instrument. After initiation of all changes in work processes, overall workload closure score increased, resulting in reduced job dissatisfaction.

Results of this pilot project reveal the complexity of nurse job satisfaction and how work-related problems increase nurse workload. Caution should be exercised when interpreting study findings because the investigators failed to specify the number of nurses participating in the project and the number of observations related to workload to determine baseline and resultant scores. Future studies using Six Sigma as a framework need to be performed to validate the effectiveness of Six Sigma as a means to improve the quality of work processes used in health care.

## CELEBRATING SUCCESSES IN CONTINUOUS QUALITY IMPROVEMENT/ TOTAL QUALITY MANAGEMENT

One of Deming's 14 principles for quality improvement is to recognize participants once performance goals are attained (Walton, 1986). In the early 1980s, the American manufacturing industry was trailing Japan. President Ronald Reagan signed a bill to investigate ways in which the government could reward organizations for productivity improvement. A decision was made to create a National Quality Award, and Congress passed the Malcolm Baldrige Quality Improvement Act (Public Law 100-107). The Malcolm **Baldrige National Quality Award** was named in honor of the acting Secretary of Commerce and amateur rodeo rider who was killed in a horse riding accident. Only two awards per category can be awarded in any year (Baldrige National Quality Program, 2004; Hart & Bogan, 1992).

The National Institute of Standards and Technology developed criteria for the award to provide meaning and legitimacy to the Baldrige Award. Baldrige quality framework consists of the following criteria known as "7 pillars": (1) leadership, (2) information and analysis, (3) strategic quality planning, (4) human resource development and management, (5) management of process quality, (6) quality and operating results, and (7) customer service and satisfaction.

The Baldrige Award process reviews organizational approaches to quality, how organizations deploy their approach, and results of the deployed approaches. Criteria for excellence in an approach means that the approach is prevention-based, has multiple evaluation/improvement cycles, uses appropriate and effective tools, techniques, and methods; is systematic, integrated, and consistently applied; is quantitatively based; and appears innovative. The organization's deployment of the program is analyzed for its use by all work groups, appropriateness of processes and activities, characteristics of the products or services offered by the organization, transactions and interactions with customers, and finally, internal processes and activities (including physical facilities and employees). The results criteria consider the following eight characteristics: (1) the absolute level of quality in the results (products, services, in health care–client outcomes); (2) comparison of results with others in the industry and world leaders; (3) quality improvement rate; (4) quality improvement breadth; (5) duration of quality improvement (maintenance of sustained gains); (6) significance of improvements to the organization's business; (7) company ability to demonstrate that the improvements made were derived from the quality approach (practices and actions); and (8) contributions of outcomes and effect on the quality improvement process.

At this time, two health care organizations have received the Baldrige National Quality Award: Saint Luke's Hospital of Kansas City (2003) and Robert Wood Johnson University Hospital in Hamilton, New Jersey (2004) (Baldrige National Quality Program, 2004).

Along with the national quality award program, individual states confer Quality Awards. Most state awards follow criteria outlined by the Baldrige National Quality Award. Winning a quality award serves as a marketing strategy for health care organizations in the United States Health Care System that relies heavily on competition to reduce health care costs (Sultz & Young, 2004).

Some institutions post baseline and improvement data in view of health team members and consumers to showcase the accomplishment of quality improvement goals. Posters highlighting goal attainment frequently recognize members of the process improvement team. Sometimes, intra-agency publications express appreciation to workers for gains in quality. Other institutions provide recognition ceremonies for nurses and other team members who achieve performance improvement goals (McLaughlin & Kaluzny, 1999; Sultz & Young, 2004).

## ✦ KEY CONCEPTS OF TOTAL QUALITY IMPROVEMENT AND OTHER QUALITY MANAGEMENT APPROACHES

**TQI** may be viewed as an organizational value and process to deliver the best possible goods and services to consumers. TQI works to improve constancy in actions while meeting (and exceeding) product and service standards. The International Organization for Standardization (ISO) is an international, nongovernmental organization composed of a network of national standards institutes of 146 countries. The goal of the ISO is to set international standards to meet business requirements as well as broader needs of a global human society. ISO standards benefit society by prompting fair trade; compatibility of technology; conformity of consumer products in terms of safety, quality, and reliability; scientific knowledge and technology for health; and guidelines to prevent global environmental contamination (ISO, 2004). The ISO outlines eight key principles for TQM known as ISO 9000. ISO 9000 assures consistency among all international efforts aimed at TQM, CQI, and TQI .The eight principles are outlined in Table 20-3 with examples of how a health care organization might follow them. Key principles of TQI consider persons who receive services and attend to persons providing services. Therefore, TQI enhances the health care delivery experience for everyone.

To summarize, all quality improvement programs focus efforts on the following four areas: (1) customer service (internal customers are those who work within an organization, and external customers are the consumers of the organization's service); (2) ways to improve the quality of key work processes; (3) development and use of quality tools

TABLE 20-3

## Key Principles of TQI Based on ISO Principles and How a Health Care Organization Might Follow Them

| TQM/ISO Principles | Examples |
| --- | --- |
| Customer focus: the goal is to delight external and internal customers | • For external customers (recipients of health care services), provide them with "the little" extras that make big differences such as customized menus, backrubs, esthetically appealing rooms<br>• For internal customers (physicians, interdisciplinary health care professionals, nursing staff members, and other supportive client services staff), create an open trusting work environment that encourages collaboration and suggestions to improve work-related processes that are studied, and if feasible, implemented |
| Leadership: the goal is to provide vision, direction and understanding of the constancy of purpose among all members of the organization | • Empower all workers by inviting them to participate in departmental strategic planning<br>• Provide education about the mission, values, goals and objectives of the organization to all workers |
| Involvement of people: all persons within the organization should feel ownership in the TQM values and processes | • Formation of nursing unit and other departmental-based quality circles<br>• Form interdepartmental and interdisciplinary quality improvement teams to improve work processes that involve more than one department or discipline<br>• Institute interdisciplinary shared governance systems for nursing and other professional disciplines |
| Process approach: desired results are more effectively accomplished when related resources and activities are defined and managed as a process | • Constant monitoring of organizational performance, comparing results with similar organizations (benchmarking), and sharing results on a regular basis with all organizational members<br>• Consistent use of client care pathways |
| Systems approach to management: leaders and persons in the organization must look outside the organization to plan how best to use physical, monetary, and human resources | • Analyzing local, regional, and global trends to plan future services<br>• Reviewing and analyzing current work processes to determine how to improve health care and health education services<br>• Staying abreast of the latest scientific advancements in disease management, illness prevention, health promotion, and health care delivery |
| Continual improvement: constant improvement becomes a permanent organizational objective | • Always looking for ways to improve delivery of health care services<br>• Continual reinforcing the importance of improving quality with staff via education, informing staff of performance results<br>• Sharing data with all organizational members who deliver specific services |

*(continued)*

## Key Principles of TQI Based on ISO Principles and How a Health Care Organization Might Follow Them (Continued)

| TQM/ISO Principles | Examples |
|---|---|
| Factual approach to decision making: actual data, current trends, and other forms of objective information serve as the basis for decision making within the organization | • Staying informed of current trends and advances in health care<br>• Using data generated by quality improvement processes to guide actions, changes and plans<br>• Piloting new equipment before making purchases |
| Mutually beneficial supplier relationships: the organization forms partnerships with external contractors based on the quality of goods and services they can provide | • Identifying vendors that provide high quality products<br>• Securing exclusive purchasing contracts with identified vendors |

Adapted from ISO (2004) and St. Luke's Hospital of Kansas City Organizational Manual.

and statistics; and (4) involvement of all persons and organizational departments that provide service to the consumer (Bohnet, Ilcyn, Milanovich, Ream, & Wright, 1993; McLaughlin & Kaluzny, 1999; Miller & Flanagan, 1993; Sultz & Young, 2004).

When performance fails to attain benchmarks (predetermined goals that encompass not only the organization's goals, but also the goals of the competing and other similar organizations), all involved persons work together to fix the work process systems, rather than blame individuals (Bohnet et al., 1993; McLaughlin & Kaluzny, 1999; Miller & Flanagan, 1993; Wilson & Porter-O'Grady, 1999).

## ⬥ TQM/CQI PROCESSES IN HEALTH CARE

TQM/CQI place consumers first. Persons providing services seek to find ways to streamline work processes. Deming proposed that the more complex work processes have more chances of error. Consistency of action reduces error rates (Koch & Fairly, 1993; Sultz & Young, 2004). McLaughlin & Kaluzny (1999) suggest that variation in work processes is 'fat' that needs to be reduced. They categorize variation into common cause (random, inherent variation attributed to how a work process is performed) and special source (nonrandom, arising from a particular source).

To determine sources of variation in a work process, TQM/CQI programs use a variety of instruments. The instruments are presented in Table 20-4. Most of the instruments (except regression analysis) diagram the steps of a given process, provide a picture for persons involved in the QI process and help identify variations and/or potential sources of error within the work process.

Once the work process has been fully described, participants in the TQM/CQI process can proceed in implementing the Deming PDCA cycle. The following is an example of how Laura, the nurse in the chapter vignette, and the nursing department where she works would use TQM/CQI to correct the problem.

*Step 1: Identify a work process to be improved*: Accuracy of warfarin administration.

*Step 2: Organize a CQI/TQM team*: Select members to serve on the team that are involved in the work process. In this case, members would include a physician who

TABLE 20-4

## Instruments Used In TQM/CQI Programs

| Instrument | Description | Advantages |
|---|---|---|
| Flow chart | Graphic representation of sequence of events required to attain a specific outcome. Specific symbols depict steps of a process (rectangle = activity, diamond-shaped polygon = decisions, triangle = wait, large circle = file, small circle = go to another point, arrows demarking direction of the overall process. | Easily identify sources of variation and easily updated to keep current |
| Fishbone diagram | A horizontal line depicts the work process with the desired outcome appearing at the far lefthand side of diagram. Inputs into the work process are represented as lines (or spines) that intersect the horizontal line draw obliquely from the base line in upward or downward directions. The diagram looks like a fish skeleton. | Great for depicting work processes during brainstorming sessions, readily stratified to show details |
| Run chart | Displays the frequency of events or a particular observation over time. Frequency counts are connected by a line. | Wonderful way to depict data alterations arising from changes and key for knowing if improvements have resulted from changes |
| Pareto chart | Displays data using a rank order. Factors with the most frequent observation appear first followed by less frequent observations. | Ability to stratify causes, identifies the top causes, helpful to prioritize changes and useful to show results of change |
| Histogram | Bar-type graph that displays the frequency of something occurring. | Ability to detect frequency of root causes in a process and useful for tracking results of changes |
| Control chart | Depicted as a run chart, but has statistically determined upper and lower limits of variation above and below the average performance | Essential to see if process remains under control |
| Scatter diagram | A point is placed across a vertical and horizontal axis to demonstrate the relationship between two variables. | Useful to see if any relationships between two variables are occurring to detect causes and to monitor the effects of changes |
| Regression analysis | Statistical testing of correlational models. | Tests hypothesis used by organizations for decision making |

Adapted from Koch, M., & Fairly, T. (1993). *Integrated quality management, the key to improving nursing care quality.* St. Louis: Mosby; McLaughlin, C., & Kaluzny, A. (1999). *Continuous quality improvement in health care* (2nd ed.). Gaithersburg, MD: Aspen.

writes warfarin orders, a unit secretary who transcribes the physician order, a pharmacist who fills the order, a courier who delivers daily doses to the nursing units, and one or two nurses who note off physician orders and administer the medication.

*Step 3: Clarify the current work process*: The team meets and diagrams out the current process from the time the order is written until the client receives the ordered medication.

*Step 4: Identify and understand all variation sources*: The team notices that there may be as few as four persons (if the nurse transcribes and gives the medication) to as many as seven persons involved in the process of daily warfarin administration. The team also notes that daily orders may be written at any time during the day and that sometimes a daily order may not be given. They analyze all the medication incident reports filed related to warfarin administration that confirm the information generated from the brainstorming session. In addition, they create a checklist for collecting data regarding administration of warfarin for 2 weeks before the next meeting.

*Step 5: Select the improvement*: The team discovered after its data collection that administration of the medication to the wrong client occurred infrequently, but delay in administration was a more prevalent quality problem. Therefore, the team decides that perhaps commonly administered dosages could be placed in the computerized medication dispensing station and a nurse will double-check warfarin with another nurse before giving it to a client. The suggestion is made to institute a bar-coding device medication administration system at a future date.

*Step 6: Implement the improvement*: The nurses obtain ordered doses from the computerized medication dispensing system, and check the doses with another nurse.

*Step 7: Check and compare results with desired outcome*: Within a month of implementing step 6, the number of incident reports filed related to warfarin administration decreases by 25%.

*Step 8: Take steps to maintain improved performance and suggest ways to further improve the process*: Proposal is made for a hospital-wide patient band/medication bar-coding system to be purchased and implemented within the next 2 years.

Using a TQM/CQI approach, Laura, the nurse, does not receive a reprimand from her manager for giving the medication to the wrong client; rather, work processes are found to contribute to her error and those made by other nurses. In health care, the professional nurse plays a pivotal role in TQM/CQI.

To recognize success in implementing the TQM/CQI project, the hospital acknowledges contributions of the QI team in the organizational newsletter. The team also posts graphs indicating reduction in warfarin administration errors in the staff lounge of the cardiac unit.

## ✦ PROFESSIONAL NURSING ROLES IN QUALITY IMPROVEMENT

As health care organizations adopt a CQI philosophy, the professional nurses may have opportunities to showcase the unique contributions they make to interdisciplinary health-care delivery while assuming leadership roles in the TQM/CQI process. Professional nurses can combine all approaches to quality improvement outlined in this chapter as they compliment each other and can be used together effectively (Institute of Medicine, 2004). Data collection by nurses related to a quality initiative (an area for improvement) serves as one of the best ways for professional nurses to understand and participate in the QI process. The following discussion outlines how nurses might use professional nursing roles to promote QI.

## The Role of Caregiver and Quality Improvement

Professional nursing continues to study the effects of nursing care on client outcomes. Client outcomes that arise directly from nursing assessment and intervention are known as **nursing-sensitive outcomes.** Display 20-1 displays nursing-sensitive outcomes that have been identified to date. Most of these outcomes have been identified through nursing research. Doran's (2003) *Nursing-Sensitive Outcomes: State of the Science* provides a comprehensive, integrative literature review of research studies addressing the impact of professional nursing care on client outcomes. When nurses use their education and clinical skills in practice, clients experience short- and long-term benefits (Doran, 2003; Institute of Medicine, 2004).

In some health care organizations, consumer surveys provide a rich source of information for how services can be improved. Some organizations may elect to collect data on staff compliance to published standards of care as a way to monitor quality of nursing care. Porter-O'Grady and Malloch (2002) suggest that quality could be posed as a value question. Quality care includes using available resources judiciously, providing services in a timely fashion, and rendering appropriate interventions. Some institutions practicing shared governance form Quality Councils that monitor the quality of nursing care services at the unit level, overall institutional level, and/or both levels. For example, a hospital is interested in determining if the nursing staff is complying with the Center for Disease Control Standards and hospital standards for changing intravenous administration tubing. Staff nurses collect information on the standard using clinical assessment and client care documentation. The process of data collection increases nurse awareness of the importance of changing IV tubing per institutional policy. After the data are tabulated, nurses receive the results. If the results reveal less than satisfactory performance, some form of staff education is implemented. If performance meets standards, some form of recognition is received.

---

### Nursing-Sensitive Outcomes

DISPLAY 20-1 ●

#### Client Outcomes

Safety from medication and other treatment-related errors

Reduced use of restraints

Functional status

Self-care

Effective symptom management

Effective pain management

Satisfaction with received health care services

Effective management of fatigue

Effective management of nausea and vomiting

Effective management of dyspnea

Early detection and effective management of postoperative complications

Reduced incidence of urinary tract infections

Reduced incidence of pneumonia

Increased incidence of successful rescue following cardiac or respiratory arrest

Reduced incidence of pressure ulcers

Reduced client/visitor falls

*Source:* the American Nurses Association. (1995). *Nursing report card for acute care settings.* Washington, DC: Author; The Institute of Medicine. (2004). *Keeping patients safe.* Washington, DC: The National Academies Press; Doran, D. (Ed.). (2003). *Nursing-sensitive outcomes: The state of the science.* Sudbury, MA: Jones and Bartlett.

# The Role of Critical Thinker and Quality Improvement

In nursing education programs, many times nursing students strive for perfection in all assignments. Sometimes faculty members hold students to a level of clinical perfection when caring for clients in clinical settings. Some nurses perceive that errors result from carelessness, inattention to detail, indifference, or lack of knowledge. Attainment of human perfection defies what it means to be human. However, when some nurses make an error, they feel ashamed.

When organizations and society punish nurses for errors, nurses may be apt to hide them. However, when nurses and health care organizations transform their thinking using concepts of QI, it is discovered that more errors occur as the result of work processes and systems rather than from individual action. Medication administration, an activity frequently performed by nurses, poses great risks to clients. More than 770,000 persons die or suffer irreversible injury because of adverse drug events (including medication errors) (Institute of Medicine, 2004). Causes of medication errors include prescription errors, increased nurse responsibility for knowing medication dosages, action and potential adverse effects, and errors in calculated dosages (Cohen, Robinson and Mandrack, 2003; Institute of Medicine, 2004). A survey conducted by Cohen and colleagues (2003) involving 775 nurses revealed that 58% of these nurses reported that error reports served as a valuable means to measure a nurse's competency with medication administration. Six hundred twelve respondents (79%) reported the belief that most medication errors occurred when nurses failed to follow the "5 rights" religiously when administering client medication. Over half (51%) reported that their personnel files contained copies of incident reports filed for medication errors they made. Four hundred eighty nurses (79%) reported that technology such as bar coding, smart IV pumps, and computerized order entry systems would decrease the rate of future medication errors. Finally, less than half of the respondents reported that they consistently initiate incident records when catching mistakes made by other nurses (37%), a pharmacist (45%), or a physician (43%).

Work-related processes identified by the respondents as contributing to medication errors included being distracted or interrupted when administering medication, having inadequate staff, caring for high numbers of clients, reading illegible medication orders, working with medications with similar names and packaging, and having incorrect dosage calculations. The Institute of Medicine (2004) reported these findings along with miscommunication, lack of patient information, infusion pump malfunctions, and problems with IV delivery (extravasations, incompatibility of medications, dilutants, and ordered fluids).

Ninety-one percent of respondents to the Cohen and colleagues survey (2003) reported that a thorough analysis of all medication-related incident reports would provide a good understanding of why medication errors occurred.

Nurses use critical thinking to develop theoretical approaches to evaluate and improve the quality of nursing care (Sidani, Doran and Mitchell, 2004). The following five key factors interact to affect client outcomes (directly or indirectly):

1. Client characteristics: personal, sociocultural and health-related factors.
2. Professional characteristics: personal (dedication, commitment, finding meaning in work), educational preparation, keeping current with new practice advances, and sociocultural factors.

3. Health care setting: physical layout, availability of supplies, organizational culture.
4. Health care interventions for client: invasiveness, risks, type, if individualized to specific client.
5. Nature and timing or attainment of expected outcomes for health care interventions.

The function of all five characteristics produce direct effects on client outcomes, thereby accounting for individual and variable responses to nursing and health care interventions. The authors also identify two form of indirect effects "...moderating and mediating" (p. 61). Moderating effects address the effectiveness of care to produce desired outcomes according.to different levels of the five factors and mediating effects explain variance based on all factor effects on the intervention provided to the client.

A nursing-specific theoretical approach to evaluate nursing care is more valuable to nurses than relying on approaches used by medicine or business. As critical thinkers, nurses who use a theoretical approach can generate questions to gather data for a holistic approach to nursing care concerns and choose instruments to consistently measure the effects of nursing care. A theoretical approach also fosters an understanding of the unique contributions nurses make in the health care setting. A consistent approach to evaluating nursing care fosters quality improvement initiates because comparisons can be tracked over time.

## The Role of Client Advocate and Quality Improvement

Nurses work endlessly to consider the client's best interests. When participating in quality improvement activities, nurses advocate for all clients. Improvements in work processes reduce care errors. Nurses who acknowledge the effects of physical and mental fatigue advocate for clients when refusing to work overtime. Nurses who provide direct client care services for time frames equal to or exceeding 12.5 hours triple the chance of making errors (Rogers, Hwang, Scott, Aiken, & Dinges, 2004). Working extra shifts also increases the chance of committing nursing care errors (Rogers et al.; The Institute of Medicine, 2004).

Despite the research evidence linking long shifts and overtime to nursing errors, some nurses volunteer for overtime shifts to fill staffing shortages. Some institutions require nurses to work mandatory overtime. Many nurses consider long hours and overtime acceptable and agree to work them despite the effects of fatigue on judgment (Leighty, 2004). Nurses who refuse extra shifts may be perceived as not being good members of the nursing care teams. However, refusing to work long hours and overtime may be the best way to prevent nursing care errors, increasing the quality of health care services while ultimately looking out for the client's best interest.

## The Role of Change Agent and Quality Improvement

Professional nurses act as change agents when they identify needed changes in work processes to improve the quality of nursing care. Change occurs rapidly in the health care arena. As new health care devices, medications, and treatment advances become available, nurses need to change practice procedures. Nurses, as stakeholders in the delivery of health care, continuously examine which rituals and routines remain applicable and determine which ones should be discarded (Porter-OGrady & Malloch, 2002).

West Florida Regional Medical Center (WFRMC) provides an example of how TQM/CQI benefits institutions and clients. In 1988, a QI team found $16,800 in lost charges from ineffective nursing documentation. They were able to change documentation protocols. WFRMC also devised a universal charting system across all units, thereby decreasing the man-hours required for performing chart audits. The obstetrical department eliminated the need for duplicate charting of vital signs by reducing the number of documentation forms. The development of a hospital-wide Pharmacy and Therapeutic Team saved approximately $200,000 annually in antibiotic administration costs by merely listing the least expensive antibiotics to use ahead of more expensive ones on the culture and sensitivity laboratory reports. The team also suggested routine monitoring of client serum creatinine levels for nephrotoxic antibiotics, which then expanded to monitoring electrolytes for clients receiving diuretics and IV fluids. These activities caught potential adverse effects of medications more quickly and resulted in earlier interventions (McLaughlin & Kaluzny, 1999). Therefore, the QI process has the potential to save lives (direct client benefits) with simultaneous cost reductions in care delivery (institution benefits with potential consumer savings if reductions are passed to insurance companies who could lower health care insurance premiums).

As leaders of a nursing care team, professional nurses must clearly communicate changes in practice procedures to all team members. Some staff members (especially those who have worked in nursing for a long time) need to learn new approaches, how to operate new machinery, and learn new skills. Replacing traditional practice may create distress for some older nurses. Successful integration of change requires that the innovation fits well with the practice setting, has congruence with staff roles, improves client outcomes, and complements values and beliefs. Empowering staff for making work-related decisions and empowering clients to assume responsibility for their health increases the chance of successful change (Porter-O'Grady & Malloch, 2002). Because change requires unlearning old ways and learning new ones, the role of counselor/teacher becomes critical.

## The Role of Counselor/Teacher and Quality Improvement

Before adopting an innovation, staff must be educated about the reasons for the innovation, changes in practice policies and how to operate new equipment (if applicable). Staff educational programs may be planned using the teaching/learning principles outlined in Chapter 18. Interdepartmental educational programs provide staff with the opportunity to network, share successes with change, and support each other.

Along with education, nurses and unlicensed care providers need emotional support during times of nonstop change. Psychological effects of change have been delineated in Chapter 19. Staffs need time to grieve for the way things have been traditionally done before they can fully embrace innovations. When the innovation process becomes tough or stuck, staff relationships may be the only glue holding the nursing care team together. Taking time to deeply listen to peers and team members fosters capturing the messages and the meanings that surround ever-continual change processes associated with TQM/CQI programs (Porter-O'Grady & Malloch, 2002).

## The Role of Coordinator and Quality Improvement

As care coordinators, nurses must assess work colleagues for their ability to perform safe, effective client care. Physical and mental fatigue impair work performance. Actual errors and near misses (errors caught just in time before they occurred) are more likely to happen when hospital nurses work longer than 12-hour stretches; work overtime, regardless of shift length; and work more than 50 hours per week (Institute of Medicine, 2004; Rogers, Hwang, Scott, Aiken, & Dinges, 2004).

As coordinators of care, professional nurses must seek ways to provide quality of care while using resources effectively. Nursing unit characteristics directly affect client outcomes. Increased nurse perception of autonomy/collaboration has been instrumental in reducing incidences of urinary tract infections and failure to rescue events. When specialized nurses provide care with continuity, lower rates of pneumonia and cardiac arrests were reported along with shorter length of hospital stays. High levels of nurse manager support have been associated with reduced levels of pressure ulcer prevalence and client mortality (Aiken, Smith, & Lake, 1994; Aiken, Clarke, & Sloane, 2000; Boyle, 2004; Haven & Aiken, 1999).

## The Role of Colleague and Quality Improvement

The American way of life values independence and self-sufficiency. Nurses frequently have a strong sense of responsibility for individual vigilance that accentuates independence and self-sufficiency. Some nurses believe that asking for help with client assignments might be viewed as a sign of incompetence. Also, these nurses are afraid of being perceived as being weak if they needed to ask for assistance with a problem (Tucker & Edmondson, 2003). However, the QI process discourages this form of thinking as all health team members have the responsibility to point out work process flaws.

When flaws are identified with work processes, QI teams are formed. Participation in the QI project team provides opportunities for nurses to network with other members of the health care team, thereby strengthening working relationships with them. During team deliberations, members of the QI team have opportunities to see and value the unique skills and approaches they bring to client health care delivery.

Continuous quality improvement requires health team competencies that differ from those that were successful in the past. Wilson and Porter-O'Grady (1999) outline the key leadership competencies required in today's health care organizations (Display 20-1). However, in organizations subscribing to TQM/CQI programs, all team members need to learn how to use these competencies. These competencies acknowledge the individual strengths of everyone who participates in a process and demands that each person use his or her specific knowledge and talents in providing health care using a multidisciplinary team approach. Changes in client care processes become the responsibility of each team member. For CQI to be effective, all health team members must develop collegial partnerships.

## ✦ SUMMARY AND SIGNIFICANCE TO PRACTICE

TQM/CQI operate on the philosophy that all things can be improved. The professional nurse plays key roles in improving the quality of health care delivery. Nurses bring a

## Leadership Competencies for All Engaged in the TQM/CQI Process

1. Acknowledging and using the inner wisdom of self and others
2. Recognizing the interconnection of everyone and everything
3. Abandoning the hierarchical approach to leadership
4. Recognizing that persons performing the work are the specialists
5. Engaging in systems thinking
6. Recognizing patterns
7. Synthesizing new ideas and processes
8. Committing to lifelong continuous learning
9. Adapting to and accepting chaos
10. Facilitating each team member's involvement and accountability
11. Empowering others
12. Being receptive to new ideas and the ideas of others
13. Facilitating group meeting and participation of everyone in organizational processes (especially decision making)
14. Coaching
15. Acting with immediacy and equality
16. Displaying technical expertise in all aspects of health care delivery
17. Practicing principles of effective relationship dynamics
18. Sharing administrative functions
19. Favoring collaboration over competition

Adapted from Porter-O'Grady, T., & Malloch, K. (2002). *Quantum leadership: A textbook for new leadership.* Gaithersburg, MD: Aspen.

unique perspective and skill set to enhance client care quality. Professional nursing interventions directly affect client outcomes. TQM/CQI processes use solid evidence to foster team decision making in health care organizations. All health team members must be invested in the TQM/CQI processes to ensure success.

## FROM THEORY TO PRACTICE

1. Do you think that the health care industry should be held to the same quality of services as that of big business and industry? Why or why not?
2. How would you have to change your practice and practice environment to strive toward attaining the same level of quality that is required of the business and manufacturing industries?
3. How does your clinical practice setting view incident reports? What are the advantages of having staff completing incident reports for quality monitoring purposes? Are you afraid to complete incident reports? Why or why not?

## WWW INTERNET EXERCISES

1. Visit the National Quality Forum website at http://www.qualityforum.org.
   Visit the Joint Commission for Accreditation of Healthcare Organizations at http://www.jcaho.org.
   Compare the information found on these websites.
   Which website do you think offers the best information for nurses? Why or why not?
   Which website offers the best health-related information for consumers? Why or why not?
2. Visit Toyota Corporation at http://toyota.com/planetkaizen./index.html. View the online presentation of Toyota's quality improvement process. If unable to access

the program, you can access the program by visiting Toyota's home page at http://www.toyota.com, then click on the words "Planet Kaizen" at the bottom of the page. What do the Japanese words *kai* and *zen* mean?

3. Visit General Electric Corporation and read about how they use Six Sigma to assure quality products and services at http://www.ge.com/sixsigma. Learn more about the concepts of Six Sigma.

## INTERNET RESOURCES

Joint Commission for Accreditation of Healthcare Organizations: http://www.jcaho.org.
National Quality Forum: http://www.qualityforum.org.
GE-Six Sigma: http://www.ge.com/sixsigma.
Toyota Plane Kaizen: http://www.toyota.com/planetkaizen/index.html.
George Group- Six Sigma-Lean: http://www.georgregroup.com.
Baldrige National Quality Program: http://www.quality.nist.gov.
See a picture and hear Dr. Juran's voice at http://www.does.org. Just click on his picture once you get to the site.
W. Edwards Deming Institute: http://www.deming.org.
Juran Institute: http://www.juran.com.
Philip Crosby Associates: http://www.philipcrosby.com.

## REFERENCES

Aiken, L., Clarke, P., & Sloane, D. (2000). Hospital restructuring: Does it adversely affect care and outcomes? *Journal of Nursing Administration 30,* 457–465.

Aiken, L., Smith, H., & Lake, E. (1994). Lower Medicare mortality among a set of hospitals known for good nursing care. *Medical Care, 32,* 771–787.

American Nurses Association (1995). *Nursing report card for acute care settings.* Washington, DC: Author.

Baldrige National Quality Program, (2004). Available at: www.quality.nist.gov/Improvement_Act.htm. Accessed July 13, 2005.

Bohnet, N., Ilcyn, J., Milanovich, P., Ream, M., & Wright, K. (1993). Continuous quality improvement: Improving quality in your home care organization. *Journal of Nursing Administration, 23,* 42–48.

Boyle, S. (2004). Nursing unit characteristics and patient outcomes. *Nursing Economic$, 22,* 111–123.

Chowdhury, S. (2002). *The power of six sigma.* Chicago: Dearborn Trade Publishing.

Cohen, H., Robinson, E., & Mandrack, M. (2003). Getting to the root of medication errors: Survey results. *Nursing, 33,* 36–46.

Crosby, P. (1979). *Quality is free: The art of making quality certain.* New York: Mentor.

DesHarnais, S., & McLaughlin, C. (1999). *Continuous quality improvement in health care* (2nd ed.). Gaithersburg, MD: Aspen.

Doran, D. (Ed.) (2003). *Nursing-sensitive outcomes: State of the science.* Sudbury, MA: Jones and Bartlett.

Duffy, J. & Hoskins, L. (2003). The Quality-Caring Model ©. *Journal of Advanced Nursing, 26,* 77–88.

Hart, C., & Bogan, C. (1992). *The Baldrige.* New York: McGraw-Hill.

Haven, D., and Aiken, L. (1999). Shaping systems to promote desired outcomes. *Journal of Nursing Administration, 29,* 14–20.

Institute of Medicine (2000). *To err is human: Building a safer health system.* Washington, DC: The National Academies Press.

Institute of Medicine. (2004). *Keeping patients safe.* Washington, DC: The National Academies Press.

International Organization for Standardization. (2004). Introduction. Available at: http://www.iso.org/iso/en/aboutiso/introduction/. Accessed July 13, 2005.

Joint Commission on Accreditation of Healthcare Organizations. (2004). *Facts about the Joint Commission on Accreditation for Health Care Organizations.* Available at: http://www.jcaho.org/about+us.jcaho-facts/htm. Accessed July 13, 2005.

Joint Commission on Accreditation of Healthcare Organizations. (2004a). *2005 Hospitals' National Patient Safety Goals.* Available at: http://www.jcaho.org/accr edited+organizations/hospitals/npsg/05_npsg_hap.htm. Accessed July 13, 2005.

Juran, J. (1989). *Juran on leadership for quality.* New York: The Free Press.

Kalisch, P. A., & Kalisch, B. J. (2004). *The advance of American nursing* (4th ed.). Philadelphia: Lippincott Williams & Wilkins.

Koch, M., & Fairly, T. (1993). *Integrated quality management: the key to improving nursing care quality.* St. Louis: Mosby.

Leighty, J. (2004). Test pilots. *Nurseweek, Heartland Edition,* (August 23, 2004), pp. 15-16.

McLaughlin, C. P., & Kaluzny, A. D. (1999). *Continuous quality improvement in health care* (2nd ed.). Gaithersburg, MD: Aspen.

Miller, S., & Flanagan, E. (1993). The transition from quality assurance to continuous quality improvement in ambulatory care. *Quality Review Bulletin, 19,* 62–65.

Mish, F. (ed.). (1994). *Merriam-Webster's collegiate dictionary* (10th ed.). (1994). Springfield, MA: Merriam-Webster.

Morgan, S. & Cooper, C. (2004). Shoulder work intensity with Six Sigma. *Nursing Management 35,* 28–32.

Ouchi, W. (1981). *Theory Z: How American business can meet the Japanese challenge.* Reading, MA: Addison Wesley.

Pande, P., Neuman, R., & Cavanagh, R. (2000). *The Six Sigma way: How GE, Motorola and other top companies are honing their performance.* New York: McGraw-Hill.

Porter-O'Grady, T., & Malloch, K. (2002). *Quantum Leadership: a textbook for new leadership.* Gaithersburg, MD: Aspen.

Rogers, A., Hwang, W., Scott, L., Aiken, L. & Dinges, D. (2004). The working hours of hospital staff nurses and patient safety. *Health Affairs, 23,* 202–212.

Sidani, S., Doran, D., & Mitchell, P. (2004). A theory-driven approach to evaluating quality of nursing care. *Journal of Nursing Scholarship, 36,* 60–65.

Sultz, H. & Young, K. (2004). *Health Care USA: Understanding its organization and delivery* (4th ed.). Sudbury, MA: Jones & Bartlett.

Tucker, A., & Edmondson, A. (2003). When problem solving prevents organizational learning. *Journal of Organizational Change Management. 15,* 122–137.

Walton, M. (1986). *The Deming management method.* New York: Putman.

Wilson, C. K., & Porter-O'Grady, T. (1999). *Leading the revolution in health care* (2nd ed.). Gaithersburg, MD: Aspen.

As a profession, nursing can count on change. Professional nurses have many nursing career options. A rewarding and satisfying career depends on the interests and passions of each individual nurse. Once nurses discover what they want to do, they can use specific career development strategies to assure success. Many nurses move from one area of professional practice to another throughout a professional nursing career. To meet the future need for professional nursing and to secure a future for the nursing profession, nurses need to examine current trends, develop future scenarios, and envision a preferred future. Once a preferred future is envisioned, then professional nurses can work together to make it reality.

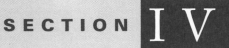

SECTION IV

# Glimpsing the Future of Professional Nursing

# CHAPTER 21

# Career Options for Professional Nurses

## KEY TERMS AND CONCEPTS

Universal Job Skills

Licensure

Certification

Advanced Nursing Practice

Graduate Nursing Education

Nurse Practitioners

General Nursing Practice

Specialized Nursing Practice

Clinical Ladders

Nurse Entrepreneurs

Certified Nurse-Midwives (CNMs)

Nursing Administration

Nursing Academia

## LEARNING OUTCOMES

By the end of this chapter, the learner will be able to:

1  Outline universal job skills.

2  Specify which universal job skills nurses possess.

3  Identify career options for nurses educated at the generalist level.

4  Explain the differences between general and advanced nursing practice.

5  Distinguish certification from advanced nursing practice.

6  Describe advanced nursing practice roles and responsibilities.

## VIGNETTE

Laura is thinking about entering the nursing profession. As she explores professional nursing, Laura finds that there are many career options within the profession. Laura interviews three nurses and finds that one nurse remained employed for over 20 years as a staff nurse at a clinical agency that was part of the nurse's undergraduate nursing program. Another nurse that she interviewed shared her experiences with a nursing career that began as a nursing assistant, followed by several years each of hospital staff nursing, school nursing, and outpatient clinic nursing. The same nurse pursued a graduate nursing degree and currently works as a nurse practitioner in a small rural clinic. The last nurse Laura interviewed was a nurse faculty member who held a nursing doctorate and seemed to enjoy research and teaching. After learning about the diverse career options in nursing, Laura decides to pursue a nursing career, but will keep her options open until she finds her niche.

Setting career goals begins with self-assessment. Ideally, career goals should match personal values and acquired skills. As outlined in the vignette, nurses have many career options without leaving the nursing profession. This chapter explores career options in professional nursing that have not been presented in previous chapters.

# UNIVERSAL JOB SKILLS

In 1992, the *Occupational Outlook Handbook* published by the United States Bureau of Labor Statistics delineated the following **universal job skills** for all types of work: (1) leadership/persuasion, (2) problem solving/creativity, (3) working as part of a team, (4) manual dexterity, (5) helping or instructing others, (6) initiative, (7) frequent contact with the public, and (8) physical stamina. Very few jobs involve all of the universal job skills. However, nursing requires all of them.

Many job skills mastered by nurses readily transfer to other fields (Waxman, 2005). The comprehensive skill set required by professional nurses may be a reason that career opportunities in nursing are quite different. Individuals rank the importance of job skills differently, and the ranking provides a clue to personal values. Personal values guide nurses in deciding in which areas to practice professional nursing.

## Questions for Reflection 21-1

1. How do I use each of the eight universal job skills in my daily professional nursing practice?
2. How do other jobs use the skills differently than nurses?
3. Why does nursing require mastery of all eight universal job skills?

# LEVELS OF NURSING PRACTICE

In the United States, state legislatures and state boards of nursing regulate practice. In Canada, provincial/territorial professional nursing associations assume responsibility for regulating professional nursing practice (except the province of Ontario where the College of Nurses of Ontario assumes this responsibility). In both countries, regulation of practice involves determining educational qualifications, setting standards of professional practice, limiting the use of the title "registered nurse," approving nursing education programs, determining the extent of continuing education and competency, disciplining professional members who endanger the public, and specifying the scope of nursing practice (McIntyre & Thomlinson, 2003; National Council of State Boards of Nursing, 2000). When nurses complete a preparatory nursing education program, (associate degree, diploma, or baccalaureate degree), successfully pass the National Council of State Boards of Nursing Licensure Examination (NCLEX), and pay nursing licensure fees, they begin professional practice as registered nurses. **Licensure** is a process of legal authorization for nursing practice. Newly licensed nurses practice as generalists initially. However, with increased nursing experience in a particular area of practice, many nurses become specialized.

Professional nurses associations recognize professional nurse competence in a particular nursing field by certification. **Certification** means that an individual meets specified requirements, which usually include specialized knowledge and skill in a specialized area of nursing practice. Most certifications in professional nursing practice require a specified number of years of experience within a specialty along with successful completion of a competency examination. Some nursing regulatory agencies use certification from professional nursing associations "as a substitute for regulatory certification" (Porcher, 1996, p. 180). However, in many cases, certification does not fulfill regulatory requirements to attain advanced practice nursing status.

**Advanced nursing practice** occurs when nurses receive **graduate nursing education** (collegiate education beyond the baccalaureate degree toward a master's degree or doctorate). In the early days of **nurse practitioners** and nurse midwifery, graduate nursing education was not required for entry into advanced nursing practice. Many states used certification as credentialing. Depending on the nature of advanced practice (nurse practitioners and midwives), additional state nursing licensure is required (Sultz & Young, 2004). In the case of nurse practitioners (who deliver primary, secondary, and tertiary health care services in collaboration with a physician), many states require that they enter into collaborative practice agreements with physicians licensed in the state of practice (Sultz & Young).

## ⬤ GENERAL NURSING CAREER OPPORTUNITIES

The nursing profession offers a wide array of opportunities. Nurses have the flexibility to focus on one area of practice or work in several practice areas. In addition, nurses may work for an organization or for themselves. **General nursing practice** encompasses areas of practice in which no additional or specialized formal education is required. **Specialized nursing practice** occurs when nurses work in a specific clinical area (such as obstetrics, oncology, and intensive care) where additional education and training are needed to meet specific client concerns or master unique clinical nursing skills. In many specialty areas of nursing practice, nurses become certified in the area of practice, which means they have mastered specific skills and possess a unique knowledge to deliver client care. When a nurse identifies a problem in practice, a potential opportunity has arisen for a new area of nursing practice. Sometimes, an identified problem leads to the development of a personal business or an entirely new health service to be offered by a large medical center. The more common areas of nursing practice are briefly summarized in this section. Detailed information about specific nursing careers is in this and subsequent chapters: advanced practice nursing (later in this chapter); nursing informatics (in Chapter 15); lobbying as a nurse (in Chapter 16), and nursing careers in community health nursing (Chapter 14).

### Acute Care or Hospital Nursing Options

The hospital nurse who provides direct client care is whom most people imagine when asked to describe a nurse. In 2000, 59.1% of employed registered nurses worked in hospitals. Of those nurses, 75% reported spending more than 50% of their time in direct client care (American Nurses Association, 2003). Recent changes in the health care delivery system have resulted in a variety of career options for nurses working in acute care.

## Staff Nursing

Nurses engaging in direct client care find themselves in a fast-paced and challenging position. Within the past decade, acuity of hospitalized clients has dramatically increased. Now, nurses frequently care for clients who once would have been admitted only to intensive care units. As complex specialized skills become requirements for various types of staff nursing (such as oncology and cardiac specialties), many nurses become certified in specialty practice areas. Experience and certification in specialty areas of practice result in highly trained experts delivering client care. As nurses develop more technical expertise in specific areas, they cannot be expected to provide expert nursing care to clients outside those areas of clinical specialties. However, because basic nursing education effectively prepares professional nurses to assume safe care responsibilities as nurse generalists, hospitals sometimes assign nurses to work outside their clinical specialty areas.

Staff nurses in acute care settings seem like circus performers. They juggle multiple tasks simultaneously. They walk tightropes when confronted with competing client care priorities, such as quality client care, cost containment, supervision of unlicensed assistive personnel, and shared governance responsibilities. They serve as ringmasters when getting clients where they need to go for diagnostic tests, surgery, or rehabilitative therapy. They soothe disgruntled clients, families, and physicians like the lion tamer who gets lions to remain calm. They assume the role of spotter when taking steps to monitor the safety of the environment for clients and staff. Finally, they act as clowns when they use humor to defray highly emotionally charged situations.

Keeping nurse experts at the client bedside poses challenges for acute care organizations. Some hospitals have designed nursing **clinical ladders** as a means to keep highly qualified and experienced nurses at the bedside. Clinical ladders reward experienced bedside staff nurses for ongoing professional development activities. Rewards include more income, and job titles denoting professional accomplishments and experience. Frequently nurses who climb clinical ladders serve as mentors or preceptors to novice nurses. Many use educational status, specialty professional nurse certification, integration of nursing research in clinical practice, and participation in shared governance activities as criteria for promotion (Cutler, 2002; Davis & Bheenucks, 2003; Robitaille & Whelchel, 2005).

### Questions for Reflection 21-2

1. What are the benefits of having clinical nursing ladders for nurses? For hospitals?
2. Would a clinical nursing ladder keep me at the bedside? Why or why not?

## Staff Development

Recent concerns related to staff competency and improving care quality have provided support for hospitals to maintain nursing staff education and training departments (sometimes called staff development). In addition to providing continuing education and staff competency verification for professional nurses, members of staff education and training departments provide consistent training for unlicensed personnel. Some hospitals require graduate degrees in nursing or education for these positions. Titles for nurses working in this field include staff educator, clinical education specialist, inservice educator, and educational specialist (Case, 1997b). Some institutions (usually smaller ones) also use the staff development personnel to plan community education programs. When a hospital is used as a clinical site for more than one nursing program, staff educators frequently coordinate clinical day availability, set up programs to verify clinical faculty competence, develop student clinical orientation programs, and keep records related to nursing program satisfaction with the agency as a clinical site.

## Utilization Review

To verify the effective use of hospital services, many hospitals and insurance companies use nurses to streamline inpatient care. In response to Medicare regulations, hospitals have developed utilization review programs. Because nurses have the education and experience to understand effective use of resources, sometimes they obtain employment as utilization reviewers. Some managed care organizations employ nurses as preadmission coordinators who prepare clients for hospital admission by coordinating preadmission testing and providing clients with education related to the usual hospital course (especially for surgical procedures). In addition, some managed care organizations use nurses as case managers who act as the client care advocate to make care-related decisions, recommend medical treatments, certify insurance coverage, and listen to customer expectations and problems.

When working as a reviewer, strong clinical background, good research skills, and well-developed skills in analysis are required. Nurses in these positions frequently serve as liaisons among the provider, physician, and consumer.

## Risk/Quality Management

Most hospitals have departments to track unusual reported incidents, identify potential liability areas, and provide staff education on the documentation and reporting of incidents, and assist staff when legal actions or malpractice suits arise. Risk management focuses on reducing institutional financial losses because of care errors and accidents. Nurses employed in risk management departments sometimes hold law degrees.

Although all nurses play a role in managing the quality of health care provided within their institutions, some larger organizations may have a centralized quality management department to assess the quality of services provided. Because a large portion of the services offered by hospitals is nursing care, nurses may be members of the quality department to monitor the quality of nursing care services rendered to customers. However, other organizations opt for a decentralized approach to quality management. In these cases, staff nurses assume a larger role in monitoring the quality of nursing care.

## Travel Nursing

With regional and seasonal shortages of registered nurses, some nurses (especially those who like variety, taking risks, and traveling) elect to travel to different inpatient institutions to practice bedside client care. Travel nurses accept staff nurse assignments in all areas of the hospital. Travel nurses may contract with a travel nurse agency or work as independent contractors. Most traveling agencies require that a nurse have 1 to 2 years of acute care experience before offering him or her a contract.

Travel nurse agencies may contract with hospitals to fill vacant staff nurse positions. The agency offers nurses positions from which to choose; assistance with housing, moving, and professional licensure expenses; and some may offer benefits (health insurance, life insurance, and retirement plans.). Terms of contracts with travel nurse agencies vary greatly. Most temporary agencies require nurses to fulfill their current contract and then wait a time before accepting a position once held as a travel nurse (Kearney, 2003). For example, conditions of a contract may state that the nurse must not accept employment at a hospital where the agency sent the nurse for 2 years after severing ties with the nursing agency.

## Extended Care Facility Nursing

The American Nurses Association (2003) reported that 152,894 registered nurses worked in extended care facilities. Most of these nurses were educated in diploma or associate degree programs.

### Elderly Long-Term Care

For many years, nurses have viewed professional nursing in long-term care institutions (nursing homes or extended care facilities) as unattractive. However, for nurses desiring to escape the fast pace of acute care nursing and establish long-term relationships with clients, long-term care (LTC) nursing provides these opportunities. In most LTC facilities, professional nurses assume supervisory roles and delegate tasks to licensed practical/vocational nurses, certified medicine aides, and other unlicensed care providers. With the push for earlier hospital dismissals, LTC facilities also currently care for younger clients. Complex care needs, such as mechanical ventilation, tracheotomy, hyperalimentation, and tube feeding have become common in such facilities. Some LTC clients are residents only long enough to complete postoperative therapy or to regain strength after a hospital stay. Thus, the professional nurse can maintain some acute care clinical skills when working in LTC. Some LTC facilities offer assisted living services. Professional nurses conduct initial periodic client assessments, screen clients for health problems, see clients when health-related problems arise, develop the client care plan, manage client medications, supervise licensed and unlicensed personnel as they provide client care, and determine staff inservice educational needs (Mitty, 2003). Instead of an institutional approach to client care, most LTC facilities view themselves as the client's home.

Some nurses find great rewards in working with the elderly. Unfortunately, some elderly clients have no families or support systems, and members of the LTC staff become their only source link to the outside world. Many elderly clients develop strong personal relationships with LTC staff. Because death is viewed as a normal part of life in LTC facilities, residents may not be subjected to many invasive procedures or become attached to technological equipment that is used only to preserve life. Most LTC facilities permit visits by hospice when death is imminent, enabling comfortable, dignified, and peaceful deaths.

With the projected increases in the elderly population needing assisted living, LTC nursing represents one of the fastest growing careers. LTC offers professional nurses the chance to make a big difference in individual lives.

### Rehabilitation Nursing

Advances in trauma care and increases in chemical dependency have resulted in an explosion of rehabilitation facilities. Likewise, insurance companies have identified that transferring clients to rehabilitation facilities after bouts of acute illness or surgery saves money. Rehabilitation units have opened as part of acute care and LTC facilities, and freestanding rehabilitation centers offer services to consumers. Some centers specialize in specific rehabilitation needs for a particular health problem, such as stroke, head injury, spinal cord trauma, chemical dependency, chronic respiratory illness, amputation, cancer survival, or blindness.

In contrast to nurses working in acute care, rehabilitation nurses participate as equal partners of an interdisciplinary health team. Rehabilitation nurses need to be cooperative team players and have excellent organizational and communication skills. There is a strong focus on client education because the goal of rehabilitation is to get the clients to care for themselves or coach someone on how to care for them. Rehabilitation nurses may become very involved with clients and families and experience great satisfaction from being part of the client's journey toward mastering an independent lifestyle. The Association of Rehabilitation Nurses offers special certification in rehabilitation nursing.

## Outpatient Nursing Opportunities

Besides acute care nursing, many nursing opportunities occur in outpatient settings. Some outpatient nursing opportunities demand specialized education and training.

### Outpatient Clinics and Physician Offices

Nurses working in outpatient clinics and physician offices usually work with clients who have less acute conditions. In 2000, ambulatory care centers employed 209,324 registered nurses. More nurses employed in outpatient settings worked part time than in any other professional nursing clinical setting (ANA, 2003). Many nurses choose these settings because the hours are better and the working conditions less stressful. Depending on the clinic or office, the professional nurse may be a specialized expert or a generalist. Some nurses work in clinic settings, where on specific days of the week a specialized clinic may be held. Clinics and offices may be located close to a hospital, in a professional office building, or in a shopping mall. Some clinics offer services 24 hours a day, 7 days a week for illnesses and injuries not requiring emergency services. The research brief presents the key responsibilities assumed by registered nurses in ambulatory cancer centers and clinics.

### Research Brief 21-1

Ireland, A. M., DePalma, J. A., Arenson, L., Stark, L., & Williamson, J. The Oncology Nursing Society Ambulatory Office Survey. *Oncology Nursing Forum, 31. OnLine Exclusive,* E 147–156.

Three hundred twenty-five oncology nurses working in ambulatory oncology care centers and offices responded to a survey to determine the most commonly performed tasks and how important it was for the registered nurse to complete them. More than two-thirds of the nurses surveyed held Oncology Certified Nurse status and baccalaureate or higher degrees in nursing.

More than 205 of the respondents administered IV medication, transfused blood, accessed and drew blood from vascular access devices, started peripheral intravenous lines, performed telephone triage, renewed prescriptions, and assisted with invasive procedures. Less than 200 of the nurses reported feeling that it was very important that the registered nurse (RN) renew prescriptions and assist with invasive procedures because these tasks could be delegated to other cancer care team members. Only 183 respondents reported that patient identification before chemotherapy administration was part of their safety policies and procedures. Most of the nurses reported that chemotherapy documentation included drug dose and name, route and site of administration, presence of blood return before administration, client education, tolerance to the infusion, body surface area calculation, and beginning and ending time.

Ninety-three percent of the respondents reported using a specific form to document telephone conversations held with clients and families. Over 93% of the nurses assumed responsibility for client education and reported that education on symptom management, treatment-related and other adverse effects were very important to include in patient education session. Forty percent of the nurses reported that the setting used a functional approach to nursing care. Less than 30% of the registered nurses reported facilitating decisions regarding movement toward and ongoing management of palliative client care. More than 40% of the nurses reported being responsible for infusion room scheduling, and 54% reported fixing any clinic scheduling problems. In addition, 74% of the RNs reported having responsibilities for completing billing tickets for third-party reimbursement and 33% of these RNs assumed responsibility for reviewing client charges for accuracy. Forty-nine percent of the RNs reported that they assumed responsibility for procuring medications for indigent clients, even though 23% reported believing that this was very important for a RN to do. Of the nurses responding, 240 RNs reported that the role of the RN in clinical trials was to follow protocols strictly.

Only 40% of the RNs reported that they stayed abreast of legislative initiatives related to nursing and cancer care. Forty-seven percent reported that their work setting had open positions. To combat the nursing shortages, the RNs reported the need to start recruiting nurses to replace them now rather than wait until later. Recruitment efforts reported included speaking to nursing students and other nurses at local hospitals. The RNs reported that nurses previously employed in critical care adapted well to oncology nursing.

Results of this study show the usual job responsibilities assumed by RNs in ambulatory oncology centers/clinics. This survey outlines specific job requirements for nurses employed in outpatient oncology settings. This information could be useful to an organization opening a new outpatient oncology center/clinic, refine oncology nurse job descriptions, and recruit new RN personnel. Because the RNs responding to the survey worked in different clinical agencies, results of this study may likely apply to many ambulatory oncology centers and clinics. Critical care nurses adapted well to the field of oncology nursing, because recruitment efforts included oncology nurse presentations at local hospitals and nursing schools, and offered flexible working hours. Additional research is needed to see if RN responsibilities would be similar in other ambulatory care settings.

## Outpatient Surgery Centers

The number of outpatient or ambulatory surgical centers has exploded within the past 20 years. Many surgical procedures do not require a postoperative hospital stay. Although these centers do not have all the resources that are available in an acute care setting, they do have emergency equipment available and policies to guide staff if life-threatening emergencies arise. Many nurses working in outpatient surgery centers have operating room experience. In this setting, some nurses admit clients, assist with surgical procedures, provide care after anesthesia has been administered, teach clients about discharge instructions, and accompany them to vehicles for the ride home. Some outpatient surgery centers have nurses call to check on client progress the day after the procedure.

## Special Care Centers

In addition to outpatient clinics and surgery centers, disease-focused centers provide expert care to persons with health problems such as diabetes, heart disease, renal failure, and cancer. Some large urban medical centers have opened breast care centers that provide a comprehensive approach to breast health. Services include screening mammography, self-breast examination education, a comprehensive library related to breast cancer, ultrasound testing, and breast biopsy. In these settings, nurses work as interdisciplinary team members to provide holistic, comprehensive client care.

### Community Nursing Centers

Nursing community centers offer primary health care services to middle- and lower-class clients at reduced cost as compared to traditional clinics and physician offices. Nurse-run centers usually have a nurse practitioner and nurses with specialized skills in health education, stress reduction, weight issues, and lifestyle management, and other wellness-focused health topics to deliver services. Community nursing centers may be located in a school or church. Nursing centers often have an affiliation with a collegiate nursing program. If required care is not available at the community nursing center, nurses make referrals and sometimes arrange for services. Depending on the funding, the nursing center may pay for services arranged within a provider network.

### Community Education

As consumers seek wellness education, professional nurses frequently find themselves volunteering for various community education groups to teach a variety of health classes. Local businesses, civic organizations, and churches frequently want to offer staff and members information regarding cardiopulmonary resuscitation, first aid, cancer self-examinations, parenting skills, babysitting, and healthy lifestyles. Some organizations request health screenings and may sponsor health fairs.

### Cardiac Rehabilitation

Within the past 20 years, most cardiac clients have received offers to participate in cardiac rehabilitation programs after undergoing cardiac catheterizations, pacemaker implants, or open-heart surgery. Persons recovering from myocardial infarctions also qualify for cardiac rehabilitation. Cardiac rehabilitation centers can be found in hospital settings, physician offices, or fitness centers. These programs rely on the expertise of professional nurses and exercise physiologists to develop and supervise a physical workout for patients with cardiac disease.

Most cardiac rehabilitation nurses have a background in critical care nursing and have Advanced Cardiac Life Support (ACLS) certification. Cardiac rehabilitation nursing responsibilities include observing cardiac monitors as clients exercise, performing periodic pulse and blood pressure measurements, assessing for signs of overexertion, and teaching relaxation and stress reduction techniques. Some cardiac rehabilitation programs use the nurse for nutritional lifestyle counseling and mental health counseling when nutritionists (or dietitians) and psychologists are not part of the program.

### Forensic Nursing

Forensic nurses provide care to victims of violent crime. Many emergency departments have a nurse who has special education in working with victims of violent crimes. Nursing care provided by forensic nurses includes the following: caring for the victim's injuries, identifying and documenting the injures (including taking photographs), determining wound patterns, collecting evidence (samples of hair, tissue, and body fluids) for future trials, and testifying in court to present and explain evidence and examination findings. Victims of violent crime benefit from having forensic nurses because the nurse knows how to approach and counsel victims of violent crime. Some emergency departments have special rape crisis or abuse crisis programs in which victims receive care from forensic nurses in specially designated rooms. In these cases, the nurse makes referrals to social workers for arranging safe living arrangements and follow-up counseling (Stevens, 2004).

## Business Opportunities

In addition to being involved with direct client care, nurses can find employment opportunities in the business sector. Business career opportunities enable nurses to make an impact on client care by bringing the care ethic to corporations that supply products and reimbursement for health care.

### Insurance and Managed Care Companies

Insurance and managed care companies use nurses for evaluating care delivered to customers. Third-party payers frequently use nurses as gatekeepers to verify that company resources have been effectively used to provide services. Responsibilities for nurses employed by companies include reviewing medical records and activities to evaluate the need for care, ensuring that the appropriate level of care was received, and determining that quality care was delivered in a timely fashion.

Along with quality management, third-party payers use nurses to staff telephones to certify insurance coverage before service delivery. Nurses who fill certification positions need a strong clinical background and an ability to grasp a global picture of all the issues surrounding care delivery. However, nurses employed in this position frequently encounter many ethical dilemmas when working with complex clinical issues and deciding when to certify care. If a wrong decision is made, the nurse may be solely accountable for it, especially if the nurse is a company manager.

### Telephone Triage and Health Care Advice Lines

Managed care companies, physician offices, clinics, and hospitals frequently use professional nurses to staff call centers devoted to determining the urgency of care, providing health information, referring clients to appropriate health care providers, scheduling appointments with health care providers, and offering health advice. Although triage and health care advice lines started out as a marketing strategy, they quickly demonstrated the ability to streamline the use of health care services, thereby reducing health care costs. Some managed care companies require that subscribers call the triage nurse to certify trips to emergency departments. Nurses use assessment and therapeutic communication skills to determine the extent of the health problems of callers. Because some clients become frequent callers, telephone triage nurses may develop long-term relationships with them. Some nurses report that they schedule time to call clients to follow up on decisions they made.

### Marketing and Sales

Companies that sell products such as pharmaceuticals, IV equipment, and monitors often hire professional nurses as sales representatives. Nurses provide credibility for product promotion, especially when they have used the product in clinical practice. Nurses also provide an insight into product improvements and future products that may be useful in client care delivery. When complex equipment is purchased, the company often provides staff education in the use of the equipment. As sales representatives, nurses know how to approach other nurses and anticipate questions and problems that the nurse may experience.

Sales representatives must be energetic and self-motivated. Because most sales representatives work from their homes and travel a lot, they work flexible hours. Much time is spent meeting with prospective customers. Knowledge related to the business world and principles of operating a home office provide needed skills for nurses entering the corporate world. Some companies provide a base salary that does not meet the salary earned from clinical practice. However, significant bonuses can be earned when commissions arrive from successful sales.

### Occupational Health and Worker's Compensation Programs

Many businesses have occupational health departments for which nurses work at managing workplace injuries, preventing work-related illnesses, screening for environmental or occupational hazards, providing employee educational services, and marketing employee health programs to other companies. Occupational health nurses frequently offer CPR training and health promotion education for company employees. They also respond to work-related injuries or medical emergencies that occur. Some companies rely on the occupational health nurse to track the progress of workers recovering from work-related injuries. Other companies use nurses employed by the worker's compensation insurance plan to monitor worker progress. Nurses often develop light-duty work programs for employees who cannot perform all regular job duties but can provide some work for the company.

### Private Consulting

When a nurse identifies a problem, an area for consulting has surfaced. As companies outsource employee services, demands for consultants increase. Health care organizations use consulting firms to prepare for accreditation visits, apply for quality awards, meet employee educational needs, engage in work redesign, and look for ways to reduce operating costs. Consultants have insider status, with which they provide special services within a system that employs them. Other consultants have outsider status; they work for a company that provides services to organizations or as an independent contractor (Norwood, 1998). For example, a hospital may employ an enterostomal therapist specifically to provide ostomy care and education for clients and families. However, when the need arises for staff education related to ostomy care, the hospital uses the enterostomal therapist to provide a staff program. Extended care facilities may use external nurse consultants for monthly client assessments or to provide client services such as foot or ostomy care. Health care consumers may use nurse consultants to assist in selecting an extended care facility for a family member, paying medical bills, or learning relaxation techniques.

The success of nursing consultants depends on personal proficiency in the area where consultation is provided; strong theoretical, business, and clinical skills; the ability to solve problems quickly; and the ability to compete with other consultants. Consulting or working as an independent contractor can be done part time until the business becomes established and profitable (Norwood, 1998).

Medical-legal nurse consultants have been in existence for many years. As our society grows more litigious, the demand for medical-legal nurse consults rises. Membership in the American Association of Legal Nurse Consultants grew from 35 in 1989 to 3,956 in 2000 (American Association of Legal Nurse Consultants, 2001). Medical-legal nurse consultants collaborate with lawyers on malpractice, litigation, personal injury, product liability, and workers' compensation and criminal cases. Nurse consultants coach attorneys on the proper use of medical terminology and save them time by gathering pertinent information on cases. Nurse consultants work with legal teams for plaintiffs or defendants. Sometimes, the nurse consultant can tell from reviewing a chart if a plaintiff has a case. They frequently serve as expert witnesses during court trials.

In recent years, many nurse consultants have become **nurse entrepreneurs.** Starting and running an independent business is a complex undertaking, which is discussed in the next section. Some nurses who have specialized education in complementary health care practices, such as massage, therapeutic touch, aroma or magnet therapy, may assume the role of nurse consultant when they actually use or help others to incorporate these practices into client care.

## ✦ ADVANCED NURSING PRACTICE CAREER OPTIONS

Nursing offers areas of advanced practice. Most advanced nursing practice careers require some education beyond the baccalaureate degree. In 2003, the American Nurses Association reported that 7.3% of registered nurses (196,279 nurses) had the education and credentials to practice as an advanced practice nurse. Of those 14,643 had the qualifications to work as a clinical nurse specialist and nurse practitioner (ANA, 2003).

### Nursing Practitioners

Nurse practitioners (NPs) provide primary health care services to consumers. Nursing care services provided by NPs include assessing client health using a holistic framework; identifying medical and nursing diagnoses; planning and prescribing treatments; managing health care regimens for individuals, families, and communities; promoting wellness; preventing illness and injury; and managing acute and chronic health conditions. The NP role surfaced during a physician shortage in the 1960s. The first NPs attended certification programs that lasted from a few weeks to as long as 2 years. NPs carved out a distinct difference in practice from the medical model by using a holistic approach to care based on nursing theory. As recognition grew, mostly related to the reduced cost of primary care and positive health outcomes for clients, NP programs in higher education settings proliferated. Currently, the American Association of Colleges of Nursing reports 321 NP programs in the United States (Rosseter, 2003).

Today, more than 95,000 NPs practice in a variety of settings (Bureau of Health Professions, 2003). Frequently, the health care system defines NP practice according to clients served, including pediatric NP, family NP, adult NP, and geriatric NP (Bureau of Health Professions). Before qualifying for direct third-party reimbursement, NPs must obtain certification. Several bodies offer certification examinations, including the American Nurses Credentialing Center, the American Academy of Nurse Practitioners and Nurses, the National Certification Board of Pediatric Nurse Practitioners, and the National Certification Corporation. Most NPs are required to renew certification every 5 years (Crutchfield, 1997; Snyder et al., 1999). This process requires documented practice and evidence of continuing education (Snyder et al.).

Within their relatively short existence, NPs have earned the respect of clients and other health team members. Recent research has demonstrated the effectiveness of NPs in primary care, health promotion, decreasing hospitalization rates, and client satisfaction. Nurse practitioners have been featured on network television news shows. In addition to demonstrating the value of their contributions to health care, NPs provide health care services to the underprivileged and persons living in underserved areas (Bureau of Health Professions, 2003; Snyder et al., 1999).

## Certified Nurse-Midwives

**Certified nurse-midwives (CNMs)** independently manage women's health care with a special emphasis on pregnancy, childbirth, postpartum care, newborn care, family planning, and well woman care. Well woman care focuses on family planning, screening for female-related cancer, and management of perimenopause and postmenopause. Certified nurse-midwife care supports the natural processes of birth, growth, development, and aging; CNMs intervene only if absolutely indicated.

Of all the advanced practice roles, midwifery is the oldest. Records of midwifery practice are documented in the Bible. As the profession of medicine arose, midwifery declined. Mary Breckenridge, who received midwifery education in Scotland, became the first practicing nurse-midwife in the United States when she established the Frontier Nursing Service in 1925. In 1932, the first American nurse-midwifery education program opened in the Maternity Center of the Lobenstein Clinic in New York City. Slow growth in nurse-midwifery occurred, and in 1955, the American College of Nurse-Midwives was established. By the 1970s, nurse-midwifery became a demand of consumers seeking a more natural approach to childbirth (Snyder et al., 1999).

The American College of Nurse-Midwives developed national accreditation for nurse-midwives in the 1970s. Currently, more than 8,000 CNMs practice and manage approximately 6% of all births in the United States. In most states, CNMs possess prescriptive authority and receive direct third-party reimbursement for services (Bureau of Health Professions, 2003).

Although they started as certificate programs, nurse-midwifery programs progressed to graduate nursing education. Forty-seven nurse-midwifery programs are housed in

American universities, and all but seven programs are incorporated into master of nursing programs.

Research evidence indicates that CNMs contribute substantially to the quality of maternal-child health care. The Bureau of Health Professions (2003) reported reduced cesarean section rates and fewer medical interventions for women at low risk when compared with women at low risk who received care from physicians. Studies report significantly lower neonatal mortality, birth weights, and infant mortality, as well as higher birth weights of infants when women were attended by CNMs. Along with improved outcomes, CNMs provide women with health care at reduced costs (Snyder et al., 1999; Bureau of Health Professions, 2003; Gaudier, 2003; Rosseter, 2003).

## Clinical Nurse Specialists

Clinical nurse specialists (CNSs) are highly skilled clinical experts in a specialized area of nursing practice and use all the steps of the nursing process to promote health, prevent complications, and manage health problems. CNSs work in many settings, including hospitals, schools, extended care facilities, homes, and community agencies. In 1954, Hildegard Peplau established the first graduate level CNS program at Rutgers University to prepare psychiatric CNSs. Today there are 78 graduate nursing programs in the United States that prepare CNSs (All Nursing Schools, 2004).

At first, CNSs primarily worked in hospitals to provide support for patients and nursing staff. However, with the advent of managed care, many hospitals enlisted CNSs to serve as case managers. Clinical nurse specialists coordinate care of highly acute patients within the hospital and have been used as discharge planners. They practice in many subspecialty fields, including pulmonary, oncology, neuroscience, geriatrics, rehabilitation, diabetes, hospice, and palliative care.

## Certified Registered Nurse Anesthetists

Certified registered nurse anesthetists (CRNAs) provide anesthesia and anesthetic-related services to health care consumers. Records of nurses administering anesthesia indicate that this was a widespread and accepted practice in the late 1800s. Mother Magdalene Weidlocher developed the first nursing course in anesthesiology in 1912. Nurses employed by St. Mary's Hospital in Rochester, Minnesota became well known for their expertise in anesthesia administration in the early 1900s. One of the Mayo brother's nurses, Alice McGaw, published several papers related to her successful administration of anesthesia to thousands of patients in the early 20th century. The formal education process for CRNAs began in 1952. The standard CRNA curriculum consists of "45 hours of professional development, 135 hours of anatomy, physiology and pathophysiology; 45 hours of chemistry and physics; 90 hours of anesthesia principles; and 45 hours of clinical and literature review conference" (Snyder et al., 1999, p. 7). Along with completing the 24-month program outlined, the nurse must administer at least 450 anesthetics before taking the certification examination.

All 50 states recognize CRNA practice. According to the American Association of Nurses Anesthetists, CRNA practice includes preanesthetic assessment; anesthetic plan development and implementation; anesthesia induction; selection, application, and insertion of noninvasive and invasive monitoring devices; anesthetic selection, acquisition, and administration; fluid and ventilatory support; administration of medications and fluids to facilitate the emergence and recovery from anesthesia; patient discharge and follow-up care after anesthesia administration; airway support and management in medical emergencies; and implementation of various acute and chronic pain treatment modalities. Despite rigorous, standardized education, approximately 80% of CRNAs practice anesthesia with a group of physician anesthesiologists. The other 20% practice independently to provide anesthesia services to outpatient clinics and rural hospitals (more than 70% of rural hospitals rely on CRNAs for anesthesia services). Certified registered nurse anesthetists receive payment for services directly from third-party payers. Finally, CRNAs assume full legal responsibility for their actions (Snyder et al., 1999).

## Registered Nurse First Assistant

Registered nurse first assistants (RNFAs) may be employed by hospitals and physicians or may work as independent contractors. Practice settings for RNFAs include hospitals, ambulatory surgical centers, and physician offices. RNFAs work collaboratively with surgeons during surgery. RNFAs prepare skin for incisions, hold retractors, assist clamping vessels, suction, perform cautery, irrigate the surgical wound beds, and close incisions. Along with working in the operating room, RNFAs collect client histories, perform preoperative assessments, make client preoperative visits, educate clients about procedures, and conduct postoperative visits (Martinkus, 2004). RNFAs are widely used in rural hospitals.

The scope of responsibility of RNFAs varies according to employment setting. RNFAs working in surgeons' offices tend to have more autonomy and responsibilities than RNFAs employed by hospitals. The Association of Operating Room Nurses (AORN) published the first official statement on RNFAs in 1984, and then structured an educational and certificate program for RNFAs in 1985. Qualifications for certification as a RNFA include current licensure as a RN, certification from the AORN as a certified operating room nurse, bachelor's degree in nursing or a master's degree in nursing with a bachelor's degree in another field of study, and 2,000 documented hours of RNFA practice with the first 120 hours being completed under the guidance of a surgeon preceptor (Martinkus, 2004).

RNFAs are reimbursed for their services at a lower rate than assisting surgeons. Medicare does not reimburse RNFAs for their services. Many receive payment from surgeons or hospitals for which they work (Martinkus, 2004).

## Nursing Administration

Most health care organizations employ nurses as administrators or managers. Positions in **nursing administration** range from departmental heads (Head Nurse or Nurse Manager) to chief nursing officers (Director of Nursing). In many hospitals, the traditional "head nurse" position has been replaced with a "nurse manager," who may have to manage more than one unit. Many hospitals require advanced degrees for management or administrative positions. Many colleges and universities offer graduate nursing education in nursing administration. Some nursing administrative personnel have opted to pursue graduate degrees in business to facilitate role performance. Complex budgetary consideration, institutional accreditation requirements, legal issues, decisions related to new care products, and staff management concerns (including having enough staff for effective care) comprise some of the key dimensions of the nurse manager role (Falter, 1997).

## Nursing Academia

Teaching the new generation of nurses provides great rewards for nursing faculty members. A career in **nursing academia** (nursing education) enables experienced nurses to share their knowledge and expertise with future professional nurses. As a faculty member, the professional nurse has opportunities to polish clinical skills, expand knowledge of clinical nursing, engage in nursing research, and participate in community service while sharing knowledge and teaching skills with future nurses. Although most nursing programs require a master's degree in nursing and recent clinical experience for faculty appointment, some associate degree and vocational nursing programs may hire a baccalaureate-prepared nurse. Most programs preparing certified nursing assistants use baccalaureate-prepared nurses as faculty. Nursing programs offering baccalaureate degrees prefer to hire faculty with nursing or educational doctorates. Most graduate nursing programs require doctoral preparation for faculty members (Case, 1997a; Valiga & Streubert, 1991).

Faculty roles vary across various educational settings. Most nursing faculty members engage in scholarly activities, teaching, and community services. State and private sponsored research universities require faculty to develop a program of nursing research. In these settings, faculty members develop research proposals, write grants to fund projects, engage in research, disseminate research findings, and fulfill teaching responsibilities. Nursing programs in the community college emphasize technical aspects of nursing, and faculty members concentrate on teaching students clinical skills. Many faculty members practice nursing outside of the academic setting to maintain clinical competence (Case, 1997a; Valiga & Streubert, 1991).

Distance learning programs pose different challenges for faculty. In addition to being content and practice experts, nurse faculty must have the knowledge and expertise to run computer hardware, use software to engage learners, work with technology support staff, and establish online student relationships. Faculty also find that they can enter course information onto websites from any computer linked to the Internet. Students can access course information and electronically submit assignments at any time. If online discussions are part of the course, students and faculty must routinely check discussion boards. With new technology, faculty must remain more flexible with online instruction; especially if the required technology fails (Ryan, Carlton, & Ali, 2004).

## Nurse Entrepreneurs

Because of the complex factors and education needed to establish and maintain an independent business, the career as nurse entrepreneur fits the description of advanced nursing practice. Most entrepreneurs follow similar career paths. Many nurses experience some form of trauma that serves as the reason for a career change. Traumatic events may be a singular event, such as reaching a personally significant age, changing marital status, having a child or children, or it may be a compilation of factors, such as job boredom, frustration with administration, unfulfilled need, or a general feeling that life is being wasted. First, such nurses discover an idea for a viable business. Frequently, the idea for a business appears while practicing professional nursing in a traditional institution. Second, the entrepreneur gathers more information about the idea to provide a solid foundation for the new business concept. Third, entrepreneurs develop the business concept by verifying the idea through the gathering of more information. The fourth step involves an initial test of the business concept for success. The fifth step consists of expanding the number and types of offered products or services. The sixth and final step involves business expansion to include organizational structures, employees, policies, and procedures (Vogel & Doleysh, 1988).

Not all nurses possess the personality characteristics needed to embark on the entrepreneurial career path. Key personality characteristics shared by successful entrepreneurs include a willingness for risk taking, self-confidence, internal locus of control, determination, perseverance, interpersonal communication skills, willingness to delay gratification, business awareness, desire for total control, ability to direct others, physical stamina, mental resilience, and a strong need for achievement. The four following steps serve as guidelines for discovering a niche for a business: (1) developing a business idea, (2) market service analysis, (3) market testing, and (4) trial run. Running a personal business requires detailed knowledge of the corporate world and governmental policies that guide small businesses (Vogel & Doleysh, 1988; Waxman, 2005).

Waxman (2005) identifies advantages and disadvantages of being a nurse entrepreneur. Advantages include a high level of autonomy, flexible working hours, constant change, meeting lots of new people, using previously untapped skills (creativity and interpersonal), and being paid high hourly rates. Disadvantages include constant change, loss of employee-based fringe benefits, having to secure accounts payable, taking risks, loss of daily contact with other nurses, no paid time off, and loss of job structure. However, nurses, especially those who enjoy working independently, find being an entrepreneur very satisfying and rewarding.

### Questions for Reflection 21-3

1. What further information about the career options presented in this chapter do I want?
2. Who would I contact to explore an appealing nursing career option?
3. What additional education or skills would I need to obtain to pursue another career option in nursing?

## ● SUMMARY AND SIGNIFICANCE TO PRACTICE

The nursing profession offers many career options to professional nurses. Nurses have opportunities to change specialty and practice areas that are not afforded to the other health professions. Many expanded and most advanced nursing practice roles require additional education. Most advanced nursing practice roles require certification. Some states require additional licensure for selected advanced practice arenas. Some nurses find that discovering one's personal niche in the profession can be challenging. However, exploring various career options helps nurses to decide what area of practice suits them best.

## FROM THEORY TO PRACTICE

1. How would I respond to Laura in the vignette if she asked me about my current nursing practice? Why would I respond in this manner?
2. Whom would I contact if I wanted to explore one of the nursing career options presented in this chapter? Why would I contact this person?

## WWW INTERNET EXERCISES

1. Visit the Sigma Theta Tau International website at http://www.nursingsociety.org. Click on the career icon found in the left margin of the website and explores areas related to career information, career mapping, and retirement planning. Did you find this information useful? Why or why not?
2. Visit the American Nurses Association website at http://www.nursingworld.org. Find information about specialty practice certification and advanced practice nursing. Was this information useful? Why or why not?

## WWW INTERNET RESOURCES

Sigma Theta Tau International: http://www.nursingsociety.org.
United States Department of Labor Bureau of Statistic *Occupational Outlook Handbook:* http://stat.sbls.gov/oco.
All Nursing Schools: http://www.allnursingshcools.com.
Nursing Spectrum: http://www.nursingspectrum.com.
American Nurses Association: http://www.nursingworld.org.
Health Web: http://www.healthweb.org.
Johnson & Johnson's Discover Nursing website: http://www.discovernursing.com.
Health Resources and Service Administration: http:/www.hrsa.gov.
Travel Nursing: http://www.travelnursing.com.
Forensic Nursing: http://www.forensicnurse.org.

## REFERENCES

All Nursing Schools (2004). Clinical Nurse Specialist Programs. Available at: http://www.allnursingschools.com/featured/clinical-nurse-specialist. Accessed March 5, 2005.
American Association of Legal Nurse Consultants. (2001). 2000–2001 Annual report. Available at: http://www.aalnc.org/annualreport/2001/. Accessed July 5, 2005.
American Nurses Association (2003). Today's registered nurse—numbers and demographics. Available at http://nursingworld.org/member/practice/fsdemogrpt.cfm. Accessed July, 2005.
Bureau of Health Professions (2003). *A comparison of changes in the professional practice of nurse practitioners, physician assistants, and certified nurse midwives: 1992-2000.* Available at: http://bhpr.hrsa.gov/healthworkface/reports/scope/scope1-2./htm. Accessed July 1, 2005.
Case, B. (1997a). Educator role. In B. Case (Ed.). *Career planning for nurses* (pp. 317–337). Albany, NY: Delmar Publishers.
Case, B. (1997b). Where are you taking your career? In B. Case (Ed.). *Career planning for nurses* (pp. 1–27). Albany, NY: Delmar Publishers.
Crutchfield, J. (1997). The nurse practitioner, nurse anesthetist, and nurse midwife. In B. Case (Ed.) *Career planning for nurses* (pp. 161–177). Albany, NY: Delmar Publishing.

Cutler, K. P. (2002). Clinical ladder protocols and nurse career development. *Long-term Care Interface, 3*, 22–32.

Davis, N., & Bheenuck, S. (2003). A professional development pathways scheme. *Nursing Standard, 17*, 40–43.

Gaudier, F. (2003). *Health encyclopedia: Special topics—Certified nurse midwife profession.* Available at http://www.henryfordhealth.org/12893.cfm. Accessed July 18, 2005.

Ireland, A. M., DePalma, J. A., Arenson, L., Stark, L., & Williamson, J. The Oncology Nursing Society Ambulatory Office Survey. *Oncology Nursing Forum, 31. OnLine Exclusive,* E 147–156.

Kearney, S. (2003). *Hitting the road: A guide to travel nursing.* Philadelphia: Lippincott Williams & Wilkins.

Martinkus, W. (2004). A cut above. *NurseWeek* (Heartland edition), (November 1, 2004), 8–9.

McIntyre, M., & Thomlinson, E. (2003). *Realities of Canadian nursing: Professional, practice and power issues.* Philadelphia: Lippincott Williams & Wilkins.

Mitty, E. (2003). Assisted living and the role of the nurse. *American Journal of Nursing, 103*, 32–44.

National Council of State Boards of Nursing (NCSBN). (2000). *Mutual recognition frequently asked questions.* Available at http://www.ncsbn.org. Accessed July 18, 2005.

Norwood, S. L. (1998). *Nurses as consultants: Essential concepts and processes.* Menlo Park, CA: Addison-Wesley.

Porcher, F. (1996). Licensure, certification and credentialing. In J. Hickey, R. Ouimette, & S. Venegoni (Eds.). *Advanced practice nursing: Changing roles and clinical applications* (pp. 179–187). Philadelphia: Lippincott.

Robitaille, D., & Whelchel, C. (2005). Take PRIDE in your clinical ladder. *Nursing Management, 36*, 16.

Rosseter, R. (2003). *Nurse practitioners: The growing solution in health care delivery.* Available at http://aacn.nche.edu/Media/FactSheets/npfact.htm. Accessed July 18, 2005.

Ryan, M., Carlton, K., & Ali, N. (2004). Reflections on the role of faculty in distance learning and changing pedagogies. *Nursing Education Perspectives, 25,* 73–80.

Snyder, M., Mirr, M. P., Lindeke, L., Fagerlund, K., Avery, M., & Tseng, Y. (1999). Advanced practice nursing: An overview. In M. Snyder & M. P. Mirr (Eds.). *Advanced practice nursing: A guide to professional development* (2nd ed., pp. 1–24). New York: Springer Publishing.

Stevens, S. (2004). Cracking the case: Your role in forensic nursing. *Nursing, 34*, 54–56.

Sultz, K., & Young, H. (2004). *Health care USA: Understanding its organization and delivery* (2nd ed.) Sudbury, MA: Jones and Bartlett.

United States Bureau of Statistics. (1992). Occupational Outlook Handbook. Washington, DC: Author.

Valiga, T., & Streubert, H. (1991). *The nurse educator in academia: Strategies for success.* New York: Springer Publishing.

Vogel, G., & Doleysh, N. (1997). *Entrepreneuring: A nurses' guide to starting a business.* NLN Publication no. 41-2201. New York: National League for Nursing.

Waxman, K. (2005). Nurse entrepreneurship: Do you have what its takes? *2005 Pathways to Success.* Hoffman Estates, IL: NursingSpectrum.

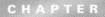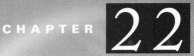

# CHAPTER 22

# Development of a Professional Nursing Career

## KEY TERMS AND CONCEPTS

Values
Career Goals
Passion
Envisioning
Vision
Vision Statement
Mission Statement
Networking
Mentoring
Linear Career Paths
Nonlinear Career Paths
Career Mapping
Professional Nursing Résumé
Curriculum Vitae
Professional Portfolio

## LEARNING OUTCOMES

By the end of this chapter, the learner will be able to:

**1** Discuss the relationship of values when setting career goals.

**2** Use a process to discover a passion for a specific area of professional practice.

**3** Compose personal vision and mission statements for professional nursing practice.

**4** Prepare a professional nursing resume.

**5** Compile a nursing resume and professional nursing portfolio.

**6** Specify strategies to develop a professional nursing network.

**7** Explain how networking and mentoring enhance career opportunities.

**8** Design a career map for a future professional career.

## VIGNETTE

Glen and Patricia work together on an inpatient oncology unit. They both started as new graduates a year ago. During a shift report, Glen mentions that he is thinking about changing jobs because he no longer enjoys his work. In response to his statement, Patricia states, "Oh, I'm sorry to hear that you don't love the patients the way I do. I just feel so satisfied if I can get one of them to smile, even for a minute or have them share how they are coping with cancer. I think that I want to spend my entire career specializing in oncology nursing."

## Questions for Reflection 22-1

1. What steps does each of these nurses need to take to establish a nursing career tailored to best meet their personal needs and desires?
2. How can other nurses support these two novice nurses as they pursue career goals?
3. Why is it important for nurses to support each other as they pursue career goals?

The responsibility for professional nursing career development lies within each nurse. As the health care delivery system changes, new opportunities for professional nursing practice arise. Professional nurses live in an exciting time in which specialized and complex skills have an impact on client care. Developing required competence for effective professional nursing practice, especially in specialty areas of practice, takes many years. As a profession, nursing offers a wide array of practice areas. Nurses decide what type of nursing they wish to pursue and where they want to practice. How a nursing career develops depends on the individual nurse. Some nurses create detailed written career plans with established timelines for implementation. Other nurses rely on seizing opportunities as they arise. This chapter outlines the importance of matching career goals with personal values, discovering ways to instill personal passion into practice, considering factors to envision a future career, developing strategies to create and implement a career map, and closing one's career with effective retirement planning.

## ● VALUES AND CAREER GOALS

Every person has an established set of values. **Values** denote what a person perceives as being important in life. Values provide guidance to persons as they interact with each other and the environment. When persons share values, communities are formed (Barrett, 1998). Even within the profession of nursing (a community), no two nurses share an identical set of values. Examples of values include truth, integrity, justice, peace, health, education, conservation, possessions, money, security, safety, career, and family. Life has many important values, and selecting which ones are the most important can be a difficult task. Identification of personal favorite activities can provide a clue to defining a personal set of values. Self-betrayal occurs when personal life behaviors fail to match a personal set of values. In early life, values are formed in families, but over time, personal values may change. Nurses learn professional values as part of socialization into the profession.

Certain areas of nursing cater to different sets of values. Nurses who value technologically complex skills tend to pursue critical care, emergency department, or perioperative nursing. Nurses who value long-term relationships and the wisdom of the elderly find great rewards in working in extended care facilities with a geriatric population. Hospice nursing provides rewards for nurses who value comfort and peace in the dying process, rather than preserving life at all costs. Nurse practitioners practice the value of health promotion. Nurses for whom the generation of knowledge is a cherished value may become nurse researchers or theorists. Unlike other professions, nursing

---

**Values Clarification Exercises**

*Step 1* Find a quiet peaceful place where you can spend some time alone free from interruption.

*Step 2* Close your eyes and answer the following question: What things in life are important to me as a person? Record the list of items you consider important.

*Step 3* Close your eyes and answer the following question: What things in life are important to me as a professional nurse? Record the list.

*Step 4* Identify the common entries found on both of your lists to identify similarities of your personal and professional values. Create a list for these results.

*Step 5* Generate a list of activities in which you engaged during the past week and include the approximate amount of time spent in each activity. Place each activity in a list according to how much time you spent on it, with the activity in which you spent the most time at the top of the list.

*Step 6* Compare this list to the list generated in steps 2, 3, and 4. This represents the congruence of how you spend your time with your set of personal and professional values.

*Step 7* Answer the following questions:

1. Am I living in accordance with my personal values?
2. Am I living in accordance with my professional values?
3. Are there any things that I could do differently to live out my personal and professional values?

---

offers many career opportunities that fit with a nurse's personal values. Most nurses use personal values when determining **career goals** (specific professional nursing accomplishments). Display 22-1 offers exercises for use when engaging in the process of values clarification.

## ● DISCOVERING YOUR PASSION IN NURSING

Chang (2000) defines **passion** as a "personal intensity, an underlying force that fuels our strongest emotions" (p. 19) and passions as "activities, ideas and topics that elicit these emotions" (p. 19). When persons perform with passion, the world becomes full of opportunities, rather than obstacles, and they focus on personal abilities, rather than limitations. All persons have the capacity to live passionate lives. Persons who live out their life's passions follow their hearts. An individual's passions change as life evolves. A life without passion becomes a life of regrets (Chang, 2000). When persons follow a career based on passion, work becomes play (Abrams, 2000). Nursing is a content-based and context-based passion because it centers on a highly specialized topic (client care) and centers on a theme that can be applied to several activities (helping others).

Chang (2000) outlines a seven-step process to develop a passion plan for living that requires feeling, thinking, and acting. The seven steps are:

1. Start from the heart: Acknowledge all emotions and desires and recognize their power. Engage in a gradual process that requires identifying things that inspire or elicit deep strong emotions. (This may mean rediscovering things from childhood.)
2. Discover all your passions.
3. Clarify the purpose of your passions: Identify the results of living out life's passions. The purpose of each passion helps to determine how it will be followed.

4. Define the actions to achieve each passion: Develop an action plan for each passion.
5. Perform with passion: Implement the action plan developed in step 4, which may require some form of risk taking.
6. Spread the passion: Share the passion and how it excites you with others and let it permeate all your interactions with others.
7. Persist in the passion: Stay the course, despite any unexpected circumstances or obstacles that may arise.

Passionate nurses provide client care from the depths of their hearts and souls. They hold to professional ideals and have no fear in confronting situations that compromise client care. Because of their excitement as they practice nursing, nursing colleagues and other members of the health care team catch their enthusiasm. Through acts of authentic caring, clients and significant others receiving nursing care from passionate nurses feel safe and important. Nurses and clients deeply connect with each other, and the fond memories of the nursing situation last a lifetime.

### Questions for Reflection 22-2

1. What are the deep emotions that surface when I engage in nursing practice?
2. What activities in clinical practice result in extremely high levels of personal satisfaction?
3. What passions, other than nursing, do I have currently in my life?
4. Why is it important to have passions or interests other than nursing in my life?

## ● ENVISIONING YOUR NURSING CAREER

**Envisioning** means picturing oneself in the future (Mish, 1994). A personal **vision** specifies a future desired state for oneself. Developing a career vision statement assumes that change in one's career will occur. The ideal professional nursing career vision would include nursing-related passions. Because nurses progress through human life transitions, personal career vision statements may be revised to address changes in physical, mental, and spiritual health status. A nurse may leave a position to stay home with children. A nurse may re-enter clinical practice because of the loss of a spouse or because children have left home. Because physical stamina declines with age, a professional nurse may decide that he or she needs to leave a particular clinical practice area and pursue one that requires less physical exertion. Reviewing personal values and strengths facilitates the development of a career vision. All visions start with dreams. When developing a personal vision, let ideas flow without inhibition. Visions may be articulated in the present or future tense. A **vision statement** is a written declaration of a desired future state and may incorporate ideas for future improvement (Barrett, 1998; Covey, 1992, 2004; Wesorick, Shiparski, Troseth, & Wyngarden, 1997).

---

**Sample Personal Vision Statement**                    DISPLAY 22-2 ◈

I envision myself to be a professional nurse who demonstrates authentic caring toward and appreciation of all living persons and things.

---

**Sample Mission Statement**                    DISPLAY 22-3 ◈

As an authentic professional nurse, my personal mission is take time to listen genuinely to clients, families, nursing colleagues, and other members of the interdisciplinary health team to provide them with the highest quality of service that is humanly possible.

---

Vision statements relate closely to mission statements. **Mission statements** specify how visions may be actualized (Barrett, 1998) or specify the meaning and purpose behind work (Covey, 1992, 2004; Wesorick et al., 1997). Florence Nightingale viewed nursing as a spiritual calling. Barrett (1995) presents the concept of "soul work" as activities to be performed by the energy field occupying a living human body. For some, professional nursing may be one way to fulfill one's life purpose. Mission statements clearly and concisely outline specific service using action verbs and the meaning behind them that comes from the heart (Wesorick et al., 1997). Mission statements related to a professional nursing career usually focus on client care. Displays 22-2 and 22-3 present a sample personal nursing vision and mission statement.

When nurses create a career vision based on passions, they commit to living out a meaningful life as they engage in activities of the soul, rather than those of the mind or head. Passionate nursing practice enables nurses to live out their life purpose of caring for others.

## ◈ NETWORKING

**Networking** consists of exchanging ideas and information among individuals, groups, or institutions (Mish, 1994). Professional networks are interconnected groups of persons who profess a certain vision or mission. Interacting with other professional nurses enables the nurse to become cognizant of career opportunities and learn about nursing care practice variances across settings. When nurses interact with each other, their professional networks expand. Strategies for the development of effective professional networks include courage and a willingness to call others, a genuine desire to help others, freely sharing information with others, distributing professional business cards, and actively participating in collaborative projects (Abrams, 2000; Case, 1997).

Opportunities for networking occur at work, school, and professional organizational and community service activities. Networking outside of the nursing community enables nurses to expand their knowledge outside the discipline of nursing, share information about professional nursing with those who are not nurses, and explore other career options. Many nurse consultants and entrepreneurs rely on networking (professional and community) to generate business (Waxman, 2005).

## Questions for Reflection 22-3

1. Why is it important to have strong peer collegial relationships?
2. What have I done during the past week to strengthen my relationships with nursing colleagues?
3. What networking opportunities are available to me as a nursing student?
4. Why is networking important in nursing education?
5. What networking opportunities are available to me as a practicing nurse?
6. Have I taken advantage of professional nursing networking opportunities? Why or why not?

## ⬤ MENTORING

For centuries, novices in various professions have sought the advice of experienced professionals. The term "mentor" has its roots in the Greek myth of Odysseus entrusting the education of his son to his friend named Mentor (Mish, 1994). In recent years, the word **mentoring** has come to denote the process of enlisting an experienced guide or trusted adviser who assumes responsibility for the professional growth and advancement of a less experienced person, called the protégé. Mentors open doors, create opportunities, and provide career role modeling for protégés while inspiring them. In nursing, mentors provide direction for persons just entering the nursing profession or a specialized area of nursing practice. Mentors provide wisdom to protégés and help them develop professional networks. Mentors often actively sponsor protégés when career opportunities in the selected field arise (Falter, 1997). In addition, protégés help mentors by serving as research assistants and sounding boards and assisting them in clarifying ideas (Malone, 1999).

Because the mentoring relationship requires personal chemistry between the involved persons, many nurses experience difficulty in finding mentors. Sometimes, novices construct barriers to establishing a mentoring relationship with a seasoned professional. Barriers that are constructed include not wanting to impose on a potential mentor's time, fear of relationship failure, and having difficulty identifying the right person to be a mentor. However, sometimes the mentoring relationship may just unfold over the course of a career. Persons become mentors for various reasons, including desiring to help another, admiring the novice's personal and professional goals and vision, being reminded of a former younger self, and having been a protégé in a successful mentoring experience (Abrams, 2000; Malone, 1999). Successful mentoring requires mutual respect, complimentary personalities, open attitudes, proper timing, and appropriate quality and quantity of guidance (Abrams).

To ease the burden of professional transition to clinical practice for new graduate nurses, some health care institutions offer mentoring or preceptor programs. Preceptor and mentoring programs provide guidance for new nurses and those changing specialty practice areas. These programs frequently ease the transition for the new graduate to independent, professional practice (Thomka, 2001; Messmer, Jones, & Taylor, 2004). Sometimes, these programs result in effective mentoring relationships. However, mentoring requires reciprocal investment in the relationship. Because most mentors have years of experience within a given field, they have much wisdom to impart to protégés (Falter, 1997). Mentoring provides mentors with the opportunity of fulfilling developmental tasks related to the productive and older professional nurse. Sometimes the mentor finds a protégé willing to continue the mentor's professional contributions as the mentor retires or loses interest in them as part of a natural career trajectory.

## Research Brief 22-1

Messmer, P., Jones, S., & Taylor, B. (2004). Enhancing knowledge and self-confidence of novice nurses: The "shadow-a-nurse" ICU program. *Nursing Education Perspectives, 25,* 131–136.

The investigators performed a pilot study involving 12 nursing students and their preceptors in a critical care nursing course. The investigators developed a critical care nurse internship program in which students shadowed nurses to gain critical care nursing knowledge and skills. Students shadowed experienced nurse preceptors and novice critical care nurses during the clinical learning activity. Students who shadowed nurses in the adult ICU completed Toth's Basic Knowledge Assessment Tool (BKAT). Students who shadowed nurses in the Neonatal ICU took the Neonatal ICU Assessment Competency Examination (NICU). Both student groups completed the Watson Glaser Critical Thinking Appraisal (WGCTA). They also completed the tools after the clinical experience and then after 1 year of critical care experience. The shadowers also kept a written log of their experiences, which were analyzed by one of the investigators. Preceptors completed the WGCTA upon selection as preceptors and 1 year after having served as a preceptor to the nursing students.

The shadowers showed statistically significant gains in their knowledge scores for critical care nursing. However, there was a slight drop (not statistically significant) in WGCTA scores after shadowers had 1 year of critical nursing experience. Thematic analysis of student logs revealed that shadowers identified that the shadowing experience increased their self-confidence and self-esteem as well as helping them socialize into the roles of ICU nurse.

There are several reasons to exercise caution when interpreting the results of this study. First, the small sample size makes it difficult to generalize findings to other nurses. Second, the WGCTA was identified as possibly not being a sensitive tool to measure critical thinking attributes required in professional nursing practice. Replication studies on the effects of similar programs to ease the transition to professional nursing practice would be useful. Additional studies also should be performed to see if shadowing programs are beneficial towards novice nurse recruitment and retention efforts by ICUs and other clinical practice settings.

## Questions for Reflection 22-4

1. What are the characteristics of an ideal mentor?
2. Why are these characteristics important?
3. If I were to select a professional nursing mentor today, whom would I choose?

# ● CAREER DEVELOPMENT STRATEGIES

Once nurses identify career directions on which to focus, they can use a variety of strategies to make their ideal career happen. Most authors addressing career development begin the process with a self-assessment of personal values followed by a period of dreaming about what a future career may look like (Bongard, 1997b; Chang, 2000; Donner & Wheeler, 2001; Malone, 1999). A career in nursing equips nurses with many life skills that can transfer to other professions. Basic nursing knowledge transfers to a variety of professional nursing specialty areas. No two nurses follow identical paths for career development.

## Career Paths

No one career planning process has been proven to be superior to others. The process may be linear or nonlinear, and nurses select which to use based on their ability to tolerate uncertainty and ambiguity (Bongard, 1997a).

**Linear career paths** require nurses to follow a sequential series of steps. For example, staff nurses working with students decide that they would like to become nursing faculty. They earn a nursing master's degree before they apply for nursing faculty positions. Once employed by a nursing program, they closely follow a tenure track system with specific criteria for advancement from instructor to full professor. Nurses who like structure and meeting designated deadlines prefer this approach to career development (Bongard, 1997b).

**Nonlinear career paths** rely on life circumstances and critical incidents that result in career changes. Nurses following nonlinear career paths frequently create careers by using their interests, outside experiences, and nursing skills. They seize opportunities as they arise. Nurses using a nonlinear approach to career development frequently create new nursing positions within a health care organization or become entrepreneurs. In today's unstable health care arena, nurses following nonlinear career paths have a better chance of professional survival, especially as health care organizations elect to eliminate nursing positions to reduce client care costs (Bongard, 1997b).

## Career Development Model

Donner and Wheeler (2001, p. 2) view career development as "an iterative and continuous" process and combine linear and nonlinear approaches to career development. They have developed a five-phase career planning and development model, which starts with scanning the environment to understand current realities and future trends in society that have implications for nursing and create possibilities for new areas of clinical practice. Donner and Wheeler emphasize the importance of periodic self-assessments and reality checks related to self-identity and how others view individual nurses. If nurses find that current employment situations do not fit with attributes discovered from self-appraisal, Donner and Wheeler suggest that it may be time to pursue an alternative career path. They also advocate for the creation of a career vision to link current status with future possibilities. Nurses may then use the career vision as a motivating source for remaining in a current practice setting or making a change. Donner and Wheeler suggest that designing a strategic career plan around the career vision facilitates attainment of career goals. Finally, once a career plan has been established, efforts should be channeled into marketing professional skills by forming an expansive professional network, developing a mentoring relationship, and further refining verbal and written communication skills.

## Career Mapping

Malone (1999) uses the term "**career mapping**" to denote a continuous process of nursing career development in which career moves unfold as a person engages in professional practice and lifelong learning. This process starts with identification of values, determining the importance of each value, and envisioning a future. The future vision creates a blueprint for personal action to make that envisioned future become reality.

To facilitate the preferred career vision, Malone suggests that nurses analyze career trends to verify societal needs for specific professional nursing services. Areas of resources for trend identification include the United States Department of Labor (Malone, 1999), the United States Bureau of Statistics, *Healthy People 2010*, the American Association of Colleges of Nursing, the National League for Nursing, and the American Nurses Association. As the number of elderly citizens increases, the demand for nurses specializing in geriatric nursing and case management also should increase (Malone, 1999).

Once nurses select a preferred career vision based on need, specialty certification serves as an important step in the career mapping process. Professional certification provides public acknowledgment of professional competence, enhances career opportunities, demonstrates the ability of the profession for self-regulation, and increases personal power (Malone, 1999). The American Nurses Credentialing Center offers 27 certification examinations across a variety of nursing practice areas (Malone, 1999). Nurses also can earn certification from a variety of nurse specialty organizations.

Malone (1999) specifies that networking seems to be a frequently overlooked step in career mapping. Along with networking with professional nursing colleagues, nurses frequently overlook the importance of networking with professionals from other disciplines. Networking with other members of the health care team and with other professionals within the community enables nurses to gain a more global perspective related to the meaning of health and the needs for future health care delivery.

In addition to networking, Malone (1999) cites the benefits of the mentoring process to the career mapping process. Personal and professional mentors serve vital roles in the career mapping process. Early career experiences with mentors help shape personal values and instill confidence in young persons to pursue their dreams.

## ⬤ MAKING A NURSING CAREER CHANGE

Nurses make career changes for a variety of reasons. Some nurses pursue part-time employment to spend more time with families or pursue outside interests. At times, nurses may become bored with a current practice area and decide to change specialties. Nurses also may experience intense value conflicts with an employer that result in an employment change. Some nurses follow partners when their employment situations change. Frequently, when nurses receive more education, they change jobs. Finally, a desire to pursue a different field of nursing sometimes provides the stimulus to return to school.

Several strategies prove useful for the nurse wishing to remain viable in today's employment market. First, keeping a current résumé enables immediate action when an opportunity for an employment change surfaces. Second, refining personal interview skills provides confidence when interacting with future employers. Third, networking with other nurses at professional organizational meetings, career fairs, conventions, and community service activities enables acquisition of key information about employment opportunities. Fourth, making lists of personal assets, strengths, and preferred professional activities helps identify the type of position best suited to the individual nurse. Fifth, exposing oneself to motivational information in print, on tape, or on videotape arms the nurse considering change with a "can do" attitude. Finally, after accepting a new position, easing out of the old one gracefully makes it easier to return if the new job fails to be better than the old one (Cardillo, 2001). Some basic skills and strategies used for marketing oneself and finding the right job are described here.

### Questions for Reflection 22-5

1. What is my ideal picture of my future nursing career?
2. How can I make this picture a reality?
3. What are the consequences of not envisioning an ideal future nursing career?

## Finding Available Nursing Opportunities

When considering changing nursing positions, nurses can use a variety of resources to locate employment opportunities. Most organizations (hospitals and integrated health systems) post internal job openings in areas accessible to employees and in human resources departments. Along with internal job postings, many organizations list employment opportunities on organizational or company websites (the Editors of VGM Career Horizons, 1996; Yate, 1998). The Internet also offers online job search commercial sites, such as Monster Board's Monster Health Care or Career Mosaic's HealthOpps (Enger, 1999). Nursing journals and periodicals contain classified advertisements with available nursing opportunities. Professional nurses learn about career opportunities from networking with nursing colleagues during professional nursing organizational events (Case, 1997; The Editors of VGM Career Horizons, 1996). In times of nursing shortages, some health care agencies turn to radio and television advertising to recruit nurses. Finally, local newspapers publish classified ads related to employment opportunities in nursing and other professional careers and nonprofessional work. Classified advertisements and website and internal organizational postings usually contain information regarding a contact person to call or instructions to follow when applying for a specific position.

## Marketing Your Skills

Employers need to verify that applicants have the correct skills to meet the demands of the position. When applying for a specific position, nurses may find that tailoring cover letters and résumés to address specific skills outlined by a position may prove to be more successful in securing a new job. Documents showcasing professional skills may be saved as computer files and edited to fit the requested skills and previous professional experience delineated by the posted job. Special care must be taken to verify that all information sent to prospective employers and clients has attractive visual appeal and no spelling or punctuation errors. Poorly constructed documents readily find their way into the trash (Bongard, 1997b; The Editors of VGM Career Horizons, 1996; Yate, 1998).

### Cover Letters

Cover letters provide a general introduction to a prospective employer or client. In addition, the letter provides an opportunity to shed light on the job applicant's personality while explaining the reasons for the contact. If the organization specifies in the advertised position a person to contact, applicants should send the cover letter to the designated person. Two forms of cover letters provide information. The traditional cover letter provides reasons for contact, expands on the rationale for applying for a position, and details how to contact the writer to set up an interview (Figure 22-1). The second form for a cover letter actually matches job requirements with acquired credentials and skills (Figure 22-2). The second cover letter format saves time for persons who screen applicants for interview invitations because they can easily read specific applicant qualifications. Typewritten or printed addresses on all materials sent to prospective employers or clients also send a better impression than handwritten ones. Finally, the cover letter signature may be the last item that the Human Resources Department reads, so applicants should pay close attention to verify that is neat and legible.

### Résumés

The résumé originated as a solution for employers who wanted to interview only qualified job applicants. Human resources persons who screen job applications find most résumés dull and boring. A good **professional nursing résumé** presents individual strengths, while showcasing special skills and professional accomplishments (Editors of VGM Career Horizons, 1996; Yate, 1998). A good résumé will get the candidate an interview, and the résumé preparation assists in interview preparation, especially for the dreaded request for applicants to "tell me about yourself." Résumé preparation also provides time for reflection about a career. All résumés strive to showcase professional achievements, attributes, and experience while minimizing any potential weaknesses, and to stimulate enough interest in the applicant to ensure an invitation for an interview (Yate).

Most persons use chronological or functional résumé formats. Of the two forms, the chronological format is used the most. Some persons opt to combine the two formats when developing a résumé (Yate, 1998). Table 22-1 outlines the chronological and functional résumé formats and highlights the strengths of each. Selection of format depends on where a person is within a career trajectory, employment experiences, and the type of opportunity being considered. Figures 22-3 and 22-4 offer examples of both types of résumés. Résumé preparation experts and publications disagree on many aspects of résumé preparation. However, they do agree on several preparation principles.

Jane Doe, RN, BSN
111 E. Lilac Avenue
Springfield, MO   65106


October 3, 2002


Mary Ashcraft, RN
Nurse Recruiter
Human Resources Department
Springfield Medical Center
803 North Maple Street
Springfield, MO   65107


Dear Ms. Ashcraft:


As I was reading the Springfield Daily News, I spotted your advertisement for a nursing position
on your oncology unit. I have recently moved to Springfield, Missouri and would like to work for
Springfield Medical Center, the premier hospital in the area. My professional nursing background
includes previous oncology nursing experience.


I am enclosing a copy of my resume so that you may review my credentials. I would appreciate
the opportunity to discuss my qualifications in person. Please call me at my home, 417-888-6464,
at any time to schedule an interview. If I am not available to take your call, please leave a
message and telephone number so I can contact you.


Thank you for reviewing my credentials. I look forward to meeting you soon.


Sincerely,


Jane Doe, RN, BSN

**Figure 22-1**
Sample cover letter.


Persons reviewing résumés in human resources departments spend little time reading individual résumés. Résumés containing more than 1 to 2 pages most likely will **not**
be read. The typical résumé receives about a 30-second review. When a job or career
objective is present, Human Resources Department employees assume that if it fails to

Jane Doe, RN, BSN
111 E. Lilac Avenue
Springfield, MO   65106


October 3, 2002


Mary Ashcraft, RN
Nurse Recruiter
Human Resources Department
Springfield Medical Center
803 North Maple Street
Springfield, MO   65107


Dear Ms. Ashcraft:


As I was reading the Springfield Daily News, I spotted your advertisement for a nursing position on your oncology unit. I have recently moved to Springfield, Missouri and would like to work for Springfield Medical Center, the premier hospital in the area. I have also read the exciting news about the current expansion of the oncology services at Springfield Medical Center.

My professional nursing background includes previous oncology nursing experience and the following summary outlines how my qualifications fit your nursing position requirements:

| Your requirements | My qualifications |
|---|---|
| * Professional nursing licensure in Missouri | * Professional nursing license in Nebraska for 6 years |
| | * Current Missouri nursing license |
| * One year's experience in oncology nursing | * Five years' experience in oncology nursing at St. Luke's Hospital, Omaha, NE |
| * OCN certification | * Current OCN certification |

I am enclosing a copy of my resume so that you may review my credentials. I would appreciate the opportunity to discuss my qualifications in person. Please call me at my home, 417-888-6464, at any time to schedule an interview. If I am not available to take your call, please leave a message and telephone number so I can contact you.

Thank you for reviewing my credentials. I look forward to meeting you soon.


Sincerely,


Jane Doe, RN, BSN

**Figure 22-2**
Sample skill-matched cover letter.

**TABLE 22-1**

## Comparison of the Chronological and Functional Résumé Formats

| | Chronological Résumé | Functional Résumé |
|---|---|---|
| Description | Lists job titles and responsibilities in chronological order | Highlights professional skills (also called skill-based résumé) |
| Components | Contact information<br>Job and career objectives<br>Career summary that highlights dates of each position<br>Education<br>Special awards or honors<br>Community service | Contact information<br>Job or career objective<br>List of skills specific for job<br>Dates of previous positions, usually at the end or in smaller type<br>Education and skills acquired from employment or community service activities |
| Situations for best use | Documentation of personal career growth<br>Continued employment in a field without too many job changes | Professional career established<br>Beginning of a career<br>Career change with the goal to focus on relevant skills<br>Stagnant or declining career<br>Returning to the workforce after a prolonged absence |
| When best not to use | Frequent job changes (every 1–2 years)<br>Just finishing school<br>Seeking a career change | No situations |
| Advantages | Showcases detailed employment history<br>Outlines specific job responsibilities and previous employers | Highlights skills, rather than employment history<br>Makes it easier for human resource personnel to determine if skills match posted job description<br>Can include skills gained from outside areas of past employment |

From: The Editors of VGM Career Horizons. (1996). *Résumés for nursing careers.* Lincolnwood, IL: VGM Career Horizons; and Yate, M. (1998). *Résumés that knock 'em dead* (3rd ed.). Holbrook, MA: Adams Media Corporation.

match the open position, the applicant does not want the position. The following suggestions make it easier for résumés to be efficiently processed:

1. Organizing categories in a logical manner.
2. Using a font size of 11 to 14 picas from an easily readable print style (Arial, Bookman, News Gothic, or Times New Roman are a few suggested font styles) and keeping the font style consistent (larger size can be used effectively to present headings).
3. Using 8 1/2-inch by 11-inch paper because employers frequently photocopy résumés for distribution to department managers and human resources files.
4. Selecting high quality, white, cream, or pastel (avoid pink) paper of 16- to 25-pound weight.
5. Limiting résumé blocks to five to seven lines.

**Jane Doe, RN, BSN**
**111 E. Lilac Avenue**
**Springfield, MO 65106**
**(417) 888-6464**

| | |
|---|---|
| **Objective** | Obtain a professional nursing position on an oncology client care unit |
| **Experience** | St. Luke's Hospital, Omaha NE<br>Oncology Unit<br>Evening Charge Nurse     **July 1997 to September 2002** |
| | University of Nebraska Medical Center, Omaha NE<br>Post Anesthesia Care Unit<br>Staff Nurse     **May 1995 to July 1997** |
| | University of Nebraska Medical Center, Omaha NE<br>East Seven (Surgical Nursing Unit)<br>Staff Nurse     **May 1994 to May 1995** |
| | Longview Extended Care<br>Licensed Practical Nurse     **May 1992** |
| **Education** | BSN, University of Nebraska     **May 1994**<br>LPN, Clarkson Technical School,<br>Omaha, NE     **May 1992** |
| **Professional Credentials** | Missouri Professional Nursing License<br>ACLS Certification<br>Oncology Nursing Society Certification<br>Oncology Nursing Society<br>American Nurses' Association |

**Professional and Personal References Available Upon Request**

**Figure 22-3**
Sample chronological résumé.

6. Using action verbs to describe current and previous job skills and responsibilities.
7. Maintaining strict alignment of margins within sections.
8. Keeping a free-flowing appearance without any noticeable breaks.
9. Having a friend or family member proofread it.

**Jane Doe, RN, BSN**
**111 E. Lilac Avenue**
**Springfield, MO 65106**
**(417) 888-6464**

**Objective:** Full-time professional nurse position on an adult oncology unit

**Skills**
- Certification in oncology nursing since June, 1996
- 5 years' experience in oncology nursing
- Experienced in insertion and removal of percutaneous intravenous central catheters
- Taught Oncology Certification Review courses on chemotherapy administration and radiation therapy for oncology staff
- Published newsletter for the local chapter of the Oncology Nursing Society
- Supervised staff of two RNs and three patient care technicians as evening charge nurse

**Education**
- BSN, University of Nebraska Medical Center, May 1994
- Oncology Certification Course, Omaha Chapter of the Oncology Nursing Society, May 1996
- 30 hours of continuing education in Oncology Nursing, May 1998 to July 2000
- LPN, Clarkson Technical School, May 1992

**Professional Credentials**
- Certification in oncology nursing by the Oncology Nursing Society
- Missouri Professional Nursing License #556087352
- Nebraska Professional Nursing License #N6670889
- Current certification in ACLS and BCLS

**Professional Organizations**
- Oncology Nursing Society (past secretary of the Omaha, Nebraska Chapter)
- American Nurses Association

**Employment History**

St. Luke's Hospital, Omaha NE
Oncology Unit
Evening charge nurse                 July 1997 to September 2000

University of Nebraska Medical Center, Omaha NE
Post Anesthesia Care Unit
Staff nurse                          May 1995 to July 1997

University of Nebraska Medical Center, Omaha NE
East Seven (Surgical Nursing Unit)
Staff nurse                          May 1994 to May 1995

Longview Extended Care
Licensed practical nurse             May 1992

**Professional and Personal References Available on Request**

**Figure 22-4**
Sample functional résumé.

Professional nurses may develop a résumé independently, seek the advice of career counselors, or have it generated by a résumé specialist. Most personal computers have the capability of accommodating résumé preparation software programs. The Internet has several electronic résumé preparation websites. State employment agencies also may have websites to assist with résumé generation. Yate (1998, p. 73) proposes using hypertext markup language to "create sharply designed and formatted résumés" that can be sent electronically to prospective employers and clients. Advances in computer software and electronic mail services enable job applicants to submit resumes via e-mail; some organizations prefer electronic submission of job application material over paper copies.

When providing contact information, the résumé should contain the person's name without any titles (unless it is a gender-neutral name), mailing address, telephone number, and electronic mailing address. If the telephone is connected to an answering machine, care should be exercised to specify this in the cover letter, and the applicant should frequently check the answering machine. Frequent reading of e-mail also should occur if potential employers use e-mail notification for establishing telephone or personal interview appointments. Applicants should refrain from using current employment addresses and telephone numbers unless they have informed current employers of their search for another job (Bongard, 1997b; The Editors of VGM Career Horizons, 1996; Yate, 1998).

Finally, résumés lose power if they contain mistakes or possess certain characteristics. Yate (1998) offers the suggestions for what should never go into a résumé:

1. Giving the document a title, such as résumé, fact sheet, or curriculum vitae.
2. Stating availability for employment.
3. Specifying reasons for leaving previous or current job.
4. Outlining references (employers have the legal obligation to obtain written consent from prospective employees before they can check references).

The résumé provides applicants with a written format to showcase professional skills and written communication abilities to prospective clients and employees. Usually, no verbal interaction occurs between the person screening the résumé and the applicant. Thus, utmost care should be taken when creating a résumé to create the best impression.

## Reference Lists

Personal and professional references do not belong on a résumé (The Editors of VGM Career Horizons, 1996; Yate, 1998). The type and number of references vary across organizations (typically three to six are required). Position applicants usually find out the number of required references when they complete an employment application. When specifying references, common courtesy suggests that applicants inform the persons whose names appear on the reference list. In addition, if persons have used more than one surname while they have been employed, this information should be included somewhere because it can make verifying references difficult if a married name is given to a reference when he/she knows the person by a maiden name (Yate).

To make the absolute best impression, nurses should submit all materials printed with the same font and using the same type of paper (including the mailing envelope if possible). This creates a uniform package and presents an image of being detail oriented (Yate, 1998).

### Curriculum Vitae

For nurses embarking on a career in academia, a **curriculum vitae** (CV) fills the need for a professional résumé. A CV specifies all professional presentations and complete citations for authored publications. Other information frequently found on a CV, but not on a résumé, includes consultation activities, details of professional organizational membership and activity participation, and listings of continuing education program attendance (Bell, 2001; Bongard, 1997b). Unlike the résumé, a CV may be many pages in length. Bongard (1997b) suggests that a professional nurse may want to develop a CV and résumé. To discover the major differences between a résumé and CV, nurses could ask a nurse faculty member to see a copy of a CV.

## Professional Portfolios

Some nursing programs have students generate nursing portfolios as part of a course or to fulfill curriculum requirements (Serembus, 2000b). Nurses returning to school may use a **professional portfolio** to earn credit for life experiences (Bell, 2001; Lettus, Moessner, & Dooley, 2001; Serembus, 2000b). Commercial artists take portfolios with them to display creative projects when they attend job interviews. Nurses who have a nursing professional portfolio may elect to take them to interviews to display evidence of creative works, publication, institutional form development, participation in program development, and other professional nursing endeavors (Bell, 2001). Sometimes (especially in academia), a professional portfolio may be required for promotion.

Portfolio components vary according to intended use. Serembus (2000a) suggests that nurses develop a comprehensive professional portfolio that can be used to develop a presentation portfolio to fit a situation, such as advancement or securing a new nursing position. Nurses should include the following information in a professional portfolio: résumé, nursing philosophy, letters of recommendation, licenses, certifications, education diplomas, transcripts, results of standardized tests for graduate study, honors, awards, professional organizational memberships, publications, photographs of presentations, continuing education program certificates, evidence of community service, and letters of appreciation (Bell, 2001; Serembus, 2000a, 2000b). Bell specifies that portfolio development provides nurses the opportunity to "reflect on" the professional actions that enabled them to learn from various experiences.

Although a professional portfolio may take lots of time to develop, it provides an opportunity to showcase professional accomplishments (Bell, 2001) and break the ice during a job interview. In addition, a job applicant can permit potential employers to review the portfolio after the interview has been completed. If a portfolio is left with the interviewer, the applicant must specify when he or she plans to retrieve it.

## Interviewing Skills

A personal interview enables potential employers or clients an opportunity to assess applicants to determine how they may fit with the organization. When an interview invitation is extended, applicants are one step closer to getting the desired position. Successful interview performance relies on adequate preparation. Table 22-2 outlines some tips for effective performance during an employment interview. Some nurses find the interview process stressful. However, interview skills improve with repeated practice. Some nurses find rehearsing with someone who assumes the role of interviewer to be an effective strategy for interview preparation. The interview allows employers and clients a chance to evaluate candidates on a personal level.

Prospective employers have legal limitations regarding specific questions they may ask during an employment interview. Some organizations have prospective employees interview with a member of the Human Resources Department, the

TABLE 22-2

## Tips for Effective Interviewing

| Tip | Rationale |
| --- | --- |
| Learn as much as possible about the organization. | Knowledge of mission and philosophy enable the ability to anticipate questions related to personal fit with the organization. |
| Dress conservatively in a business suit or well-tailored dress, not uniform or scrubs. | Present a professional appearance. The employment interview rule is to dress one level above the position being considered. |
| Avoid wearing fragrances, smoking, or filling your car's gas tank right before the interview. | Fragrances create impressions. Heavy perfumes may trigger allergies, and the smell of smoke emphasizes the habit. |
| Rehearse the employment interview with a friend or family member. | Allay interview nervousness and anxiety. |
| Bring nursing license and certification requirements with you. | Prospective employer may want to copy these for your file. |
| Prepare a set of questions related to the agency and position. | Asking questions may generate information to continue or stop pursuing the position. Questions also reveal interest. |
| Be armed with information related to the local market salary, bonus, and job expectations. | Verification that position is aligned with current market. |
| Arrive 5–10 minutes before scheduled time. | Extra time provides time to relax immediately before the interview, allays potential anxiety related to tardiness, and demonstrates punctuality. Arriving too soon may make the interviewer feel rushed with a previous appointment. |
| Look busy while waiting—read a magazine, look over a list of questions, or review your résumé. | Interviewer may accompany previous appointment to waiting area, and making use of waiting time creates a positive first impression. |
| Do not bring friends or relatives to the interview site. | Concern for them may keep you from being focused on the interview. Potential perception of lack of self-confidence. |
| Greet the interviewer with direct eye contact and a firm handshake. | Business etiquette dictates use of firm handshake when first meeting someone, and eye contact denotes assertiveness in Western culture. |
| Do not chew gum. | Disrupts articulation of words, and chewing motion creates an unprofessional appearance. |
| Always ask a question if asked if you have any questions. | Denotes interest in organization and also that you are focused on the interview. |
| Be honest and forthcoming with all answers. | Dishonesty or perceptions of covert information provide reasons for interviewer not to continue the job application process. |
| If asked about why you left previous places of employment, describe situation specifically using positive terms. | Chances are that if applicants speak negatively about previous employment experiences, they will do this when they quit this organization. |
| Wait for the interviewer to address salary, hours, and working conditions. | Usually not covered in the first interview. However, these must be discussed before accepting a position. |

## Tips for Effective Interviewing (Continued)

| Tip | Rationale |
| --- | --- |
| Limit answers to each question to three statements and share something about yourself related to the question. | Targeted and brief answers facilitate the interview process. |
| Come prepared to address professional experiences and include information related to teamwork. | The trend is toward behavior-based interviewing, in which applicants are expected to share specific examples of how they executed various aspects of professional nursing and evidence of working in teams. |
| Carry a briefcase to store evidence of accomplishments, extra résumés, reference letters, and reference list. | Briefcases keep materials neat and project an air of professionalism. |
| Conclude the interview with a question related to the next step of the interview process. | Communicates continued interest in pursuing the position. |
| Write a thank you note to the interviewer as soon as possible after the interview. | Shows appreciation and highlights courtesy as a personal strength; also provides one last opportunity to highlight a personal strength. |

Source: Bongard, B. (1997b). Managing your career. In B. Case (Ed.), *Career planning for nurses* (pp. 69-73). Albany, NY: Delmar Publishers.

department manager, and staff department members before an employment offer is extended. Nurses who inquire about the hiring process during the initial interview can prepare themselves for any future interviews. In times of nursing shortages, employers offer large sign-on bonuses and other amenities to attract qualified nurses. When applying for positions with attractive bonuses and incentives, nurses should be aware of the risks associated with such enticements. Some incentives require nurses to sign contracts agreeing to a specified time commitment for employment. If nurses do not abide by conditions for the incentives, they usually must reimburse the employer for all or a portion of funds received.

### Follow-Up Communications

After the interview, applicants who send a thank you note by the morning after the interview have extended common courtesy toward the interviewer. Manners mean a lot to organizations that value customer service and teamwork. A follow-up thank you note also gives applicants a chance to summarize interview highlights and to make a final positive impression.

## ✦ SUMMARY AND SIGNIFICANCE TO PRACTICE

Development of a meaningful nursing career requires an open attitude, periodic self-assessment, lifelong learning, creativity, and courage. Along with personal characteristics, nurses rely on others for effective career development. Nursing provides an opportunity to live out the spiritual need to help others. Nurses help clients when engaging in client care and education activities. They help each other through professional networking and mentoring. To live out a preferred career vision, professional nurses must develop a plan and market their personal and professional skills to make the vision become reality.

Steps followed in changing a nursing career provide nurses with the opportunity for self-evaluation and marketing professional skills and personal strengths. When seeking a new position in nursing, nurses must capitalize on the wide set of job skills they have acquired through their previous professional experiences. Nurses sometimes fail to market themselves as fully as they should, in fear of being viewed as cocky or boastful.

## FROM THEORY TO PRACTICE

1. Review the vignette at the beginning of the chapter and answer the following questions:
   - What advice would you give to Glen as he looks for ways to change his nursing career?
   - Why is this advice important?
   - Why do you suppose that Pat is content in her current nursing position?
   - What are the positive and negative consequences of staying in a nursing position for a long time?
2. Develop a professional nursing résumé and compile a professional nursing portfolio. Analyze both projects. Are you on target to meeting your desired career goals? Why or why not?
3. Determine a nursing career goal. Design a career map to meet your desired career goal.

## WWW INTERNET EXERCISES

1. Develop a brief professional nursing résumé using the 10-Minute Resume Website http://www.10minuteresume.com. Print the résumé and then compare it to one you generate using a computer software program. Visit the website the Résumé Resource Center (http://www.resumestore.com) and find how much it would cost to purchase a nursing and other types of résumés and cover letters. Would it be worth it to you to pay for a professionally generated resume and cover letter? Why or why not?
2. Visit the Nursing Spectrum website at http://www.nursingspectrum.com. Click any of the entries under Jobs/Employers. Read about job openings, information on travel nursing and prospective employers. Scroll down the page until you find the Career Management section where underneath the heading, click on the words "Managing Your Career". On the next screen you will find information career changes, self-marketing, and preparing for employment interviews. Select and read one entry on Career Fitness, On-the-job Fitness, Job Transition Fitness, and Attitude Fitness. Summarize each entry read and specify the reasons why or why not you thought that this is useful information.

## WWW INTERNET RESOURCES

1. For available professional nursing positions: Visit specific places where your would like to be employed, a local newspaper website, or a general job posting site such as http://www.monster.com.

2. For help with resume preparation:
   http://www.10minuteresume.com or http://www.resumestore.com.
3. Nursing Spectrum: http://www.nursingspectrum.com.
4. Sigma Theta Tau International: http://www.nursingsociety.org.
5. The American Nurses Association: http://www.nursingworld.org.

## REFERENCES

Abrams. S. L. (2000). *The new success rules for women*. Roseville, CA: Prima Publishing.

Barrett, R. (1998). *Liberating the corporate soul, building a visionary organization*. Boston: Butterworth-Heinemann.

Bell, S. K. (2001). Professional nurse's portfolio. *Nursing Administration Quarterly, 25*, 69–73.

Bongard, B. (1997a). Creating your own job: Using nonlinear strategies to reach your career goals. In B. Case (Ed.), *Career planning for nurses* (pp. 87–103). Albany, NY: Delmar Publishers.

Bongard, B. (1997b). Managing your career. In B. Case (Ed.), *Career planning for nurses* (pp. 59–86). Albany, NY: Delmar Publishers.

Cardillo, D. (2001). Knowing when it's time to move on. *Nursing Spectrum, 2*, 20.

Case, B. (1997). Where are you taking your career? In B. Case (Ed.), *Career planning for nurses* (pp. 1–27). Albany, NY: Delmar Publishers.

Chang, R. (2000). *The Passion plan*. San Francisco: Jossey-Bass Publishers.

Covey, S. (1992). *Principle-centered leadership*. New York: Simon & Schuster.

Covey, S. (2004). *The 8th habit: From effectiveness to greatness*. New York: Free Press.

Donner, G. J., & Wheeler, M. M. (2001). Taking control of your career and your future. *Excellence in clinical practice, 2*, 2.

The Editors of VGM Career Horizons. (1996). *Résumés for nursing careers*. Lincolnwood, IL: VGM Career Horizons.

Falter, E. J. (1997). The nurse-manager-to-executive track. In B. Case (Ed.), *Career planning for nurses* (pp. 203–217). Albany, NY: Delmar Publishers.

Lettus, M. K., Moessner, P. H., & Dooley, L. (2001). The clinical portfolio as an assessment tool. *Nursing Administration Quarterly, 25*, 74–79.

Malone, B. L. (1999). Career mapping: Visioning your future. In C. A. F. Anderson (Ed.), *Nursing student to nursing leader: The critical path to leadership development* (pp. 290–301). Albany, NY: Delmar Publishers.

Messmer, P., Jones, S. & Taylor, B. (2004). Enhancing knowledge and self-confidence of novice nurses: The "shadow-a-nurse" ICU program. *Nursing Education Perspectives, 25,* 131–136.

Mish, F. (Ed.) (1994). *Merriam Webster's Collegiate Dictionary,* (10th ed.). Springfield, MA: Merriam-Webster.

Serembus, J. F. (2000a). Pocket full of miracles: A professional portfolio can be a powerful force in your career advancement. *American Journal of Nursing, 100*, 67.

Serembus, J. F. (2000b). Teaching the process of developing a professional portfolio. *Nurse Educator, 25*, 282–293.

Thomka, L. A. (2001). Graduate nurses' experiences of interactions with professional nursing staff during transition to the professional role. *The Journal of Continuing Education in Nursing, 32*, 15–19.

Waxman, K. (2005). Nurse entrepreneurship: Do you have what its takes? *2005 Pathways to Success,* Hoffman Estates, IL: Nursing Spectrum.

Wesorick, B., Shiparski, L., Troseth, M., & Wyngarden, K. (1997). *Partnership council field book*. Grand Rapids, MI: Practice Field Publishing.

Yate, M. (1998). *Résumés that knock 'em dead* (3rd ed.). Holbrook, MA: Adams Media Corporation.

# CHAPTER 23

# Shaping the Future of Nursing

## KEY TERMS AND CONCEPTS

Future

Vision

Possible Future

Plausible Future

Probable Future

Preferable Future

Scenarios

Evidence-based Nursing Practice

Multistate Licensure Compact

## LEARNING OUTCOMES

By the end of this chapter, the learner will be able to:

1 Compare and contrast the terms "possible future," "plausible future," "probable future," and "preferable future."

2 Identify professional nursing implications for presented future scenarios.

3 Outline strategies for professional nurses to plan for the future.

4 Specify key considerations for future nursing education.

5 Discuss the role of nursing scholarship in the future of the nursing profession and health care.

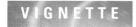
VIGNETTE

Jane is a registered nurse who just received word that the hospital where she has worked for 15 years is closing. Reasons for closing the hospital include declining economic forces in the community, less demand for services, increased competition for clients among health care providers, high unemployment, inability to meet financial demands, inadequate wiring and space to support new technology, inability to find replacement parts for building infrastructure, difficulty attracting and keeping enough nursing staff, and movement of physician practices to the more affluent suburbs. Jane wonders why she did not see the closure coming. Because Jane has worked for the past 10 years on the day shift in the postpartum unit, she knows that her work hours and special area of practice most likely will change. As Jane thinks about the situation, tears form in her eyes, and she wonders how she could have better prepared herself for the future she faces.

Carol Sando, RN, DNSc, authored this chapter in the fourth edition.

**? Questions for Reflection 23-1**

1. How can I prepare myself so that I maximize the use of my knowledge, skills, and talents as a professional nurse?
2. Where would I like to be in the nursing profession 10 years from now?
3. What steps do I need to take to accomplish my future career vision?
4. What are the consequences for me as a professional nurse if I fail to consider what changes may occur within health care and the nursing profession in the next decade?

Humans have attempted to predict the future for many centuries. Pyramids in Egypt contain hieroglyphics that predict the future of the human race. Ancient Greek philosophers attempted to predict the future. Various religious texts, such as the Bible and Koran, contain prophecies. Fortune-telling has sustained the passage of time, despite an era in Western culture that highly values scientific evidence. Various aspects of human life confirm that the future repeats the past, such as the predictability of the changing of the seasons and recurrence of cultural holidays. When catastrophic events occur (such as terrorist attacks or natural disasters), many persons express the belief that some powerful external force is behind such situations. Recent technological advances have resulted in the development of sophisticated forecasting models and programs to aid humans in preparing for the future. However, because of the random nature of the universe, even the best forecasting methods cannot determine the future.

Throughout many generations, humans have come to realize that the only thing upon which they can rely is change. People age as time passes. Dramatic environmental and societal changes have influenced human health, health care delivery, professional nursing practice, nursing education, and nursing scholarship. Many of the forces influencing changes have been presented in detail in preceding chapters. Because the forces influencing professional nursing intertwine, an effort has been made to avoid redundancy. This chapter focuses on the future as a concept and outlines potential future scenarios so that the nursing profession and individual nurses can plan to meet the challenges during the early 21st century and beyond.

## ✦ A CONCEPTUAL APPROACH TO THE FUTURE

Depending on the context in which it is used, the word **"future"** means "that is to be, . . . relating to or constituting a verb tense expressive of time yet to come, . . . existing or occurring at a later time, . . . the time that is yet to come, . . . what is going to happen" (Mish, 1994, p. 475). Whatever the definition, unless time ceases, the future will arrive soon.

Futurists use a variety of methods to forecast the future. Minkin (1995) proposes using a format that identifies and analyzes trends and determines implications of them before making predictions. Other futurists have used similar approaches in forecasting future trends with some success; these approaches include the writings of Naisbitt (1996), Aburdene and Naisbitt (1992), Naisbitt and Aburdene (1990), Johnson and White

(2000), and Toffler (1970, 1990). Other futurists, such as Thomas Alva Edison, started with a **vision** (the concept of electric lighting) and then took steps to make the vision a reality. In terms of the future, the meaning of vision expands to include forecasting or prophecy.

Scholarly debate has occurred about the ability of mankind to shape the future. Minkin (1995) says the future is the only part of life that persons can change from actions or inaction. Sullivan (1999, p. 5) identifies two relevant assumptions about the future. "First, the future is uncertain. ... Second, we choose and create major aspects of the future by what we do or fail to do." However, many religious faiths hold the belief that the future unfolds as part of a grand plan by a higher power.

Henchley (1978) specifies the following four possible ways of looking at the future. Henchley's approach considers the wildest possible ideas to probable concepts based on human history and trends.

The **possible future** considers all potential things that may occur, including the wildest ideas that even violate current scientific laws (Henchley, 1978). Examples include unpredicted catastrophes, such as the catastrophic earthquake and tsunami disaster on December 26, 2004; potential, coordinated, multiple worldwide terrorists attacks; and a large meteor hitting and destroying the planet. Science fiction media and doomsday prediction exercises serve as sources for the possible future.

The **plausible future** focuses on what may occur based on current trends that may be combined to describe a range of potential futures (Henchley, 1978). Examples include increasing tensions between the United States and other nations, developing clean sources of energy, increasing disparity of incomes between the rich and poor, and increasing global pollution by human beings.

The **probable future** presents a picture of what most likely will happen, with the future being primarily a mirror to the present with little or no actual change. Examples would include continued financial strain on health care providers and consumers in the absence of a reformed health care system and continued advances in technology and science, increasing the complexity of life and health care decisions.

The **preferable future** proposes the desired state for the future. Development of a preferred vision requires development of common visions, shared values, and strategic plans among many groups of persons. The preferable future starts by identifying a vision and taking steps to make the vision reality. Indeed, this future results from deliberate actions or inaction. Examples of this would include the unification of all health care providers (including third-party payers), consumers, and elected officials to develop a realistic comprehensive health care reform program and alleviation of culturally-biased health care delivery by actively recruiting the best and brightest of all cultural groups into the health care professions.

**Scenarios** are forecasts, "a model of an expected or a supposed sequence of events" (Mish, 1994, p. 1612). They raise awareness of the wide range of possible implications of external forces, sensitize people to potential threats and opportunities, and allow examination of alternative options for action. The scenarios presented in this chapter barely skim the issues that affect the future of professional nursing. Some of the presented scenarios are controversial. The scenarios without reference citations represent the author's predictions of what could possibly happen.

# ● FUTURE SCENARIOS FOR SOCIETY AND HEALTH CARE

Many forces that shape the future remain uncontrollable by the human race. Humans have yet to find ways to control acts of nature, such as weather patterns, earthquakes, certain epidemics, and famines. However, humans control governments, laws, and policies. Unfortunately, professional nurses have limited societal status and resources to become highly influential in the determination of laws, policies, and regulations. Professional nurses rely on building coalitions with more influential members of society and creating a solid united front to create change. The following scenarios related to society and health care primarily contain factors that remain out of the control of professional nursing.

## The Aging American Population Changes the Nature of Society

By the year 2030, the number of elderly Americans is projected to double, resulting in the need for increased nurses to provide health care services to them. (Burggraf & Barry, 2001; Institute for the Future, 2003). More home health nurses will be needed because increasing numbers of elderly will live at home and need help with activities of daily living and management of complex drug regimens. Nurse geriatric consultants will help caregivers cope with the declining health of the elderly. Finally, nursing research will need to be conducted to determine needs and trends of the aging population (Burggraf & Barry, 2001).

Clinical issues projected to arise will be prevention of infectious diseases (especially human immunodeficiency virus—sexually active seniors may refrain from condom use when pregnancy is not a potential consequence of intercourse, along with the development of antibiotic-resistant bacteria). In addition, strategies for reversing the aging process may appear. Biotechnology also may create spare body parts and tissue transplants and implanted computer chips for disabled persons. Finally, gene therapy, herbal therapies, and more drugs will be used to cease or reverse the aging process or maintain sexual potency (Burggraf & Barry, 2001).

Frequently, the elderly with resources exhaust them to pay for health care services. As people age, they consume more health care services (Wolf, 2003). By 2030, 20% of the American population will be over the age of 65 years and fewer than 50% will have defined pension plans. Forecasters predict that a possible intergenerational conflict may arise. Younger workers may revolt against paying high Social Security taxes to support the elderly (Institute for the Future, 2003). In the author's version of a worst case and possible scenario, American values will change, and the social obligation of the aged will be to die so that resources are conserved for use by the young. Laws are passed to make euthanasia and assisted suicide legal, and the elderly who do not want to be a burden to their children or society willingly end their lives.

For the financially solvent elderly, specialized extended care facilities will be built to provide individualized care to persons with common disabilities, diseases, and ethnic heritage. Because some elderly will live with children, the family unit will become intergenerational. As working adults serve as primary caregivers for the aged, geriatric day care programs will increase. The stress of caring for a debilitated aging adult will result in exhausted and depressed caregivers, resulting in neglect or some type of abuse. Caregiver programs will be developed to provide social and emotional support for them. Geriatric education, mental health and respite care services will be available only for those who can pay for them. Legislation to provide funding for aging services, caregiver programs, medical care, and tax credits for home care giving will be enacted (Burggraf & Barry, 2001). In this possible scenario, children and young adults gladly assume responsibility for caring for aging parents and relatives in their homes.

In contrast, a plausible scenario is that the elderly maintain control of the government because of their history of political activism, increased numbers, and financial stability. The elderly would exert great pressure on policy makers to increase the level of federal and local support for health care (Institute for the Future, 2003).

However, the probable scenario would be that the elderly might enjoy improved health from advances in medical science, remain a strong lobbying group, and demand increased governmental support for life and health care needs. In this scenario, society and governmental support for the health care of the elderly would remain similar to that of current systems.

Finally, in the preferred scenario, the aging population makes health-promoting lifestyle choices (starting in middle adulthood) and develops strong ties with younger persons. Persons of all ages work together to develop policies related to health care delivery that provides equal access to services for all who need it. The affluent elderly engage in volunteerism and willingly assume financial responsibility for having life needs met, leaving public resources for the elderly and other societal members who cannot pay for basic life needs, including health care.

## Questions for Reflection 23-2

1. How can the nursing profession prepare for the increased numbers of elderly who will need future nursing services?
2. What are the possible consequences for the nursing profession if it fails to address the aging population issue?

## Global Terrorism

Before September 11, 2001, the United States considered itself immune to multiple terrorist attacks or acts of war. However, some persons forewarned of a coordinated terrorist attack plan (National Institute of Medicine and the National Research Council, 1999). According to Dickey and Power (2001), Islamic extremists possess a profound hatred of America and have a 100-year plan for world conquest. The plan calls for removal of a United States presence from Muslim nations and replacement of moderate governments with Islamic fundamentalist governments. The Internet links terrorists and provides evidence for them about the global Westernization that fuels their hatred. Hatred of America could become more widespread, as could global efforts to crush the nation, which some perceive as wealthy and selfish. (Note that most Muslims are against violence and world conquest.) Since the attack on the United States, terrorists launched attacks on public transportation systems in Spain immediately prior to a national election.

According to a 1999 study conducted by the National Institute of Medicine and the National Research Council, terrorist organizations use the basic freedom enjoyed by Americans to infiltrate public and private institutions. They become invisible by developing friendships with American citizens. The higher education system provides the members of terrorist organizations with the knowledge and expertise to develop plans for attacks based on science and technology. Unfortunately, technology may be used by people (or machines) to release powerful weapons, such as designer pathogens with cures known only to the aggressor. In addition, technological progress may result in the development of nanotechnology, biotechnology, and robotics that may have the capability to destroy the human race while leaving buildings and physical infrastructures intact. Knowing that United States citizens depend on power sources for health, safety, and business, terrorists target power plants and oil pipelines. Because of the fear of eliminating the rights of states and individuals, the American government has failed to develop a federal disaster plan that could be immediately implemented in the event of a thermonuclear, chemical, or biomedical attack (National Institute of Medicine and the National Research Council, 1999).

In response to the multiple hijackings and destruction of the World Trade Center in New York (resulting in more than 2,000 civilian fatalities from 80 different nations), the United States declared war on terrorism. United States military forces were deployed to areas around the globe to launch an attack on terrorists harbored in Afghanistan. A war in Iraq was launched because of *reported* links of the Iraqi government to terrorist groups and the presence of weapons of mass destruction. Other countries, including Australia, Japan, Ukraine, Latvia, the Czech Republic, Italy, South Korea, Norway, Poland, Protugal, Romania and Great Britain, joined the war on terrorism. As in all wars, much environmental destruction occurred, and many persons have been injured or have died.

At the writing of this chapter, the results of the war on terrorism remain unknown. However, the use of many resources for fighting results in fewer resources available to fight hunger, disease, illiteracy, and poverty. A possible scenario is that continued bombing and battles result in many civilian casualties, which may lead to more countries considering the United States a nation striving to conquer the world to force democratic and capitalistic values on all persons.

However, a more plausible scenario results in the strengthening of the coalition of countries engaging in the war on terrorism. In this scenario, the United States declared war on terrorism. In this scenario, the United Nations (UN) becomes the place where strategic plans are made to rid the world of terrorist acts initiated by well-organized groups with global networks. The UN also develops a global response plan to chemical and biological attacks. However, acts of terrorism performed by individuals remain unpredictable, and the persons responsible for such acts remain elusive.

Unfortunately, the probable scenario results in a future not much different from that of today. The United States and certain allies develop stronger ties, and the war on terrorism lasts for many years. In response to identified biological attacks, the United States stockpiles medications and vaccines for future use, if needed. Most Americans refuse to be intimidated by terrorist threats and continue with their usual life practices, such as working, shopping, and attending sporting and other recreational events. A few anxious citizens stockpile supplies needed to prepare themselves in anticipation of a terrorist attack using nuclear devices. The government makes efforts to stimulate the economy while spending vast amounts of money to preserve homeland security. Less money becomes available to provide services to the poor and to repair infrastructure (roads, sewage systems, power plants). American citizens live with minor inconveniences, such as having to arrive earlier and wait longer in lines when traveling by commercial airlines. Health care workers are asked to register voluntarily to serve as members of federal, state, or local medical response teams (Veenema, 2003).

## Questions for Reflection 23-3

1. How can the nursing profession be ready to confront the effects of terrorist acts?
2. Why is being prepared for the effects of terrorism important to the nursing profession?

## Obesity and Health Care

Currently, 65% of Americans are overweight and, of those, 33% of the overweight are obese. Obesity is linked to type II diabetes. Recent studies project that diabetes will develop in one in three Americans born in the year 2000 before they die. Ancient humans survived as hunter-gatherers and efficient storage of energy promoted the survival of the human race. However, in modern times, Americans (and citizens of other developed nations) engage in a sedentary lifestyle and have unrestricted access to high-caloric foods (Institute for the Future, 2003; United States Department of Health & Human Services [USDHHS], 2000; Lazar, 2005). Besides diabetes, being overweight and obese contribute to the development of degenerative arthritis, hypertension, heart disease, stroke, gall bladder disease, sleep apnea, respiratory difficulties, and certain forms of cancer (USDHHS).

A possible scenario related to the problem of obesity is that science discovers ways to turn off the "thrifty gene," blocks chemicals responsible for hunger, and develops an effective weight loss pill that has few and insignificant adverse effects (Millett & Kopp, 1996). In addition, scientists realize that individual genetics determine how foods are metabolized and used by the body. Nutritional counseling based on individual genetic profiles becomes widespread (Underwood & Adler, 2005). A forecast by the author related to obesity includes government support to obese and overweight citizens for the following weight reduction efforts: prescription drugs for weight loss, memberships to health clubs, and psychological counseling. In return, governments impose taxes on "junk" food (unless the citizen is underweight), and initiate tax surcharges on obese citizens to defray projected increased health care costs. Many people lose weight and adopt a healthy lifestyle (to avoid increased taxes), which results in reduced demand for secondary and tertiary health care services.

A plausible scenario related to the incidence of obesity developed by the author reads as follows. In developed nations, affluent citizens keep getting larger and larger. They have access to unlimited food, engage in sedentary jobs, fail to exercise, and find comfort in passive entertainment (watching movies or television and spending endless hours engaged in computer activities). Health problems, once thought of as afflictions of aging, occur at younger ages (Trossman, 2005). Young, educated citizens find themselves incapable of performing any manual labor. They rely on housekeepers and gardeners to maintain a home or they live in condominiums or apartments where building and ground maintenance is provided. Because of their size and health problems, the young adults quickly find themselves unable to work because of their health, resulting in an increased incidence of worker disability. The obese young *and* the elderly consume health care services to the point of exhaustion. Nurses caring for the obese clients sustain more back injuries (Trossman, 2005). Nursing becomes one of the most dangerous professions because of the high incidence of permanent disability arising from work-related injuries.

A probable scenario related to increased obesity is that some obese and overweight persons recognize the impact of weight on their energy level, feelings of well-being, and health. Corporate America recognizes the problem and works to capitalize on the obesity epidemic. Numerous weight reduction products are developed and marketed to consumers. Obese and overweight consumers turn to science in hopes that it will discover a painless, quick way to lose weight. Persons with an external locus of control blame others for their weight. However, persons with an internal locus of control take steps to reduce their weight. Legislative efforts to pass regulations and laws protecting consumers from poor eating habits, knowing all unhealthful food ingredients in available foodstuffs, warning consumers about fraudulent weight reduction plans, and taxing "junk" food fail. Persons receive education on healthy lifestyles. Some persons (many who need psychological counseling) need the advice of health care providers and lose weight. However, others persons continue the cycle of temporary weight loss followed by weight gain. Persons (nurses and unlicensed care providers) caring for obese health care consumers have access to technological and other assistive devices to prevent work-related injuries (Trossman, 2005).

However, the preferred future would mean that more (ideally all) persons would adopt a healthy lifestyle. Health care professionals provide worldwide education programs that address the health hazards of being obese and overweight. Success at getting the message occurs. People lose lots of weight. They consume only the number of calories to maintain healthy body weight and follow the recommendations of getting 30 minutes of vigorous exercise daily (USDHHS, 2000). Health care dollars are spent on health promotion, resulting in increased savings because of reduced consumption of secondary and tertiary health care services.

### Questions for Reflection 23-4

1. How does obesity affect the health of health care consumers and nurses?
2. What are the potential adverse effects of caring for obese clients for nurses?
3. What are possible ways to minimize the health hazards for nurses working with obese clients?
4. What safety devices are present in my current clinical practice setting for nurses to use when caring for obese clients?
5. Do I use the safety devices available to me? Why or why not?

## Genetic Research

Findings from the Human Genome Project will have profound effects on society. Genes for various diseases have been discovered, and eventually these discoveries will lead to new detection and treatment techniques. Genetic testing may result in determining suitable marriage partners, safe insurance risks, individualized diets, and human evolution. Persons also may receive genetically designed medication to prevent or treat illnesses. In addition, persons known to be at risk for a particular affliction may begin screening for a particular disease earlier in life than would be recommended for the general population (Institute for the Future, 2003).

The completion of human genome mapping and the results of future genetically based research provide the foundation for various scenarios. A possible scenario comes from the movie *Gattaca*, (Sony Pictures, 1997) in which individuals receive genetic testing at birth to determine their future lives. The state selects the profession (or work), education, and genetic composition for all citizens. Marriage is no longer needed because new human life is created using artificial insemination in women genetically designed to thrive during pregnancy and childbirth. Individuals lose the freedom to choose their destiny.

However, a plausible scenario would be that persons would be genetically tested at birth to determine potential health risks. For the person with the genetic disposition to cancer, screenings would begin earlier in life than would be recommended for the general population. Drug companies would use genetic research to design effective medications against previously incurable forms of illness. In addition, genetically designed medications for individuals would enhance disease prevention and treatment efforts (Garcia et al., 2001; Check & Rogers, 2001; Offit, 1998). The cost of health care escalates as individually designed drugs increase costs for production and create more medications. Only the affluent have access to genetically designed medications. However, persons requiring earlier and more frequent disease screenings receive them (Institute for the Future, 2003).

Finally, the probable scenario proposes that pharmaceutical companies and health care providers will use information generated from human genetic research to find treatments for and ways to prevent illness. Persons with familial tendencies for particular diseases will be offered genetic testing to determine optimal screening, prevention, and treatment modalities. Genetic testing will be performed only with voluntary consent (Check & Rogers, 2001; Offit, 1998). In the case of genetic research, the probable scenario most likely is the preferred scenario.

### Questions for Reflection 23-5

1. What impact will advances in genetic research have on the nursing profession?
2. What additional knowledge and skills will be needed by nurses in the future because of advances in genetic research and genetically based health care?
3. What are the potential hazards for consumers who undergo genetic testing?
4. What are the potential benefits of having a genetic health profile performed on all persons?

# ● FUTURE SCENARIOS FOR HEALTH CARE DELIVERY

Projecting existing trends, Bezold (1996) developed four scenarios that describe radically different potential pictures of the health care delivery system at the start of the 21st century: the business-as-usual, hard times, buyer's market, and healthy healing communities scenarios.

## Business-as-Usual Scenario

The probable, business-as-usual scenario assumes continued technological ingenuity, sophisticated communication, and high levels of consumption. Although most Americans are better off, the percentage of poor continues to rise. Health care reform has been left to the states, which in turn leave it to the marketplace. Advances in biomedical knowledge and technology make it possible to forecast, prevent, and manage illnesses earlier and more successfully. High-tech interventions such as performance-enhancing bionic implants and organoids (a new organ or organ part grown outside the body and then implanted) are widely available to those who can pay for them. Hospitals become smaller and their numbers decline, reducing the number of hospital beds by two thirds in two decades. Health care delivery becomes more efficient, so health care's percentage of the gross national product (GNP) stabilizes at 15% (Bezold, 1996). The extension of the current environment additionally devalues the role of professional nursing and results in fewer persons entering the profession, and practicing nurses continue to seek employment outside of hospital settings. The nursing shortage continues to worsen.

## Hard Times Scenario

This possible scenario assumes that times are tough for the economy as a whole and for health care. Although health care costs currently have stabilized at 15% of the GNP, 44 million persons (11 million of them children) in the United States do not have health insurance (USDHHS, 2000). As unemployment increases, citizens pressure the federal government to create universal access to a frugal basic package of care. Health care innovation slows dramatically, as do heroic measures to prolong life. A two-tier health care system emerges for the health "haves" and "have nots."

Nursing care of acutely ill clients would be important in this scenario, but nurses would be poorly paid and have little prestige. Consequently, most nurses would be from lower socioeconomic groups and from foreign countries. Some consumers of nursing services might have less confidence in receiving care from a foreign nurse, especially when the consumer may not understand the nurse's instructions because of her or his accented speech. Clients who could pay would be cared for in the home by private duty nurses (Bezold, 1996).

To streamline the use of limited resources, Herzlinger (2004) suggests that government-financed and insurance-covered health treatments would be limited to those with an established history of successful outcomes, based on reliable scientific evidence and documented emphasis on promoting client comfort. Nurses would rely on standardized protocols for specific health care problems or concerns to shorten the time required for attaining the desired health outcomes. Standardized protocols would be followed by nurses and physicians for treating specific client health problems. Standardized protocols would reduce costs while enhancing client outcomes. Consumers with knowledge and resources would become empowered to act as equal partners with health care professionals. However, consumers without knowledge and or resources might not be able to access needed health care services.

## Buyer's Market Scenario

In this preferred scenario, Bezold (1996) and Herzlinger (2004) propose that the responsibility for health and health care expenditures has been returned to the consumer. Insurance coverage includes a tax to help pay for the cost of care given to the poor. Health care providers are certified by the state on the basis of knowledge and competence. Health care providers, especially nurses, use evidence-based guidelines for practice. Competition for health care consumers becomes fierce, and health care organizations work to delight consumers. People rely less on health care providers and have better tools for changing their lifestyles and preventing or managing illnesses. Consumers, rather than the third-party payers, choose from various types of providers and treatments. Because health becomes a highly valued aspect of human life, consumers seek health care for illness prevention, rather than disease treatment (Herzlinger, 2004).

This scenario offers real potential for nursing to achieve greater power and influence. Nursing practice based on scientific evidence elevates the level of professionalism for nurses. Nurses present solid evidence for optimal staffing patterns for positive client outcomes. Because nurses are seen by society as professionals who have altruistic concerns for clients and have reasonable workloads, more persons choose to enter the profession. Nurses develop independent practices and demonstrate superiority in primary health care delivery. By accessing consumers directly, nurses would have a major role in promoting health. Education would emphasize ways of teaching consumers how to promote individual, family, and community health.

## Healthy, Healing Communities Scenario

This preferred and probable scenario involves a focus on "healing the body, mind, and spirit of individuals and communities" (Bezold, 1996, p. 38). Neighbors look out for each other, and people work together to eliminate problems such as drugs, teenage pregnancy, and the effects of poverty. However, as information makes workers more productive (or replaces workers altogether), unemployment grows to 25%. Health care organizations help to make communities environmentally and financially sustainable with the help of unpaid volunteers. Health promotion efforts begin in early childhood. Older persons find rewarding ways to contribute to the community, reducing disability and the time spent in long-term facilities. Advanced technologies lead to a comfortable life for most people, and bionics, robotics, smarter homes, and more caring neighborhoods allow disabled elderly individuals to remain in their homes. Consumers are involved in decision making regarding their health. The emphasis is on wellness and the development of full human potential, with rejection of anonymity, artificiality, manipulation, and unnecessary size or complexity.

Nurses would be full partners with consumers in this scenario, helping people with self-care and health promotion activities while providing information to support fully informed decision making. Older persons would be valued and would be cared for at home. Various information sources to support health would be available at home through computer networks. Nurses would be recognized as highly educated professionals, whose contribution would be valued for its effectiveness.

## Implications for Nursing Related to the Health Care Scenarios

Through advocacy of the principles outlined in its failed agenda for health care reform (American Nurses Association [ANA], 1991), nursing has a vision to help shape its future. "Nursing offers just what the American health consumer hopes for" (Porter-O'Grady, 1994, p. 38). The ANA develops an annual legislative agenda to assure that issues that affect professional nursing practice are addressed in ways to promote the health of American citizens while protecting the interests of nursing. If nurses communicate and act effectively as a cohesive group with consumers, legislators, and other policy makers to influence decisions affecting health care delivery, the result will be enhanced opportunities for authority, regardless of which scenario dominates the delivery system. Otherwise, the agendas of others will take precedence, and professional nursing and nurses will be at risk (Milstead, 1999).

## ✦ EVOLVING HEALTH CARE NEEDS AND HEALTH CARE DELIVERY

Demonstrable shifts are occurring in the causes of mortality associated with infectious diseases, chronic diseases and diseases associated with life stress. For example, acquired immunodeficiency syndrome (AIDS) and related illnesses remain a major cause of death and disability in young adults. In recent years, the incidence of new AIDS cases has declined only in white homosexual males. Increased rates have been observed among women and heterosexuals who fail to practice safe sex. Influenza and pneumonia are still the sixth highest cause of death in children 1 to 14 years of age, but the leading cause of death in childhood, unintentional injuries, is preventable. Recent increases in childhood asthma cases have been noted. Indiscriminate use of antibiotics has resulted in the development of antibiotic-resistant organisms. Homicide and suicide are major causes of death in adolescents and young adults (ages 15 to 24 years). Diseases such as coronary heart disease, cancer, diabetes, chronic liver disease, and unintentional injuries are the top causes of death in Americans between 25 and 65 years of age and have been associated with lifestyle choices. Infant deaths have been linked to prenatal smoking, alcohol, drug use, and malnutrition (USDHHS, 2000).

Every indication is that these trends will continue, if not accelerate, concomitant with an ever-increasing lifespan and the rapid pace and increasingly technological emphasis of modern life. Infections, violence, and lifestyle-related diseases fall within the realm of nursing expertise. In recent years, many persons have become interested in assuming responsibility for their health. Persons with computers frequently consult resources on the Internet to learn about health conditions and healthy lifestyle patterns. Health conscious consumers often ask nurses about the quality of health information from the Internet and various forms of media. When nurses provide consumers with valid and reliable information, they assume leadership in helping people prevent illness and experience optimal health.

In the past, hospital admittance often was prescribed because nursing care was needed. Until fairly recently, common reasons for hospital admittance included diagnostic laboratory testing, routine care, or rehabilitation, in addition to treatment of illness. Increasingly, the high cost and highly specialized medical technology associated with hospital admittance have led to the use of hospitals primarily for diagnosis and attempted cure of serious acute illnesses and acute treatment of chronic disease. When clients become physically stable, they are transferred to other settings (extended care or rehabilitation centers) or sent home to recover.

Minor illness and disease prevention increasingly are provided through separately contracted ambulatory care in clinics, physicians' offices, and people's homes. Many times, nurse practitioners assume the role of primary health care provider. Sometimes, home health nurses serve as the physician's eyes and ears when homebound clients cannot travel to ambulatory care settings. These represent opportunities for professional nurses to assume more responsibility, provide effective health care services, and demonstrate the value of the nursing profession to consumers and other health care professionals.

The current organization of the health care delivery system focuses on clients contracting with physicians for care, while nursing is supplied by the hospital as part of a package of services. Recent expansion of the use of nurses as primary care providers has resulted from federal legislation that provided Medicare and Medicaid reimbursement for nurse practitioners. Unfortunately, the current health care system remains focused on medical cure and chronic disease stabilization. Health maintenance organizations attempted to change the target of health care to health promotion. However, this effort proved to be more expensive than anticipated (Kleinke, 1998).

The future of the health care delivery system has yet to be determined. The establishment of integrated health care networks, with a large acute care facility located in an urban area with small hospitals, ambulatory care settings, and clinics, seems to be a future trend. In the future, the system could move toward either increased centralization or increased decentralization of services (Kleinke, 1998). The decentralized model, comprising a number of laterally linked components separate from a large urban acute care center, could facilitate entrepreneurial nursing delivery systems, such as independent nursing practices and partnerships between nurses and various other health care professionals.

Some systems are building point-of-service networks to broaden consumer choice and embracing "disintegration" (Goldsmith & Goran, 1996; Kleinke, 1998). With direct third-party reimbursement from private or federal insurers, nurses could contract directly with clients for the provision of nursing services. Through contractual agreements, nurses could provide essential professional services as autonomous providers, rather than as employees. In recent times, some physicians have opted to become employees of large integrated health care systems, resulting in a decline of control over medical practice (Kleinke).

However, given the power, influence, and control of the medical–hospital industry, it is unlikely the health care delivery system will be completely restructured in the near future. Some hospitals have moved toward centralization of services in care centers that include ambulatory services as well as inpatient care. This model accentuates the current status of most nurses as employees and further consolidates the financial control of health care by hospitals and physicians. The challenge for nursing would be to gain autonomy within the system. For this, nurses would need equality with other health professionals, which can be accomplished only through comparable educational qualifications and an equivalent allocation of authority.

The movement toward prospective payment is bound to become the standard for third-party reimbursement by private and public agencies, for physicians and other professionals, and for hospitals and other care institutions. Nursing must actively promote the cost benefits and care outcomes of having educated, highly skilled professional nurses in the system, or the trend toward replacement of registered nurses (RNs) by unlicensed workers and workers who are less qualified and paid less will be accelerated.

The nursing profession must emphasize the cost-effectiveness of competent care and assume the initiative in documenting the unique contribution of nursing to the restoration of well-being and prevention of illness in clients. Nursing's "ability to articulate specific and refined costs of nursing activity and compare them to achieved outcomes will have a direct relationship to the ability of nurses to render measurable, achievable, and cost-effective care" (Porter-O'Grady, 1986, p. 205). Research efforts in recent years have demonstrated that outcomes of client care are improved when they receive care from professional nurses (Aiken, Clarke, Sloane, 2000; Aiken, Smith & Lake, 1994; Haven & Aiken, 1999; Doran, 2003). One positive aspect of prospective payment is the potential for clear labeling of the distinct contribution made by nursing to the restoration of well-being, which promotes the valuing of nursing services by the public.

Porter-O'Grady (1986) predicted that nursing would shift away from dependent, illness-fixed, delegated, and narrowly defined roles that include institutionally defined and prescribed care and safety responsibilities in direct-care, physician-dominated, interruptive functions. Some professional nurses have proven that they have immense skill and expertise in fulfilling the role of case managers. In some ways, professional nursing remains subservient to physicians and institutional administration. Efforts to contain costs have enabled acute care facilities to embrace unlicensed care providers who receive training to perform tasks that once fell within the realm of professional nursing practice. Advanced practice nurses in some states must enter into contractual arrangements with physicians, in which the physician assumes responsibility for client care decisions; some states still refuse to grant advanced practice nurses prescriptive privileges.

Kreuger-Wilson and Porter-O'Grady (1999) forecast that professional nurses will have the ability and opportunity to lead the health care revolution. They advocate for the development of a multidisciplinary health care team in which each professional member brings a unique perspective and expertise to a client care situation. New nursing roles will be interdependent and health-based while having flexible applications. Nurses will work collaboratively with administration to assume control of professional practice in acute and extended care facilities. Nurses with deep commitment to professional practice will participate in multidisciplinary shared governance.

In the community, nurses will be held accountable for health outcomes and developing prescriptions for health maintenance and promotion. Teleconferencing, personalized client health cards, and telemonitoring currently provide support to community and home health nurses and use of these devices will become more widespread. Functions will be multidisciplinary, aimed toward prevention or correction, and defined by standards. However, if most professional nurses are not educated in baccalaureate programs, they will lack the required knowledge, skills, and experience to practice autonomously outside of the confines of the hospital or other institutions (Hadley, 1996).

**Questions for Reflection 23-6**

1. How do you think the current health care system will look in 10 years?
2. What knowledge and skills will be needed for effective nursing practice in 10 years?
3. How can nurses best prepare for the future health care delivery system?
4. What can the nursing profession do to help members prepare for the challenges in the future health care delivery system?

# ⬤ THE FUTURE OF PROFESSIONAL NURSING PRACTICE

Hadley (1996, p. 6) describes five challenges that nursing faces:

1. Demonstrating that nurses provide cost-effective, high-quality care that can be measured.
2. Adopting uniform licensure and educational requirements for the profession and establishing simpler, fewer titles.
3. Overcoming the mentality of an oppressed minority.
4. Accepting job insecurity.
5. Sustaining a commitment to lifelong professional learning.

Since Hadley published the challenges, some progress has been made. The following discussion outlines current progress and future ways for professional nursing to meet Hadley's identified challenges facing the nursing profession.

## Evidence-Based Nursing Practice

Nursing research findings, quality improvement data results, and clinical experience provide the foundation for evidence-based nursing practice. **Evidence-based nursing practice** uses the best available source of information to enable cost and clinically effective client care. Systematic nursing research and detailed evaluations of health care interventions provide strong evidence that nurses can use as foundations for practice. In the past, nurses performed many tasks based on tradition and ritual. Evidence-based practice enables nurses to determine the effects of newly developed technology, alternative and complementary treatments, and the differences professional nurses make in client care outcomes (Dempsey & Dempsey, 2002). Nurses are doing a better job at producing and disseminating information about their impact in the delivery of high quality care (Aiken, Clarke, & Sloane, 2000; Aiken, Smith, & Lake, 1994; Doran, 2003; Haven & Aiken, 1999). However, more needs to be done to inform the public and policy makers of the substantial contributions professional nurses make to health care.

Evidence-based practice enables nurses to be taken more seriously by other health care providers and society. Scientific justification for nursing actions raises the level of professional practice. In addition, evidence-based practice may serve as the vehicle for the nursing profession to clearly delineate a definition for the term "nursing."

## Multistate Compacts for Nursing Licensure in the United States

Despite the recommendation by the Pew Health Professions Commission (1995) for the health care professional regulation to remain controlled by individual states, the National Council of State Boards of Nursing (NCSBN, 2000) has initiated an effort for a mutual recognition model for professional nurse registration. Under mutual recognition, RNs could practice nursing across state lines, provided that the states participated in the mutual recognition compact.

The interstate compact helps states with shortages of professional nurses by allowing nurses from bordering states to practice without needing to obtain additional nursing licenses. Electronic- and telecommunication-based nursing practice frequently crosses state borders. The nurse would obtain licensure in the state of legal residence. To protect the integrity of individual State Nurse Practice Acts (SPA), the professional nurse would abide by the SPA where the client receives care (NCSBN, 2000, 2001).

The advantages of a single professional nursing license would facilitate interstate practice, improve tracking of nurses with disciplinary problems, increase cost effectiveness, simplify the nursing licensure process, eliminate duplicated listing of licensed nurses, and enhance interstate commerce. In addition, interstate licensure simplifies the licensing process for nurses who are employed by traveling nursing agencies (NCSBN, 2000).

Although multistate professional licensure may seem appealing, several disadvantages surface. State Boards of Nursing would need to raise licensing fees for professional nurses to accommodate for revenue generated by nurses who hold more than one state nursing license. Nurses with a disciplinary action record may not be able to obtain a fresh start in professional nursing after recovering from chemical addiction or after meeting the discipline requirements of a state board of nursing. Multistate licensure also would enable nursing agencies to provide professional nurses to institutions where nurses decide to engage in collective bargaining or strikes to improve working conditions.

To maintain state control of professional nursing licensure, individual states must pass state legislation to participate in the **multistate licensure compact.** By 2005, efforts to enact legislation have been successful in 18 states (Arizona, Arkansas, Delaware, Idaho, Iowa, Maine, Maryland, Mississippi, Nebraska, New Mexico, North Carolina, North Dakota, South Dakota, Tennessee, Texas, Utah, Virginia, Wisconsin) but have failed in others (NCSBN, 2004). Some failures have been the result of poor communication between State Boards of Nursing and State Nurses Associations. In some states, participation in a multistate compact is prohibited by the state constitution, thereby creating another obstacle for multistate nursing licensure compact legislation.

## The Demise of the Profession

The demise of the nursing profession is a possible future scenario. Within 10 years, 40% of working RNs will be 50 years old or older (Horrigan, 2004). Since 1996, associate degree nursing programs continue to graduate more nurses than other programs (Hopkins, 2001; Horrigan). Associate degree nursing programs focus on the technical aspects of nursing practice. If the trend continues, the nurses providing care to elderly, infirm, and disabled patients will be fewer, less educated, and older. Since 1985, more than 50% of new nurses educated in the United States have graduated from associate degree nursing programs (Hood & Leddy, 2003; NCSBN, 2004a; NCSBN, 2005) As a way to prepare for the nursing shortage, some states are considering expanding the scope of practice of emergency medical technicians to include providing services that currently fall within the scope of professional nursing practice in emergency departments and intensive care units.

To combat the projected shortage, the federal government has increased funding for persons interested in pursuing a career in nursing. Hospitals are offering tuition reimbursement plans to recruit new nurses to fill vacancies (Henriksen, Page, Williams, & Worral, 2003). Along with federal initiatives, the Robert Wood Johnson Foundation has funded a variety of projects to develop a strong, highly educated and diverse nursing workforce (Newbergh, 2005). However, despite these efforts, the United States Bureau of Labor Statistics projects a shortfall of more than 623,000 RNs in 2012 (Horrigan, 2004). Unless the nursing profession can recruit and retain new members, professional nurses may not be available to care for clients. This will result in reduced client functional status. Clients will be unable to provide self-care. Pain and other symptoms will not be controlled as effectively. Finally, more clients will sustain injury as they receive health care services (Doran, 2003).

## Nursing Gains Clout in Health Care

A more optimistic approach to and preferred scenario for the future of professional nursing would be that the profession becomes cohesive, provides solid evidence for contributions made to health care, and is valued by society and other health professionals. Nurses have fought with each other for generations on issues such as entry-level education for professional practice, collective bargaining, defining professional nursing practice, and control of professional practice (for example ANA versus NCSBN and staff nurses versus nurse administrators). Professional nurses work to safeguard the public against threats to health. As nurses provide solid evidence for the contributions they make to health care, society and other health team members will realize the value of professional nurses. Nurses have assumed the role of client advocate for many decades by protecting consumers from unscrupulous care providers and from serious treatment errors. The movement toward a multidisciplinary health team approach to client care provides nurses with an opportunity to showcase their knowledge and expertise.

### Questions for Reflection 23-7

1. What nursing knowledge areas need further development?
2. What is the current state-of-the-art knowledge on areas that need additional development and refinement?
3. How can nursing research affect the nursing profession and clinical practice?
4. How do I feel about a multidisciplinary approach to health and health care research?
5. What are the advantages of a multidisciplinary approach to health and health care research?
6. What are the disadvantages of a multidisciplinary approach to health and health care research?

When nurses demonstrate specialized knowledge and expertise that make differences in client care outcomes, society will greatly value the profession. Nurses will enjoy greater autonomy and higher salaries. Then, the profession of nursing will have no difficulty attracting the best and brightest young persons to the profession.

## ● THE FUTURE OF NURSING EDUCATION

The knowledge base and technology used in providing nursing care will continue to increase, as will nurses' need for skill and ability in: (1) intensely acute aspects of client care, (2) diagnostics and decision making, (3) use of complex computer systems and technology in clinical practice, (4) client teaching, (5) coordination of and delegation to less-skilled workers, (6) collaboration with clients and health care professionals to improve the quality of health, (7) understanding and using research to provide a strong scientific base for nursing practice, and (8) communicating to the public and health care providers the unique contributions nurses make to health care.

In the future, more than ever, nurses will need a broad-based education, assertiveness skills, technical competence, and the ability to deal with rapid change. However, research and technology may provide the instruments nurses require for defining professional nursing, demonstrating that professional nursing care affects client care outcomes, and marketing professional nursing to the public.

Since the 1960s, there has been an intensive national effort to promote the baccalaureate degree as the entry level for professional nursing. In that time, although there has been an increase in the number of nurses prepared at the baccalaureate level, there also has been a dramatic increase in the percentage of nurses prepared at the associate degree level. More than 70% of currently practicing nurses are prepared at the technical level of nursing. In the United States, education for entry into professional nursing can occur at one of four levels: the associate degree, the baccalaureate degree, the master's degree, or the doctoral degree. Thus, there are at least four different patterns of education that create nurses with different levels of knowledge and expertise. In addition, the multiple entry levels into nursing create confusion for health care consumers who consider that all nurses are alike.

The current pattern of more professional nurses entering the profession with associate degrees rather than baccalaureate degrees may continue. As a profession, nurses have been closely associated with upward mobility, especially for women. Most associate degree programs are located in community colleges, making them financially and geographically accessible. Demand can readily be met by an increased supply of licensed workers in a short time. Associate degree–prepared nurses offer basic skills required for safe client care in highly controlled acute, subacute, and extended care facilities (Balik, 1998). As the complexity of professional nursing increases and nursing care moves to the community, where delivery settings have many uncontrolled variables, associate degree–prepared nurses may lack theoretical knowledge to deliver safe, effective nursing care in these settings. The PEW Task Force on Accreditation of Health Professions Education (1998) proposed an educational ladder for RNs with associate degrees. Some nursing programs have developed creative approaches to advancing the level of nursing education. Examples of these programs include the RN to master's degree in nursing and the RN to nursing doctorate.

Before their baccalaureate studies, many RN students perceive nursing education at the baccalaureate level as additional and partially redundant, rather than as different and enriching. Little incentive for professional education is provided by the delivery system, which lacks differential salary structures or clearly articulated differences in job expectations. Licensure as an RN after associate degree education has reinforced this model.

Some propose that education for entry to professional nursing be moved to the master's level, rather than the baccalaureate level. This level of education would prepare the student for a combination of specialized and generalized practice appropriate for the developing delivery system. All students would need previous general education and possibly a bachelor's degree for entry into nursing, which would strengthen the liberal arts and science base for practice, prepare an educated person, encourage recruitment of students from other fields, and raise the status and authority of the profession. This model for nursing education probably would include the associate degree or baccalaureate degree for nursing assistants and the master's degree for licensed professional nurses.

Currently there are four doctoral programs leading to a Doctor of Nursing (ND) degree. Three of these consider the ND as the first professional degree. One program offers the ND as a post–master's degree that has multiple program entry points (Standing & Kramer, 2003). Aydelotte (1992, p. 470) summarizes the possible problems of this type of program:

- The goals of the program are not understood.
- The differences between the ND and other doctoral programs in nursing, such as the PhD or DNSc, are not perceived.
- Employers expect the ND graduate, as an entry-level practitioner, to perform in traditional nursing roles.
- The "nursing and health communities" hesitate "to accept general professional nursing knowledge as meriting a practice doctorate" (Aydelotte, p. 470).

The purpose of the ND degree program is to prepare a generalist in professional nursing. The student enters the program as a nonnursing college graduate. Following the program, the ND graduate would continue into a master's degree program as preparation for specialized practice and into a PhD or DNSc program as preparation for research and advanced role specialization (Aydelotte, 1992; Standing & Kramer, 2003).

Arguments for a nursing doctorate as the degree for entry into professional nursing practice include the following (Aydelotte, 1992, pp. 447–478):

1. The content for professional nursing practice and socialization for the role merit doctoral preparation.
2. An entry-nursing doctorate would clearly differentiate between technical and professional programs and roles.
3. Educational preparation for nursing would be on an educational level with other health professionals (e.g., medicine, pharmacy, and clinical psychology). Credentials are important to status and influence.
4. Reorganization of health care systems will require mature, articulate professionals "who command attention because of their knowledge base and skill" (p. 477).

However, considering the continued resistance to any upgrading of the current educational preparation for licensure, it is unlikely that either the entry master's or the entry doctorate model will achieve widespread acceptance in the near future.

A fourth possibility is that the baccalaureate degree will finally become the entry-level credential for professional practice and be recognized as such with the appropriate licensure, as is the case currently in South Dakota. Most major nursing organizations, including the ANA and the National League for Nursing, have endorsed this goal. An increasing number of nurses are seeking baccalaureate education and the credentials to practice at the professional level.

The nursing profession needs to better articulate and publicize (both internally and to the public) the contributions of professionally educated practitioners to health promotion and restoration and illness prevention. This book has identified the knowledge base and values that characterize the professional nurse in the hope that this will be the first step toward acceptance of scholarship and demonstration of professional competence in practice. If the baccalaureate or a higher degree does become the entry level for professional practice, the associate degree probably might become the accepted credential for nursing assistants, who could perhaps receive licensure as a technical nurse.

Regardless of which model is accepted, all educational programs must continue to modify their curricula to include changes in the theoretical and technical database for nursing. For example, computer technology is making an enormous impact on discovery, communication, information storage, and instructional techniques. Some nursing programs provide online distance education as the primary means for program instruction. Recent strides have been made in increasing the computer literacy of nursing students, professional nurses, and nursing faculty. However, not all schools include computer courses in their curricula. In addition, little attention has been paid to the moral implications of a computerized society that engenders feelings of isolation associated with impersonal communication and invasion of privacy.

For many years, there has been criticism of the basic model for nursing education. With its emphasis on behavioral objectives, "education is directed toward the preparation for a 'job' rather than for life as a professional" (Aydelotte, 1992, p. 469). To foster professionalism in nursing, critics of current educational processes propose the following changes in professional nursing programs: (1) emphasis on intellectual skills, rather than on mechanistic and technical abilities; (2) a learning environment that incorporates caring, compassion, and values; (3) attention to pattern recognition and the role of intuition in addition to "rules;" (4) active involvement in learning, rather than passive transmission of knowledge; (5) more attention to professional socialization and ethics; (6) content relevant to emerging needs and the redesign of the delivery system; and (7) concern with the process, not just with content.

All nurses need to be familiar with areas such as "health care economics, management of human resources, community needs assessment, peer governance, health care agencies, systems management, cost control, cost-effectiveness, strategies, and cost accounting" (Porter-O'Grady, 1986, p. 216), as well as policy development, information management, ethical decision making, technology use, and other areas of developing knowledge (Sullivan, 1999). The continuing development and testing of the theory will lead to knowledge that must be integrated into educational curricula.

To create a nursing profession to meet the needs of a multicultural population, nurse educators must work to recruit students from a variety of cultural backgrounds. However, more importantly, nurse educators must work to retain students from minority backgrounds once they are enrolled in nursing education programs. Special educational support systems may be required for remediation of reading and writing skills (especially for students who speak English as a second language). Curricular content and educational materials must include information regarding American and international cultural differences. Professional nurses from various cultural backgrounds can help faculty in the recruitment and retention of a culturally diverse student population. Finally, culturally diverse students rely on faculty of similar backgrounds for an effective connection within nursing programs. However, until faculties become culturally diverse, current faculty members need to make special efforts to connect with minority students to help them succeed in nursing education and perhaps attract them to the world of nursing academe (Sullivan & Clinton, 1999).

As the multidisciplinary health team approach to health care delivery grows, nurses will need education related to other health care providers and information on how to work as a team. In an ideal world, all members of the health care team should learn together, beginning with the first day of their professional education. Faculty from all respective disciplines also would learn and work collaboratively to prepare students to grasp individual discipline content while assessing interdisciplinary processes during carefully designed and conducted seminars.

## ✦ THE FUTURE OF NURSING SCHOLARSHIP

Within the past two decades, nursing research has received increased support from professional nurses and policy makers. The National Institute for Nursing Research (NINR) celebrated its tenth anniversary in 1996 as part of the National Institutes of Health. The NINR provides grant funding for nurse researchers. Results of funded nursing research are disseminated at annual NINR meetings (Grady, 1999).

In addition, nursing research–based protocols have been developed for client care in the areas of skin management, cognitive impairment, culturally relevant care, pain, and chemotherapy-induced nausea and vomiting. Nursing research findings frequently cross health care disciplines. As interdisciplinary approaches to health care demonstrate improved client outcomes, nurses will be asked to participate in multidisciplinary research efforts.

Rapid development in nursing theory and research during the past 20 to 25 years points to a promising outlook for the future. Nursing needs to develop and explicate theories to predict nursing outcomes. Increasingly, nursing research has validated models and theories for nursing care to provide foundations for care. If this trend continues, nursing will develop a unique knowledge base to fulfill the criteria defined for a profession.

## ✦ SUMMARY AND SIGNIFICANCE TO PRACTICE

Although the future cannot be predicted with great accuracy, nurses can accurately predict that health care delivery and the nursing profession will change. Visualizing several possible futures and identifying a preferred future enable nurses to shape the future of professional practice. Some projected changes threaten professional practice unless nurses provide scientific evidence of the benefits of nursing care, earn consumer confidence in their abilities as primary health care providers, receive recognition of the contributions they bring to the multidisciplinary health care team, and assume responsibility for creating a preferred future. The preferred future is one in which health care consumers and providers value the contributions nurses bring to the multidisciplinary health care team while working as informed, professional partners to assure safe, compassionate health care that is accessible to all and relevant to meeting the evolving health care needs of a global society. Every single professional nurse bears the responsibility to make the preferred future become a reality.

## FROM THEORY TO PRACTICE

1. Reread the vignette at the beginning of the chapter. What assumptions did Jane make regarding her nursing career? How did these assumptions create a future problem for her? What advice would you give Jane to help her deal with her situation? What are Jane's possible reactions to the advice that you would give her? Specify reasons for each possible reaction that you identify.
2. Make a list of the scenarios in this chapter that seem implausible and those that you do not agree with. Conduct a literature search to substantiate your viewpoints on the list of identified scenarios. Develop a more realistic scenario.
3. What actions can you take to promote a preferred future for the nursing profession? Why are these actions important?

## WWW INTERNET EXERCISES

1. Visit the home page of Sigma Theta Tau International at http://www.nursing society.org. On the home page, click on the words "About Us." On the next screen, you will see the heading "Society Supported Initiatives"; click on the word "ARISTA" and on the next screen, click on the Executive Summary Report. Do you think that the preferred future outlined in this document is desirable? Why or why not? How can you contribute to the preferred future of the nursing profession outlined in this online document?
2. Visit the home page of the American Association of Colleges of Nursing at http://www.aacn.nche.edu. Scroll down the page and find the heading "Nursing Shortage Resource." Click and read information contained in the documents "About the Nursing Shortage" and "Strategies for Addressing the Nursing Shortage." What can we do collectively as a profession to alleviate the nursing shortage? What can you do as an individual to alleviate the nursing shortage? What are the potential consequences of inaction in this future crisis for health care and the nursing profession?
3. Visit the American Nurses Association at http://www.nursingworld.org. On the home page, click on "Nursing Issues/Programs." On the next menu, click on "Agenda for the Future." Do you agree with ANA initiatives for the future? Why or why not? What contributions can you make to fulfill the plan outlined in *Nursing's Agenda for the Future?*

## INTERNET RESOURCES

Sigma Theta Tau International: http://www.nursingsociety.org.
American Nurses Association: http://www.nursingworld.org.
National League for Nursing: http://www.nln.org.
American Association of Colleges of Nursing: http://www.aacn.nche.edu.
Institute for the Future: http://www.iftf.org.
National Institute of Health Future of Stem Cells: http://stemcells.nih.gov/
then click on "stem cell information" type in the search terms to learn about the latest health research on a topic of interest.
Institute for Alternative Futures: http://www.altfutures.com.
The Bootstrap Institute: http://www.bootstrap.org.
Discover Nursing: http://www.discovernursing.com.

## REFERENCES

Aburdene, P., & Naisbitt, J. (1992). *Megatrends for women*. New York: Villard Books.
Aiken, L., Clarke, S., & Sloane, D. (2000). Hospital restructuring: Does it adversely affect care and outcomes? *Journal of Nursing Administration 30*, 457–465.
Aiken, L., Smith, H., & Lake, E. (1994). Lower Medicare mortality among a set of hospitals known for good nursing care. *Medical Care, 32*, 771–785.
American Nurses Association (1991). *Nursing's agenda for health care reform*. Kansas City: Author.
Aydelotte, M. K. (1992). Nursing education: Shaping the future. In L. Aiken & C. Fagin (Eds.), *Charting nursing's future: Agenda for the 1990s* (pp. 462–484). Philadelphia: J. B. Lippincott.
Balik, B. (1998). The impact of managed care and integrated delivery systems on registered nurse education and practice. In E. O'Neil & J. Coffman (Eds.), *Strategies for the future of nursing* (pp. 41–63). San Francisco: Jossey-Bass.
Bezold, C. (1996). Your health in 2010: Four scenarios. *The Futurist, 30*, 35–39.
Burggraf, V., & Barry, R. (2001). What the future holds for gerontology. *Nursing, 31*, 52.
Check, E., & Rogers, A. (2001). Solving the next genome puzzle. *Newsweek, 69*, 52–53.
Dickey, C., & Power, C. (2001). A spreading Islamic fire. *Newsweek 69*, 36–37.
Dempsey, P. A., & Dempsey, A. D. (2000). *Using nursing research: Process, critical evaluation, and utilization* (5th ed.). Philadelphia: Lippincott Williams & Wilkins.
Doran, D. (Ed.), (2003). *Nursing-sensitive outcomes: State of the science*. Sudbury, MA: Jones and Bartlett.
Garcia, C., Wildund, R., Arca, M., Zoliani, G., Fellin, R., Mialoi, M., & Calandra, S., Bertolini, S., Cossu, F., Grishin, N., Barnes, R., Cohen, J., & Hobbs, H. (2001). Autosomal recessive hypercholesterolemia caused by mutations in a putative LDL receptor adaptor protein. *Science, 292*, 1394–1398.
Goldsmith, J. C., & Goran, M. J. (1996). Managed care mythology: Supply-side dreams die hard. *Healthcare Forum Journal, 39*, 42–47.
Grady, P. A. (1999). The future of nursing research. In E. J. Sullivan (Ed.), *Creating nursing's future: Issues, opportunities, and challenges* (pp. 259–270). St. Louis: Mosby.
Hadley, E. H. (1996). Nursing in the political and economic marketplace: Challenges for the 21st century. *Nursing Outlook, 44*, 6–10.
Havens, D., and Aiken, L. (1999). Shaping systems to promote desired outcomes. *Journal of Nursing Administration, 29*, 14–20.
Henchley, N. (1978). Making sense of the future. *Alternatives, 7*, 24–26.
Henriksen, C., Page, N., Williams, R., & Worral, P. (2003). Responding to nursing's agenda for the future: where do we stand on recruitment and retention? *Nursing Leadership Forum, 8*, 78–84.
Herzlinger, R. (2004). *Consumer-driven health care*. San Francisco: Jossey-Bass.
Hood, L., & Leddy, S. (2003). *Leddy and Pepper's conceptual bases of professional nursing* (5th ed.). Philadelphia: Lippincott Williams & Wilkins.
Hopkins, M. E. (2001). Critical condition. *NurseWeek, 2*, 15–19.
Horrigan, M. (2004). Employment projections to 2012: Concepts and context. *Monthly Labor Review (127)*, 3–22.
Institute for the Future (2003). *Health & health care 2010* (2nd ed.). San Francisco: Jossey-Bass.

Johnson, T., & White, A. (2000, February/March). Six business principles for the 21st century. *Civilization, 61*(2), 57.

Kleinke, J. D. (1998). *Bleeding edge: The business of health care in the new century.* Gaithersburg MD: Aspen.

Krueger-Wilson, C., & Porter-O'Grady, T. (1999). *Leading the revolution in health care: advancing systems, igniting performance* (2nd ed.). Gaithersburg, MD: Aspen.

Lazar, M. (2005). How obesity causes diabetes: Not a tall tale. *Science, 307*, 373–375.

Millett, S., & Kopp, W. (1996). The top 10 innovative products for 2006: Technology with a human touch. *The Futurist, 30*, 16–20.

Milstead, J. A. (1999). *Health policy & politics: A nurse's guide.* Gaithersburg, MD: Aspen.

Minkin, B. H. (1995). *Future in sight.* New York: Macmillan.

Mish, F. (Ed.) (1994). *Merriam Webster's Collegiate Dictionary* (10th ed.) Springfield, MA: Merriam-Webster.

Naisbitt, J. (1996). *Megatrends Asia.* New York: Simon & Schuster.

Naisbitt, J., & Aburdene, P. (1990). *Megatrends 2000.* New York: Penguin.

National Council of State Boards of Nursing (NCSBN). (2000). *Mutual recognition frequently asked questions.* Available at: http://www.ncsbn.org.pdfs/FrequentlyAskedQuestions.pdf. Accessed July 20, 2005.

National Council of State Boards of Nursing (NCSBN). (2001). *Mutual recognition information.* Available at: http://www.ncsbn.org. Accessed July 20, 2005.

National Council of State Boards of Nursing (NCSBN), (2004). *Nursing license compact implementation.* Available at: http://www.ncsbn.org/nlc/rnlpvncompact_mutual_recognition_nurse_.asp. Accessed July 20, 2005.

National Council of State Boards of Nursing (2004a). *2003 NCLEX statistics.* Available at: http://www.ncsbn.org/pdfs/Table_of_Pass_Rates_2003.pdf. Accessed July 20, 2005.

National Council of State Boards of Nursing (2005). *2004 NCLEX statistics.* Available at: http://www.ncsbn.org?pdfs/Table_of_Pass_Rates_2004.pdf. Accessed July 20, 2005.

National Institute of Medicine and the National Research Council. (1999). *Chemical and biological terrorism.* Washington, DC: National Academy Press.

National League for Nursing. (1997). *Nursing DataSource 1997, Volume 1. Trends in Contemporary Nursing Education.* New York: National League for Nursing Press.

Newbergh, C. (2005). The Robert Wood Johnson Foundation's commitment to nursing. In S. Isaacs, & J. Knickman (Eds.), *To improve health and health care, volume VIII* (pp. 73–98). San Francisco: Jossey-Bass.

Offit, K. (1998). *Clinical cancer genetics: Risk counseling and management.* New York: John Wiley.

PEW Health Professions Commission. (1995). *Critical challenges: Revitalizing the health professions for the twenty-first century.* San Francisco: University of California, San Francisco Center for the Health Professions.

PEW Health Professions Commission (1998). Recreating Health Professional Practice for a New Century. San Francisco: University of California, San Francisco Center for the Health Professions.

Porter-O'Grady, T. (1986). *Creative nursing administration: Managing participation into the 21st century.* Rockville, MD: Aspen.

Porter-O'Grady, T. (1994). Building partnerships in health care: Creating whole systems change. *Nursing and Health Care, 15*, 34–38.

Standing, T., & Kramer, F. (2003). The ND: Preparing nurses for clinical and educational leadership. *Reflections on Nursing Leadership, 29*, 35–37, 44.

Sullivan, E.J. (Ed.), (1999) *Creating nursing's future.* St. Louis: Mosby.

Sullivan, E. J., & Clinton, J. F. (1999). Achieving a multicultural nursing profession. In E. J. Sullivan (Ed.), *Creating nursing's future: issues, opportunities, and challenges* (pp. 317–333). St. Louis: Mosby.

Toffler, A. (1970). *Future shock.* New York: Random House.

Toffler, A. (1990). *Powershift: Knowledge, wealth, and violence at the edge of the 21st century.* New York: Bantam Books.

Trossman, S. (2005). Obesity on the rise. *The American Nurse, 37*, 1, 4.

United States Department of Health and Human Services. (2000). *Healthy People 2010, Volumes 1 & II.* Washington, DC: Author.

Underwood, A., & Adler, J. (2005). Diet and genes. *Newsweek, CXLV*, 39–48.

Veenema, T. (Ed.) (2003). *Disaster nursing and emergency preparedness for chemical, biological and radiological terrorism and other hazards.* New York: Springer Publishing.

Wolf, G. (2003). Coming of age in health care: Changes, challenges, choices. *Reflections on Nursing Leadership 29*, 32–34, 44.

# INDEX

Pages followed by *f* indicate figure; those followed by *t* indicate table.

## A

Academic careers, 602
Access to health care, 450
Accountability
  autonomy and authority, 321–323
  checklist, 338–340
  in era of cost containment, 336–338
  in future, 338
  professional. *See* Professional accountability
  responsibility and answerability, 320–321
Acquired immunodeficiency syndrome (AIDS),
      effect on health care systems, 248
Acute care nursing
  career options in, 589–592
  risk/quality management, 591
  staff development, 590–591
  staff nursing, 590
  travel nursing, 591–592
  utilization review, 591
Adaptation Model (Roy), 115–117, 156, 477–478
Administrative personnel, 601–602
Advanced practice nursing, 251, 257
  career options, 598–603
Advocacy
  meaning of, 527–528
  as principle of communication, 197
  teaching–learning and, 494–496
Aesthetic knowledge, 97–98
Affirmations, 220
Agency for Health Care Research and Quality
      (AHRQ), 450–451
Aging population, effect on health care systems,
      248, 631–632
Alcohol abuse, 248
Alternative delivery systems, 252–253
American Association of Colleges of Nursing
      (AACN), 28
American Medical Association (AMA), 237
American Nurses Association (ANA), 28–29,
      440–441
Analytical epidemiology, 381
Ancient civilizations and nursing, 40–44
Anesthetists (CRNAs), 600–601
Anonymity, 270
Answerability, accountability as, 320–321
Anxiety
  communication and, 187–188
  effect on client readiness for learning,
    500–501
Armed forces nursing, 396–397

Art of influencing public policy, 455
Art of lobbying, 440–441
Assessment
  community, 376
  comprehensive environmental, 366–368
  cultural, elements of, 305–306*t*
  nursing, based on ethnicity, 312–313*t*
  in nursing process, 145–146
Assimilation, global, 292–298
Associate degree programs, 18, 55, 645
Assyria, ancient history of nursing, 42
Attitudes
  conveyed about employing agency, 332
  healthy, 213
  in helping relationship, 181–182*t*
  toward personal health care, 249–250
Authority, accountability as, 321–323
Autonomy
  accountability as, 321–323
  and self-regulation, 26
Awareness, in Leddy's Human Energy Model,
    129

## B

Babylonia, ancient history of nursing, 41–42
Baccalaureate programs, 29, 54–55, 335–336,
    645–647
Baldrige National Quality Award, 571–572
Barriers
  to effective collegial cooperation, 547
  to research utilization, 279–281
Behavior change
  health strengths, 212
  lifestyle, strategies for, 213–215
  lifestyles and health, 211–212
  models for, 208–211
Being there, presence as, 177*t*
Benchmarking, 570
Benner's Novice-to-Expert model, 13–15, 497
Berlo's communication model, 170–171
Body language, 174
Budgeting skills, 536–538
Burnout, stress and, 218–219
Business-as-usual future scenario, 637
Business opportunities
  insurance and managed care companies, 596
  marketing and sales, 597
  occupational health and worker's
    compensation programs, 597
  private consulting, 597–598
  telephone triage and health care advice lines,
    596–597
Buyer's market future scenario, 638